The Harmonic Mind

The Harmonic Mind

From Neural Computation to Optimality-Theoretic Grammar

Volume 1. Cognitive Architecture

Paul Smolensky and Géraldine Legendre

A Bradford Book
The MIT Press
Cambridge, Massachusetts
London, England

First MIT Press paperback edition, 2011

This book was set in Book Antiqua, Bernhard Modern BT, and Garamond by the authors.

Library of Congress Cataloging-in-Publication Data

Smolensky, Paul, 1955–
The harmonic mind: from neural computation to optimality-theoretic grammar / Paul Smolensky and Géraldine Legendre.
p. cm.
"A Bradford book."
Contents: Vol. 1. Cognitive architecture.
Includes bibliographical references and index.
ISBN 978-0-262-19526-3 (hc : alk. paper) -- 978-0-262-51619-8 (pb.)
1. Neural networks (Computer science) 2. Natural language processing (Computer science) 3. Artificial intelligence. I. Legendre, Géraldine, 1953– II. Title.

QA76.87.S623 2006
006.3'2—dc22

2005054385

The MIT Press is pleased to keep this title available in print by manufacturing single copies, on demand, via digital printing technology.

To Natalie Rabinowitz Smolensky, Eugene Smolensky,
and Joshua Legendre Smolensky

for all you have given us

Contents

Volume 1. Cognitive Architecture

Part I
Toward a Calculus of the Mind/Brain: An Overview

Volume 2. Linguistic and Philosophical Implications

Part III
Optimality Theory: The Cognitive Science of Language

Part IV
Philosophical Foundations of Cognitive Architecture

Contributors

Lisa Davidson
Department of Linguistics
New York University

Paul Hagstrom
Department of Modern Foreign Languages & Literatures
Boston University

John Hale
Department of Linguistics
Michigan State University

Kristin Homer
Aurora, Colorado

Peter Jusczyk
deceased

Géraldine Legendre
Department of Cognitive Science
Johns Hopkins University

Donald W. Mathis
Department of Cognitive Science
Johns Hopkins University

Yoshiro Miyata
Department of Media Arts and Sciences
Chukyo University

Alan Prince
Department of Linguistics
Rutgers University

William Raymond
Department of Psychology
University of Colorado at Boulder

Paul Smolensky
Department of Cognitive Science
Johns Hopkins University

Melanie Soderstrom
Cognitive and Linguistic Sciences
Brown University

Antonella Sorace
Theoretical and Applied Linguistics
University of Edinburgh

Suzanne Stevenson
Department of Computer Science
University of Toronto

Bruce Tesar
Department of Linguistics
Rutgers University

Marina Todorova
Department of Cognitive Science
Johns Hopkins University

Anne Vainikka
Department of Cognitive Science
Johns Hopkins University

Colin Wilson
Department of Linguistics
UCLA

Preface

The goal of this book is twofold: to present a proposal for a cognitive architecture—with particular attention to the language faculty—and to instantiate a formal, aggressively interdisciplinary conception of cognitive science. The cognitive architecture centrally involves mathematics that will be unfamiliar to many in an interdisciplinary audience. To maximize accessibility, the ideas are presented at multiple levels of formal elaboration: the introductory chapters should be accessible to all, with elaborations for specialists relegated to later chapters. Also to promote ease of access, numerous expository boxes offer concise but substantial summaries of relevant background material from several disciplines.

At many colleges and universities, interdisciplinary groups of faculty, postdocs, and students meet to learn about and discuss work in cognitive science outside their own disciplines. Such a group provides a good model for this book's intended audience. The more introductory chapters and background boxes are written to be accessible to those with little training in the relevant field. Other chapters are written to provide experts with substantial results. The same examples are used in many chapters to facilitate the progression from more basic to more sophisticated treatments.

To maximize usability, this book is constructed to function when only a subset of the chapters are read. Increasing the extent to which chapters are self-contained introduces an unavoidable but hopefully acceptable degree of recapitulation, especially of the basic ideas that play a major role in multiple chapters.

Chapter 1 (Section 7) presents the specifics concerning the expository boxes, the interdependence of the chapters, the various disciplines they draw upon, and their inherent accessibility; it also gives a chapter-by-chapter summary of the entire book. The interrelatedness of the chapters is recalled in the introductions to the four parts of the book and in the abstracts to individual chapters; the abstracts attempt in particular to situate the content of each chapter in the big picture, sketched in the final section of Chapter 2: the ICS map. A table of contents for each chapter also identifies the topics discussed in that chapter.

To aid in navigating the book, the footers at the bottom of each page contain information concerning the location of the chapter's figures, tables, boxes, sections, and numbered items. The page on which, say, Figure 5 appears has 'Figure 5' at its foot; this label persists in the footers of subsequent pages until the appearance of Figure 6. The item numbered '(55)' in Chapter 5 is referred to in other chapters as 'Chapter 5 (55)'; 'Section 5:5.5' refers to Section 5.5 of Chapter 5. In our use of cross-references, we have done our best to optimize the conflicting demands of (1) readability and (2) precision in the use of terminology and reference to explicit principles.

In preparing these volumes, we have received much inspiration from the new generation of students who are training to become genuine cognitive scientists. For them, we offer this book as one conception of their emerging field.

Preface

Acknowledgments

Our deepest appreciation goes to our coauthors, especially Alan Prince, for all we have learned from them, for the great satisfaction we have derived from working with them, for their permission to include some of our joint research here, and for their patience with the excruciatingly long process of completing this book. Most of this joint work was already complete in the December 2000, prior to the subsequent additions which expanded the work by 50%.

For many helpful comments on a large part of the manuscript, we are grateful to Mark Johnson and especially to Matt Goldrick. We have benefited from the detailed feedback of students in seminars devoted to earlier drafts, at Johns Hopkins University in 2001 and 2002 and at Stanford University in spring 2002. We are extremely grateful to Tom Wasow, who not only gave us his own detailed critiques of nearly every chapter, but also painstakingly transmitted copious comments from the participants in his Stanford seminar. It was largely in response to this input that we undertook major revisions that culminated in the final draft of February 2004.

The multidisciplinary research discussed in these volumes connects with a vast heterogeneous literature of which the nearly 1,000 references included here barely scratch the surface. We regret that we were not able to do better, but the care and feeding of the manuscript became overwhelming; since we prepared camera-ready copy ourselves, managing the figures, formatting, typesetting, and copyediting became all-consuming. The erratic citation profile is one of the side effects of the intricate derivational history of a work built by folding together and attempting to homogenize materials written over a span of two decades.

For crucial help in preparing the manuscript, we thank Rebecca Hanna, Victoria Chan, Rachel Gawron, Emily Mosdell, and Joshua Legendre Smolensky. We are also extremely grateful to Josh for the original cover artwork, inspired by several trips as a threesome to the Vancouver area where we discovered a common love for and a desire to understand this unique form of native American art.

The manuscript benefited greatly from the painstaking copyediting of Anne Mark, whose heroic efforts extending over a year displayed her legendary skill at finding errors of every conceivable sort, from arrows in figures to typos in French to dates of references. Any remaining errors—and departures from perfect editorial consistency—are our own responsibility, and likely the result of oversights in implementing Anne's corrections.

At MIT Press we thank Tom Stone for sharing our vision for this work. For their help in bringing the book to press, we thank Sandra Minkkinen, Yasuyo Iguchi, and especially Margy Avery. We owe the index to the strenuous efforts of Holman Tse. For their encouragement and help with publication early on (starting in 1992), we warmly thank Amy Pierce Brand and Tammy Kaplan.

We are most grateful to our faculty and student colleagues in the uniquely stimulating environment of the Department of Cognitive Science at Johns Hopkins. The untimely loss in 2001 of our friend and collaborator Peter Jusczyk has been a terrible blow to us, as to so many others; we are thankful for the time we had to learn from him.

For partial support of the research reported here, we gratefully acknowledge NSF grants IRI-8609599, ECE-8617947, IST-8609599, BS-9209265, IRI-9596120, IIS-9720412, DGE-9972807, and BCS-0446954.

A work of this size has a large impact on family life. We might not have survived the experience with sane minds were it not for all the family members who supported us throughout this endeavor.

For allowing us to forget about the book and for providing much-needed relief with noisy gatherings à la française, fine food, and wine galore, we thank the faraway Legendre family.

For sharing our hopes and travails during the endless gestation of these two volumes, we thank Natalie and Gene Smolensky.

We reserve our most heartfelt thanks for Josh, a real mensch, who made this book possible by allowing it to intrude on our family from the day he moved to Baltimore as a seven-year-old (1994) to the day he left for college (2005).

Part I

Toward a Calculus of the Mind/Brain: An Overview

The picture we will paint can be sketched roughly like this. The human mind/brain is a computational system with two very different formal descriptions. At a lower, more fine-grained level of description, this computational system is connectionist: a massively interconnected network comprising billions of slow, simple processing units, all operating simultaneously. Each unit possesses a numerical activity level; information is encoded in patterns of activity over large groups of units. Connectionist networks are a formal characterization of neural computation, at approximately the level of networks of nerve cells.

In the human mind/brain, higher cognition—such as abstract thought—is possible because the connectionist computer is specially organized. This special structure entails that key large-scale, global properties of the connectionist network constitute a powerful higher-level virtual machine, a machine that performs symbolic computation: rule-governed manipulation of complex structures that are built of abstract symbols. This symbolic computer is a formal characterization of mental computation, at approximately the level of concepts.

Explicit mathematical bridges link the continuous, numerical, lower-level description of brain to the discrete, structural, higher-level description of mind. Both descriptions are essential for characterizing the meaningfulness and the effectiveness of cognition; they are formally united in the Integrated Connectionist/Symbolic Cognitive Architecture (ICS). This unification, we argue, strengthens both connectionist and symbolic cognitive theory. In the domain of language, the connectionist foundations of ICS lead ultimately to a new symbolic formalism, one that furthers the theory of universal grammar: Optimality Theory (OT). OT offers a new conception of what it is that the grammars of all human languages share; it also provides a new formal characterization of exactly how they differ. Furthermore, OT strengthens the ties between linguistic theory and the study of language acquisition and language use.

The integration under ICS of connectionist and generative theories of grammar—and of connectionist and symbolic theories of cognition generally—helps to unify cognitive science along several dimensions: the methodological divergence among research traditions inherited from the disparate sciences of cognition, the apparent incoherence of the substantive content of cognitive theory derived from these divergent traditions, and the metatheoretical schism separating philosophies of science centered on specific models from those centered on general, formal principles.

Each chapter in Part I introduces one of the four parts of the book. Chapter 1 is an overview of the book as a whole, as is Part I itself, at a more detailed level. Chapter 2 introduces Part II, which articulates the principles that define ICS and derives their formal consequences. Chapter 3 introduces Part IV, which explores the implications for cognitive explanation of ICS's integration of connectionist and symbolic computation. Chapter 4 introduces Optimality Theory, the topic of Part III, where OT is applied in depth to a range of problems in the cognitive science of language.

1 Harmony Optimization and the Computational Architecture of the Mind / Brain

Paul Smolensky and Géraldine Legendre

What type of computer is the human mind/brain? The answer we propose is this: the mind is a symbol-manipulating computer, an abstract virtual machine realized in a brain performing connectionist computation. This characterizes the core of *higher* cognition, the particularly challenging and important realm of cognitive faculties operating in domains like abstract reasoning and language—faculties that are highly developed only in the *human* mind/brain. In this chapter, after reviewing the basics of symbolic and connectionist computation, we characterize our proposed Integrated Connectionist/Symbolic Cognitive Architecture (ICS) in the most general terms. We then discuss the structure of the book in detail and preview illustrative results from all other chapters.

Contents

When you get to the fork in the road, take it.
— Yogi Berra

1 Symbols and Neurons: What Type of Computer Is the Mind/Brain?

In the last half-century, cognitive science has made remarkable progress on the problem of understanding cognition. This problem has been fertile ground for intellectual investigation for two millennia, under many names and from many diverse perspectives. The recent progress on this very old problem derives largely from the foundational hypothesis of modern cognitive science: *cognition is computation.* This hypothesis permits the rigorous analysis of cognition—even at its most abstract—through a formal characterization of cognitive calculation. But computation is a rich notion that can be formalized in many ways. So the fundamental hypothesis of cognitive science—cognition is computation—immediately gives rise to the fundamental question of human **cognitive architecture**: just what *type* of computation is cognition? This is the most basic question addressed in this book.

The question of what type of computer we have in our heads gets its urgency from a tension in cognitive science that is immediately apparent from the customary definition of this discipline: the scientific study of the **mind/brain**. What on earth is a mind/brain? The term may, of course, be used as a kind of hedge, to blur whether the object of inquiry is a biological organ or a much more elusive entity, the mind, whose structure is not inherently physical but somehow much more abstract. In this book, however, 'mind/brain' is no equivocation: the theory developed here aims to characterize the notion mind/brain formally, rendering it an object suitable for scientific investigation.

What type of computer is the mind/brain? The tension implicit in this question arises because the type of computer that the brain appears to be has little in common with the type of computer that the mind has long been taken to be. A brain is a massively parallel computer consisting of billions of processors (neurons). These processors manipulate numbers (neural activation levels). The quantitative internal interactions within the computer (the efficacy of synaptic connections between neurons) change in response to the statistical properties of the computer's experience. While there is still much uncertainty in these matters, for the purposes of understanding cognition, this kind of **connectionist**—or **parallel distributed processing** (**PDP**)—system appears to be the most fruitful general characterization of neural computation at the present time. A connectionist cognitive architecture seems virtually inevitable from the perspective of neuroscience (Churchland and Sejnowski 1992).

But a very different kind of computational architecture has provided the most fertile hypothesis for the theory of **mind**. Not just in contemporary cognitive science, but implicitly since antiquity, the fundamental hypothesis has held that the mind is a serial computer that manipulates discrete structures built of abstract symbols.

For example, contemporary articles in the journal *Artificial Intelligence* provide highly sophisticated versions of a conceptualization of the mind that comes to us from at least as far back as Aristotle, through the mediation of logicians such as Boole, Frege, Tarski, and Turing. It is this conception of mind that led to the invention of the modern digital computer. And this same view has also framed a body of research which appears to show that a key component of higher cognition is the ability to reason by manipulation of complex symbolic expressions according to logic-like rules (Newell and Simon 1963; Pylyshyn 1984; Fodor and Pylyshyn 1988).

The point is reinforced by contemporary articles in theoretical linguistics journals, which provide in-depth theories of aspects of the human language faculty. These analyses represent modern formalizations of conceptions of grammar going back more than two millennia to Pāṇini in ancient India. The extremely broad and deep research literature in linguistics provides a wealth of evidence for the hypothesis that a central component of human cognition is the ability to produce and interpret linguistic forms by manipulating intricate symbolic expressions in accord with rules of grammar (Chomsky 1986; Frank 1998; Pinker 1999).

Going well beyond language and reasoning, modern computational work in higher visual perception, action planning, problem solving, and most other higher cognitive domains has similarly gained great explanatory leverage by analyzing cognition as arising from the manipulation of complex, abstract, symbolic structures. Such a **symbolic cognitive architecture** seems inescapable from the perspective of research on higher mental functions.

In short, the (symbolic) computational architecture of the mind appears to be utterly unrelated to the (connectionist) computational architecture of the brain.

Because virtually all research in cognitive science must be conducted within some (at least implicit) computational architecture, the current schizophrenia concerning the fundamental nature of that architecture has put the field in a state of crisis. The depth to which individual researchers are committed to—and invested in—either a symbolic or a connectionist computational architecture is evident in the vehemence with which this issue is debated in a multitude of cognitive science venues. Concerning the respective roles played in cognition by symbolic and connectionist computation, several radically different philosophical positions have been articulated; indeed, developing and arguing for one such position is a primary goal of this book. Several of these philosophical stances are outlined below in Box 8, after additional groundwork is laid.

To draw out the tension between the different computational architectures seemingly characterizing the brain and the mind, in the following two sections we briefly review some of the fundamental concepts of connectionist and symbolic computation. Readers familiar with these topics may wish to skim to Section 4, where we frame the resolution of this tension that we propose and develop in this book.

2 Connectionist Computation

The brain can be studied from a range of perspectives. For example, the neuroscientist's basic question we take to be this: what is the function of each component of the nervous system? But we take the cognitive scientist's question concerning the brain to be quite different:

(1) The neural question for cognitive science

How are complex cognitive functions computed by a mass of numerical processors like neurons—each very simple, slow, and imprecise relative to the components that have traditionally been used to construct powerful, general-purpose computational systems? How does the structure arise that enables such a medium to achieve cognitive computation?

A fruitful approach to this difficult problem is the mathematical modeling strategy: hypothesize a set of equations that abstractly describe the dynamics of numerical variables characterizing neural states, and analyze the consequent collective properties of these states to determine whether they can yield particular cognitive functions. This strategy places strong constraints on the equations posited: on the one hand, they must be simple enough to make possible the analysis of the collective properties of networks with millions of neurons; on the other hand, they must be complex enough that the resultant collective properties actually suffice to compute interesting cognitive functions. Mathematical models of neural computation with this delicately balanced degree of complexity are **connectionist networks.**[1]

Here, as in any scientific domain, the mathematical modeling strategy implicitly adopts two working hypotheses concerning the simplifications it requires. The first is that, for the purposes of the cognitive computations under investigation, the characteristics of neural computation that are formalized in these models are, overall, more important than the characteristics that are omitted. The second working hypothesis is that once the computational consequences of simpler characteristics are mathematically understood, further characteristics of neural computation can then be added, to incrementally broaden and deepen the understanding afforded by the theory. Evidence of the fertility of these hypotheses is provided by numerous contributions of connectionist modeling to brain theory; these are evident in the articles appearing in *Neural Computation* and the many other journals devoted to computational neuroscience research. (The relation of connectionist networks to the brain is discussed in Box 6, following relevant considerations concerning symbolic theory.)

Despite the simplifications involved in connectionist modeling, at present the collective properties of large networks can usually be analyzed only to a very limited degree. This poses special challenges for the use of such networks as vehicles for explanation in cognitive science (McCloskey 1992). (With respect to language, some of

[1] A tiny sample of relevant literature: Kohonen 1977; Hinton and Anderson 1981; Rumelhart, McClelland, and the PDP Research Group 1986; Hertz, Krogh, and Palmer 1991; Smolensky, Mozer, and Rumelhart 1996; Abbott and Sejnowski 1999; Bechtel and Abrahamsen 2002.

these challenges are taken up in Chapter 22.)

Connectionist theory per se is the topic of Chapters 5–10 and so our discussion here will be brief. (See also the example connectionist network described in Box 1.)

Connectionist networks are large, interconnected collections of simple parallel computing elements, each of which carries a numerical **activation value** that it computes from the values of neighboring elements in the network, according to some simple numerical formula. The network elements or **units** ("model neurons") influence each others' values through connections ("model synapses"); each connection carries a numerical strength or **weight**. The influence of unit i on unit j is the activation value of unit i times the weight—strength—of the connection from i to j. Thus, if a unit is active (has a positive activation value), its influence on a neighbor's value is positive if its weight to that neighbor is positive ("excitatory"), and negative if its weight is negative ("inhibitory").

In a typical connectionist network, input to the system—say, the letters of a word W—is provided by imposing (**clamping**) activation values on the **input units** of the network; these numerical values represent some encoding or **representation** of the input. The activation on the input units propagates along the connections until some set of activation values emerges on the **output units**; these activation values encode the output the system has computed from the input—say, the pronunciation of the word W. Mediating between the input and output units there may be **hidden units** that do not participate directly in the representation of either the input or the output.

The interpretation of a network state can be characterized in terms of its elements or properties. Whether an interpretation possesses a given element or property x (say, a particular letter) might be determined by the activity of a single network unit; this is a **local representation** of x. Alternatively, the presence of x may be determined by the **pattern of activity** over a set of units—a **distributed representation**, in which the activity of a single unit is part of the representation of many alternative elements x (see Box 2).

The particular computation performed by the network in transforming the input pattern of activity to the output pattern depends on the set of connection strengths; these weights are usually regarded as encoding the system's **knowledge**. In this sense, the connection strengths play the role of the program in a conventional computer. In the networks introduced in Chapter 6 and developed formally in Chapters 7–10, the connection strengths are computed by the analyst and provided directly to the network. Often, however, connectionist networks program themselves; that is, they have autonomous procedures for tuning their weights to eventually perform some specific computation. These **learning algorithms** often depend on training in which the network is presented with sample input-output pairs from the function it is supposed to compute.

Formal analysis of connectionist computation employs many branches of mathematics. Most central to this book are **vector**, **matrix**, and **tensor algebra**. The list of activation values of all connectionist units constitutes a network's **activation vector**;

the array of weight values of all connections constitutes its **weight matrix**. Vectors can be added together, and they can be multiplied by matrices; this sort of **linear algebra** is generalized in the **tensor calculus**, where for our purposes a tensor is just another structured collection of numbers over which algebraic operations are defined. Chapter 5 (especially Boxes 1 and 2) provides a simple introduction to linear and tensor algebra and explains how tensors are useful in providing networks with the structure needed to compute complex functions like those of symbolic computation, characteristic of much of human higher cognition. The basic ideas introduced in Chapter 5 are developed formally in Chapters 7–8.

As introduced in Chapter 6 and developed in detail in Chapter 9, formal analysis reveals that many connectionist networks perform **optimization**: they compute those activation values for hidden and output units that, together with the given activation values of the input units, maximize a measure of self-consistency or **well-formedness** called **Harmony** (see Box 3). The Harmony of a network state can be interpreted as the degree to which the state satisfies a set of "soft" **constraints** implemented in the network's connections. Thus, when the network achieves a state of maximal Harmony, it has optimally satisfied these constraints (see Box 4).[2]

In another application of optimization, powerful connectionist learning procedures have been developed by formally analyzing learning as an optimization process: minimizing the error made by the network on its training sample, for example. The power of optimizing connectionist learning procedures has enabled much important research on the question of what knowledge can, in principle, be inductively learned from the statistical structure of experience—formal exploration of the empiricist epistemological program. In this book, however, our focus is on the *nature* of knowledge, rather than its origin. (Chapters 17 and 18 do address learning of phonology and syntax, respectively, but the research reported there does not employ connectionist learning, nor empiricist theory more generally. Chapter 21 does use statistical learning, in the design of a grammar-learning network with a priori knowledge of specific linguistic principles.)

At present, the importance of connectionism for the theory developed in this book is largely unrelated to learning or empiricism. What is crucial are the connectionist proposals that mental representations are encoded in activation vectors, that mental processes are encoded in weight matrices, and that optimization is central to cognition. These connectionist characterizations of neural computation, we will argue, have many important implications for cognitive science, quite independently of further principles regarding learning that in the future will no doubt prove critical.

To begin to appreciate the significance of the basic connectionist principles of computation, it is helpful to contrast them with the types of principles that have traditionally been employed in the study of the mind—those of symbolic computation, the topic of the next section.

[2] Some key contributions are Hopfield 1982, 1984; Cohen and Grossberg 1983; Hinton and Sejnowski 1983, 1986; Smolensky 1983, 1986; Geman and Geman 1984; Ackley, Hinton, and Sejnowski 1985; Golden 1986.

Box 1. An example connectionist network

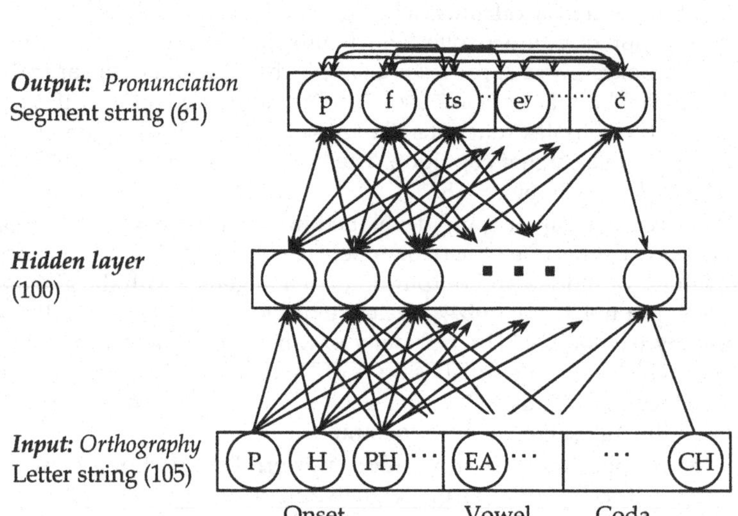

This network (Plaut et al. 1996) learns to pronounce monosyllabic English words. In brief (and simplifying somewhat), the network works as follows. The spelling of a word is presented to the network by setting (**clamping**) the values of its 105 input units, which are divided into three groups. The first group represents the **orthographic onset** of the word: the consonants preceding the first vowel-letter. For each letter sequence spelling a single sound (a **grapheme**) that can appear in an English onset, there is a corresponding unit. So if the first two letters are *PH*, the activation value of the *PH* grapheme unit is set to 1 (active), as are the activations of the *P* and the *H* units. The second group of input units provides a corresponding graphemic representation of the first vowel sequence, and the third input group, a corresponding representation of the **orthographic coda**, the final portion of the word (primarily consonants, but also possibly including a final *E*). The layer of input units supports a **local representation** of individual letters and a (modestly) **distributed representation** of letter strings: the representation of *PHONE* involves the activity of multiple units, each of which participates in the representation of multiple strings.

Once the input activation values—constituting the **input vector**—have been clamped, activation flows from them up to a layer of 100 **hidden units**; this layer functions as internal scratch paper for the network's calculations. Activation then flows up from the hidden units to the output units, which host a representation of a pronunciation for the word. The output representation is similar to the input representation, except that in the place of letters there are units of speech, **segments** (e.g., *č*, the sound spelled *CH* in *CHURCH*).

Activation in the output layer flows around within the layer, as well as back down to the hidden layer. The presence of closed loops of connections, enabling activation to continually circulate, makes this a **recurrent** network. The equation governing the activation spread is that of an **additive net**; in Section 9:3.2.3.5, it is shown that the equation used in the network simulation is equivalent to $da_\gamma/dt = f(\iota_\gamma) - a_\gamma$, where a_γ is the activation value of unit γ, $f(\iota) \equiv 1/[1+e^{-\iota}]$ is a nonlinear "squashing" function that limits activation values to the range from 0 to 1, and ι_γ is the **input activation** that unit γ receives from the units connected to it. With $W_{\gamma\beta}$ denoting the **weight** of the connection to unit γ from unit β, this input to γ is $\iota_\gamma = W_{\gamma 1} a_1 + W_{\gamma 2} a_2 + \cdots \equiv \Sigma_\beta W_{\gamma\beta} a_\beta$, the weighted sum of the activations of those network units that have connections to γ. (Networks of this general form were among the first to be shown to optimize the well-formedness measure we call **Harmony** (Cohen and Grossberg 1983), although the Plaut et al. network does not impose the condition of symmetrical connectivity, $W_{\gamma\beta} = W_{\beta\gamma}$, which is required to guarantee Harmony maximization in recurrent nets.)

This network contains 26,582 connections. Fortunately, the network programs itself, determining a set of weights for all these connections that allows it to pronounce English words. This is done through the modification for continuous-time networks (Pearlmutter 1989) of a learning algorithm for recurrent networks called **back-propagation through time** (Rumelhart, Hinton, and Williams 1986). This is a **supervised** learning algorithm: the network is given examples of the correct outputs for a **training set** of inputs. Thus, during training, the input units are clamped for the spelling of an English word, and the network is given the output unit values encoding the correct pronunciation. The learning algorithm changes the weights slightly so that the next time that input is received, its output will be a little closer to the correct output. (To simulate efficiently the effect of receiving more training with words of higher frequency in English, larger weight changes are made for words with higher frequency.) The learning algorithm minimizes a measure of the network's total error on its training set. If the training set provides an adequate sample of all possible inputs, the weights learned ought to generalize appropriately to novel inputs the network has never seen before (e.g., pseudowords like *POOT*).

For Plaut et al.'s network, the training set consisted of 2,998 words, each presented 1,900 times during learning. The resulting weights produced correct pronunciations for 99.2% of the training words. To assess the generalizations learned by the network and compare them with human generalizations, the net was tested on nonword inputs. Given *POOT*, for example, the network produced a pronunciation rhyming with *foot* (not *boot*), in violation of a set of English spelling-to-sound correspondence rules that define the **regular** pronunciation. The regularity of the network's output for nonwords depended upon the regularity of English words with similar spelling (**neighbors**). The network's pronunciation of nonwords was regular for 93.0% of those nonwords for which the neighbors were regular, but only 62.8% for nonwords with some irregular neighbors. For human subjects pronouncing the same nonwords, Glushko (1979) reported corresponding values of 93.8% and 78.3%. The network simulated other aspects of human performance as well: pronunciation was faster (i.e., the network reached a stable output in less simulated time) for high-frequency English words than for low-frequency words (Forster and Chambers 1973); pronunciation was slower the more neighbors a word had whose pronunciations were inconsistent with its own (Glushko 1979; Taraban and McClelland 1987; Jared, McRae, and Seidenberg 1990); and this slowing effect was stronger for lower-frequency words (Seidenberg et al. 1984).

The internal structure of the network was probed to assess the degree to which the network had acquired knowledge of subword spelling-to-sound correspondences (like $PH \rightarrow f$) as opposed to whole-word correspondences. Plaut et al. develop a complex picture of the network as an intersecting set of **componential attractors**; we can only sketch this rich notion here. Inputs of the form $PH\!-\!-$ put the network in an initial state that is attracted to a final state in which the output pronunciation has the form *f*––. This type of attractor controls those dimensions of the network's state space that include the orthographic and phonological onsets; it functions like a *PH*-to-*f* spelling-to-sound correspondence rule. Along other dimensions, analogous attractors control the vowel and coda correspondences. An input *PHONE* lies in the intersection of three such attractors, which together govern the overall input-to-output mapping. These intersecting attractors yield regular input-to-output mapping not only for the actual English words that, during learning, gave rise to them: they also do so for novel letter sequences like *PHAT*. (Furthermore, comparable structure in the networks studied by Brousse and Smolensky (1989) was shown to enable rapid learning of new inputs that share the combinatorial structure of the training set.) The regularities leading to componential attractors are only partial in English, however. Woven through the grid of componential attractors are other attractors responsible for irregular pronunciations. This type of partial decomposition of inputs into constituent parts for dealing with regularities in combinatorial domains bears an intriguing relation to the symbolic combinatorial strategy discussed in Section 3.

Box 2. Distributed representations

Distributed representations are central to connectionist computation for several types of reasons; some of them are summarized here.

Empirical considerations

"Sensory and motor variables are typically represented by a population of broadly tuned neurons" (Zhang and Sejnowski 1999). That is, a sensory or motor neuron is typically active over a rather broad range of values for a stimulus or response variable about which it carries information. Values of such a variable can be systematically distinguished by considering the differential responses of an entire population of neurons. Such distributed representations—or **population codes**—in the brain have received a great deal of empirical and theoretical attention from neuroscientists in recent years. Examples abound in the neuroscience literature (e.g., Churchland and Sejnowski 1992; Abbott and Sejnowski 1999).

A prominent case is the coding of movements in monkey motor cortex (Georgopoulos et al. 1982). A motor neuron has a preferred direction of movement for which it fires at its greatest rate, but it fires also for a wide range of directions surrounding its preferred direction. In fact, the activity for a direction θ is essentially proportional to the cosine of the angle between θ and the cell's preferred direction. The population code for a particular direction θ is a widely distributed activity pattern for which θ is the vector average of all the preferred directions of active neurons, each direction weighted by the level of activation of the corresponding neuron.

Another well-studied case is the encoding of spatial location in the **place cells** of the rat hippocampus (O'Keefe and Nadel 1979). Within a particular environment, a place cell is active when the rat is located in a particular region of space; this region is the cell's **place field.** (Activity is further modulated by other factors such as speed and direction of movement.) Each place field covers a relatively large portion of the environment. A particular location is however quite accurately encoded in the activity pattern of the entire population of place cells. The simultaneous activity of 25–30 neurons recorded in freely moving animals contains sufficient information to enable recovery of the encoded position with an uncertainty as low as two times the theoretical minimum; furthermore, the recovery operation can itself be done in an extremely simple network (Zhang et al. 1998).

Experiments in the form of computer simulations show that when connectionist networks learn their own internal representations in hidden units, these representations are generally heavily distributed (e.g., Sanger 1989; Churchland and Sejnowski 1992). If learning methods for connectionist networks are in the same general computational class as those at work in building actual neural representations (see Box 6), we should expect distributed representation to be just as ubiquitous in the brain as indeed it appears to be (for examples, see Churchland and Sejnowski 1992).

Theoretical considerations

When the items being represented are characterized by many features—when they inhabit a high-dimensional **content space** C—encoding accuracy is typically increased when neurons are more broadly tuned (Hinton, McClelland, and Rumelhart 1986; Zhang and Sejnowski 1999; cf. Pouget et al. 1999). Here's an intuitive explanation; for simplicity, assume all units are binary, with activity either 0 or 1. Call an item in C a **content point,** c, and the portion of C for which neuron β responds its **field.** If β is a sensory neuron, its field is a **receptive field,** and a stimulus c is characterized by a set of sensory features; if β is a place cell, its field is a place field and c is a location; and so on. In distributed representations, fields are relatively large and overlapping; in local representations, small and nonoverlapping. For a local representation, the single active unit β tells us only that the content point c being represented is somewhere in the field of β; thus, to achieve high accuracy, this field must be small. But in a high-dimensional space *C*, it takes an enormous number of small fields to cover the entire space: to make 10 distinctions on each of *d* dimensions, 10^d fields are required—exponential growth in *d* (the infamous "curse of dimensionality").

With larger, overlapping fields, many fewer units are required to achieve the same accuracy. To take an extreme case of distribution, suppose each unit has activity 0 or 1, its field is the region within *C* where the *k*th dimension has a particular value *v*, and all other dimensions have any value whatever. With 10 distinct values *v*, each such region covers 1/10th of the entire space. With such units for each of the *d* dimensions *k*, there are 10*d* units in all. Now in the representation of *c*, the total pattern of activity specifies one of 10 values for each dimension *k*; thus, this distributed representation has the same accuracy as the preceding local representation, which required 10^d units.

This amounts to the simple observation that with *n* binary units, there are only *n* possible representations if only one unit can be active, but there are 2^n representations if any number of units can be active. With only *n* distinct representations, the accuracy of a local representation is limited to 1/*n*th of the total space *C*, whereas for distributed representations, each activation pattern can denote one of 2^n distinct regions. Put differently, with *n* binary units, the number of elements that can be given distinct encodings is *n* with local representations, but 2^n with distributed representations.

In the case of motor control, it can be shown formally that broadly tuned neurons with cosine response functions—exactly as seen in monkey motor cortex—form an encoding that minimizes average errors in producing forces (Todorov 2002).

While distributed representations are advantageous for accurately representing a single element, they are more problematic for representing multiple elements simultaneously. With local representations, if two units are active, this indicates the presence of two items, each represented by one of the active units. But if it takes a pattern of activation over an entire population of units to specify a single item, how can two items be represented? This will prove to be a crucial question for the theory developed in this book; it is explicitly addressed in Chapter 5 (3).

Distributed representations encode a similarity relation between representations: two activity patterns are similar to the extent that each unit has similar activation levels in the two patterns. Local representations are all totally dissimilar to one another in this sense. Two similar representations will be treated similarly in the processing within a network, since processing is simply based on the activation levels of each unit. In this respect, distributed representations are the numerical counterpart of the symbolic notion of **distinctive features**. Rather than being formalized as an atomic symbol, equally different from all others, in phonological theory a speech sound like [m] is formalized as a pattern of feature values: [+nasal, +labial, −vocoid, …] (Box 12:2). The sound [n] is similar: it has all the same feature values as [m], except for the single value [−labial]. The phonology treats [n] and [m] similarly since phonological behavior is determined solely by feature values, nearly all of which are identical for [n] and [m].

Box 3. Harmony optimization in neural networks

With the following simple network, Harmony optimization in connectionist networks can be illustrated quite explicitly:

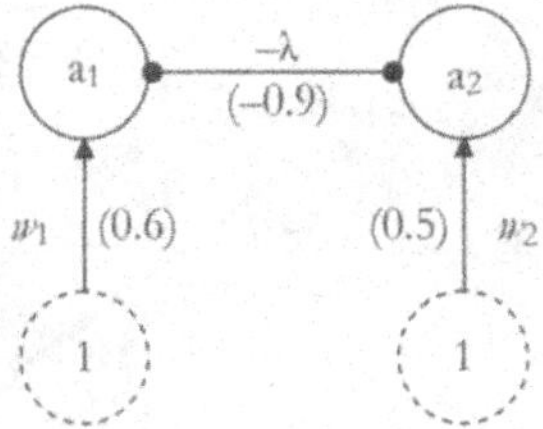

There are two dynamic units—solid circles—which inhibit each other with a strength of $\lambda = 0.9$. Each receives activation from an input unit—a dashed circle—with activity fixed at 1. The left dynamic unit thus receives input activation $1 \cdot w_1 = 0.6$ from the left input unit. The other dynamic unit receives input activation 0.5. The dynamical equations describing activation flow in this net are those of the **additive network** of Section 9:3.2.3.5 (and Box 1 above):

$$\frac{da_1}{dt} = -a_1 + w_1 - \lambda a_2 \qquad \frac{da_2}{dt} = -a_2 + w_2 - \lambda a_1$$

In Chapter 9, this dynamics is shown to maximize the following Harmony function (see also Section 6:1):

$$\begin{aligned} H(\mathbf{a}) &= a_1 W_{11} a_1 + a_1 W_{12} a_2 + \cdots - \tfrac{1}{2}\left(a_1^2 + a_2^2 + \cdots\right) \\ &= \sum_{\alpha\beta} a_\alpha W_{\alpha\beta} a_\beta - \tfrac{1}{2} \sum_\alpha a_\alpha^2 \\ &= a_1 w_1 + a_2 w_2 - \lambda a_1 a_2 - \tfrac{1}{2}\left(a_1^2 + a_2^2\right) \end{aligned}$$

The time course of activation and Harmony for this network are graphed below:

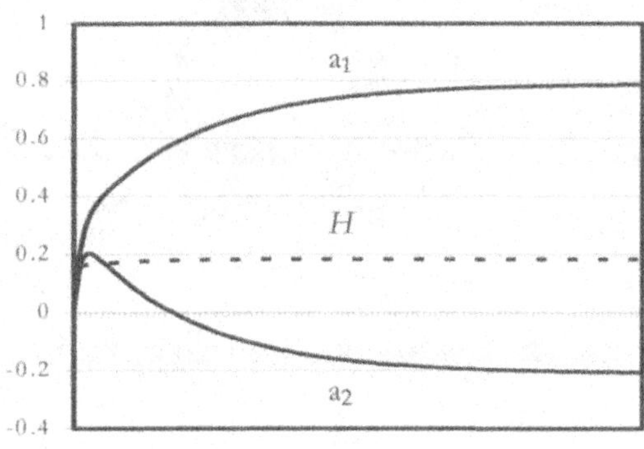

The activation vector $\mathbf{a} = (a_1, a_2)$ asymptotically approaches (0.79, –0.21); in the final state, a_1 is positive, because unit 1 has greater input, and a_2 is negative, despite unit 2's positive input, because it is inhibited by unit 1. The Harmony value steadily (**monotonically**) increases to the value 0.2.

The time course or **trajectory** of the activation vector is plotted below in a two-dimensional **activation state space**, with a_1 and a_2 serving as the coordinate axes:

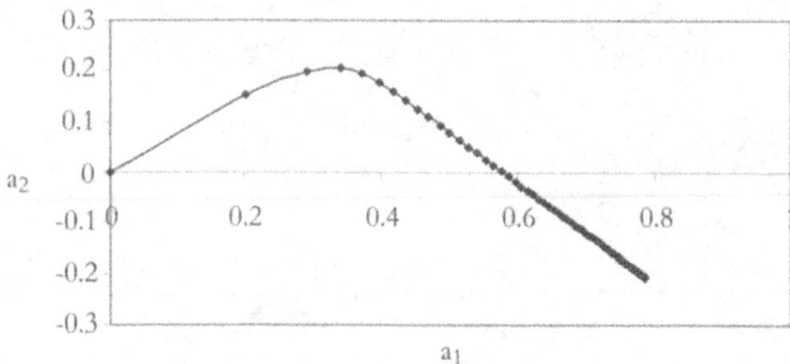

(The complete activation space has two additional dimensions, one for each input unit; but since the input units have fixed values 1, they don't need to be plotted.)

In the 3-D graph that follows, the Harmony function is plotted as a surface above the activation state space: the height of the surface above a point in the horizontal plane with coordinates (a_1, a_2) is the Harmony of the network state in which the dynamic units have those two activation values. The trajectory above is redrawn in the horizontal plane below, and is lifted up to the surface to show the Harmony values as activation flows through the network and the network state moves along its trajectory. The trajectory shows typical **hill-climbing** optimization behavior: it ascends up the Harmony surface, converging to a maximal (peak) value.

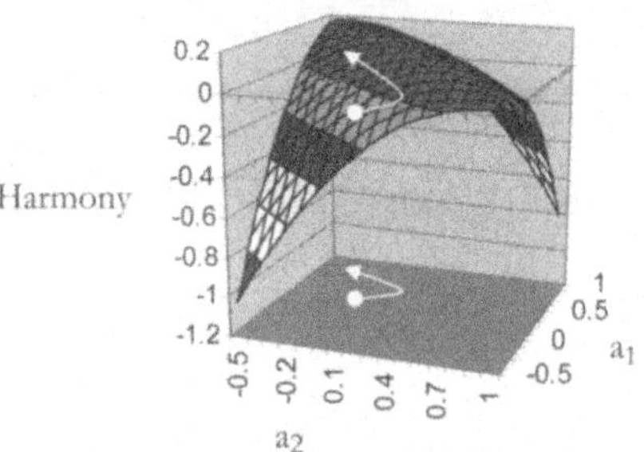

Box 4. Optimization over microconstraints in neural networks

To illustrate how Harmony maximization in a neural network can be understood as optimization over constraints, we return to the simple network of Box 3.

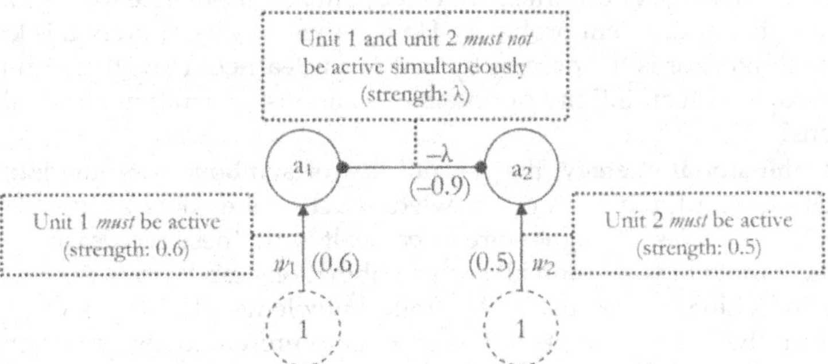

The diagram above gives a verbal characterization of the constraint encoded in each connection of the net. Because the connection between the two dynamic units is inhibitory (has a negative weight), activation in one unit inhibits or lowers the activation in the other unit. The result toward which this process is directed is a state in which, if one unit is active, the other unit is inactive—that is, a state satisfying the constraint 'Unit 1 and unit 2 must not be active simultaneously'. The connection to the first dynamic unit from the first input unit is positive, so it carries positive activation, exciting unit 1 (i.e., increasing its activation level); this process is directed toward a state satisfying the constraint 'Unit 1 must be active'. The same applies to unit 2.

The key observation is that *these three constraints* **conflict**. That is, *there is no state that satisfies them all.* How is this conflict adjudicated? This is where the *strengths* of the constraints figure crucially. The strength of each constraint is encoded in the numerical value of the corresponding connection weight. The strongest constraint of all, with strength 0.9, requires that unit 1 and unit 2 not be simultaneously active; so if this strongest constraint prevails, one unit will be active, the other inactive. If unit 2 is the active one, this state will satisfy the constraint requiring that unit 2 be active, but violate the constraint requiring that unit 1 be active. This is not optimal because this satisfies the weaker constraint (strength 0.5) while violating the stronger one (strength 0.6). The optimal state will instead have unit 1 active and unit 2 inactive. And indeed in the final state of this network, $a_1 = 0.79$ (active) and $a_2 = -0.21$ (inactive). These particular numerical activation values define the optimal compromise among the conflicting constraints, with these particular numerical strengths and this particular dynamics.

3 Symbolic Computation and the Combinatorial Strategy

While theories of brain have taken as their starting point hypotheses concerning neural *processes*, theories of mind have tended to develop from analysis of mental *function*. In recent times, functional characterizations of the mind emphasize its remarkable **productivity**: the ability to correctly process an unbounded set of possible inputs. For instance, knowledge of arithmetic or algebra makes it possible to solve a virtually unlimited number of different problems. How is this possible? Surely this knowledge is not itself infinite, nor is the process by which it is learned. How then can it be used to correctly cope with an infinity of possible situations, generating an infinity of correct solutions?

The **combinatorial strategy**, the central idea of symbolic computation, assumes that in such cases, a finite store of knowledge determines how a finite set of basic pieces—digits, variables, '+' signs—are to be dealt with; these pieces can be *combined* in an infinite variety of ways, and all such combinations can be processed by processing all the individual pieces using the finite knowledge. The types of pieces, and ways in which they may combine to form mental representations, are determined by the particular symbolic computational system being considered (Fodor 1975; Gleitman and Liberman 1995; Anderson and Lebiere 1998).

This idea is extremely general and has been applied to all domains of higher cognition. The central case—the best developed, and the most directly relevant to the work in this book—is the domain of language. This section illustrates the combinatorial strategy via the problem of processing sentences; at the same time, several basic linguistic concepts are introduced that will be employed later in the book (see also the boxes listed under 'Linguistics Background' in Table 3). Symbolic computation per se is not the topic of any subsequent chapter, but rather is presumed background knowledge; so we will now develop a specific example in some detail in an attempt to convey the general ideas. The perspective we adopt is that of a discipline squarely centered in symbolic cognitive science: generative linguistics. This view focuses heavily on features of language that may not be the most salient from other perspectives. Such differences are addressed in Box 5, via a series of 'Frequently Unasked Questions' concerning language and linguistics, intended for those unfamiliar with generative linguistics.

3.1 The combinatorial strategy illustrated: Sentence processing

A remarkable property of the human mind, surely worthy of explanation by a cognitive theory, is this: a sentence such as

(2) *The cake I baked for Josh didn't seem to please him*

—and trillions of others like it—can be readily produced and understood by normal adults competent in English (Chomsky 1965). Understanding such a sentence involves many things, but at the very least, it entails knowing who did what to whom.

Box 4

A little investigation shows this to be a surprisingly complex matter. In the particular case of sentence (2), for example, acts of baking and pleasing are involved; comprehension requires, among many other things, coming to know the facts in (3).

(3) Who did what to whom?

a. It was I (rather than Josh) who baked the cake.

b. What did *not* happen was the pleasing (rather than the baking).

c. The thing found not pleasing was the cake I baked (rather than me or Josh).

d. The one not pleased was Josh (rather than me).

e. Etc., etc., etc.

How can the ability to produce and understand an enormous range of sentences like (2) be *explained*? That is, what principles could be assumed of the mind, such that it would logically follow from these principles that the mind can competently produce and comprehend all such sentences?

The explanation developed by the symbolic theory of mind rests on a general theory of mental processes, employing a version of the combinatorial strategy described in (4).

(4) The combinatorial strategy (process level)

a. The mind can *analyze* a sentence like (2) into parts that are related in specific ways to each other and to the sentence as a whole.

b. These relationships are relatively few in number, and each contributes in a fixed way to allowing the whole to be processed via its parts.

For now, 'combinatorial strategy' will refer to this process-level version; in the theory we propose in this book, the general combinatorial strategy will be employed at a different level (see Section 3.4).

The combinatorial strategy can be applied to sentence (2) as follows:

(5) Combinatorial strategy applied to (2): first step

The sentence (2) as a whole is analyzed (decomposed) into two parts:

a. *The cake I baked for Josh didn't seem to please him*

= *SUBJECT PREDICATE*

The parts are[3]

b. SUBJECT = *the cake I baked for Josh*

c. PREDICATE = *didn't seem to please him*

This analysis of (2) can be written as follows:

d. [$_{\text{Sentence}}$ [$_{\text{SUBJECT}}$ *The cake I baked for Josh*] [$_{\text{PREDICATE}}$ *didn't seem to please him*]]

Alternatively, this same analysis can be diagrammed as a **tree**:

[3] 'Subject' and 'predicate' refer to traditional notions, independent of any contemporary syntactic theory.

e.

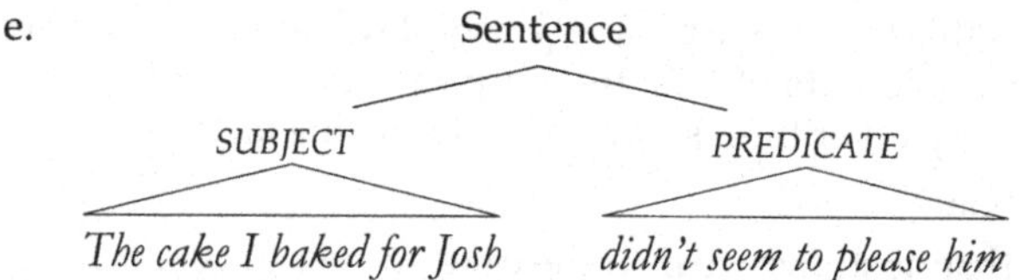

The combinatorial strategy requires much more analysis of this type before a sentence as complex as (2) can be understood, but when this analysis is complete, the subject-predicate relationship (along with the other relationships identified during the analysis) can be used to explain how the mind knows who did what to whom (3).

The combinatorial strategy's principle that the mind analyzes (2) into the combination of two **constituents,** ***SUBJECT*** and ***PREDICATE,*** allows this strategy to decompose the explanation of the mind's ability to process (produce and comprehend) (2) into three subproblems.

(6) Problem decomposition, (process-level) combinatorial strategy

To explain how the sentence (2) as a whole is correctly processed,

a. explain how the mind analyzes the sentence as a whole into its constituent parts (i.e., how it performs **parsing**),
b. explain how the mind processes individual constituents,
c. explain how the mind reassembles the processed constituents.

Now the second subproblem, (6b), is to process each individual constituent. Here it is important to note that each constituent part of (2) is basically the same type of object as the sentence we started with: a phrase. Exploiting this, the combinatorial strategy (**recursively**) uses the *same* approach to explain how constituents are individually processed: the constituents are themselves analyzed into (sub)constituents. For example, **embedded** within the first constituent of (2),

SUBJECT = the cake I baked for Josh ,

are two (sub)constituents, a ***MODIFIER*** (relative clause) and its ***HEAD***:

HEAD = the cake

MODIFIER = I baked for Josh .

Since the *MODIFIER* is itself a kind of sentence, it in turn has the following two (sub-sub)constituents:

SUBJECT = I

PREDICATE(gapped) = baked ___ for Josh .

Missing from this predicate is the thing baked, *the cake*; we have indicated this missing part with the **gap** '___' positioned where *the cake* would be if it were present. This gap is important because it indicates that the *HEAD* (*the cake*) is the thing baked, rather than the thing doing the baking. (Compare this with *the chef that ___ baked the cake for Josh,* where the different location of the gap, before *baked* rather than after it, indicates that now the HEAD = *the chef* is the one doing the baking.)[4]

When the constituents of this sentence are put back together, it is important that the mind identify the HEAD = *the cake* of the SUBJECT = *the cake I baked for Josh* as the thing that satisfies the PREDICATE = *didn't seem to please him*; this is how the mind knows that it was the cake, rather than me or Josh, that didn't please.

3.2 Other constituent relations

The symbolic theory's combinatorial strategy assumes that the mind recognizes the sentence (2) to be a whole that is related in specified ways to its parts, which may themselves be smaller wholes related in specified ways to their still smaller parts; the ability of the mind to process (2) is explained by its ability to analyze (2) into these parts and to process the whole by appropriately processing the parts (see Figure 1). Clearly, this decomposing into parts—parsing—must eventually stop, at which point the strategy must face the problem of explaining mental competence with the **primitive** or **atomic** parts—those that cannot themselves be further analyzed into constituents. Competence with the (finitely many) atomic parts is explained in symbolic theory by rote memorization: for (2), the properties of the words *bake, Josh,* and so on, are simply assumed to be stored directly in the hearer's memory.

In addition to the part-whole relationships discussed so far, other relationships are crucial in processing (2). One is the possible **coreference** connecting *him* to *Josh*: *him* can refer to the same boy referred to by *Josh,* but not, for example, to the entities referred to by *I* or *the cake.* This relationship is often notated by writing *the cake I baked for Josh$_i$ didn't seem to please him$_i$*—**coindexing** the pronoun *him* and the proper noun *Josh* with the index *i*. Yet another relation—**scope**—connects *not* (contracted in *didn't*) to the embedded predicate *please him*; this relation is needed to recognize that it was the pleasing (rather than the baking) that did not happen.[5]

Thus, the combinatorial strategy explains the mind's competence with sentences like (2) from the assumption that the mind analyzes (2) into some **symbolic structure** in which are encoded, among other things, all the relationships discussed above, which we have called 'subject', 'predicate', 'head', 'modifier', 'gap', 'coindexation', 'scope', and so forth. Such a structure as a whole is often notated along the lines of (7), where the gap is denoted by 't' rather than '___' (we have simplified considerably

[4] Sometimes, as here, whether the head is the "do-er" or the "do-ee" can be determined by the word meanings together with real-world commonsense knowledge. But the kind of general theory we are discussing must deal adequately with all sentences, including those where only structure, not content, can determine the respective roles of the participants: for example, *the president who Bush insulted ___ yesterday* versus *the president who ___ insulted Bush yesterday.*

[5] The predicate *seem to please* is inside the scope of *not*; the predicate *bake* is outside. The reverse is true in *the cake I didn't bake for Josh seemed to please him.* Whether in (2) it is the seeming or the pleasing that didn't happen—*didn't seem to please him* versus *seemed not to please him*—is an example of the many subtleties of scope that arise in natural language. Scope is a central concept in syntactic theory and applies not just to negation, but to many other **operators** as well: an operator takes a phrase that is its scope and alters it into a related phrase. In (2), *not* takes the phrase *seem to please him* and produces a phrase with the negated meaning, *not seem to please him*; Chapter 16 addresses the ***wh*-operator** that takes a declarative sentence like *x didn't seem to please him* and creates the question *what didn't seem to please him?*

relative to most actual proposals in the contemporary literature on sentence structure). In this tree structure, we have labeled phrases by their type or **syntactic category**: **S** (sentence), **NP** (noun phrase), **VP** (verb phrase), **PP** (prepositional phrase), **V** (verb), and so on. The drawing in (7) is incomplete: the constituents beneath triangles (e.g., *seem to please him*) are themselves further decomposed into subconstituents that are not shown.

Figure 1. Sentence interpretation via the combinatorial strategy

Interpret: *the cake I baked for Josh didn't seem to please him*

PARSE

SUBJECT

PREDICATE

Interpret: *the cake I baked for Josh*

Interpret: *didn't seem to please him*

PARSE

HEAD

MODIFIER

Interpret: *the cake*

Interpret: [*that*] *I baked* ___ *for Josh*

PARSE

SUBJECT

PREDICATE (*gapped*)

Interpret: *I*

Interpret: *baked* ___ *for Josh*

Interpret: *Josh*

Memory retrieval

/dʒaʃ/
Type: Human
Sex: M
Age: 18
Sport: Fencing

For sentences, as we showed in the previous section, the relevant kinds of part-whole relationships include the relationship of the subject of a sentence to the sentence as a whole, and the relationship of the predicate to the sentence as a whole, as well as the relationships linking heads, modifiers, and gaps to the larger constituents of which they are parts. (Particular instantiations of the combinatorial strategy differ

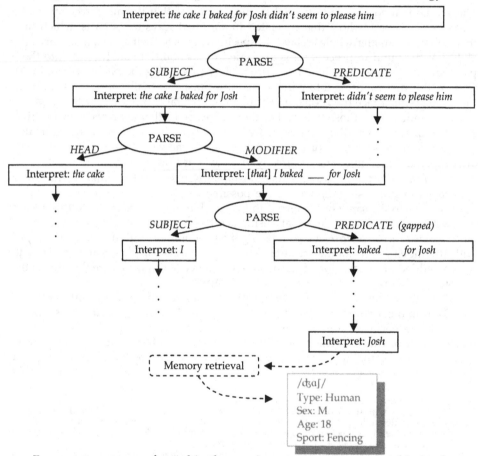

in exactly how they proceed to analyze (2) into its parts; we have just been considering one of many possibilities here.)

(7)

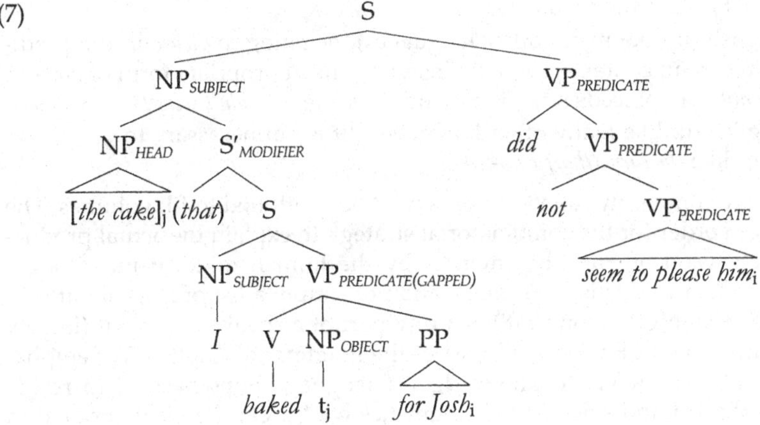

It is important to remember that (7) is just one way of *drawing a set of relationships* between wholes and their parts. The hypothesis of the combinatorial strategy is that the mind somehow contains encodings of these constituents and their relationships; these collectively form an abstract symbolic structure—a mental representation—that we may choose to draw in one way or another solely for our analytical (and typographical) convenience.

Particular instantiations of the combinatorial strategy adopt different notations and different formal analyses of sentences like (2), but when such details are put aside, the various instantiations clearly have a great deal in common, such as the relationships discussed above, in one guise or another. Also differing from one linguistic theory to another is whether a particular relationship is seen as part of the *meaning* (**semantics**) or of the *form* (**syntax**) of the actual sentence (2). But regardless of such details, what is important for our purposes is that an enormous range of research in cognitive science—from syntax and semantics in linguistics, to philosophy of language, to formal logic, to artificial intelligence and computational linguistics, to cognitive modeling of human language processing—shares a commitment to the combinatorial strategy for explaining the processes that underlie mental competence in language, and many other combinatorial domains such as reasoning and planning. It is therefore appropriate to consider the combinatorial strategy to be one of the central defining commitments of symbolic (or **structural**) approaches to cognitive theory.

3.3 Grammatical and lexical knowledge; argument structure

As applied to explaining human linguistic competence, the combinatorial strategy must assume that a speaker competent in English has a variety of types of knowledge; a few examples are illustrated in (8).

(8) Knowledge of English required for producing sentence (2)

a. In declarative sentences of English (unlike many other languages), the *subject* must *precede* the predicate.

b. In English (unlike many other languages), negating *to please* in the predicate (in certain contexts) requires inserting the appropriate form of *do*; and while *not* may precede *seem*, it may not precede *do*: *didn't seem to please him.*

c. In English (unlike many other languages), it is not necessary to use *that* in phrases like *the cake (that) I baked.*

This list of what are commonly called "rules" could be continued to fill volumes. The point here is that in order for the combinatorial strategy to explain the actual production and comprehension of English sentences by the human mind, it must be assumed that all this knowledge is *in the mind,* and not simply a list of facts about sentences of English. The information in (8) is a tiny part of a speaker's *implicit* (largely unconscious) knowledge of English—all part of the **grammar** of English. We emphasize that here 'grammar' refers to knowledge of language hypothesized to reside within every speaker's mind—not within linguistics books. On the view adopted in this book, the primary job of the grammar of English is not to determine whether a given sequence of words is grammatical or ungrammatical; rather, it is to pair meanings with the exact forms of the English sentences that express them. Thus, it is the grammar in this sense that allows a speaker with the appropriate meaning in mind to utter *the cake I baked for Josh didn't seem to please him* rather than the jumble of English words that would emerge in the absence of grammatical knowledge.[6]

Complementing grammatical knowledge is the **lexical** information a speaker has. Such information pairs the sound sequence /ʤɑʃ/ 'Josh' with a particular boy; this is the memorized knowledge assumed by the combinatorial strategy to explain how speakers understand primitive linguistic constituents. Other types of lexical knowledge are also important. To produce (2), for example, the English speaker must know that when using the verb *to please*—as opposed to its close relative *to like*—the person experiencing the emotion must be the (direct) OBJECT of the verb, and the stimulus (the cake) must be its SUBJECT: compare *the cake pleased Josh* with *Josh liked the cake.* In these examples, *the cake* and *Josh* are the **arguments** of the verb; the **argument structure** of the verb determines the linkage (or **mapping**) between the **semantic roles** (experiencer vs. stimulus) and the **syntactic roles** (SUBJECT vs. OBJECT) of the verb's arguments. (Precisely how to characterize knowledge of argument structure is a central challenge of the theory of the syntax-semantics interface; it is the topic of Chapter 11 and Section 20:2.) It is lexical information such as argument structure that governs how a particular word fits into the combinatorial structure of English sentences, making the link between the combinatorial strategy's primitive elements and the complex constituents they combine to create.

[6] The difference between the conceptions of language as a set of external words and sentences or as a system of knowledge internal to the speaker's mind has long been emphasized by Chomsky—for example, in his distinction between E-language (external) and I-language (internal; Chomsky 1986).

Box 5. Language, linguistics, and grammar:
Frequently unasked questions

The research on language presented in this book employs the view of language illustrated in Section 3, which is the perspective adopted by one of the best-developed components of symbolic cognitive theory, generative linguistics. This theory is framed by the combinatorial strategy of explanation. The generative viewpoint may hold some surprises for those new to it. In the following answers, we attempt to articulate the outlook of generative linguistics on basic questions about language that reflect presuppositions that seem to be widely held, if infrequently expressed.

Q1. "Why are linguists always making such a big deal about language learning? What's so hard about learning words?" *Unasked question: Isn't language learning basically just word learning?*

A1. There it is, the classic image of language learning: Mommy pointing and gleefully proclaiming *doggie!* Little wonder there is often scant appreciation for the problem of language acquisition. But according to the combinatorial strategy, the main action in language concerns not the *atoms* of combination—such as words—but their *patterns of combination*—grammar. It is not so much individual words, but the structures that are built with them, that make human language unique. And while there are important crosslinguistic tendencies to be found among individual words, it is in the principles of their combination that we see the real flowering of the idea that abstract universal principles are a window into the inner workings of the human mind. The history of words, their nuances of meaning and usage—these are fascinating topics, but not central to what defines language in the symbolic theory of cognition: richly productive principles governing the construction of complex combinations of atomic units. It is the question of how such abstract principles get into the minds of such young children that makes the problem of language acquisition so compelling.

Q2. "Well, suppose I grant that grammar is key to what makes human language special. But what's so hard about learning word order?" *Unasked question: Isn't grammar basically just word order?*

A2. In syntax, the primary relation between parts *X* and *Y* of complex structures is not *X precedes Y* but *X is embedded within Y*. Here, *X* and *Y* are *phrases*, not words: see (7) and Figure 1. And phrases are abstract entities; phrase boundaries must be computed by the hearer, and learners must learn how to parse sentences into phrases at the same time they are learning the grammar that governs how phrases embed within one another. This is no easy task, to say the least. Word order is certainly one aspect of syntax, but not a particularly important one. One reason is that word order is a *surface* property of language, and one of the major discoveries of modern linguistic theory is that surface properties are often less important than aspects of sentence structure hidden beneath the surface—phrase structure, for example. This hidden structure is crucial for identifying the general principles governing the systematic patterns of combination, not only within a single language, but also across different languages.

Q3. "OK, maybe learning grammar—syntax—is hard. But these complexities don't arise in phonology; learning how to recognize words is just a pattern-matching problem that doesn't seem particularly special or difficult." *Unasked question: Isn't phonology just the knowledge of how to recognize a word by its sounds?*

A3. Phonology is a component of grammar, and thus, like syntax, is primarily concerned with patterns of combination and systematic patterns of distribution of linguistic elements. The individual speech sounds forming the atoms of combination—**segments**—have internal properties that are important, but in phonology, their importance derives from their implications for how sounds *combine.* The articulatory and acoustic properties of individual segments, which figure importantly in speech recognition, are more the province of **phonetics** than of phonology. Understanding how people identify sounds, and their combinations into words, is a fascinatingly difficult problem—but phonology has little to say about it. Phonology is to speech recognition as ethology is to animal recognition: how people recognize a goose may be an interesting problem, but ethology has little to say about it. Phonology studies the social and mating habits of speech sounds: it turns out that they form family units, **syllables**, with well-defined roles for different family members; syllables travel in pairs, **metrical feet**, in which one member is dominant (**stressed**). There is a taxonomy of different types of feet (**iambic**, **trochaic**), and of different ways they organize (**stress systems**) into larger groups (**prosodic words**).[7] Learning all this is special and difficult for essentially the same reason that syntax is: the generalizations that must be learned involve hidden structure, for which direct surface evidence is weak or nonexistent. Only by analyzing the complex patterns of sound combination in a given language is it possible to learn how to identify syllables, feet, and so on, and to learn the hidden properties internal to sounds that govern their modes of combination.

Q4. "Suppose it's true that grammar learning is special and difficult, both for syntax and phonology. But how can linguists effectively study language while ignoring its raison d'être: communication?" *Unasked question: Isn't communication the crux of language?*

A4. The purpose of language is communication, so one can't possibly study language without focusing primarily on the demands of communication ... or so it might seem. But even animals with minuscule intellectual capacity communicate. What is so remarkable about human language is not *that* it lets us communicate, but

[7] In an iambic foot, the second member is stressed; in a trochaic foot, the first. Foot theory is actually quite rich. A foot can sometimes consist of a pair of **moras** rather than a pair of syllables. A mora (μ) is a unit of syllable weight: **heavy** syllables contain two moras, **light** syllables only one. The definition of a heavy syllable varies across languages: it may require a long vowel, or a diphthong, or a final consonant. Feet consisting of more than two syllables—for example, three syllables or an unbounded number of syllables—have also been proposed (see, e.g., Hayes 1980; Burzio 1994).

what it lets us communicate: elaborately structured propositions, commands, and questions with a potentially extraordinary degree of intricacy. This is possible because of the way language allows us to *form new, arbitrarily complex combinations.* Again, we're back where we started: it's not that we can communicate an atomic message through an atomic word that defines what is special about human language (*run!*)—it's that we can communicate complex, combinatorially structured meanings by means of complex, combinatorially structured expressions. This defines exactly the central province of two components of grammar: syntax and semantics.[8] These grammar components do in fact address the crux of human communication—how complex meanings get expressed with complex signals. Furthermore, the complexity of human language involves an important grammatical component even down at the level of the atoms of communication—words (or more properly, the smallest meaning-bearing elements within words, **morphemes**). For communicating the full range of human messages requires many thousands of words, and this is made possible by the combinatorial structure *internal* to words: the regular patterns by which a small set of atomic sounds combine to form an enormous set of words. And this is exactly the province of the third principal component of grammar: phonology.

3.4 Explaining the productivity of cognition

The combinatorial strategy reduces the problem of explaining mental competence with wholes to the problem of explaining competence with their parts, and then, recursively, with the subparts of the parts, and so on. The most direct approach to employing the combinatorial strategy in cognitive science is the one we have taken to define the symbolic theory of cognition. In this approach, the combinatorial strategy is applied at the *process level*. That is, this theory postulates that *internal to the mind of the cognizer* there exist a parsing process that decomposes inputs into parts, individual subprocesses that process the parts individually, and further processes that assemble the results into an integrated output.

To say that in symbolic theory, these parsing and memory processes are 'internal to the mind of the cognizer' is to say that internal properties of this system of processes are relevant to predicting corresponding properties of the cognizer's mental behavior. For example, suppose that according to the decomposition into subprocesses proposed by a symbolic theory $\mathcal{T}_{sym}$, one specific task T_1 requires all the particular subprocesses required by another specific task T_2, plus additional subprocesses.[9]

[8] The semantic component of grammar does not figure centrally in this book, but it's worth briefly mentioning that the theme running through these unasked questions applies to semantics as well. The core of linguistic semantics concerns not the meanings of individual words, but the principles governing how atomic meanings *combine* to form complex meanings. The semantics of individual words—**lexical semantics**—is also a part of linguistic semantics; but again, of central interest is how properties of the meanings of individual words govern those words' patterns of combination.

[9] For example, T_1 and T_2 might consist of performing the same general task upon two different inputs I_1 and I_2, where I_1 requires repeating some type of subprocess more times than does I_2.

Then theory $\mathcal{T}_{\text{sym}}$ predicts that T_1 will require at least as much time as T_2 to complete. $\mathcal{T}_{\text{sym}}$ also predicts that any brain damage that impairs T_2 must also impair T_1.[10] To articulate such predictions less crudely, and spell out the assumptions underlying them, is a significant job in itself; it will be taken up in Chapter 23. It is a primary task of that chapter to show how the theory developed in this book employs the combinatorial strategy at a *functional* level, but *not* at the process level. This means symbols and rules do not fill all the roles assigned to them by symbolic theory—but they retain enough of their status to support functional-level explanation of cognition. It is not symbolic but only connectionist computation that characterizes the causal interactions constituting cognitive processing.

As already discussed, a great virtue of the combinatorial strategy, a virtue the proposed theory will inherit, is that it yields a solution to one of the central problems of cognitive science: the problem of cognitive **productivity** (or **generativity**).

(9) The problem of cognitive productivity

Cognitive science must provide a formal description of a computational system with a finite store of knowledge that can be proved to have unbounded competence (such as that needed for language processing).

For instance, according to symbolic theory, the finite store of knowledge in the speaker's mind includes the memorized properties of the finite number of English lexical items and the finite (recursive) algorithm for parsing wholes into parts. This finite store can then be used to interpret or produce any of an infinite set of sentences.

We will take a **combinatorial computational system** to be a formal set of representations, and procedures for manipulating them, that instantiates the principles of the combinatorial strategy. The representations of such a system must allow the encoding of the kinds of structural relationships needed by the strategy; the procedures must allow the kinds of decomposition of wholes into parts required for combinatorial parsing, and the kinds of building of wholes out of parts required for producing combinatorial structures.

On this characterization, combinatorial computational systems may operate in a variety of ways. For example, the processing of sentence (2) might involve a step-by-step process of parsing, in which the sentence as a whole is first parsed into constituents SUBJECT and PREDICATE, and then one of these is parsed into its own (sub)-constituents, and so on. This would be a **serial** combinatorial system, the type familiar from traditional computing in general, and characteristic of symbolic cognitive theory (Jurafsky and Martin 2000).

Alternatively, (2) might be processed by a **parallel** combinatorial system, in which the structural relations involving all parts of the sentence, and all levels of embedding, are simultaneously computed. A principal contribution of the research presented in this book is an explicit formal proposal for how such parallel combinatorial

[10] $\mathcal{T}_{\text{sym}}$ further predicts that if a task T_3 is executed just before T_1 is executed, T_3 will facilitate or interfere with T_1, depending on whether the common subprocesses produce the same or different results in the two tasks.

systems can be constructed (in connectionist networks; Chapters 5, 7, and 8).

A final possibility, of course, is that a combinatorial computational system might combine serial and parallel processing—as is apparently the case for the human mind (Townsend and Bever 2001).

Having reviewed in this section and the last the basic ideas of symbolic and connectionist computation, we now consider how these cognitive architectures relate to the human mind/brain. It is in this context that the fundamental issue of "neural plausibility" can best be addressed; see Box 6.

Box 6. On connectionism and "neural plausibility"

The neural question for cognitive science is easily confused with the cognitive question for neuroscience (see (1) of the text). The cognitive question for neuroscience asks for the cognitive significance of biological components; to address it, a mathematical model must be sufficiently faithful to the neurobiology to capture the role of each component in its biological system.

But the neural question for cognitive science is very different. Cognitive science seeks a computational description of the mind, and a computational description by definition reduces complex operations to combinations of simple operations; the simplest of these operations define the cognitive architecture (see Section 23:2.2.2). So the neural question for cognitive science is, what are the primitive operations made available by the brain, to which complex cognitive functions must be reduced by computational theories? For this purpose, it is the *simplicity* rather than the *complexity* of neural operations that is critical. We want to ensure that the primitive operations of our cognitive architecture are within, not beyond, the computational abilities of biological neural networks. (For further discussion, see Section 23:1.1.)

Thus, the neural question for cognitive science is a question about *computational systems*, not about *biology*. It must therefore be situated in the landscape of computation. This brings us to the starting point of the argument, which proceeds via five propositions.

(1) It is reasonable to believe that there are natural categories of computational systems.

A major achievement of the theory of computation—codified in the Church-Turing thesis—is the demonstration that although the notion of effective procedure can be naturally formalized in a variety of ways, the alternatives are all essentially equivalent (Haugeland 1985). The same functions can be computed by each of them; procedures specified in one formalism can be mechanically translated into any other formalism. This collection of mutually equivalent computational systems defines a natural category, one that can be broken down into natural subcategories each of which can also be formalized in multiple ways (e.g., the Chomsky hierarchy, Box 6:1). We can call this the **Church-Turing** computational class.

The primitive operations defining the computational architectures of systems in the Church-Turing class include recognizing the type of a discrete symbol, writing a symbol to a discrete storage location, rewriting a symbol within a string of symbols, concatenating individual symbols to form complex structures, binding a symbol as the value of another symbol serving as a variable, changing an internal control state, and selecting the next operation on the basis of the identity of a symbol. Church-Turing architectures rely fundamentally on the discreteness of symbol types, the localization of information to individual symbols, and the strictly sequential control of operations (Box 23:1).

(2) It appears that neural computation is continuously numerical, distributed, and massively parallel; it falls in a computational class quite different from the Church-Turing class.

The activation of a neuron, on the time scale of tens of milliseconds, is a continuously varying rate of **firing**—propagation of action potentials. The information encoded in neural activity is distributed over many neurons (see Box 2). Neurons operate in parallel, and indeed the average firing rate of a population of neurons firing simultaneously is an important measure of neural computation.

There are many examples of neural systems with these properties. Their central importance is not diminished by the existence of other modes of neural operation, nor by neural descriptions at other scales of space and time (e.g., those sufficiently fine-grained to reveal the underlying discrete nature of much neural activity). Under no explicit analysis does the computational architecture of the brain come close to resembling the sequential, symbolic primitive operations of the Church-Turing class. In lieu of the discrete, local, and massively serial Church-Turing architecture, the brain—in significant part—provides a continuous, distributed, and massively parallel architecture. This type of architecture defines a natural computational class we can call the **CDP** class (continuous, distributed, and parallel). This class includes neural systems, under appropriate descriptions.

(3) Connectionist networks are simple representatives of the CDP computational class.

Connectionist networks are by design members of the CDP class in which the fundamental properties of continuous, distributed, and massively parallel computation are given extremely simple instantiations. It is reasonable to believe that the CDP class is like essentially every other formal class: the simplest cases exhibit, albeit in simple form, many of the core phenomena characteristic of the entire class. Understanding these phenomena in the simplest cases is a prerequisite to understanding their counterparts in more complex cases.

(4) Therefore, it is reasonable to believe that by studying connectionist computation, we will learn about the types of properties shared by members of the computational class that includes the brain.

The bottom line, then, is this.

(5) Within a connectionist architecture, computational reduction of cognitive theories to primitive operations yields a microtheory that is a simple representative of the computational class including neural computation. Such reduction is thus a major step toward understanding the reduction of cognition to neural computation. In contrast, reduction within a symbolic architecture yields a microtheory that is not even in the same general class as neural computation; such reduction is of little relevance to understanding how cognition can arise in a brain.

4 THE PROPOSED SOLUTION

We now return to the fundamental tension that frames the research presented in this book. What type of computation is cognition? Connectionist "brain" computation—massively parallel numerical processing? Or symbolic "mind" computation—rule-governed manipulation of combinatorially complex, discrete, abstract symbol structures? The answer we develop here is this: it is both. What makes a mind/brain, what gives rise to human cognition, is a complex dynamical system that is a massively parallel numerical computer at a lower level of formal description—a level closer to the biophysical—and, at the same time, a rule-governed processor of discrete symbolic structures at a higher level of description—a level considerably more abstract than the biophysical, but nonetheless governed by formal laws, and related to the lower-level description by precisely defined mathematical mappings.

This resolution of the tension between brain-as-numerical-computer and mind-as-symbolic-computer is easy enough to state in vague terms. Indeed, in mainstream materialist cognitive science, the proposal that the mind is a symbol-manipulating computer has always carried with it the presumption that this computer is the description—albeit at a highly abstract level—of the *brain*, which, of course, has an entirely different description at the level of individual cells (Hofstadter 1979). What has changed in recent years is that there is now a neural-level description of the brain that also describes it as a kind of computer: a numerical connectionist computer. This description abstracts away from much biological detail, but to a significantly lesser degree than does the description of the brain as a symbol-manipulating computer (see Box 6). Thus, the question we can now ask is, can the description of (mind/) brain-as-connectionist-computer be connected—with mathematical precision—to the description of mind(/brain)-as-symbolic-computer?

Our task in this book is to develop formal proposals for exactly how to make such a connection (see also Marcus 2001; Townsend and Bever 2001). These proposals assume that the connectionist computer is a description of the mind/brain at a lower level, while the symbolic computer is a description *of one and the same system* at a higher, more abstract level. Developing these proposals with formal precision poses a conceptual and technical challenge of some magnitude. The tools we bring together to meet this challenge come from several intellectual quarters.

First, the idea that a computational system can simultaneously admit rather different formal descriptions at lower and higher levels is one that has already been aggressively developed in computer science: at a lower level, bits are flipping between 0 and 1 at a furious rate, and at a higher level, on a considerably slower time scale, abstract folders are opening and closing on an abstract desktop (see Figure 2a). One **virtual machine**, a folder-manipulator, is running on top of a different lower-level machine, a bit-manipulator. Put differently, the virtual machine is a higher-level abstraction implemented in the primitive bit-manipulator. Despite the mysterious connotations of the term 'virtual', there is nothing imprecise here at all: the higher-level description is entirely formally well-defined—encoded, in fact, in precise computer programs that define the higher-level virtual machine, translating it precisely into the formal description of the lower-level machine.

Figure 2. Levels of analysis

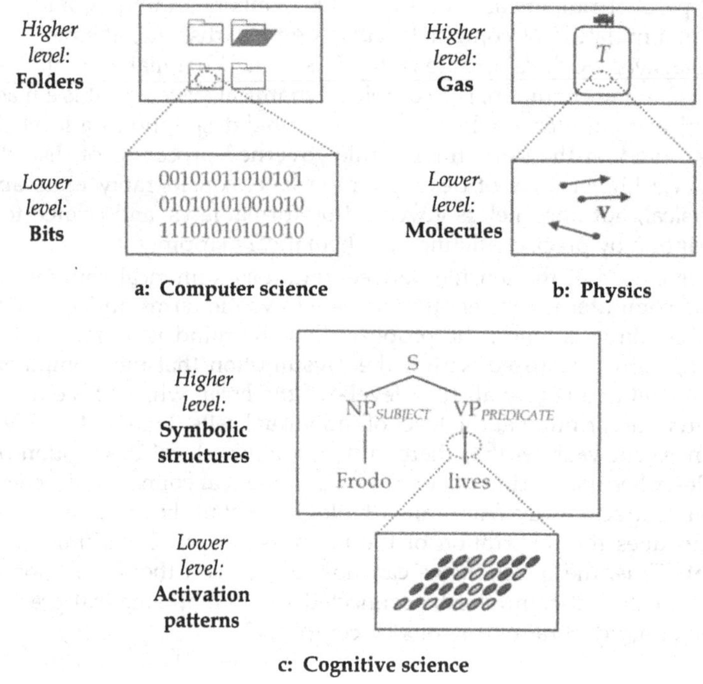

a: Computer science

b: Physics

c: Cognitive science

But our challenge here is qualitatively different from that of relating higher- and lower-level virtual machines in computer science. For in conventional computer science, the two levels of virtual machines are the *same type* of computer: discrete, serial, symbol-manipulating machines (Box 23:1). The exact vocabulary of symbols and manipulations varies across levels in a traditional computer, but this is conceptually and technically quite different from the cognitive case, where the lower-level machine is a noisy, massively parallel numerical computer, and the higher-level virtual machine a rule-governed symbolic computer. Traditional computer science provides tools for technically characterizing the higher-level machine, but not the lower-level one.

On the other hand, continuous mathematics—for example, as employed in mathematical physics—provides tools for the analysis of brain-type connectionist computation. And as in computer science, in physics the idea of rather different formal characterizations of one and the same system at lower and higher levels is a familiar one. A gas—a continuous, extended system defined by properties like volume, pressure, temperature (T), and entropy—is a higher-level description of a system that on a lower level is described as a collection of discrete, point-like atoms individually possessing none of these properties but others instead, such as velocity ($\mathbf{v}$) (Figure 2b; Reif 1965).

In the work presented in this book, ideas and techniques developed in mathematical physics and in computer science are brought together to construct a formal characterization of a mind/brain as a computational system that is parallel and numerical when described at the lower level, but, when described at a higher level, is symbolic in crucial respects (Figure 2c).

The exact type of symbolic system that will result from the shift to a higher level is not, however, an altogether familiar one in cognitive or computer science. For example, it is in key respects *not* sequential, and as a result, the role of the rules in the higher-level computational system is in many respects novel. The "psychological reality" of the rules and symbols in the new computational architecture is somewhat reduced relative to traditional symbolic theories of mind. Yet the role of symbols and rules in explaining the crucial properties of higher cognition is an essential one. For this reason, the new architecture we develop here is called the **Integrated Connectionist/Symbolic Cognitive Architecture (ICS)**: in this architecture, connectionist and symbolic computational descriptions each play an essential role in overall cognitive explanation (see Box 7). ICS does not represent either an eliminativist or an implementationalist position on the relation between connectionist and symbolic computation (see Box 8), but a novel intermediate position that we attempt to articulate most completely in Chapter 23.

Like symbolic theory, the ICS theory we develop in this book employs the combinatorial strategy for explaining the productivity of cognition. Crucially, however, unlike symbolic theory, the new theory employs this strategy not at the level of process but only at the level of function. In ICS, there are two crucial ways of decomposing representations: one is **functionally relevant**, the other **process-relevant**. These two decompositions correspond to two different levels of structure: ICS is a **split-level** cognitive architecture (Cummins and Schwarz 1991).

At the functional level, the relevant decomposition of representations is into constituents, in ICS just as in symbolic theory. Representations are interrelated in the way the combinatorial strategy requires, and this is what provides the explanation of cognitive productivity. The decomposition of representations into constituents is also what determines the *meaning* of representations.

But in ICS, the relationships among representations required by the combinatorial strategy are not established in a serial, constituent-by-constituent process. There is no step-by-step algorithm defined over constituents that describes the moment-by-moment workings of cognition: the latter requires algorithms that are defined via the process-relevant decomposition, which decomposes a representation not into its constituents, but into its *activation values*. The dynamics of cognition must be described by connectionist algorithms.

To preview one implication of the split-level structure of ICS, suppose one input I_2 consists of a subset of the constituents of another input I_1. Then use of the combinatorial strategy to explain the processing of I_1 will require more deductive steps for the *cognitive scientist*. But in ICS, it does not follow that processing I_1 must take longer for the *cognizer*: the time required to process an input is determined by the number of steps of activation spreading required by a connectionist network to compute its output. This need not correlate with the number of constituents processed.

In ICS, then, combinatorially structured, symbolic *representations* are central, but these are not processed by symbolic *algorithms* defined over that combinatorial structure. Working out the explanatory implications of the novel status of symbols in ICS will require most of Chapter 23.

Box 7. Symbolic structures in neural networks

In the cognitive architecture developed in this book, ICS, mental representations are symbol structures when formally described at a high, abstract level, and are distributed activation patterns when described at the lower level of connectionist units. As a simple illustration, the phonology of the word *cat* is often described in theoretical linguistics by a symbol structure consisting of a syllable (written σ) with two constituents. The first is the **onset**, which contains the single consonant sound *k*. The second is the rest of the syllable, the **rime**, which in turn is composed of two (sub)constituents, the **nucleus** and the **coda**. In this structure, the nucleus consists of a single segment, the vowel *æ*, and the coda consists of the single consonant segment *t*. The tree diagram below denotes this symbol structure and the chart shows how it might be reduced in ICS to a pattern of activation over a set of 14 connectionist units.

The activation pattern realizing this symbol structure is shown on the lowest horizontal line of the chart, labeled [$_\sigma$ k [æ t]]. The area of each of the 14 circles represents the activation value of one of the 14 units. This pattern is in fact the result of superimposing (adding together) the four activation patterns represented on the top four horizontal lines of the chart. Each of these patterns realizes one of the symbols in the structure. The first realizes the symbol σ filling the role of tree root (denoted r_ε); the second, the symbol *k* filling the role of left-child-of-root (denoted r_0), and so on.

Figure 2 *Box 7*

Each of these patterns is in turn built up of an activation pattern realizing the symbol (e.g., *t*) and an activation pattern realizing its role (e.g., r_{11}; right-child-of-right-child-of-root). We will not illustrate this further level of structure here, but the operation binding these two patterns together—the **tensor product**—is illustrated in Box 2:1 and developed in detail in Chapter 5.

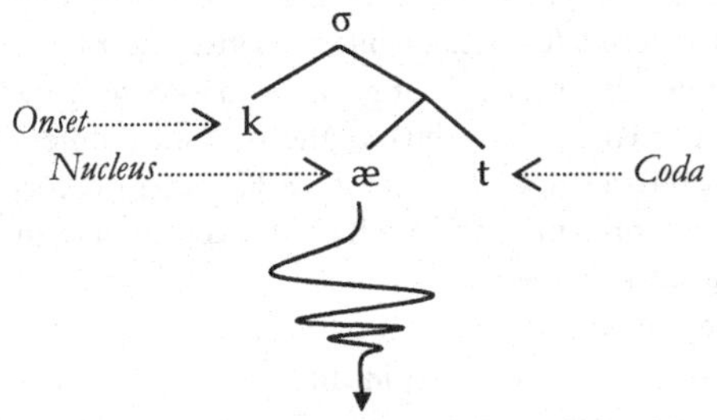

Activation patterns: *cat* and its constituents

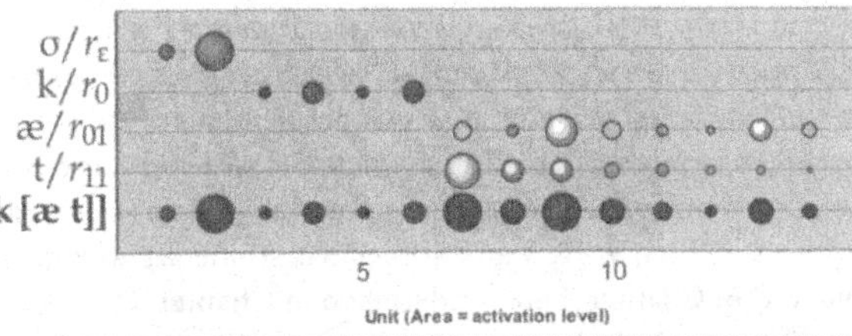

Box 8. The relation between connectionist and symbolic computation

According to the **eliminativist** position, the science of the mind/brain must eliminate mentalist notions such as beliefs, goals, and symbols from scientific discourse, replacing them with appropriate concepts from neuroscience. To the extent that connectionist theory can stand in for brain theory, this position states that connectionist theory should ultimately eliminate symbolic theory from cognitive science. A guiding eliminativist metaphor from physical science puts symbolic and connectionist theory in correspondence with Aristotelian physics and modern physics: the latter has utterly eliminated the former from science. The symbolic conception of the mind is seen as prescientific, its concepts being as irrelevant as quintessence to the ultimate scientific theory, which is to be stated entirely in neural terms.

At the opposite extreme, the **implementationalist** position asserts that symbolic theory is an exact scientific account of cognition at a suitably abstract level of analysis and that neuroscience must ultimately explain how symbols and rules are literally implemented in the brain. According to the guiding implementationalist metaphor, the mind truly is a symbolic computer implemented in the brain: just as we can develop exactly correct symbolic algorithms for digital computers without concern for how they might actually be implemented in a particular physical computer that executes them, so we can develop correct symbolic theories of mental computation that are not influenced by how they may happen to be implemented in neural "wetware." An analogy from physics might be this: symbolic theory is to connectionist theory as Keplerian theory is to Newtonian gravitational theory. The former describes the orbits of the planets in geometric terms (ellipses), while the latter describes the movement over time of the planets under the influence of gravitational force. Newtonian theory provides a way of deducing Keplerian orbits as the necessary outcome of gravitational dynamics. Newtonian physics does not eliminate Keplerian theory: it provides more general and fundamental principles from which the correctness of Keplerian physics can be formally deduced and thereby explained; it shows how Keplerian orbits are "implemented" in temporal dynamics.

The cognitive architecture developed in this book, ICS, represents a novel intermediate position that integrates the eliminativist insight that cognition reflects its neural realization with the implementationalist insight that symbolic computation captures important aspects of the structure of cognition, despite its apparent neural implausibility. The ICS position is not eliminativist, because it maintains a crucial role for symbolic theory in cognitive science; it is not implementationalist, because the symbolic theory proposed is novel, shaped by its neural realization, and because only symbolic *representations*, and not symbolic *algorithms* for manipulating them, are claimed to be cognitively relevant. The involved and somewhat subtle argumentation behind these claims is previewed in Chapter 3 and undertaken in Chapter 23.

A partial analogy between ICS theory and physics, which even suggests some of the particular mathematical principles proposed in ICS, is this: symbolic theory is to connectionist theory as classical Newtonian mechanics is to quantum mechanics. Quantum mechanics does not "implement" classical mechanics, because quantum mechanics gives rise to macroscopic effects inconsistent with classical physics (e.g., superconductivity), and entails a different metaphysics (concerning uncertainty, for example). Despite such profound differences, however, quantum mechanics is a microtheory which entails that, to an excellent degree of approximation, classical physics is a valid macrotheory. Quantum mechanics does not eliminate Newtonian physics from science; on the contrary, by providing a precise (yet approximate) reduction of Newtonian theory, the quantum microtheory delimits and explains the validity of the Newtonian macrotheory. The analogy to ICS theory is only partial, however; relative to the physics case, the ICS microtheory, based in connectionist computation, has a considerably more extensive impact in reshaping the symbolic macrotheory. The substantial revision of symbolic grammatical theory resulting from ICS theory would be analogous to quantum mechanics yielding major revisions of Newtonian theory.

5 The Evidence

The evidence in favor of the new cognitive architecture is of two general types, one deriving from the more conservative aspects of ICS, the other from the more innovative aspects.

5.1 Prior evidence

Our proposal is conservative in the sense that it integrates two previously developed computational accounts of the mind/brain, one at the mind level, the other at a level significantly closer to a biophysical description of the brain. In the broadest sense, the evidence previously amassed in support of *both* these two different computational accounts may now be taken as evidence in favor of the integrated account. The reward for successfully unifying the connectionist and symbolic architectures is the opportunity to take the best of two very different worlds.

ICS posits mental representations for higher cognitive domains that are describable, at a high level, as complex symbol structures; thus, ICS is supported by the wealth of psychological, linguistic, and computational evidence for symbolic representations in higher cognitive domains ranging from higher-level vision and planning to language and reasoning. At the same time, the mental representations posited by ICS theory are also describable, at a lower level, as the numerical activation values of a large collection of simple parallel processing units; thus, ICS is generally supported by the neurophysiological evidence that information is so represented in the brain. Obviously, it is exactly in order to accrue both these types of evidence that we have chosen to tackle the serious obstacles that must be overcome if symbolic and neural-network theories of cognition are to be formally unified.

Of course, the preceding remarks provide only a crude first approximation to the empirical ledger—it is the burden of considerable future research to construct a much more articulated analysis of what previously garnered evidence survives as support for the unified theory. But the point remains that the integrated theory has access to a wide range of evidence, of the kinds already developed in the existing sciences both of the brain and of the mind—a broader empirical range than does any framework that rejects across the board as irrelevant, or obsolete, either neural or symbolic theory. This point is significant because such rejectionist approaches have attracted large followings in the fields of neural and cognitive science. Within mind-centered research, it is tempting to adopt the implementationalist position and dismiss issues of neural computation as too low-level to be cognitively relevant; in brain-centered research, it is easy to embrace the eliminativist position and view issues of mental computation as rendered moot by reduction to biology. By contrast, in proposing ICS, we assume responsibility for ultimately confronting the empirical and theoretical issues central to both mental and neural computation; relevant evidence is to be found at all of the levels of organization constituting the mind/brain.

5.2 Novel evidence

The second kind of evidence in favor of ICS—the kind we most explicitly develop in this book—derives from the aspects of the architecture that are not conservative, but novel. The novel elements are usefully viewed as being of two types: the top-down and the bottom-up. In the top-down category are ways in which connectionist computation is made more powerful—in both the computational and the explanatory sense—in order to meet the strong constraint that it serve as the lower-level platform for what emerges as symbolic computation at a higher level of description. This sort of evidence is developed primarily in Part II (computational power) and Part IV (explanatory power).

In the bottom-up category are ways in which the symbolic theory we develop is either restricted or enriched relative to previous proposals for symbolic cognitive architectures. Because the symbolic level emerges from a lower-level connectionist substrate, it is simplified in certain respects: for example, long, "massively serial" computations are replaced by one-shot, massively parallel symbolic computations. At the same time, however, some connectionist computational properties can percolate up to the symbolic level, enriching it with novel concepts.

The central such property addressed in this book is **optimization**. Connectionist computation in many cases computes representations that optimize well-formedness or **Harmony**, as noted in Section 2 and illustrated in Boxes 3–4. Optimization turns out to provide many novel conceptual and technical tools for formally characterizing, at the symbolic level, speakers' knowledge of their native language. Chapters 11–21 (including all of Part III) develop the bottom-up evidence deriving from the novel aspects of the ICS framework: contributions to the theory of human language.

Our focus on language derives from several sources. Language has always played a special role in cognitive science, and it poses a special challenge for a connectionist-grounded theory. The theory of symbolic computation is intimately bound to the theory of formal languages; and language-like representations have played a critical role in cognitive theory since its inception. Chomsky's seminal work on the grammars of formal languages and on the formal grammars of natural languages has always defined a central place in the field, and his arguments for the combinatorial, recursive character of human knowledge of language have been taken to generalize to much of higher cognition, implicating structured, symbolic mental representations with a strongly language-like character. Confronting the challenges of language is thus especially important for a comprehensive theory attributing a central role to mental representations that are not inherently language-like, such as the distributed, numerical representations of connectionist computation. And among the mind-centered research programs in cognitive science, that concerned with developing a theory of knowledge of language—grammatical theory—has achieved a singular level of success; the ability to advance grammatical theory further is thus an acid test of any general theory claiming to address cognitive organization at the mental level.

Can ICS exploit aspects of connectionist computation to actually contribute to grammatical theory? To address this question, we develop two approaches to grammar based on the connectionist-derived proposal that well-formed or **grammatical** mental representations are **optimal** symbolic structures. This proposal proves to have pervasive consequences for grammatical theory; many of these consequences are explored in this book, and we will argue that they provide both conceptual and empirical evidence in favor of the general research program.

The optimization-based grammar formalisms we develop are conceptually similar but technically quite different. The first, **Harmonic Grammar (HG)**, is most closely tied to a connectionist substratum and employs numerical optimization (Legendre, Miyata, and Smolensky 1990a, b, c, 1991; Smolensky, Legendre, and Miyata 1992). The second, **Optimality Theory (OT)**, employs nonnumerical optimization (Prince and Smolensky 1991, 1993/2004; see also McCarthy and Prince 1993a, b, 1995; Archangeli and Langendoen 1997; Dekkers, van der Leeuw, and van de Weijer 2000; McCarthy 2002). OT has been applied to virtually all facets of phonology, the component of grammar governing speech sounds and their combination (McCarthy 2004). It has also been applied to many aspects of the theory of syntax (Barbosa et al. 1998; Legendre, Vikner, and Grimshaw 2001; Sells 2001). More recently, OT approaches to semantics and pragmatics have been developed (Hendriks, de Hoop, and de Swart 2000; Blutner and Zeevat 2003). OT has from its inception been applied to language learnability and acquisition (Tesar and Smolensky 1993, 1998, 2000; Boersma 1998; Stemberger and Bernhardt 1998). A variety of computational properties of the theory have also been formally analyzed (Tesar 1995; Frank and Satta 1998; Prince 2002).

In both HG and OT, optimization amounts to this: each possible symbolic linguistic structure can be evaluated by a set of **well-formedness constraints**, each of which defines one desirable aspect of an ideal linguistic representation (e.g., 'A sentence must have a subject'). These constraints are highly general and, as a result, highly conflicting. Typically, no structure meets all such constraints, and a means is needed for deciding which constraints are most important: the well-formed or grammatical structures are the ones that **optimally satisfy** the constraints, taking into account the differing strength or priority of constraints.

In HG, the connectionist notion of constraint **weighting** is used for this accounting: the priority of each constraint in the grammar is encoded in a numerical strength, and an optimal structure maximizes the total weight of all satisfied constraints, the Harmony of the structure (see Box 9). Since the optimal structure will typically violate some constraints, HG constraints are **soft**; with traditional **hard** grammatical constraints, no violation is tolerated in a well-formed structure.

In OT, for empirical reasons discussed most explicitly in Chapter 20, a more restrictive type of constraint interaction is employed: the constraints are ranked in a **strict domination hierarchy**, each constraint having complete priority over all constraints ranked lower in the hierarchy. An optimal structure may violate a given constraint $\mathbb{C}$, but only if that permits the structure to better satisfy some constraint ranked higher than $\mathbb{C}$ (or if there simply are no structures that satisfy $\mathbb{C}$). The constraints of OT are in this sense **minimally violable.**

Box 9. Optimization over macroconstraints in neural networks

Box 4 illustrates how neural network computation can be interpreted as optimization over constraints. The constraints being optimized there correspond to individual connections in the network. Since such networks are the microlevel description of the mind/brain in ICS theory, these constraints are **microconstraints**. The constraints defining grammars, however, are **macroconstraints**, part of the symbolic macrostructure of the mind/brain. These symbolic macroconstraints are realized in neural networks as distributed patterns of connection strengths—assemblies of microconstraints—just as the symbols themselves are realized as distributed patterns of unit activations.

As discussed in detail in Chapter 13, a basic grammatical constraint of syllable structure is NOCODA, which demands that a syllable not have a coda—roughly, that the syllable not end with a coda-filling consonant, but rather with a nucleus-filling vowel (see the syllable structure tree in Box 7). While a word like *me* satisfies NOCODA, *cat* violates it. The offending final *t* in coda position is displayed in the phonological tree structure for the word *cat* illustrated in Box 7 and repeated in the figure below. This macrolevel symbol structure is realized at the microlevel by the activation pattern shown in Box 7; the last eight units of this pattern are reproduced here on the diagonal circles labeled $\mathbf{a}_{[_\sigma k\ [æ\ t]]}$. (As always, the area of a circle denotes the activation level of the unit.) The question now is, how is the macrolevel constraint NOCODA realized at the microlevel?

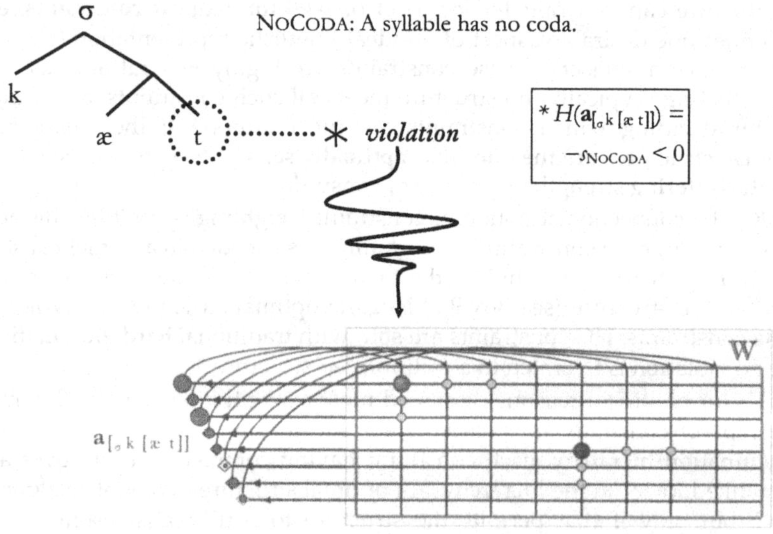

ICS constraints are realized as connection weight matrices, a distributed version of Box 4. Here, the network contains the 14 units used in Box 7 to realize *cat.* Each of these units is connected to all of the units. The entire pattern of weights of these connections is the realization of NOCODA. Since this constraint only involves the last 8 units of the network, only these are shown in the diagram. The grid shows the connections between every pair of units; activation flows out of a unit on the arching lines, down the vertical lines, and then back along a horizontal line. At the grid point where this activation transits from a vertical to a horizontal line, there is a dot, the area of which denotes the strength of that connection. (Thus, the second circle in the first column displays the weight from the first unit shown to the second.)

The activation pattern shown is the one realizing *cat,* which does have a coda; the Harmony value of this pattern is negative, given these connection weights. In fact, the activation pattern for *any* syllable containing a coda will yield negative Harmony. This is just what it means to say that this connection pattern realizes NOCODA.

The scale of the numerical values of the connections determines the strength of the NOCODA constraint: s_{NoCoda}. Doubling the magnitude of all weights, for instance, will double the negative Harmony of activation patterns realizing coda-containing syllables, thereby doubling the strength s_{NoCoda}. (The weight matrix **W** illustrated here is one special case of a general analysis contained in Chapter 10 for realizing symbolic constraints in connection strengths.)

Analogous to the weight matrix illustrated above for NOCODA are other weight matrices realizing other constraints. Superimposing (adding together) all these weight matrices gives a total weight matrix that realizes the entire set of constraints—the grammar. Now if activation spreads through the network under a dynamics such as that specified in Box 3, the network will construct a Harmony-maximizing activation pattern. If all this is set up correctly, such a Harmony-maximizing pattern will realize an optimal symbol structure—a linguistic representation that is grammatical according to the grammar realized in the weight matrix.

5.3 Strict domination

Moving from HG's optimization via weighted constraints to OT's optimization via strict domination hierarchies is a move from graded numerical computation to discrete symbolic computation. OT crucially employs the notion of violable constraint, a departure from previous symbolic theories of grammar: well-formed representations in OT typically violate many constraints. But the interaction among constraints in OT – the determination of which must be violated to form a well-formed structure in a given situation – has the kind of rigidity associated with symbolic rule systems. It may well be a hallmark of *grammatical* knowledge that the interaction of principles is rigidly discrete.

It is worth considering the possibility, however, that the resolution of conflicting information by strict domination hierarchies is a characteristic of *higher cognition generally.* In a groundbreaking series of empirical and computation studies, Gigerenzer,

Todd, and the ABC [Adaptive Behavior and Cognition] Research Group (1999) show that strict domination is applicable to decision making and estimation in a wide variety of domains—from high-school dropout rates, mortality, and the attractiveness of men and women, to rainfall, house prices, and professors' salaries. Knowledge is characterized as a series of **cues** each of which, like a grammatical constraint, favors some choices over others. The preferences of the full set of cues typically conflict. But the cues differ in their **validity**—the extent to which their preferences are correlated with decision outcomes. Cues can be thought of as ranked, those with higher validity dominating those with lower validity. In deciding between two alternatives, the cues are consulted from the top of the hierarchy; those cues that do not prefer one of the choices over the other are passed over until the highest-validity cue is found that has a preference. That one cue's preference determines the final choice; no lower-ranked cues are consulted. Such a procedure is **noncompensatory**: success on some cues cannot compensate for failure on a stronger cue.

This decision procedure is in fact identical to grammatical optimization in OT; it is called **Take the Best** (Gigerenzer and Goldstein 1999). Preliminary empirical studies suggest that in rapid decision-making, people may use Take the Best or a procedure similar to it (Rieskamp and Hoffrage 1999). This experimental evidence concerns conscious decision-making, however; other studies are needed that address unconscious processes like those involving grammatical knowledge.

Is it *rational* to make decisions on the basis of a single cue? In a series of computational studies, the ABC Group compares Take the Best with a decision procedure corresponding to HG optimization: **multiple linear regression**, in which all cues are used, each contributing to the decision in proportion to its own numerical strength (strengths being empirically determined by a relatively computationally expensive statistical estimation procedure) (Gigerenzer and Goldstein 1996; Czerlinski, Gigerenzer, and Goldstein 1999). Remarkably, averaged over 20 diverse decision-making tasks, Take the Best *outperforms* linear regression in its ability to generalize to new problems. Linear regression beats Take the Best by more than 1% in only 3 of 20 tasks—and in none of these is the margin more than 3% (Martignon and Laskey 1999). Thus, at least across a considerable range of environments (Martignon and Hoffrage 1999), if the complexity of decision procedures is taken into account, the use of the Take the Best procedure—much simpler and much less demanding of cue-evaluation—appears to be rational indeed.

5.4 Universals

An OT grammar is a set of constraints defining the preferred characteristics of linguistic representations, priority-ranked in a strict domination hierarchy. Conceivably, then, OT grammars could differ in two respects: the constraints they contain, and the ranking of these constraints. It turns out that if a fixed set of constraints is reranked, surprisingly different patterns of optimal structures result. Indeed, a fundamental hypothesis of OT is that human grammars differ *only* in ranking. The constraints themselves are the same across languages—they are strictly **universal**. The recent linguistics literature offers much evidence in favor of this hypothesis, in many parts of both the phonological and syntactic components of human grammar.

Thus, the optimization perspective enables OT to provide a novel and strong answer to two of the most central questions of linguistic theory: what do the grammars of all human languages have in common, and how may they differ? What human grammars share is a common set of violable constraints; grammars may differ only in how these constraints are ranked, that is, in how conflicts among these constraints are resolved.

The origin of these universal constraints is very much an open question, one on which OT itself is silent. The universality of these constraints may be a consequence of their biological origin: they may be genetically encoded, manifest somehow in the structure of the brain. Alternatively, the constraints may arise through learning in childhood, a consequence of universal functional pressures like the architecture of the human vocal tract and perceptual system, or the task demands of communication. Indeed, OT research in both phonology and syntax has strengthened connections between such functional considerations and formal grammatical principles. The origin of universal constraints is still principally the domain of speculation, but Chapter 21 explores whether, and how, a biologically plausible genome could possibly encode OT constraints; a demonstration system—a toy OT nativist **Language Acquisition Device**—is constructed.

5.5 Optimality Theory and the cognitive science of language

In addition to shedding new light on the issue of linguistic universals, the optimization perspective provides OT a novel approach to the relation between grammatical *knowledge* ("competence") and *use* of that knowledge ("performance"), between language-particular knowledge and its acquisition, and between grammatical knowledge and its neural realization (see Section 4:4). These long-standing problems in linguistic theory previously allowed little general formal progress.

Grammatical knowledge can be taken to be knowledge of the constraint hierarchy; use of that knowledge then consists in determining, under various conditions, which linguistic structures optimally satisfy the constraint hierarchy.

In ICS, the optimizing structure of OT grammars is realized by connectionist networks that perform Harmony maximization. Additionally, OT's characterization of grammar via optimization offers some progress toward an important goal of linguistics: connecting limitations on the space of possible human grammars to the problem of language acquisition. Finally, OT provides a first glimpse of how grammar might conceivably be biologically realized. In Chapters 12, 17, and 18, we discuss early and recent research on the learnability and acquisition of OT grammars; in Chapters 19, 20, and 21, research on the use of OT grammars and their neural and genetic encoding.

It is important here to emphasize a point made in Section 3: the well-formedness constraints of a grammar are not concerned narrowly with issues of declaring sentences 'grammatical' or 'ungrammatical'. Rather, they are the prime determinant of the mapping between linguistic expressions and their interpretations—loosely, between form and meaning. That is, when used, grammatical knowledge determines the expression of a given interpretation (**production**), or the interpretation of a given expression (**comprehension**): these are the central questions of language processing, not arcane issues of grammaticality of interest only to grammarians. In this book, for example, OT's theory of grammar will be shown to provide novel answers to the range of questions given in (10).

(10) Questions addressed via OT's theory of grammar

a. How can the expression of a given interpretation be efficiently computed—given that optimality computation generally involves comparing an infinite number of possible expressions, and that optimization problems in general are computationally intractable? (Chapter 12)

b. How, in principle, can a learner acquire a grammar, which depends crucially on knowing where hidden linguistic structure lies in learning data (e.g., phrase boundaries)—given that the location of such structure must be computed from the unknown grammar? And how, even given hypothesized hidden structure for learning data, can a learner converge on a constraint ranking that yields this hidden structure—given that the connection between constraint ranking and grammaticality is as complex and nontransparent as it is in OT? (Chapter 12)

c. What principles govern the structure of syllables, and how can these principles formally account for the observed range of variation in syllables across the world's languages? (Chapter 13)

d. What general principles govern the spread of phonological features, as in vowel harmony systems where the features of a vowel may spread throughout an entire word? (Chapter 14)

e. How may semantic roles and syntactic roles correspond in active voice, passive voice, and antipassive voice sentences? (Chapter 15)

f. What shared principles explain how to express information questions in the languages of the world, including Chinese, Bulgarian, and English, which respectively place at the front of the sentence no, every, or only one question phrase (e.g., *what*; *which book*)? (Chapter 16)

g. What must be the character of the earliest infant grammars, if any possible adult grammar is to be learnable? Can we produce relevant experimental evidence probing the phonological grammars of infants? Do adult grammars experimentally display the expected residue of early grammars? (Chapter 17)

h. Can universal syntactic principles account for the grammatical development evident in children's earliest sentences, including the quantitative differences in their use of alternative structures? (Chapter 18)

i. In syntax, is it possible for the grammar ("competence theory") to *be* the human online parser ("performance theory")—both being understood as a single system for the simultaneous optimal satisfaction of violable constraints? Can such an approach perspicuously explain a body of experimental facts concerning the difficulty people experience in online sentence processing? (Chapter 19)

j. Does the OT conception of universal grammar enable explicit models of how innate knowledge of substantive grammatical principles could conceivably be realized in a connectionist Language Acquisition Device encoded in an abstract genome? (Chapter 21)

Our claim, of course, is not that we have definitive and correct answers to all these questions; the point is rather that, in all these cases, OT enables possible answers to these questions to be formulated precisely, and then rigorously evaluated against empirical or computational criteria of adequacy. Far from constituting a system solely for distinguishing grammatical from ungrammatical sentences, OT's theory of grammar very directly provides substantial leverage on a wide range of questions about language that are of central interest for cognitive science. And this leverage is a direct consequence of OT's connectionist-derived characterization of the mapping between forms and meanings determined by a grammar: the correct form-meaning pairs are those that optimally satisfy a conflicting set of well-formedness constraints with differing strengths.

5.6 Philosophical arguments

A final type of evidence we consider is philosophical (Part IV); it arises from the union of top-down and bottom-up theory development. From the "top," we get a central problem—explaining the productivity of cognition (9)—and a general approach to its solution—the combinatorial strategy (4). From the "bottom," we get a means for realizing combinatorial structure in neural networks, a novel instantiation of the combinatorial strategy that provides a new, and in some senses deeper, explanation of cognitive productivity (Chapter 23).

The overview of the book provided below in Section 7 summarizes a number of theoretical and empirical results supporting the proposed cognitive architecture; another still briefer summary may be found in Chapter 3 (12). At a more general level than that of any particular results, we hope that, taken as a whole, the book provides some evidence for the value of an approach to cognitive science that is grounded in neural computation, yet centered on formally articulated general cognitive principles.

6 Recapitulation

Let us summarize. In our judgment, a great deal of cognitive explanatory power has been demonstrated for a hypothesis that can be loosely stated as in (11).

(11) Symbolic cognitive architecture (rough formulation)

Mental representations are complex structures built of abstract symbols. Mental processes are symbolic algorithms manipulating these structures to compute recursive functions.

In short: *Cognition is symbolic computation.*

We believe that particularly compelling evidence for this hypothesis exists within the cognitive domain of language, the arena we focus upon in this book.

At the same time, we believe it is important to give serious consideration to theoretical work in neuroscience which suggests that a very different computational architecture holds at the neural level. Obviously, the theory of neural computation is in its infancy, and its contribution must take the form of highly provisional working hypotheses. Until a better alternative comes along—a theory of neural computation that is more biologically informed but equally general in scope, tractable for mathematical analysis, and fruitful for modeling cognitive faculties—we consider a connectionist formulation of the neural computational architecture, along the lines of (12).

(12) Parallel distributed processing cognitive architecture (rough formulation)

Mental representations are patterns of numerical activation levels over a set of processing units (abstract neurons). These units perform massively parallel numerical computation via a set of numerically weighted interconnections (abstract synapses); this constitutes mental processing. Learning is the determination of correct weights via statistical analysis of experience.

In short: *Cognition is massively parallel numerical computation.*

Reconciling these two hypotheses is thus a pressing imperative for advancing the science of the mind/brain. To this end, we explore the following hypothesis:

(13) Vertically Integrated Connectionist/Symbolic Cognitive Architecture (ICS) (rough formulation)

At a lower level of analysis, the mind/brain is a computer with a connectionist architecture. Parts of this architecture are organized so that they give rise, at a higher level of analysis, to a virtual machine with a (perhaps novel type of) symbolic architecture. In higher cognitive domains where symbolic theory has been successful, this symbolic architecture governs central aspects of the phenomena.

In short: *Cognition is massively parallel numerical computation, some dimensions of which are organized to realize crucial facets of symbolic computation.*

Here, 'vertically integrated' is intended to distinguish the proposed type of integration—between a higher- and a lower-level description of a single system—from other approaches to combining connectionist and symbolic computation, in which a connectionist system and a symbolic system sit side by side as two distinct components of a hybrid system. Note that (13) refers to 'central aspects' of cognitive phenomena; this leaves open the possibility that language and other higher cognitive domains have a central skeletal structure of the basic phenomena governed by symbolic principles, while surrounding phenomena go beyond the limits of the symbolic theory. Exploring this possibility is an important future project for the ICS research program.

The first major task of this book is to refine the fundamental hypothesis (13) to make it formally well defined; the second task is to assemble evidence concerning its utility for cognitive science. The first steps toward incrementally refining the hypothesis are undertaken in Chapter 2; subsequent steps toward formalization are taken in Chapters 5 and 6, with more complete analysis and exemplification being relegated to later chapters. Much of the remainder of the book addresses evidence for the fertility of the basic hypothesis (13), evidence derived from the perspectives of computer science, theoretical linguistics, psycholinguistics, neuroscience, and the philosophy of mind.

7 Overview of the Book

This book examines cognitive architecture, grammar, and cognitive explanation.

7.1 Structure of the book

The first general topic of the book is cognitive architecture: ICS is defined by a set of explicit principles, and analyzed formally. These principles are introduced in Chapter 2 and developed in detail in Part II, Chapters 5-12. Chapters 5 and 6—in many respects the key chapters of the book—constitute an attempt to provide an intuitive introduction to the formalism needed to frame the principles more precisely and to analyze their consequences. The formal articulation of the principles in Chapters 5 and 6 is then more fully developed in later chapters, where cognitive implications are also discussed. Initial evidence for the validity of ICS is offered from two cognitive perspectives. From the computational perspective, it is argued that the architecture provides an innovative and powerful unification of connectionist and symbolic computation, achieving the difficult goal of a computationally adequate hypothesis of how symbols and rules might be naturally realized in PDP connectionist networks (Chapters 5-10). From the linguistic perspective, it is argued that new insights into the nature of certain types of grammatical knowledge are made possible by two novel grammar formalisms derived from fundamental principles of ICS, Harmonic Grammar (Chapter 11) and Optimality Theory (Chapter 12).

The single most important outgrowth of ICS research is Optimality Theory, our second general topic. Chapter 2 introduces ICS theory, focusing on components other than OT, while Chapter 4 is a self-contained introduction to OT, with some discussion of its connection to the rest of ICS theory. Chapter 12 is a systematic presentation of OT. Part III of the book, Chapters 13-21, is devoted to OT's contributions to the cognitive science of language. In Chapters 13-19, OT is considered primarily independently of the rest of ICS. Empirical evidence for the validity of OT is offered from the perspectives of both theoretical linguistics (Chapters 13-16) and psycholinguistics

Table 1. Types of questions addressed

General topics	Representative central questions
Part I: Overview	
Integrated Connectionist / Symbolic (ICS) Cognitive Architecture	Conceptually, how do connectionist and symbolic cognitive theory relate? What general principles govern this relation?
Unity of cognitive science	Methodologically, how do model- and principle-centered research in cognitive science relate?
Optimality Theory (OT)	What kind of computational system is knowledge of language (grammar)?
Part II: The ICS Cognitive Architecture	
Relating connectionist and symbolic computation	Technically, how do connectionist and symbolic computation relate?
High-level analysis of connectionist computation	What general principles govern the collective, high-level computational properties of connectionist networks?
Connectionist-based grammar formalisms	What grammar formalism follows from applying such principles to language?
	Can such a connectionist-based grammar formalism—Harmonic Grammar—give new insight into syntax-semantics interaction?
Universal grammar: computational principles	What new principles arise in answer to the question: what is it, precisely, that all human grammars share, and how, precisely, may they differ?
Part III: Optimality Theory	
Universal grammar: computational and substantive principles	What are the substantive universal principles governing syllables, simple clauses, questions, and other linguistic structures?
Acquisition of grammar Language processing Neural realization of universal grammar	What implications does the computational structure of grammatical knowledge have for its use, acquisition, and realization at the neural and genetic levels?
Part IV: Philosophical foundations of cognitive architecture	
Linguistic explanation: connections and rules; models and theories	What are the relations between model- and principle-based connectionist and generative approaches to language?
Connectionism, symbolic theory, and levels of analysis	What are the respective explanatory roles of symbolic rules and connectionist networks in cognitive explanation?
Cognitive productivity: Explanations and algorithms	What general computational properties of human cognition explain the productivity of higher cognition?

(Chapters 17–19); this evidence concerns both phonology (Chapters 13, 14, and 17) and syntax (Chapters 15, 16, 18, and 19). Chapters 20 and 21 focus on the connection between OT and ICS, relating OT with HG and with connectionist computation. Chapter 21 presents speculative initial attempts to bring OT down not only to the level of abstract neural networks, but further, to a new, still lower level of description—the level of what we call the **abstract genome**. This exercise explores the possibility in principle of genetically encoded knowledge of OT grammatical principles.

The third general topic addressed in this book is the philosophical foundation of cognitive architecture. The discussion of this topic builds directly on the work presented in Parts II–III addressing OT and the remainder of ICS theory; it is previewed in Chapter 3. Some general methodological considerations are also taken up in Chapter 3, where three types of integration are distinguished and related to the ICS research program. Part IV, Chapters 22–23, examines several foundational issues in some detail. Focusing on questions of explanation, Chapter 22 discusses how and why ICS research integrates two approaches to the study of language that are typically regarded as irreconcilable: connectionism and generative linguistics. Chapter 23 offers further evidence for ICS from the philosophical perspective. It is argued that ICS constitutes progress toward reducing mind theory to brain theory, providing a novel, and in some ways deeper, explanation of the productivity of cognition.

At a very general level, it is our hope that, as a whole, the book builds a reasonable case for the value of a conception of cognitive science that seriously undertakes multidisciplinary integration in the context of formal, principle-centered theory. The multidisciplinary mix inherent in this research program makes it particularly important to distinguish the types of questions being asked, and the types of answers being sought, in the various parts of the book. As a first step, Table 1 provides some representative general questions focused upon in the four parts.

The research methods used to address questions like those in Table 1 are drawn from several disciplines; these are identified in Table 2, where section numbers indicate localized use of a method and '✓' indicates dispersed use of the method throughout the chapter. 'Comp' refers to computational analysis, construed to include mathematical methods used in the analysis of both connectionist and symbolic systems. 'Ling' refers to both the theoretical and the empirical aspects of formal linguistic analysis, while 'Phil' refers to philosophical analysis, primarily involving the philosophy of mind and the philosophy of science. 'Psych' refers narrowly to data from cognitive psychology and psycholinguistics, data obtained both in controlled experiments and in naturalistic recordings. Finally, 'Neuro' refers narrowly to specific empirical findings of neurobiology. Contributions of psychology and neuroscience to the research program represented here are fundamental and extensive; these fields are the source of the connectionist conception of cognitive architecture. Psychology has played an essential role in the development of the symbolic cognitive architecture as well. These fundamental contributions are not registered in Table 2 simply because they are all-pervasive; the final two columns thus indicate only those points where rather specific psychological or neurobiological data make localized contributions.

Table 2. Research methods employed

		Chapter	Comp	Ling	Phil	Psych	Neuro
Part I	**1**	Overview	✓	✓	✓		
	2	ICS principles	✓	✓			
	3	Foundational implications			✓		
	4	OT introduction		✓			
Part II	**5**	Representation and processing	✓				
	6	Optimization and grammar	✓	2–3			
	7	Symbols as activation vectors	✓			4, 6	3, 5
	8	Tensor product representations	✓				
	9	Optimization in neural nets	✓				
	10	HGs for formal languages	✓				
	11	HG: Syntax/semantics	3	✓			
	12	OT principles	2–3	✓			
Part III	**13**	Syllable structure		✓			
	14	Features; constraint conjunction		✓			
	15	Grammatical voice		✓			
	16	*Wh*-questions		✓			
	17	Phonology acquisition		✓		✓	
	18	Syntax acquisition		✓		✓	
	19	Sentence processing		✓		✓	
	20	OT–HG connection	1, 3	1–2			
	21	Genomic encoding of OT	✓	✓			✓
Part IV	**22**	Connectionist grammar		✓	✓		
	23	Levels and ICS explanation			✓		

The chapters are sequenced so that reading them in numerical order will optimize logical coherency; many subsets of chapters, however, also form logically coherent threads. The dependency structure is roughly as shown in Figure 3, where a line joining two chapters indicates a recommendation that the higher chapter be read before the lower chapter; dashed lines indicate desirable but dispensable prerequisites. Roman numerals demarcate the four parts of the book. An asterisk on a chapter number, *N**, indicates that Chapter *N* will likely be challenging to a reader with very limited background in the general topic area—challenging, but hopefully approachable. A double asterisk, *N***, suggests that Chapter *N* is by and large directed to area specialists. In the chapters with no asterisks, we have tried to make nearly all of the chapter accessible to a general cognitive science audience.

We have also tried to increase the accessibility of the asterisked chapters to non-specialists through expository boxes; several have already been presented above. A few boxes address material that is tangential to or an extension of the content of the chapter; others present concrete examples of concepts presented more abstractly in the text. Most, however, attempt to give extremely concise, self-contained introductions to the background material required for the chapter. Needless to say, many important topics and subtleties won't fit into those tiny nutshells, so we ask the forbearance of specialists for the sometimes severe simplifications we make and the many corners we cut. Table 3 lists the boxes in the book, grouped by general area.

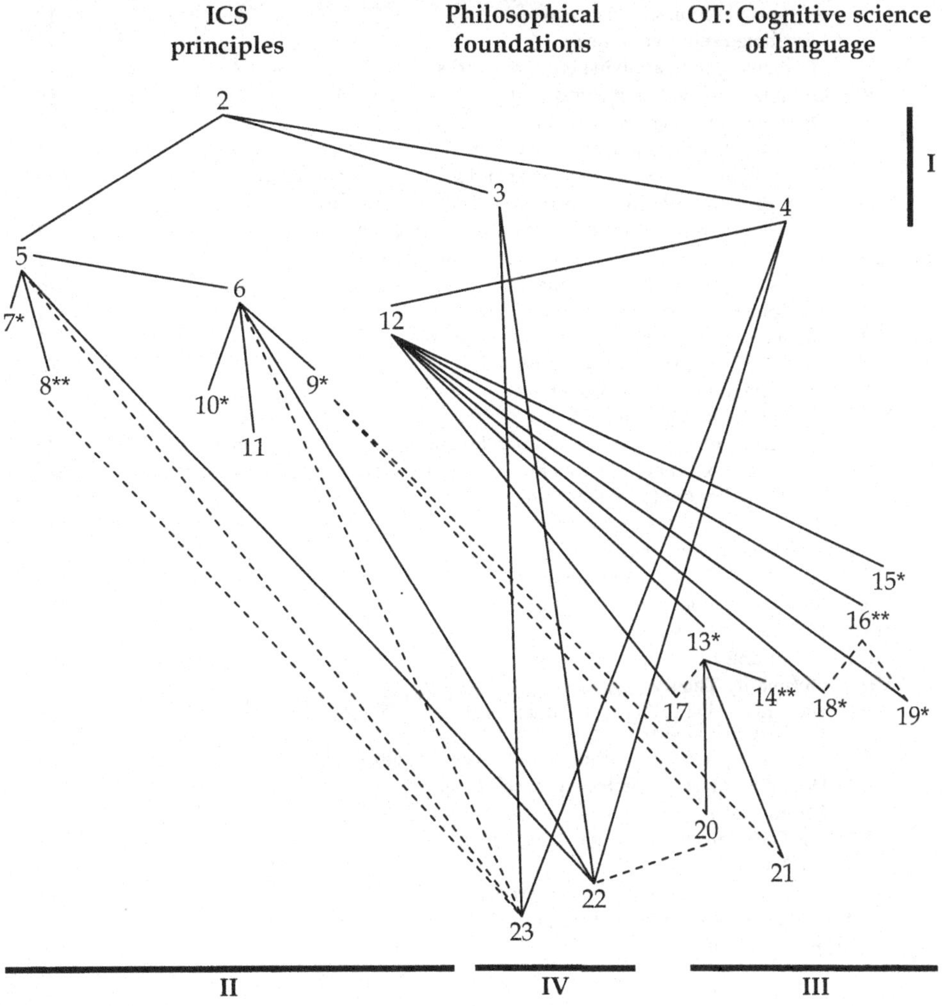

Table 3. Expository boxes

Box		Page*
	Computational and mathematical background	
5:1	Vectors and matrices: Linear algebra	150
5:2	Linear algebra of connectionist networks	157
6:1	Formal languages and abstract automata: The Chomsky hierarchy, Turing machines, and all that	210
23:1	Reducing symbolic computation to primitives: *Symbols all the way down*	*506*
23:4	$\mathcal{C}$-$\mathcal{N}$ isomorphism in arithmetic computers I	*523*
23:5	$\mathcal{C}$-$\mathcal{N}$ isomorphism in arithmetic computers II	*526*
23:6	$\mathcal{F}$-$\mathcal{C}$ isomorphism in arithmetic computers	*539*
	Connectionist background and the connectionist component of ICS theory	
1:1	An example connectionist network	10
1:2	Distributed representations	12
1:3	Harmony optimization in neural networks	15
1:4	Optimization over microconstraints in neural networks	17
1:6	On connectionism and "neural plausibility"	29
1:7	Symbolic structures in neural networks	34
1:8	The relation between connectionist and symbolic computation	35
1:9	Optimization over macroconstraints in neural networks	40
2:1	Symbol structures as activation patterns – $\mathrm{Rep}_{\mathrm{ICS}}$ illustrated	69
2:2	A simple grammar in a connectionist weight matrix	73
2:3	Processing with a simple grammar	76
3:1	The split-level architecture of ICS	104
8:1	Uniqueness of constituent decomposition exemplified	291
8:2	Extraction of constituents exemplified	293
23:8	Impairment to parts versus wholes	*575*
	Linguistics background	
1:5	Language, linguistics, and grammar: Frequently unasked questions	25
11:1	Syntactic and semantic factors in verb-argument structure: Split intransitivity	421
12:1	The X′ Theory of phrase structure	466
12:2	Rudiments of phonological theory	473
14:1	Vowel harmony	*32*
15:1	Case, thematic roles, and grammatical voice	*163*
16:1	Information questions: Semantic and syntactic structure	*186*
16:2	Multiple *wh*-questions	*189*
16:3	Constraints on *wh*-questions	*192*
	Optimality Theory	
13:1	Universal syllable theory: Ordinal construction of C/V and onset/coda licensing asymmetry	*18*
14:2	Why does proving such simple results get so complex?	*73*
14:3	Deriving power hierarchies from self-conjunction	*123*
	Foundations	
23:2	The Fodorian challenge to connectionism	*513*
23:3	Is ICS productive?	*518*
23:7	Explanation by mental representation	*545*
23:9	Competence and the limits of performance	*578*

* Italic numbers refer to Volume 2.

7.2 Chapter-by-chapter summary of the book

To better convey a sense of the scope of the book, we close this chapter by briefly stating one or two main claims of each of the remaining chapters. (Asterisks mark more specialized or technical chapters, as in Figure 3.)

Part I: Toward a Calculus of the Mind/Brain: An Overview

2 **Principles of the Integrated Connectionist/Symbolic Cognitive Architecture (ICS)**—*Paul Smolensky and Géraldine Legendre.* A set of principles define a cognitive architecture for higher cognition that can be formally characterized at two levels of description: at a lower level, as a parallel distributed processing network; at a higher level, as a symbolic computational system with novel properties derived from its lower-level connectionist realization.

3 **Foundational Implications of the ICS Architecture: Unification in Cognitive Science**—*Paul Smolensky and Géraldine Legendre.* ICS theory potentially resolves the deadlock between eliminativist and implementationalist views of the mind/brain relation, and enables progress toward bridging three distinct kinds of divisions in cognitive science: the computational gulf between lower and higher cognition, the methodological divergence across cognitive disciplines, and the rift between model-based and principle-based philosophies of science.

4 **Optimality: From Neural Networks to Universal Grammar**—*Alan Prince and Paul Smolensky.* One novel organizing principle of the symbolic description of ICS is optimization; this sheds new light on a number of central problems in the theory of universal grammar, significantly enhancing its explanatory power.

Part II: Principles of the Integrated Connectionist/Symbolic Cognitive Architecture

5 **Formalizing the Principles I: Representation and Processing in the Mind/Brain**—*Paul Smolensky.* General yet precise principles determine how activation vectors and connection matrices may realize mental representations and processes in neural networks. A central idea is the use of the vector operation of the tensor product to bind together activation patterns realizing variables with activation patterns realizing their values.

6 **Formalizing the Principles II: Optimization and Grammar**—*Paul Smolensky and Géraldine Legendre.* In the ICS framework, general principles governing computation in connectionist networks, together with central insights from generative grammar, lead to new, optimization-based, symbolic grammatical theories: Harmonic Grammar and Optimality Theory.

7 **Symbolic Computation with Activation Patterns***—*Paul Smolensky and Bruce Tesar.* The tensor product operation for binding connectionist variables to values provides the core of a family of structured connectionist representations with great diversity, including several proposals in the connectionist and computa-

tional neuroscience literatures that appear entirely unrelated to tensor product representations.

8 **Tensor Product Representations: Formal Foundations****—*Paul Smolensky*. A general formal isomorphism can be established between sets of symbolic structures and spaces of activation vectors: fundamental symbolic operations correspond to linear operations on these vector spaces. This vectorial means of realizing symbolic structure enables systematic analysis of a number of particular representations proposed in the connectionist literature; graceful degradation as capacity limits are reached; analysis of the capability of networks to store symbolic structures; realization of recursive structure in distributed representations; finite encoding of highly parallel, distributed networks that realize a formally characterized set of infinitely productive and arbitrarily complex recursive symbolic functions; and distributed realizations of harmonic grammars, including grammatical constraints.

9 **Optimization in Neural Networks: Harmony Maximization***—*Paul Smolensky*. The simplest Harmony function, introduced in Chapter 6, can be generalized so that a large variety of networks may be analyzed as performing Harmony maximization. In one class of networks, the Harmony function can be viewed as encoding the network's model of the probability distribution of representations of alternative states of an environment.

10 **Harmonic Grammars and Harmonic Parsers for Formal Languages***—*John Hale and Paul Smolensky*. Despite their simplicity, the soft rules of a harmonic grammar can specify strict formal languages of any complexity in the Chomsky hierarchy, including those generated by Turing machines. This establishes one general measure of the computational power of ICS. Harmonic grammars explicitly yield connectionist parsers for formal languages.

11 **The Interaction of Syntax and Semantics: A Harmonic Grammar Account of Split Intransitivity**—*Géraldine Legendre, Yoshiro Miyata, and Paul Smolensky*. ICS principles entail a grammar formalism, HG, that can be realized in isomorphic connectionist networks at two levels: a lower-level network employing distributed representations and a higher-level network with local representations. The latter directly implements a set of HG soft constraints. The strengths of these constraints can be determined by an appropriate connectionist learning algorithm. The acceptability judgments of a large set of French sentences exhibit very general tendencies concerning syntax-semantics relations, but the formal power of HG is needed to allow such soft syntactic and semantic constraints to interact sufficiently strongly to account for the complex overall pattern.

12 **Optimality Theory: The Structure, Use, and Acquisition of Grammatical Knowledge**—*Paul Smolensky, Géraldine Legendre, and Bruce Tesar*. Applying HG to crosslinguistic typology led Prince and Smolensky (1993/2004) to new principles: universality of constraints and strict priority ranking. The result, OT, can be characterized by a set of general grammatical principles that apply equally to

phonology and syntax, strengthening the explanatory power of universal grammar in a number of respects. Under certain general assumptions, algorithms can be developed that efficiently compute the optimal output for a given input, even though the space of competing outputs may be infinite. Effective learning algorithms can be defined for determining the language-particular aspects of a target grammar.

Part III: Optimality Theory: The Cognitive Science of Language

13 **Optimality in Phonology I: Syllable Structure***—*Alan Prince and Paul Smolensky.* A classic concrete illustration, from the original OT manuscript (Prince and Smolensky 1993/2004), shows how OT can advance the theory of universal grammar: Jakobson's (1962) typology of the inventories of basic syllable types in the world's languages is explained by the reranking of a set of simple constraints defining the structural well-formedness (or markedness) of syllables and the faithfulness of pronunciations to their fixed lexical forms.

14 **Optimality in Phonology II: Harmonic Completeness, Local Constraint Conjunction, and Feature Domain Markedness****—*Paul Smolensky.* A simple extension of basic OT is proposed, in which constraints can interact conjunctively: multiple constraint violations within a single local domain have heightened effects. This is shown formally to be necessary and sufficient for generating a general pattern, instantiated for instance in vowel harmony systems: vowel features tend to spread through a word, but fail to do so if that would result in multiple local constraint violations within a single feature domain.

15 **Optimality in Syntax I: Case and Grammatical Voice Typology***—*Géraldine Legendre, William Raymond, and Paul Smolensky.* The first application of OT outside phonology demonstrates how OT enables extremely simple, rampantly violated constraints to formally yield strong predictions. Reranking a set of basic constraints on the mapping between semantic and syntactic roles in simple transitive and intransitive clauses predicts an empirically sound typology of possible clauses in the active, passive, and antipassive voices and explains the typology of basic intransitive case-marking systems.

16 **Optimality in Syntax II: *Wh*-Questions****—*Géraldine Legendre, Colin Wilson, Paul Smolensky, Kristin Homer, and William Raymond.* A general framework for OT syntax naturally explains a central feature of syntax that seems at odds with the basic structure of OT: the language-dependent inexpressibility or ineffability of certain meanings (e.g., questions). From fundamental principles governing operator-variable relationships in *wh*-questions, a set of constraints can be developed that explains the basic crosslinguistic typology of these questions. Relativized Minimality effects are explained with constraints defined in terms of neither relativization nor minimality.

17 **Optimality in Language Acquisition I: The Initial and Final States of the Phonological Grammar**—*Lisa Davidson, Peter Jusczyk, and Paul Smolensky.* A subtle

OT principle, Richness of the Base, has important implications for language acquisition. Learnability requirements entail that early grammars must take a certain general form. Consequent predictions concerning phonological knowledge in infants are experimentally confirmed. Implications for the adult English phonological grammar are examined with experimental studies that suggest an Extended Richness of the Base principle.

18 **Optimality in Language Acquisition II: Inflection in Early French Syntax*—** *Géraldine Legendre, Paul Hagstrom, Anne Vainikka, and Marina Todorova.* The simple elaboration of the basic OT framework employed in Chapter 17 enables formal accounts of the development of the earliest syntax in French-learning children, including the relative frequencies of alternative clause structures.

19 **Optimality in Sentence Processing***—*Suzanne Stevenson and Paul Smolensky.* Using syntactic constraints from theoretical linguistics, sentences can be parsed one word at a time by using the normal "competence" grammar in the interpretive direction. This provides accounts for a range of experimental psycholinguistic data concerning the relative difficulty of different sentence structures in online sentence comprehension.

20 **The Optimality Theory–Harmonic Grammar Connection**—*Géraldine Legendre, Antonella Sorace, and Paul Smolensky.* HG is the link between OT and its connectionist foundations. Numerical Harmony maximization realizes OT optimization when constraint strengths grow exponentially as the hierarchy is mounted. A case study in syntax reexamines in light of OT the argument structure phenomena that were analyzed within HG in Chapter 11. A case study in phonology addresses the remarkable syllabification system of Berber, reducing the OT account of Prince and Smolensky 1993/2004 to a harmonic grammar, and reducing this in turn to a connectionist syllable-parser.

21 **Abstract Genomic Encoding of Universal Grammar in Optimality Theory—** *Melanie Soderstrom, Donald W. Mathis, and Paul Smolensky.* As a step toward more explicit computational theories for grounding the innateness debate, a notion of abstract genome is developed and used to design a connectionist Language Acquisition Device that realizes genetically encoded knowledge of the universal principles of the OT syllable theory presented in Chapter 13.

Part IV: Philosophical Foundations of Cognitive Architecture

22 **Principle-Centered Connectionist and Generative-Linguistic Theories of Language**—*Paul Smolensky.* OT represents a new connectionist approach to the study of language, one based on general computational principles rather than particular network models. This approach has certain explanatory advantages and engages constructively with the problems and research methods of generative linguistics; it also interfaces well with model-based connectionist research.

23 **Computational Levels and Integrated Connectionist/Symbolic Explanation—** *Paul Smolensky.* The computational level of ICS is crucially split into two sub-

levels, the higher corresponding to symbolic functional descriptions of the mind, the lower to physical descriptions of the brain. The symbolic functional level explains types of data ranging from specific error rates during phonological production to the general productivity of cognition. But the temporal and spatial structure of cognitive processes cannot be modeled by high-level, symbolic algorithms: this requires low-level, connectionist algorithms. Symbolic representations are essential for explaining cognitive function, including the meanings of mental states; connectionist algorithms are essential for explaining the moment-by-moment causal dynamics that constitute cognitive processing.

References

ROA = Rutgers Optimality Archive, http://roa.rutgers.edu

Abbott, L., and T. J. Sejnowski, eds. 1999. *Neural codes and distributed representations.* MIT Press.

Ackley, D. H., G. E. Hinton, and T. J. Sejnowski. 1985. A learning algorithm for Boltzmann machines. *Cognitive Science* 9, 147–69.

Anderson, J. R., and C. J. Lebiere. 1998. *The atomic components of thought.* Erlbaum.

Archangeli, D., and D. T. Langendoen. 1997. *Optimality Theory: An overview.* Blackwell.

Barbosa, P., D. Fox, P. Hagstrom, M. McGinnis, and D. Pesetsky, eds. 1998. *Is the best good enough? Optimality and competition in syntax.* MIT Press and MIT Working Papers in Linguistics.

Bechtel, W., and A. Abrahamsen. 2002. *Connectionism and the mind: Parallel processing, dynamics, and evolution in networks.* Blackwell.

Blutner, R., and H. Zeevat, eds. 2003. *Pragmatics in Optimality Theory.* Palgrave Macmillan.

Boersma, P. 1998. *Functional phonology: Formalizing the interactions between articulatory and perceptual drives.* Holland Academic Graphics.

Brousse, O., and P. Smolensky. 1989. Virtual memories and massive generalization in connectionist combinatorial learning. In *Proceedings of the Cognitive Science Society 11.*

Burzio, L. 1994. *Principles of English stress.* Cambridge University Press.

Chomsky, N. 1965. *Aspects of the theory of syntax.* MIT Press.

Chomsky, N. 1986. *Knowledge of language: Its nature, origin, and use.* Praeger.

Churchland, P. S., and T. J. Sejnowski. 1992. *The computational brain.* MIT Press.

Cohen, M. A., and S. Grossberg. 1983. Absolute stability of global pattern formation and parallel memory storage by competitive neural networks. *IEEE Transactions on Systems, Man, and Cybernetics* 13, 815–25.

Cummins, R., and G. Schwarz. 1991. Connectionism, computation, and cognition. In *Connectionism and the philosophy of mind,* eds. T. E. Horgan and J. Tienson. Kluwer.

Czerlinski, J., G. Gigerenzer, and D. G. Goldstein. 1999. How good are simple heuristics? In *Simple heuristics that make us smart,* eds. G. Gigerenzer, P. M. Todd, and the ABC Research Group. Oxford University Press.

Dekkers, J., F. van der Leeuw, and J. van de Weijer, eds. 2000. *Optimality Theory: Phonology, syntax, and acquisition.* Oxford University Press.

Fodor, J. A. 1975. *The language of thought.* Harvard University Press.

Fodor, J. A., and Z. W. Pylyshyn. 1988. Connectionism and cognitive architecture: A critical analysis. *Cognition* 28, 3–71.

Forster, K. I., and S. M. Chambers. 1973. Lexical access and naming time. *Journal of Verbal Learning and Verbal Behavior* 12, 627–35.

Frank, R. 1998. Structural complexity and the time course of grammatical development. *Cognition* 66, 249–301.

Frank, R., and G. Satta. 1998. Optimality Theory and the generative complexity of constraint violability. *Computational Linguistics* 24, 307–15. ROA 228.

Geman, S., and D. Geman. 1984. Stochastic relaxation, Gibbs distributions, and the Bayesian restoration of images. *IEEE Transactions on Pattern Analysis and Machine Intelligence* 6, 721–41.

Georgopoulos, A. P., J. F. Kalaska, R. Caminiti, and J. T. Massey. 1982. On the relations between the direction of two-dimensional arm movements and cell discharge in primate motor cortex. *Journal of Neuroscience* 2, 1527–37.

Gigerenzer, G., and D. G. Goldstein. 1996. Reasoning the fast and frugal way: Models of bounded rationality. *Psychological Review* 103, 650–69.

Gigerenzer, G., and D. G. Goldstein. 1999. Betting on one good reason: The take the best heuristic. In *Simple heuristics that make us smart*, eds. G. Gigerenzer, P. M. Todd, and the ABC Research Group. Oxford University Press.

Gigerenzer, G., P. M. Todd, and the ABC [Adaptive Behavior and Cognition] Research Group. 1999. *Simple heuristics that make us smart*. Oxford University Press.

Gleitman, L. R., and M. Liberman, eds. 1995. *An invitation to cognitive science*. Vol. 1, *Language*. 2nd ed. MIT Press.

Glushko, R. J. 1979. The organization and activation of orthographic knowledge in reading aloud. *Journal of Experimental Psychology: Human Perception and Performance* 5, 674–91.

Golden, R. M. 1986. The "brain-state-in-a-box" neural model is a gradient descent algorithm. *Mathematical Psychology* 30–31, 73–80.

Haugeland, J. 1985. *Artificial intelligence: The very idea*. MIT Press.

Hayes, B. 1980. A metrical theory of stress rules. Ph.D. diss., MIT.

Hendriks, P., H. de Hoop, and H. de Swart, eds. 2000. Special issue on the optimization of interpretation. *Journal of Semantics* 17, 185–314.

Hertz, J., A. Krogh, and R. G. Palmer. 1991. *Introduction to the theory of neural computation*. Addison-Wesley.

Hinton, G. E., and J. A. Anderson, eds. 1981. *Parallel models of associative memory*. Erlbaum.

Hinton, G. E., J. L. McClelland, and D. E. Rumelhart. 1986. Distributed representation. In *Parallel distributed processing: Explorations in the microstructure of cognition*. Vol. 1, *Foundations*, D. E. Rumelhart, J. L. McClelland, and the PDP Research Group. MIT Press.

Hinton, G. E., and T. J. Sejnowski. 1983. Optimal perceptual inference. In *Proceedings of the IEEE Computer Society Conference on Computer Vision and Pattern Recognition*.

Hinton, G. E., and T. J. Sejnowski. 1986. Learning and relearning in Boltzmann machines. In *Parallel distributed processing: Explorations in the microstructure of cognition*. Vol. 1, *Foundations*, D. E. Rumelhart, J. L. McClelland, and the PDP Research Group. MIT Press.

Hofstadter, D. R. 1979. *Gödel, Escher, Bach: An eternal golden braid*. Basic Books.

Hopfield, J. J. 1982. Neural networks and physical systems with emergent collective computational abilities. *Proceedings of the National Academy of Sciences USA* 79, 2554–8.

Hopfield, J. J. 1984. Neurons with graded response have collective computational properties like those of two-state neurons. *Proceedings of the National Academy of Sciences USA* 81, 3088–92.

Jakobson, R. 1962. *Selected writings I: Phonological studies*. Mouton.

Jared, D., K. McRae, and M. S. Seidenberg. 1990. The basis of consistency effects in word naming. *Journal of Memory and Language* 29, 687–715.

Jurafsky, D. S., and J. H. Martin. 2000. *Speech and language processing: An introduction to natural language processing, computational linguistics, and speech recognition*. Prentice-Hall.

Kohonen, T. 1977. *Associative memory: A system-theoretical approach*. Springer.

Legendre, G., Y. Miyata, and P. Smolensky. 1990a. Can connectionism contribute to syntax? Harmonic Grammar, with an application. In *Proceedings of the Chicago Linguistic Society 26*.

Legendre, G., Y. Miyata, and P. Smolensky. 1990b. Harmonic Grammar—a formal multi-level connectionist theory of linguistic well-formedness: An application. In *Proceedings of the Cognitive Science Society 12*.

Legendre, G., Y. Miyata, and P. Smolensky. 1990c. Harmonic Grammar—a formal multi-level connectionist theory of linguistic well-formedness: Theoretical foundations. In *Proceedings of the Cognitive Science Society 12*.

Legendre, G., Y. Miyata, and P. Smolensky. 1991. Unifying syntactic and semantic approaches to unaccusativity: A connectionist approach. In *Proceedings of the Berkeley Linguistics Society 7*.

Legendre, G., S. Vikner, and J. Grimshaw, eds. 2001. *Optimality-theoretic syntax*. MIT Press.

Marcus, G. F. 2001. *The algebraic mind: Integrating connectionism and cognitive science*. MIT Press.

Martignon, L., and U. Hoffrage. 1999. Why does one-reason decision making work? A case study in ecological rationality. In *Simple heuristics that make us smart,* eds. G. Gigerenzer, P. M. Todd, and the ABC Research Group. Oxford University Press.

Martignon, L., and K. B. Laskey. 1999. Bayesian benchmarks for fast and frugal heuristics. In *Simple heuristics that make us smart,* eds. G. Gigerenzer, P. M. Todd, and the ABC Research Group. Oxford University Press.

McCarthy, J. J. 2002. *A thematic guide to Optimality Theory.* Cambridge University Press.

McCarthy, J. J., ed. 2004. *Optimality Theory in phonology: A reader.* Blackwell.

McCarthy, J. J., and A. Prince. 1993a. Generalized alignment. In *Yearbook of morphology,* eds. G. Booij and J. van Marle. Kluwer.

McCarthy, J. J., and A. Prince. 1993b. Prosodic Morphology I: Constraint interaction and satisfaction. Technical report RuCCS-TR-3, Rutgers Center for Cognitive Science, Rutgers University, and University of Massachusetts at Amherst. ROA 482, 2001.

McCarthy, J. J., and A. Prince. 1995. Faithfulness and reduplicative identity. In *University of Massachusetts occasional papers in linguistics 18: Papers in Optimality Theory,* eds. J. Beckman, L. Walsh Dickey, and S. Urbanczyk. Graduate Linguistic Student Association, University of Massachusetts at Amherst. ROA 60.

McCloskey, M. 1992. Networks and theories: The place of connectionism in cognitive science. *Psychological Science* 2, 387–95.

Newell, A., and H. A. Simon. 1963. GPS: A program that simulates human thought. In *Computers and thought,* eds. E. Feigenbaum and J. Feldman. McGraw-Hill.

O'Keefe, J., and L. Nadel. 1979. The hippocampus as a cognitive map. *Behavioral and Brain Sciences* 2, 487–533.

Pearlmutter, B. A. 1989. Learning state space trajectories in recurrent neural networks. *Neural Computation* 1, 263–9.

Pinker, S. 1999. *Words and rules: The ingredients of language.* Basic Books.

Plaut, D. C., J. L. McClelland, M. S. Seidenberg, and K. Patterson. 1996. Understanding normal and impaired word reading: Computational principles in quasi-regular domains. *Psychological Review* 103, 56–115.

Pouget, A., S. Deneve, J.-C. Ducom, and P. E. Latham. 1999. Narrow versus wide tuning curves: What's best for a population code? *Neural Computation* 11, 85–90.

Prince, A. 2002. Entailed ranking arguments. Ms., Rutgers University. ROA 500.

Prince, A., and P. Smolensky. 1991. Notes on connectionism and Harmony Theory in linguistics. Technical report CU-CS-533-91, Computer Science Department, University of Colorado at Boulder.

Prince, A., and P. Smolensky. 1993/2004. *Optimality Theory: Constraint interaction in generative grammar.* Technical report, Rutgers University and University of Colorado at Boulder, 1993. ROA 537, 2002. Revised version published by Blackwell, 2004.

Pylyshyn, Z. W. 1984. *Computation and cognition: Toward a foundation for cognitive science.* MIT Press.

Reif, F. 1965. *Fundamentals of statistical and thermal physics.* McGraw-Hill.

Rieskamp, J., and U. Hoffrage. 1999. When do people use simple heuristics, and how can we tell? In *Simple heuristics that make us smart,* eds. G. Gigerenzer, P. M. Todd, and the ABC Research Group. Oxford University Press.

Rumelhart, D. E., G. E. Hinton, and R. J. Williams. 1986. Learning internal representations by error propagation. In *Parallel distributed processing: Explorations in the microstructure of cognition.* Vol. 1, *Foundations,* D. E. Rumelhart, J. L. McClelland, and the PDP Research Group. MIT Press.

Rumelhart, D. E., J. L. McClelland, and the PDP Research Group. 1986. *Parallel distributed processing: Explorations in the microstructure of cognition.* Vol. 1, *Foundations.* MIT Press.

Sanger, D. 1989. Contribution analysis: A technique for assigning responsibilities to hidden units in connectionist networks. *Connection Science* 1, 115–38.

Seidenberg, M. S., G. S. Waters, M. A. Barnes, and M. K. Tanenhaus. 1984. When does irregular spelling or pronunciation influence word recognition? *Journal of Verbal Learning and Verbal Behavior* 23, 383–404.

Sells, P., ed. 2001. *Formal and empirical issues in optimality-theoretic syntax*. CSLI Publications.

Smolensky, P. 1983. Schema selection and stochastic inference in modular environments. In *Proceedings of the National Conference on Artificial Intelligence* 3.

Smolensky, P. 1986. Information processing in dynamical systems: Foundations of Harmony Theory. In *Parallel distributed processing: Explorations in the microstructure of cognition*. Vol. 1, *Foundations*, D. E. Rumelhart, J. L. McClelland, and the PDP Research Group. MIT Press.

Smolensky, P., G. Legendre, and Y. Miyata. 1992. Principles for an integrated connectionist/symbolic theory of higher cognition. Technical report CU-CS-600-92, Computer Science Department, and 92-8, Institute of Cognitive Science, University of Colorado at Boulder.

Smolensky, P., M. C. Mozer, and D. E. Rumelhart, eds. 1996. *Mathematical perspectives on neural networks*. Erlbaum.

Stemberger, J. P., and B. H. Bernhardt. 1998. *Handbook of phonological development from the perspective of constraint-based nonlinear phonology*. Academic Press.

Taraban, R., and J. L. McClelland. 1987. Conspiracy effects in word pronunciation. *Journal of Memory and Language* 26, 608–31.

Tesar, B. B. 1995. Computational Optimality Theory. Ph.D. diss., University of Colorado at Boulder. ROA 90.

Tesar, B. B., and P. Smolensky. 1993. The learnability of Optimality Theory: An algorithm and some basic complexity results. Technical report CU-CS-678-93, Computer Science Department, University of Colorado at Boulder. ROA 2.

Tesar, B. B., and P. Smolensky. 1998. Learnability in Optimality Theory. *Linguistic Inquiry* 29, 229–68.

Tesar, B. B., and P. Smolensky. 2000. *Learnability in Optimality Theory*. MIT Press.

Todorov, E. 2002. Cosine tuning minimizes motor errors. *Neural Computation* 14, 1233–60.

Townsend, D. J., and T. G. Bever. 2001. *Sentence comprehension*. MIT Press.

Zhang, K., I. Ginzburg, B. L. McNaughton, and T. J. Sejnowski. 1998. Interpreting neuronal population activity by reconstruction: Unified framework with application to hippocampal place cells. *Journal of Neurophysiology* 79, 1017–44.

Zhang, K., and T. J. Sejnowski. 1999. Neuronal tuning: To sharpen or broaden? *Neural Computation* 11, 75–84.

2 Principles of the Integrated Connectionist / Symbolic Cognitive Architecture

Paul Smolensky and Géraldine Legendre

The Integrated Connectionist/Symbolic Cognitive Architecture (ICS) is defined by four general principles that are informally introduced here. These principles relate the aggregate properties of connectionist representations and processes with symbolic representations and processes, and identify optimization as a central organizing principle that spans the levels of both the connectionist and the symbolic descriptions. The informal versions of the four principles presented here provide the foundation for more formal development of these principles in Part II. Section 8 presents an extended summary of a 'big picture' of ICS research as it currently stands. This section constitutes an **ICS map**, which situates and relates the work discussed in all the chapters in Parts II–IV.

Contents

Our task in this chapter is to articulate the fundamental working hypothesis of the Integrated Connectionist/Symbolic Cognitive Architecture (ICS). This hypothesis was formulated roughly in Chapter 1 (13) as *Cognition is massively parallel numerical computation, some dimensions of which are organized to realize crucial facets of symbolic computation.* We now unpack this into four subhypotheses, which will be developed and explored throughout the remainder of this book. In Section 8, we illustrate rather concretely how these principles apply to a cognitive function, sentence comprehension.

1 SYMBOLIC STRUCTURES AS PATTERNS OF ACTIVATION

In integrating connectionist and symbolic computation, the most fundamental issue is the relation between the different types of representations they employ. The ICS hypothesis concerning this relation is our first principle, P_1, informally stated in (1).[1]

(1) **P_1. Rep$_{ICS}$**: Cognitive representation in ICS
Information is represented in the mind/brain by widely distributed activity patterns—activation vectors—that, for central aspects of higher cognition, possess global structure describable through the discrete data structures of symbolic cognitive theory.

According to this principle, at a lower level of description, a mental representation is a pattern of numerical activity levels over a large number—call it *n*—of connectionist units (e.g., Hinton, McClelland, and Rumelhart 1986; Churchland and Sejnowski 1992; Abbott and Sejnowski 1999). The list of all *n* activation values constitutes a **vector** in an *n*-dimensional vector space. The mathematics of vector spaces allows us to treat this list of activations—that is, the **activation pattern**—as an entity in its own right: an element in a higher-level description of the system, in fact (recall Figure 1:2c). (Throughout the book, the terms 'activation' and 'activity' are used interchangeably.)

In Chapter 5, we will introduce some of the relevant vector space concepts for working with this higher-level description; these are needed in order to be precise about what it means in Rep$_{ICS}$ for a set of activation patterns—a set of vectors—to possess appropriate global structure (1). For a first picture, consider the following crude analogy. Imagine a marching band in the halftime show of a football game. At the lower level of description, there are a large number of musicians, each marching around and gyrating in a peculiar fashion. But at the higher level, the same system can be seen as realizing now letters, now a static image, now a moving picture—all the while exhibiting a large-scale organized swaying synchronized to the music.

[1] In the form developed in ICS theory, this principle emerged in the late 1980s and early 1990s through a number of lines of research, the most directly relevant including work by Dolan and Dyer (1987), Smolensky (1987; 1990, et seq.), Pollack (1988; 1990), Dolan (1989), and Plate (1991; 1994). Much additional relevant literature is discussed in Chapters 7–8.

A major contribution of the research program presented in this book is the demonstration that a collection of numerical activity vectors *can* possess a kind of global structure that is describable as a symbol system. But unfortunately, unlike the case of the marching band, the global structure of spaces of activation vectors is not a kind of higher-level organization that our perceptual systems give our awareness direct access to. We need the imaging device provided by the appropriate mathematics to see the higher-level structure of activation patterns.

This mathematics is quite accessible; it is introduced intuitively in Chapter 5. That chapter presents a step-by-step development of these ideas, presuming only knowledge of high-school algebra and geometry. Two central notions introduced there are the vector operations of **addition** (denoted '+' or 'Σ') and the **tensor product** (denoted '⊗'). The formal statement of the principle RepICS that is developed in Chapter 5 (40) is previewed in (2) and illustrated in Figure 1 and Box 1.

(2) **RepICS(HC)**: Integrated representation in higher cognition

a. In all cognitive domains, when analyzed at a lower level, mental representations are defined by the activation values of connectionist units. When analyzed at a higher level, these representations are distributed patterns of activity—activation vectors. For central aspects of higher cognitive domains, these vectors realize symbolic structures.[2]

b. Such a symbolic structure **s** is defined by a collection of **structural roles** $\{r_i\}$ each of which may be occupied by a **filler** $\mathbf{f}_i$; **s** is a set of **constituents**, each a **filler/role binding** $\mathbf{f}_i/r_i$.

c. The connectionist realization of **s** is an activity vector

$$\mathbf{s} = \Sigma_i\, \mathbf{f}_i \otimes \mathbf{r}_i$$

which is the sum of vectors realizing the filler/role bindings. In these **tensor product representations**, the pattern realizing the structure as a whole is the superposition of patterns realizing all of its constituents.[3] And the pattern realizing a constituent is the tensor product of a pattern realizing the filler and a pattern realizing the structural role it occupies.

[2] The intended distinction between 'representation' and 'realization' can be illustrated with the sound sequence for *cat* and its mental encoding:

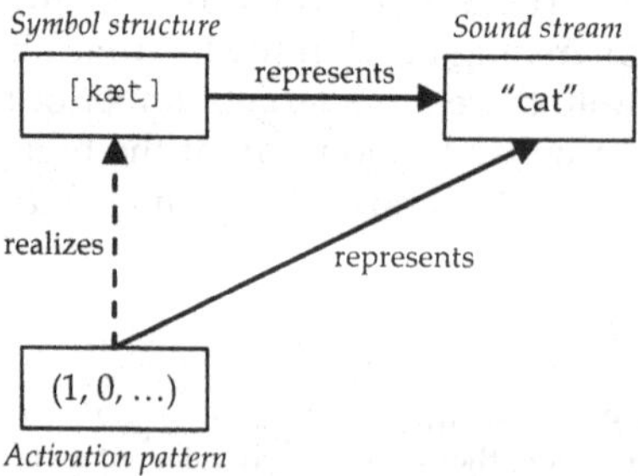

[3] For symbol structures realized in activity vectors, the whole is literally the sum of the parts.

d. In higher cognitive domains such as language and reasoning, mental representations are recursive: the fillers or roles of **s** have themselves the same type of internal structure as **s**. And these structured fillers **f** or roles *r* in turn have the same type of tensor product realization as **s**.

Figure 1. Realizing symbol structures as activity vectors

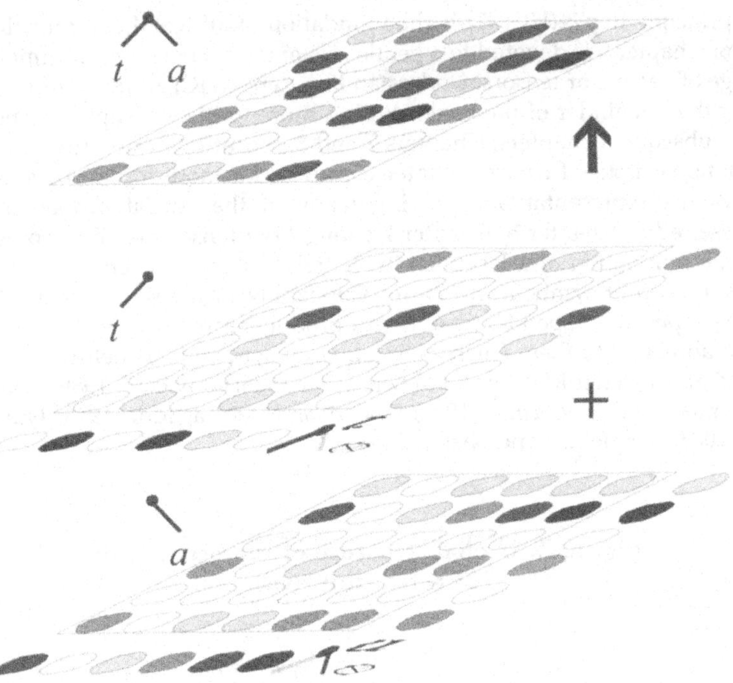

In Figure 1, different shades of gray are used to indicate activity levels of network units (circles). The top plane shows a pattern of activity realizing the microtree

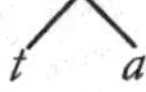

The pattern in the top plane is produced by taking the activation pattern realizing *t* in the left position (middle plane) and adding it to another pattern realizing *a* in the right position (bottom plane).

Previewing the development of Chapter 5, an example of the global structure referred to in (1) is illustrated in Figure 2. This figure illustrates the systematic arrangement, in a four-dimensional space, of a collection of activation patterns (vectors)

over a group of four network units. These patterns realize a simple symbol system containing two-symbol strings such as **AB**, **BA**, and so on. The four coordinates *x*, *y*, *z*, *w* of the point labeled **AB** give the activity values of the pattern realizing the symbol string **AB** (each cube represents a different value of *w*). As explained in Section 5:1.2.2, the four locations of the realizations of **AA**, **AB**, **AC**, and **AD** have the same interrelations as those of **BA**, **BB**, **BC**, and **BD**. This is but one example of how the organization of the space of symbol structures is mirrored in the organization of the space of activity patterns realizing those symbol structures.

The principle Rep_{ICS}(HC) (2) is the foundation of all ICS theory; for this reason, the bulk of Chapter 5 is devoted to a gentle, systematic exposition, assuming no prior knowledge of vectors or tensors. Understanding Rep_{ICS}(HC) at this intuitive level will suffice for the remainder of the book. While a more formal conception is not needed to follow subsequent chapters, Chapters 7 and 8 permit interested readers to pursue representational issues further. Chapter 8 provides a more formal development of tensor product representations, proving many of the crucial properties that are merely asserted in Chapter 5. Chapter 7 shows how tensor product representations provide the foundation of a large family of tightly related schemes for the connectionist realization of symbolic structure. This family includes a number of schemes that were proposed independently of tensor product representations and that seem to be clearly unrelated to them (such as 'binding by synchronous neuronal firing'—see Section 7:5 and von der Malsburg and Schneider 1986; Gray et al. 1989; Eckhorn et al. 1990; Hummel and Biederman 1992; Shastri and Ajjanagadde 1993; Hummel and Holyoak 2003; Wendelken and Shastri 2003).

Figure 2. Global structure of representations in activation space

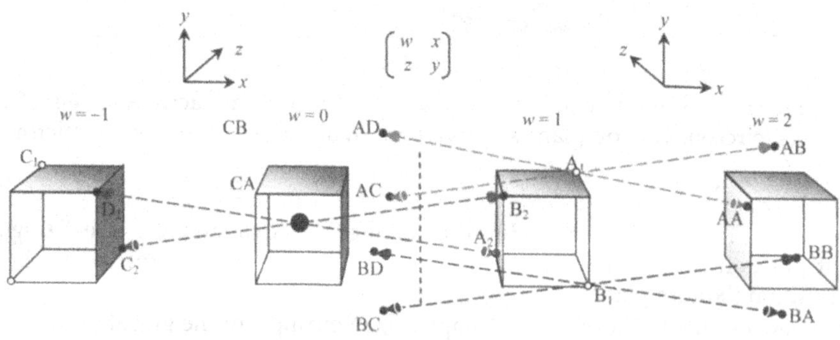

Figure 2

Box 1. Symbolic structures as activation patterns—Rep$_{ICS}$ illustrated

Consider extremely simple trees consisting of a root node dominating a pair of child nodes, where at each of these three positions, there may reside a single symbol from the alphabet {**A**, **B**, **X**, **Y**}. For example, one tree is [$_X$ **A B**] with **X** at the root (top) position, **A** at the lower left, **B** at the lower right.

These trees will be realized as patterns of activity over a set of 12 connectionist units, as shown in Figure A.

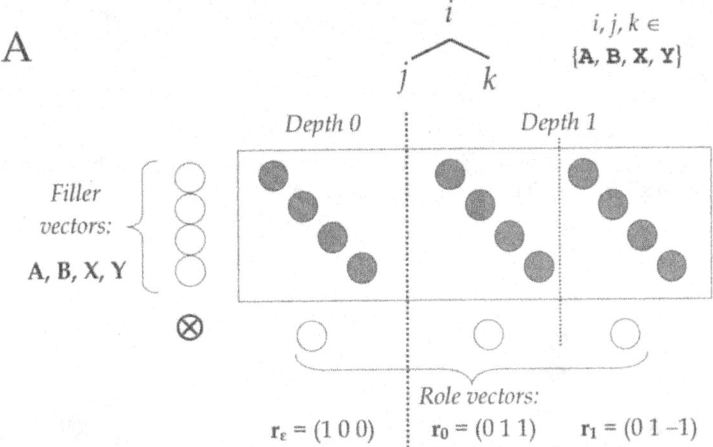

The 12 units supporting the representation are the dark circles in the rectangle; the other, unfilled, circles are imaginary units that are useful for understanding the actual representation. The **binding** of a symbol—say, **Y**—to a role—say, the root position r_ε—is denoted **Y**/r_ε; the realization of this binding is the **tensor product** vector $\mathbf{Y} \otimes \mathbf{r}_\varepsilon$. **Y** is an activation pattern realizing **Y**—a **filler vector**, which is to be imagined to reside in the stack of four imaginary units to the left of the rectangle. In this example, we take this vector to be (1 −1 1 −1) and draw it as shown in Figure B, with black circles denoting activity 1, white circles −1, and gray circles 0.

$\mathbf{r}_\varepsilon$ is the **role vector** realizing the role of root position; it is to be imagined on the three imaginary units beneath the rectangle. $\mathbf{r}_\varepsilon$ resides in the portion of this pool of units devoted to depth 0 in the tree, and is the single number 1; the two units for depth-1 roles are both 0. By the definition of the tensor product, the activity of the unit within the rectangle in row α and column β is the activity of the filler unit in row α times the activity of the role unit in column β; this product is indicated for two units with the dashed lines. (The three 'columns' are separated by vertical dotted lines.)

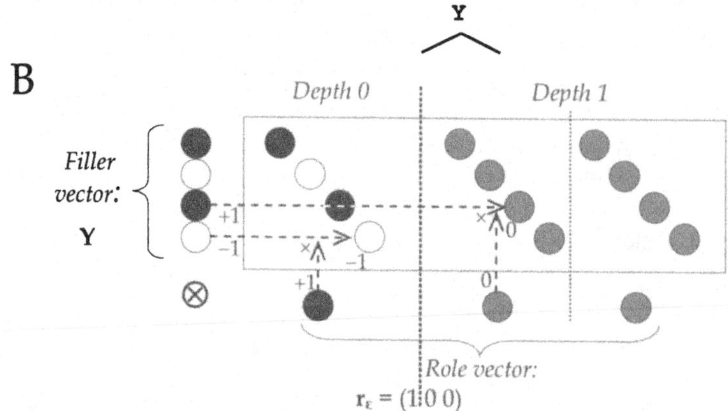

To realize **A** at the right daughter node, the relevant role is r_1, which in this example is realized as (0 1 −1). The pattern for **A** is taken to be (1 1 −1 −1); see Figure C.

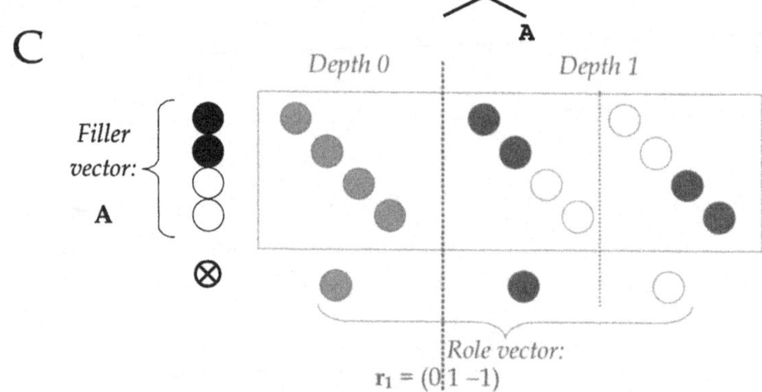

To realize the tree in which **Y** dominates the pair **B A**—that is, [$_{\mathbf{Y}}$ **B A**]—we superimpose (add) the previous two patterns (for **Y**/r_ε and **A**/r_1) and then add a third vector realizing **B**/r_0 (defined analogously to **A**/r_1). The result is the pattern shown on the top horizontal line of Figure D (the 12 units making up the representation are drawn as a horizontal line, in their left-to-right sequence within the rectangle). The area of a circle indicates the magnitude of the activation of the corresponding network unit; white denotes negative values, black positive.

This display also shows the activation pattern realizing the tree [$_{\mathbf{X}}$ **A B**] (second horizontal line), as well as the patterns for smaller structures, such as **X** in root position (bottom line), **A** in left daughter position (fifth line from the bottom, labeled '**A** –'), and the pair of daughter nodes [**B A**] with no label at the root (third line from the top). Activation patterns realizing more complex structures are built up by superimposing the patterns realizing their constituents (which are themselves built up in the same way). As shown in this figure (and Figure 2), the set of vectors realizing these structures has a high degree of **systematicity**.

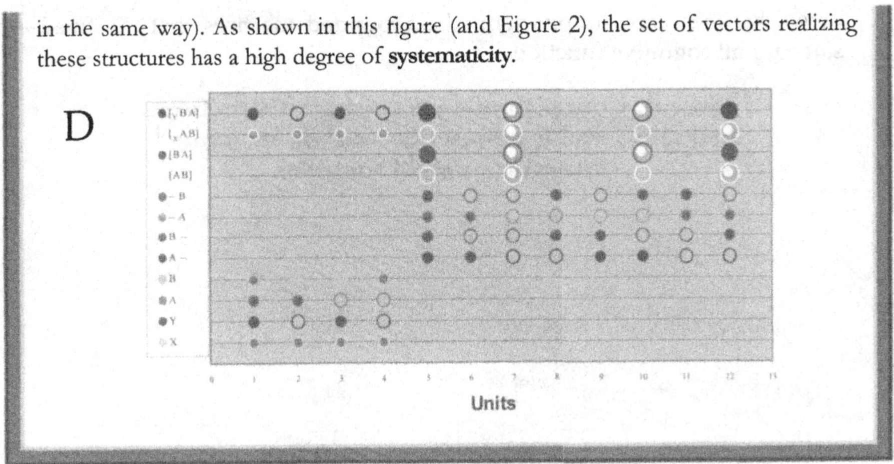

2 SYMBOLIC OPERATIONS AS PATTERNS OF CONNECTIONS

The mental representations characterized by our first principle Rep_{ICS} are of course only useful if they can be appropriately manipulated to support cognition. These **mental processes** are the subject of the second ICS principle, P_2 (Smolensky, Legendre, and Miyata 1992). This principle parallels P_1 (1) closely.

(3) **P_2. Proc_{ICS}**: Cognitive processing in ICS
Information is processed in the mind/brain by widely distributed connection patterns—weight matrices—which, for central aspects of higher cognition, possess global structure describable through symbolic expressions for recursive functions of the type employed in symbolic cognitive theory.

Chapter 5 provides an intuitive introduction to the mathematical tools that allow us to formally characterize the global structure of connection patterns in connectionist networks that compute symbolic functions. This mathematics—tensor calculus—concerns vectors and their manipulation; it is discussed in further detail in Chapter 8. (4) gives a preview of the resulting formal principles: Chapter 5 (63) and Chapter 8 (108), (132).

(4) **Alg_{ICS}(HC,W)**: Recursive processing
Central aspects of many higher cognitive domains, including language, are realized in weight matrices with **recursive structure**. That is, feed-forward networks and recurrent networks realizing various cognitive functions have weight matrices with these respective forms:

Feed-forward: $\mathbf{W} = \mathbf{I} \otimes \underline{\mathbf{W}}$ Recurrent: $\mathbf{W} = \underline{\mathbf{W}} \otimes \mathbf{R}$

In either case, $\underline{\mathbf{W}}$ is a finite matrix of weights that specifies the particular cognitive function. **I** and **R** are the **recursion matrices** for feed-forward and recurrent networks: these are simply-defined unbounded matrices that are fixed—the same for all cognitive functions.

Figure 3. Connectionist processing of structured activation-vector representations via structured connection-weight matrices

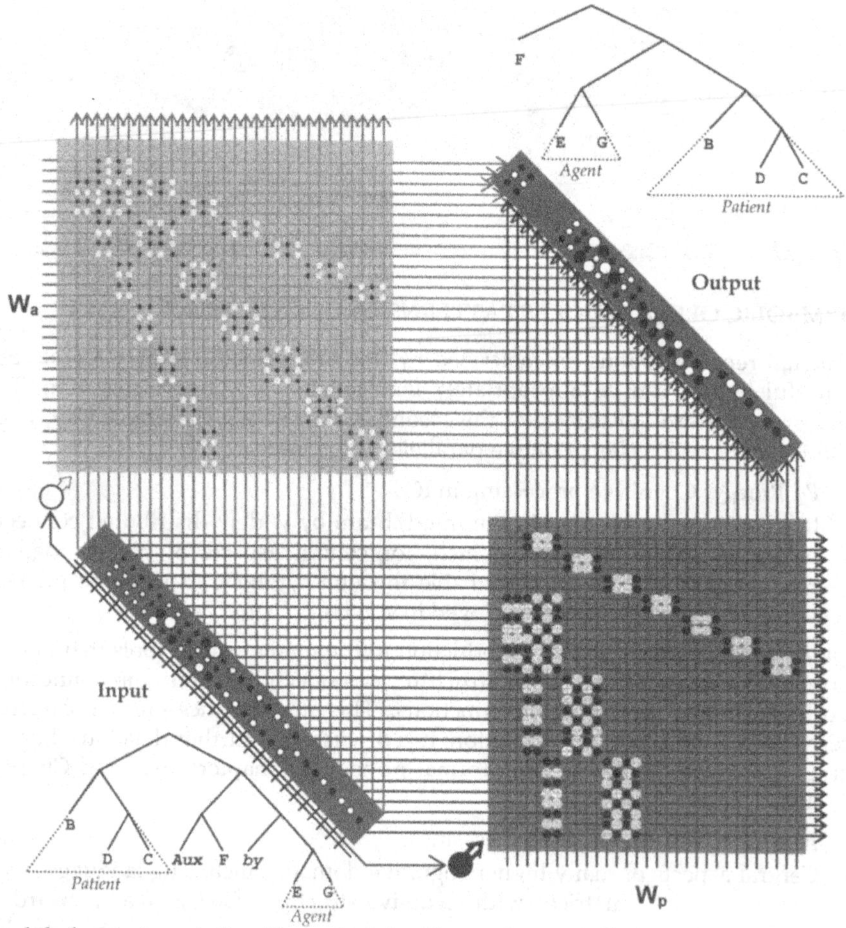

The global structure defined by principle (4) entails, we will show, that a connectionist network defined by this type of weight matrix can be described at a higher level as computing a particular recursive function (which depends on $\underline{\mathbf{W}}$). The input-output mapping of such a function *could* be specified by a sequential symbolic program, but such a program would not describe how the network *actually computes* the function: it employs massively parallel, numerical computation, with all parts of the input and output symbol structures being processed at once. This is illustrated in Figure 3, in which the global structure of the weight matrix (the large gray squares) is even somewhat discernible to the naked eye. (See also Box 2.)

Box 2. A simple grammar in a connectionist weight matrix

Consider the following extremely simple formal grammar:

$\mathcal{G} \equiv \{\mathbf{X} \rightarrow \mathbf{A}\ \mathbf{B},\ \mathbf{Y} \rightarrow \mathbf{B}\ \mathbf{A}\}$

This grammar generates a language containing only two, extremely simple, trees:

$$\mathcal{L}_{\mathcal{G}} = \left\{ \begin{array}{c} \mathbf{X} \\ \wedge \\ \mathbf{A}\quad\mathbf{B} \end{array} , \begin{array}{c} \mathbf{Y} \\ \wedge \\ \mathbf{B}\quad\mathbf{A} \end{array} \right\}$$

More compactly, $\mathcal{L}_{\mathcal{G}} = \{[_{\mathbf{X}}\mathbf{A}\ \mathbf{B}],\ [_{\mathbf{Y}}\mathbf{B}\ \mathbf{A}]\}$. Suppose these trees are realized in a 12-unit connectionist network as shown in Box 1. Suppose this network is fully connected: each unit is connected to all units (including itself). As we will show in Chapter 8 (139), the 12×12 matrix of weights of these connections can realize the grammar $\mathcal{G}$. For this grammar, the only non-zero weights are those on connections linking a unit in the depth-0 pool of 4 units with a unit in the depth-1 pool of 8 units; thus, in the following diagram of the network, the connections shown form a 4×8 matrix (inside the dashed rectangle: each dot marks one connection weight). The network is symmetric: every connection passes activation equally in both directions. In the diagram, one direction is shown by the solid arrowheads (from 4 units to 8), and the reverse direction is shown with hollow arrowheads.

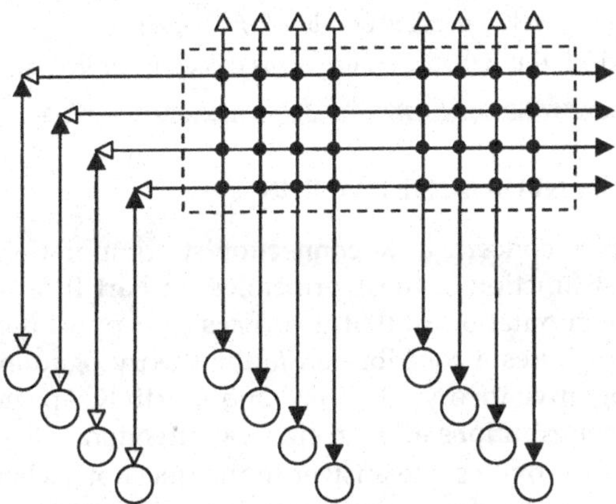

The 4×8 matrix of weights is displayed below, with the area of each circle showing the magnitude of the corresponding weight (white denotes negative weight; black, positive; 0 weights have area 0 and are not seen).

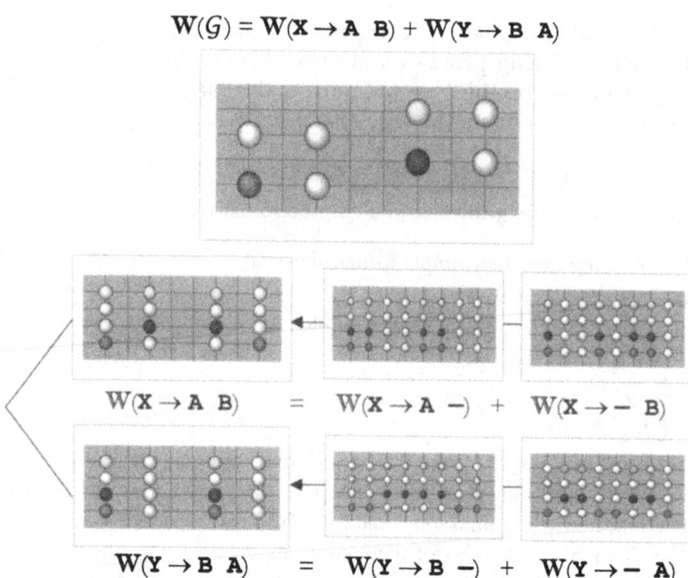

This weight matrix has the following global structure. The complete weight matrix **W**(𝒢) (top rectangle) is the sum of two matrices (leftmost rectangles below), each realizing one of the rules of 𝒢: **W**(**X** → **A B**) and **W**(**Y** → **B A**). Each of these matrices is in turn the sum of two matrices, one for each "half" of the rule; **W**(X → **A B**) is the sum of the "left half" weights **W**(**X** → **A** –) and the "right half" weights, **W**(**X** → – **B**). Each of these matrices is in turn the product of two vectors—for example, **W**(**X** → **A** –) is the product of a vector determined by **X** and a vector determined by **A**—but this level of detail is best left for Chapter 8.

The sense in which this network realizes 𝒢 is discussed in Box 3.

3 Optimization in Neural Networks

The first two principles concern how connectionist computation realizes symbolic computation. The first function of these principles (in Part II of the book) will be to enrich connectionist computation so that it suffices to support higher-level symbolic descriptions. This constitutes a contribution *to* the theory of connectionist computation *from* symbolic cognitive theory. The third and fourth ICS principles, to which we now turn, constitute contributions in the reciprocal direction.

The third principle provides one answer to the question, what higher-level characterizations can be provided for the computations performed in connectionist networks? This question is of central importance to ICS, in which symbolic computation is identified with higher-level formal descriptions of connectionist computation. The characterization of connectionist computation provided in the next principle—as a kind of optimization—will be informally introduced in Chapter 6 and formally developed in Chapter 9.[4]

(5) P_3. **HMax**: Harmony Maximization

a. (Harmony Maximization, general) In a number of cognitive domains, information processing in the mind/brain constructs an output for which the pair (input, output) is **optimal**: processing maximizes a connectionist well-formedness measure called **Harmony**. The Harmony function encapsulates knowledge as a set of conflicting soft constraints of varying strengths; the output achieves the optimal degree of simultaneous satisfaction of these constraints.

b. (Harmonic Grammar) Among the cognitive domains falling under Harmony Maximization are central aspects of knowledge of language—grammar. In this setting, the specification of the Harmony function is called a **harmonic grammar.** It defines a function that maps:

input → output = parse(input).

Part (a) of this principle (see Boxes 1:3 and 1:4) was developed primarily outside the domains of higher cognition; a prototypical domain is perception (e.g., Marr and Poggio 1976; Geman and Geman 1984). In visual perception, the input might be a set of pixel intensity levels in an image; this is encoded as a set of activation values over an array of units in a connectionist network. Activation flows from these input units and eventually settles into a stable activation pattern over the whole network; part of the network, the output units, then encodes a perceptual interpretation of the image, in which, say, each pixel is assigned a depth in three dimensions, and a degree of reflectance and illumination. The connections in the network encode perceptual constraints—for example, that the depths/reflectances/illuminations assigned to two neighboring pixels must differ only infinitesimally. Each activation pattern in the network can be assigned a numerical Harmony value that measures the degree to which the perceptual constraints are satisfied. Activation spread in the network maximizes Harmony: it constructs a final pattern of activation with a maximal Harmony value. Thus, the construction of a perceptual interpretation of a stimulus is construed as the problem of finding the interpretation that best satisfies a set of numerically weighted constraints defining the Harmony function.

Part (b) of the principle extends its scope to higher cognition—in particular, to grammar (see Box 1:9). An input to a grammatically determined function is, for example, a sequence of words; the output is a structural analysis—a **parse**—of that input—for example, e.g., a tree structure grouping words into simple phrases, these phrases into larger phrases, and so on, as illustrated in Chapter 1 (7). Harmony Maximization asserts that the grammatical output, the correct structural analysis, is

[4] This principle is due to a number of neural network researchers in the early 1980s (Hopfield 1982, 1984; Cohen and Grossberg 1983; Hinton and Sejnowski 1983, 1986; Smolensky 1983, 1986; Golden 1986, 1988). The application to language (5b) was developed in the late 1980s (Lakoff 1988; Goldsmith 1990; Legendre, Miyata, and Smolensky 1990a, 1990b, 1990c).

the parse tree that maximally satisfies a set of constraints defining a Harmony function. These constraints *are* the grammar — a harmonic grammar. (See Box 3.)

Box 3. Processing with a simple grammar

Consider the simple grammar $\mathcal{G}$, and the network realizing it, described in Box 2. Use of this grammar in processing includes two modes: top-down and bottom-up.

In top-down processing, the input is either **X** or **Y** at the root of a tree, and the output is the entire tree in the language $\mathcal{L}_G$ that has this root symbol. The plot labeled '**X** → **??**' shows the result of clamping the pattern for **X** in the four depth-0 units: ½(1 1 1 1). Activation flows through the connections shown in Box 2, according to the activation dynamics given in Box 1:3. When the network activation pattern has stabilized, the eight depth-1 units hold the pattern ¼(1 0 −1 0 0 1 0 −1). This is the pattern realizing the symbol sequence **A B**: the pattern in the fourth row from the top of Box 1. And indeed **A B** is the correct completion of a tree with **X** at the root.

The display below '**X**→ **??**' shows the activity pattern on the eight depth-1 units over time, which increases vertically: each horizontal row shows the pattern at one time. The pattern builds up steadily from zero to the final, correct pattern. The corresponding graph shows how the magnitude of the activation value of a non-zero unit β, $|a_\beta|$, grows in time. It also shows that during processing the Harmony value H steadily increases to its final value (0.5).

Top-down processing: X → ??   A B = (1 0 −1 0 0 1 0 −1)/4

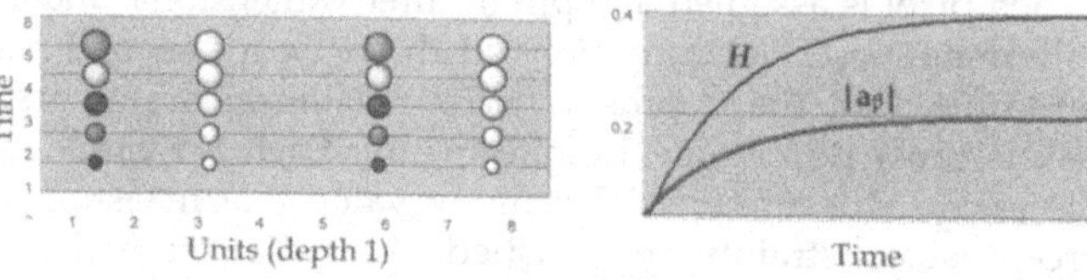

Bottom-up processing: A B → ?   X = (1 1 1 1)/2

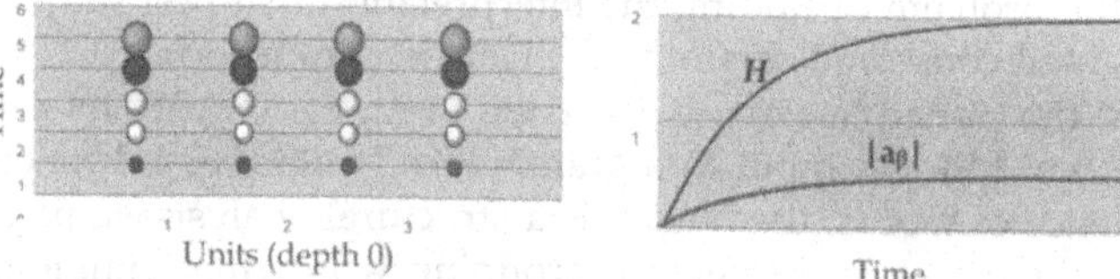

In bottom-up processing, the input is at depth 1: a string (sequence) of terminal symbols (e.g., **A B**). The output is the full grammatical tree with this terminal string; computing this tree involves filling in **X** at the root node, that is, parsing this string as category **X**. In the network, the pattern for **A B** is clamped on the eight depth-1 units; activation flows to the four depth-0 units, which steadily build up their activation values from zero. The display under '**A B → ?**' shows how the activation pattern on the four depth-0 units builds up over time; the increase in activation value $|a_\beta|$ is plotted on the corresponding graph. The final activation pattern is (1 1 1 1)/2, the pattern for **X**; the network has correctly parsed the string. As shown in the graph, during parsing the Harmony H steadily increases to its final value (2.0).

Importantly, Harmony H can be viewed here in two complementary ways. On the one hand, the correct output is defined as the representation that maximizes Harmony, given the input: this is a nondynamic, "competence grammar" view of H as a static object that defines grammatical outputs. On the other hand, the dynamics of the network that *uses* this grammar is a computational process that incrementally optimizes Harmony, steadily increasing H during processing until the final, H-maximizing state is reached. The dynamics is hill-climbing in H (Box 1:3): H specifies the processing algorithm—it provides a "performance theory." Thus, H unifies these competence and performance perspectives, the static and dynamic views of knowledge of language. (In more complex situations, the dynamic process computes only a **local** Harmony maximum, while the grammar designates the **global** Harmony maximum as the well-formed output: this competence/performance discrepancy is discussed in Section 6:2.4.)

4 Optimization in Grammar I: Harmonic Grammar

Once the previous principles are formalized, in Chapter 6 we will be able to deduce the structure of the Harmony function defining a harmonic grammar. For now, this theorem can be roughly summarized as in (6).

(6) **HG**. Harmonic Grammar soft constraints

The Harmony of a structure **s** with constituents $\{\mathbf{c}_i\}$ is determined by **soft constraints** of the following form:

$\mathbf{c}_i$ and $\mathbf{c}_j$ must not both occur in a single structure (strength: W_{ij})

Perhaps not surprisingly, given that Harmonic Grammar (HG) can be realized in basic connectionist networks, this result (6) shows how extremely simple this grammar formalism is.

This simplicity suggests that HG is a highly impoverished formalism, unlikely to be up to the demands of real language. But despite the highly restrictive nature of HG rules, in Chapter 10 it will prove possible to demonstrate the result in (7).

(7) HG expressiveness for formal languages

Any formal language can be specified by a harmonic grammar.

That is, HG affords, in an appropriate sense, the computational power of traditional sequential symbol-rewriting rule systems—power equivalent to that of Turing machines in the functions they can compute. This is a measure of the degree to which the power of symbolic computation has been realized in connectionist computation in ICS. (A concise introduction to formal languages and Turing machines is provided in Box 6:1. For an extremely simple example of a formal language, see Box 2 above.)[5]

With respect to natural languages, HG in fact appears to provide the power needed to account for the complex interaction of semantic and syntactic constraints determining French intransitive verbs' argument structure—the verb-specific relations linking the semantic and syntactic roles of the verb's argument. (The notion of argument structure was introduced in Section 1:3.3.) This result is summarized in Section 6:2.4, and is the topic of Chapter 11.

5 Optimization in Grammar II: Optimality Theory

The final principle of ICS brings together two currents of research, one representative of connectionist cognitive theory, the other a centerpiece of symbolic cognitive theory. The former strand is the HG conception of grammars as optimizing systems of soft constraints; the latter is the theory of universal grammar as developed within the generative grammar tradition. The result is a new type of symbolic grammatical theory, introduced in Section 1:5: Optimality Theory (OT; Prince and Smolensky 1991, 1993/2004). The connectionist underpinnings of OT provide it with novel characteristics, and new explanatory power, relative to previous generative formalisms. As in HG, all grammatical constraints evaluate linguistic structures simultaneously—in parallel; also, they are 'soft' or violable, and of differing strengths. Rather than formalizing strength numerically, however, OT introduces the notion of **strict domination hierarchy**. All constraints are ranked in this hierarchy, from strongest to weakest; each constraint is stronger than all lower-ranked constraints combined.

Furthermore, OT introduces the strong principle that the constraints in grammars are universal: literally the same in all human languages. What leads to crosslinguistic variation is only differences in the dominance hierarchies constituting the grammars of different languages—differences in the ranking of the same set of universal constraints. To summarize:

(8) **P_4. OT** (Optimality Theory)

Grammar contains a core consisting of a set of universal violable constraints that apply in parallel to assess the well-formedness of linguistic structures. The conflicts between these constraints are resolved via language-specific strict domination hierarchies.

Chapter 4 provides an introduction to OT, with examples of universal constraints, domination hierarchies, and the nonnumerical computation of Harmony Maximization. A systematic introduction to OT is presented in Chapter 12, and the entirety of Part III explores its application to multiple facets of the cognitive science of language.

[5] From a wide range of perspectives, the relation between the computational power of neural-network-like systems and that of Turing machines has been the topic of much literature (see, e.g., Smolensky, Mozer, and Rumelhart 1996; Siegelmann 1999; Hadley 2000; Cleland 2002; Copeland 2002, 2003).

6 UNIVERSAL GRAMMAR, UNIVERSAL GRAMMAR, AND INNATE KNOWLEDGE

A principle central to OT is the universality of grammatical constraints (and of the linguistic structures they evaluate). This is an important respect in which OT is more restrictive than HG—a most welcome restriction. In the HG analysis presented in Chapter 11, the constraints employed are intended to embody universal tendencies, but the emphasis is on capturing difficult interactions within a single language. Language-particular analysis plays an important role in OT, as it does in all grammatical theory; but OT places a strong emphasis on explaining crosslinguistic patterns—**typology**—via the reranking of a fixed set of hypothesized universal constraints.

We do not take OT to be committed on the question of the *origin* of the universality of grammatical constraints, however. We certainly do not accept an equation between universality and innateness; rather, we take this connection to be a wide-open empirical question. We do, however, share the commitment of generative grammar to the reality of language universals, and we do take it as an important goal of cognitive theory to explain the origin of these universals (see Chapter 22). We do not reject out of hand the hypothesis that universals have innate origin, although we believe that this hypothesis requires considerably stronger empirical support than is currently available. Furthermore, even if true, this hypothesis leaves two large questions unanswered: How can such abstract knowledge possibly be encoded genetically? And is there any functional explanation for why such a genetic endowment might have evolved? (The first question is taken up in Chapter 21; we have nothing to contribute concerning the second question at this point.)

At the same time, we feel the force of Chomsky's arguments from the **poverty of the stimulus** (e.g., Chomsky 1965). These arguments, in our view, place the bar extremely high for competing theories claiming that knowledge of language can be induced from experience with little or no a priori bias encoding a kind of innate knowledge of universal linguistic principles. It seems to us still quite unclear whether the current generation of empiricist learning methods, including connectionist learning algorithms, can clear this bar. On the other hand, it is little (or no) explanation of universals to simply assert that they are somehow in the genome; moreover, this hypothesis seems to be disturbingly untestable at present (see Chapter 21).

Thus, while 'Universal Grammar' denotes a body of *innate* knowledge in the Chomskyan lexicon, the more modest 'universal grammar' will denote for us the collection of principles common to the world's languages, knowledge of which, we presume, is psychologically real in native speakers (see Chapter 1). So while we take principles of universal grammar to be "in the head," we would like to be clear that at this point we are quite uncommitted about how that knowledge got there.

Table 1. Treatment of ICS principles

Topic	Principles	Proposal	Chapter	Part
Overview: ICS; OT; philosophical implications	All	Integrated Connectionist/ Symbolic Architecture	2: Informal introduction to ICS principles 3: Integration in cognitive science 4: Informal introduction to OT	I
Connectionist realization of symbolic computation	P_1: Rep_{ICS} P_2: $Proc_{ICS}$	Tensor product networks	5: Formalizing Rep_{ICS}, $Proc_{ICS}$ 7: Structured connectionist representations 8: Formal analysis of tensor product representations	II
High-level analysis of connectionist processing	P_3: HMax HG = Rep_{ICS} + HMax	Harmony maximization	6: Formalizing HMax; HG 9: Formal analysis of Harmony maximization	II
Numerical optimization in grammar	HG	Harmonic Grammar (HG)	10: Formal languages 11: Syntax/semantics interaction in French intransitive verbs	II
Universal grammar in cognitive science: typology, acquisition, and processing	P_4: OT	Optimality Theory (OT)	12: Formal introduction to OT	II
			13: Phonology I: Syllables 14: Phonology II: Features; constraint conjunction 15: Syntax I: Case and voice 16: Syntax II: *Wh*-questions 17: Phonology acquisition 18: Syntax acquisition 19: Online sentence processing	III
	OT, HG	OT realized in connectionism	20: OT-HG relations 21: Genomic encoding of OT	III
Foundations of cognitive architecture	All	ICS explanation	22: Integrating connectionism and generative grammar 23: ICS computational levels: Bridging mind and brain	IV

7 Treatment of ICS Principles in the Book

The four principles of ICS introduced in this chapter are discussed throughout the book, at several levels of technical detail. The principal treatments of each principle are indicated in Table 1.

8 The Big Picture: An ICS Map

The preceding sections of Chapters 1 and 2 sketch a high-level overview of ICS theory. In this section, we outline in some technical detail the 'big picture' of the ICS research program as it currently stands, indicating how the parts of the picture contributed by individual chapters fit together. This section will be referred to in later chapters as the **ICS map**; it is intended as a reference to be consulted when each new chapter is read, to help situate the research described in that chapter in the bigger scheme of the overall research program. Thus, in this section it is necessary to refer to theoretical constructs that are developed later in the book. It is infeasible to define all these terms here; they can be treated as temporary placeholders until the chapters developing them are read.

For this purpose, we will imagine an ICS treatment of the human sentence processor. We say 'imagine' because key bits of the picture must be filled in by future research before there is a sufficiently complete set of results to allow the construction of a comprehensive theory—a theory that reduces syntactic and semantic processing of complex sentences to the level of neural computation. (A critical part of such a theory is presented in Chapter 19: OT is used to explain—on the basis of grammatical structure—the real-time parsing preferences of the human sentence processor, as revealed by a substantial body of empirical studies.)

We start with the large-scale structure of the language-processing system. A particular such structure is not (yet) specified within ICS theory. So for purely expository purposes, to minimize distractions, let's assume a very simple structure for the relevant part of the system: a syntactic module receives a string of words as input and produces as output a grammatical parse for this string; this parse tree is then sent as input to a semantic module, which produces a meaning—a semantic interpretation—as output. Readers are cordially invited to imagine instead their favorite modular or nonmodular structure. The suggested two-module structure is suited for present purposes because it provides a simple and natural setting for discussing both of the fundamental modes of neural computation developed within ICS theory: the syntactic module illustrates the realization of symbolic OT grammars in recurrent networks, while the direct translation of a syntactic tree to a semantic expression illustrates the realization of recursive symbolic functions in feed-forward networks.

Imagine that the system has already processed the classic string *the horse raced past the barn* (Bever 1970). A syntactic representation has been constructed in the syntax module; it is a tree structure realized in a connectionist pattern of activity. That tree has been mapped by the semantic module to some semantic representation such as

∃e, x.raced(e;x) & horse(x) & ... — this can be glossed 'there is an entity *x* participating in an event *e* such that *e* is a racing event and *x* is a horse, and ... [during the event the horse moves from one side of a barn to the other]'. Obviously oversimplified, but sufficient here.

Then another word, *fell*, is received. This word cannot be accommodated within the current parse: the new word is a main verb and the existing parse already has a main verb, *race*. Reparsing is required, with *raced* reanalyzed as the passive participle of a relative clause that has been reduced: *the horse [that was] raced past the barn*. This entire phrase is then parsed as the subject of the main verb *fell*: *the horse [that was] ... fell*. This new tree structure has a new interpretation, in which the event referred to by the sentence is an event of falling rather than of racing.

We will now walk through a fairly detailed ICS picture of this process, breaking the discussion down into six parts. Each part consists of a diagram and a discussion of the diagram in the context of the general questions and results that underlie the illustration. The diagrams build up to the final one, Figure 9.

In addition to results achieved to date, this discussion mentions a few of the more immediate open problems for the ICS research program. The intention is to guide the reader by indicating not only the key results to look for in this book, but also potential results that are not be found here.

8.1 Representations: Form

The most basic elements of a cognitive theory are its representations; we discuss for the moment only the representation in the syntactic module. This is a pattern of activity over network units, which for concreteness we will take to be a realization of a syntactic parse tree. The results involved here are extremely general, and the tree structure could be replaced by any of a wide range of symbolic representations. The situation is schematized in Figure 4. In (9), the particular example illustrated in Figure 4 is described. This is to be viewed as a concrete case of a general solution to a general problem. This problem is stated in (10), while (11) summarizes the results concerning this problem that are developed in ICS research and that are central to its account of higher cognition. Some of the most important aspects of the problem that remain open at this point are mentioned in (12); together, (11) and (12) suggest the current frontier of ICS research on the general problem.

In this section, much of the model structure shown in diagrams like Figure 4 is depicted solely for expository concreteness; these bits have not been the subject of ICS research per se. Rather, research has focused on finding general solutions to the general problems identified below.[6] The chapters in which the results are principally discussed are indicated in square brackets. The circled numbers in Figure 4 are cross-references to the text (9) discussing the figure, and similarly throughout this section.

[6] In this respect, ICS research is 'principle-centered' rather than 'model-centered'; see Section 3:2.3 and Chapter 22.

Figure 4. Representations: Form

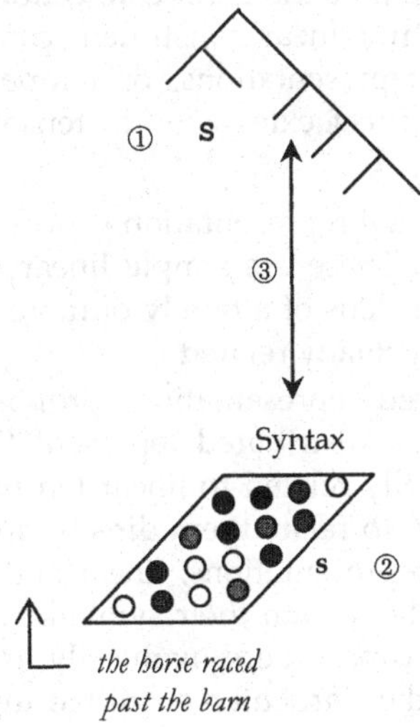

(9) Illustration (Figure 4)
Object of study: $S \equiv$ the syntactic component of the mental representation resulting from processing *the horse raced past the barn*
① In a symbolic formalism: a tree structure **S** describing S
② In a connectionist network: a distributed activation pattern **s** describing S
③ **s** is the tensor product realization of **S**.

The parse tree **S** schematically illustrated in Figure 4 symbolically encodes the analysis of *the horse raced past the barn* as a complete sentence, in which the main verb is *raced*. The activation pattern **s** is a connectionist encoding of the same analysis; these are two formal descriptions of the same mental representation S.

(10) General problem. Representations: Symbolic ↔ connectionist
Find general formalisms for precisely realizing symbolic representations of cognitive theory in distributed, vectorial connectionist representations.

The foundation for integrating symbolic and connectionist computation must be a general formal relationship between the very different systems of representation they employ.

(11) Results
a. Representations: Symbolic ↔ linear connectionist
Tensor product realization maps symbolic structures decomposed into filler/role bindings into activation vectors; constituents simply add ③ [Chapters 5 and 8; (2) above].

b. Representations: Linear connectionist ↔ nonlinear connectionist
Seemingly very different methods for connectionist realization of symbolic structure, employing nonlinear constituent combination, or more space-efficient distributed representations, or temporally extended activation patterns, are in fact direct extensions of tensor product representations [Chapter 7].

The core of the ICS theory of mental representation is provided by tensor product realizations of symbolic structure. These are simple linear representations. But these simple representations are the nucleus of a family of more complex, nonlinear representations to which they can be formally related.

While the kinds of structured representations proposed in symbolic cognitive theory and the kinds of nonlinear distributed representations proposed by connectionist models can each be formally related to linear tensor product representations, it's not yet clear how, in general, to relate them directly to each other (12a). And all these distributed connectionist representations, linear and non-linear, share a property that sharply distinguishes them from their symbolic counterparts: the meaning of representational constituents cannot be dynamically assigned in real time in response to the requirements of the particular cognitive input currently being processed (12b).

(12) Open problems. Representations: Symbolic ↔ nonlinear connectionist
a. Find tractable general formalisms for directly relating symbolic and nonlinear connectionist representations, and general methods for analyzing such representations.
b. Find something like dynamic distributed memory allocation, so that a connectionist representational space does not need to be laid out all at once prior to computation—rather, the representational contents of patterns evolve dynamically during a computation in response to the particular demands of the current input. (This is not representational adaptation during *learning*, but during input → output *computation*, on a much shorter time scale.)

8.2 Representations: Well-formedness; computational perspective

Syntactic representations have a special property: they are grammatically well-formed. The ICS picture is sketched in Figure 5; (13) elaborates.

(13) Illustration (Figure 5)
Object of study: well-formedness of S = the syntactic component of a mental representation, as in (9)
① A tree structure **s** describing S
② A distributed connectionist activation pattern **s** describing S
③ The tree structure **s** is **well-formed** according to some symbolic grammar $\mathcal{G}$ (e.g., a rewrite-rule system or an OT constraint hierarchy)

④ A set of soft constraints expressing $\mathcal{G}$ as a harmonic grammar – $\text{HG}_{\mathcal{G}}$ – according to which **s** is well-formed
⑤ A systematic formal mapping from a rewrite-rule or OT grammar $\mathcal{G}$ to an equivalent harmonic grammar $\text{HG}_{\mathcal{G}}$
⑥ A weight matrix $\mathbf{W}_{\mathcal{G}}$ according to which **s** is a maximal-Harmony tree realization
⑦ Equivalence: the activation patterns that are maximal-Harmony tree realizations with respect to $\mathbf{W}_{\mathcal{G}}$ are those of the optimal trees according to $\text{HG}_{\mathcal{G}}$ and hence of the optimal trees according to $\mathcal{G}$.
⑧ The representation *S* is computed by maximizing Harmony; in processing the last word *barn,* the network state climbs to the top of the Harmony landscape, moving from a previous state (a) to a final state (b) that maximizes Harmony: *S*.

Figure 5. Computation of well-formed representations

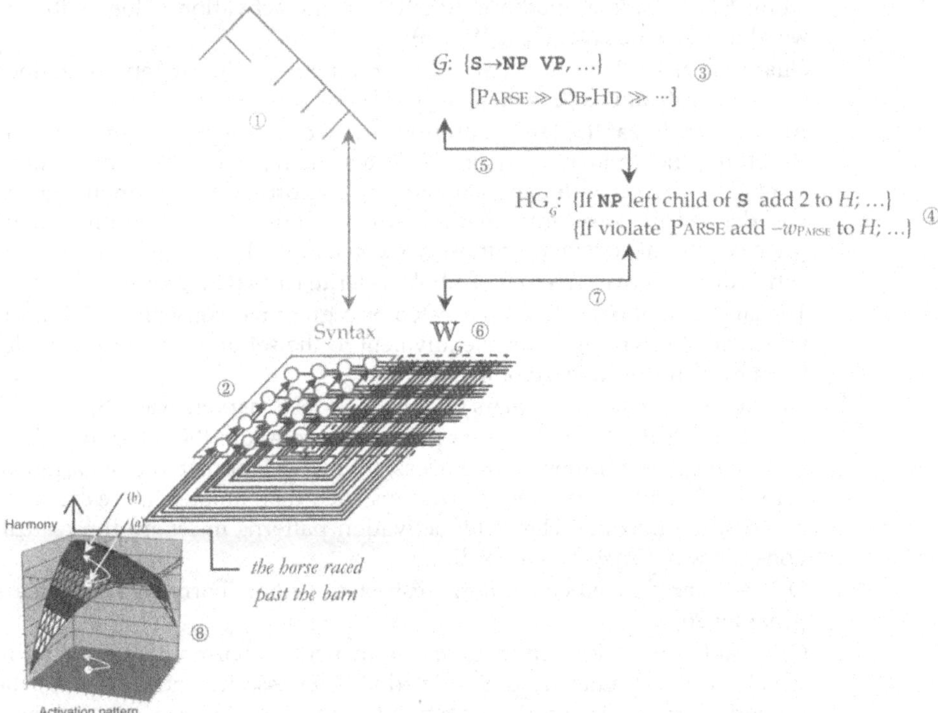

The syntactic representation *S* is well-formed according to a grammar that is characterized in ICS theory at three levels of description: at the highest level, as a symbolic grammar $\mathcal{G}$ ③; at the lowest, as a matrix of connection weights $\mathbf{W}_{\mathcal{G}}$ ⑥; and in between, as a harmonic grammar $\mathrm{HG}_{\mathcal{G}}$ ④, which numerically evaluates relative well-formedness or Harmony. The network performs optimization, moving to the representation of maximal Harmony ⑧. In making this formally explicit, we indicate the general problem in (14), the technical progress to date on the problem in (15), and some open technical problems in (16). The technical concepts and issues involved are developed in the indicated chapters in Part II.

(14) General problem. Symbolic grammar G ↔ WG of recurrent net
Find a general means of realizing a symbolic grammar in the weight matrix of a recurrent network.

(15) Results

a. **W** ↔ optimizing a quadratic Harmony function *H*, for harmonic networks [Chapters 6 and 9]
In the class of recurrent harmonic networks, processing maximizes Harmony *H*, which is a quadratic function of the activation values with the weights as coefficients ($\Sigma_{\alpha\beta}\, a_\alpha W_{\alpha\beta}\, a_\beta$).

b. Quadratic *H* ↔ 2nd-order harmonic grammars for linear representations over tree realizations [Chapters 6 and 11]
Among the linear (≡ tensor product) network realizations of symbolic structures, the optima of a quadratic *H* are the representations that realize symbol structures with maximal Harmony according to a harmonic grammar defined by constraints that are at most 2nd-order in the constituents (each constraint considers at most two constituents).

c. 2nd-order HGs over trees ↔ symbolic rewrite rules [Chapter 10]
The language of parse trees generated by a grammar consisting of context-free symbol-rewriting rules is equivalent to the set of optimal trees as defined by a 2nd-order harmonic grammar.

d. 2nd-order harmonic grammars over trees ↔ **W** [Chapters 6 and 8]
Given one of the following, it is possible to compute the other: (i) a 2nd-order harmonic grammar $\mathcal{G}$ over trees; (ii) the weight matrix of a harmonic network $\mathcal{N}$ with linear tree-realizations such that, among the realizations of trees, the maximal-Harmony activation patterns in $\mathcal{N}$ are the realizations of the optimal trees according to $\mathcal{G}$.

e. OT ↔ unrestricted-constraint, restricted-weight harmonic grammars [Chapter 20]
Optimality-theoretic grammars are equivalent to harmonic grammars in which the constraints are unrestricted (not necessarily 2nd order) but the numerical strengths of the constraints are restricted (to exponentially growing values, implementing OT's strict domination interaction).

f. Symbolic rewrite-rule or 2nd-order OT grammar ↔ restricted-weight 2nd-order harmonic grammar ↔ quadratic *H* of a harmonic network ↔ har-

monic network weight matrix **W**
Chain together above results.

(16) Open problems

a. Given a rewrite-rule, 2nd-order OT, or harmonic grammar over trees, and a harmonic network $\mathcal{N}$ with linear realizations of those trees, find a weight matrix **W** for $\mathcal{N}$ with a Harmony function such that the optimal trees according to the grammar are realized by activation patterns that maximize Harmony over *all* states of $\mathcal{N}$, including those that are *not* realizations of trees.

a. Explain the emergence of OT's strict domination constraint interaction—and local conjunction [Chapter 20]—from network-level principles.

b. Determine the status at the network level of OT constraints that are not second-order.

8.3 Well-formedness: Empirical perspective

The adequacy of a formal account of well-formed syntactic mental representations, such as the grammatical formalisms discussed in the previous subsection, is ultimately an empirical question. This question includes the central empirical problem of theoretical linguistics: to explain the general well-formedness patterns observed in the world's languages, and, at least as important, the patterns *not* found in human languages (18). The same general problem applies to both phonological and syntactic well-formedness. Examples of empirical problems addressed in this book, and the results, are listed in (17) and (19). The set of such empirical problems needing attention is virtually limitless (20). As shown by ② and ③ in Figure 6, in most of the ICS research reported in this book, linguistic data are accounted for via grammatical analysis, rather than connectionist modeling ❶. (Such filled circled numbers mark elements that are *not* part of ICS theory.)

(17) Illustration (Figure 6)

① Data: preferred partial parse trees of sentences processed one word at a time, as deduced from psycholinguistic data on patterns of processing difficulties [Chapter 19]
Other examples of data treated: well-formed complete sentences [Chapters 11, 15, 16, and 20] or well-formed syllabifications [Chapters 13, 14, and 20]

② OT ↔ data on real-time parsing preferences
An OT grammar explaining *preferred* partial parses as *optimal* partial parses [Chapter 19]

③ Another example: HG ↔ data on well-formed (complete) sentences [Chapter 11]
A harmonic grammar explaining acceptability of verbs in various constructions from a set of crosslinguistically motivated soft constraints

❹ Network ↔ data on well-formed sentences
Although a commonly traveled route for connectionist research on language, this is the path not taken in most of the ICS research reported here [Chapters 3 and 22]; the work in Chapter 11 does employ this route in part, however

Figure 6. Empirical tests of representational well-formedness

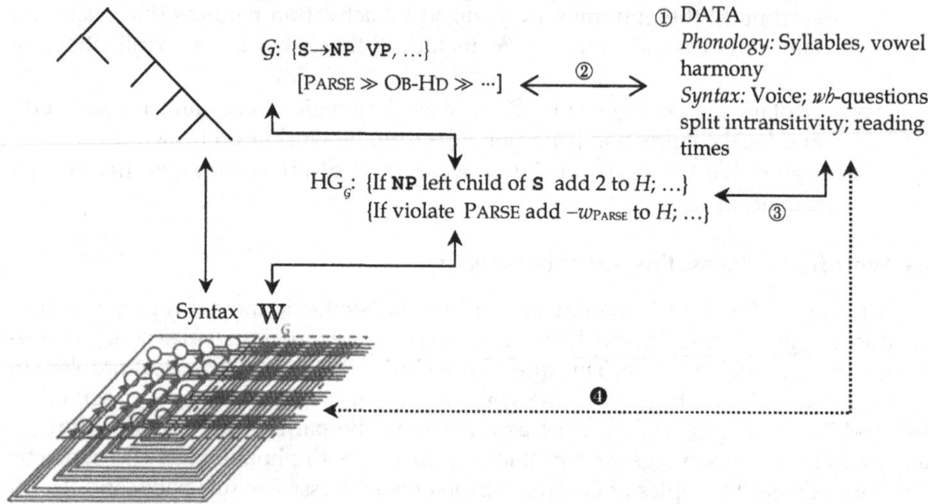

(18) General problem. Data ↔ grammars
What are the grammatical principles that determine the well-formed linguistic representations of all human languages, and what exactly do these principles predict as the typological space of all possible patterns connecting the forms and meanings of expressions in a language?

(19) Results
a. HG ↔ acceptability judgments [Chapter 11]
The grammar formalism of HG sheds light on the complex data of split intransitivity phenomena.
b. OT ↔ universal typologies of phonological and syntactic systems [Chapters 4, 12–16, 19, 20]
The grammar formalism of OT enables empirically sound characterizations of the typological spaces of possible syllable structure inventories, vowel harmony systems, grammatical voice systems, information questions, online attachment preferences, and split intransitivity patterns.

(20) Open problems
Unbounded. (But note that the existing OT literature does address an ex-

tremely broad set of problems. See Chapter 12 for sources, especially the online Rutgers Optimality Archive, http://roa.rutgers.edu.)

8.4 Functions

Utilizing the concept of well-formedness, grammars specify an important type of cognitive function: the outputs of this function are the grammatical or well-formed representations. The syntactic component of the mental representation of a sentence has been our working example. Now we shift attention to the cognitive function mapping the syntactic parse tree to its semantic interpretation. For concreteness, we are assuming here that a semantic representation can be described at a sufficiently abstract level as an expression of symbolic logic; equivalently, many other symbolic semantic representations could be substituted. Of main concern for development of ICS is the realization of such functions in connectionist networks. Figure 7 portrays the ICS picture, with the various elements labeled in (21). A version of the general research problem addressed here is formulated in (21); a few technical results and open questions are listed in (23) and (24).

Figure 7. Computing cognitive functions

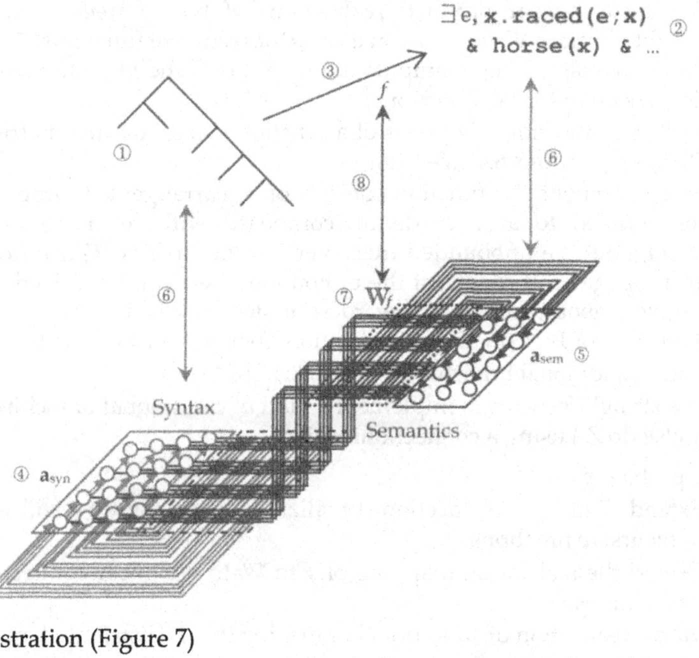

(21) Illustration (Figure 7)

① Syntactic structure $\mathbf{s}_{\text{syn}}$ for *the horse raced past the barn* (a tree)

② Semantic structure $\mathbf{s}_{\text{sem}}$ for *the horse raced past the barn* (a predicate calcu-

lus expression)
③ Symbolic interpretation function mapping $\mathtt{s}_{syn}$ to $\mathtt{s}_{sem}$
④ Activation pattern $\mathbf{a}_{syn}$ realizing $\mathtt{s}_{syn}$
⑤ Activation pattern $\mathbf{a}_{syn}$ realizing $\mathtt{s}_{sem}$
⑥ Tensor product realization mapping $\mathtt{s}_{syn} \leftrightarrow \mathbf{a}_{syn}$; $\mathtt{s}_{sem} \leftrightarrow \mathbf{a}_{sem}$
⑦ Weight matrix $\mathbf{W}_f$ for a feed-forward network, mapping $\mathbf{a}_{syn}$ to $\mathbf{a}_{sem}$
⑧ Systematic mapping $f \leftrightarrow \mathbf{W}_f$ between symbolic functions like f and weight matrices like $\mathbf{W}_f$

(22) General Problem. $\mathbf{W}_f \leftrightarrow$ symbolic function f
Find a class $\mathscr{F}$ of symbolic (recursive) functions that approximates as closely as possible the set of cognitive functions, and a systematic mapping that takes any function f in $\mathscr{F}$ and produces a weight matrix $\mathbf{W}_f$ for a feed-forward network that computes f (i.e., if f maps $\mathtt{s}$ to $\mathtt{t}$, then $\mathbf{W}_f$ maps $\mathbf{s}$ to $\mathbf{t}$, where $\mathbf{s}$ and $\mathbf{t}$ are the activation patterns realizing symbol structures $\mathtt{s}$ and $\mathtt{t}$ according to a given realization mapping).

(23) Results
a. Symbolic PC functions $\leftrightarrow \mathbf{W}_f$ over linear representations [Section 8:4.1.8]
For linear (tensor product) realizations of binary trees, a mapping to weight matrices $\mathbf{W}_f$ for any f in a set $\mathscr{F}$ of recursive functions generated by the fundamental tree-manipulating operations: the **PC** functions (Realization Theorem for PC Functions)
b. Finite specification properties of a function f in $\mathscr{F}$ and the matrices $\mathbf{W}_f$ realizing f [Sections 8:4.1.7–4.1.8]
Every symbolic PC function consists of a rearrangement around the tree root limited to a finite depth, composed with recursive propagation throughout the unbounded tree; every weight matrix $\mathbf{W}_f$ is a finite matrix $\underline{\mathbf{W}}_f$ propagated throughout the unbounded network by a fixed, extremely simple unbounded **feed-forward recursion matrix I** (Finite Specification Theorem for PC Functions; Realization Theorem for PC Functions)
c. Local conditional branching [Section 8:4.3]
It is straightforward to implement a kind of conditional branching ('if X do Y else do Z') using a connectionist unit.

(24) Open problems
a. Extend $\mathscr{F}$ (and its connectionist realization mapping) to a still wider class of recursive functions.
b. Extend the realization mapping of f to $\mathbf{W}_f$ to nonlinear connectionist representations.
c. Find a realization of conditional branching that is distributed, not local.

8.5 Processing

Characterizations—at two levels of description—of several aspects of the syntactic and semantic components of the mental representation resulting from processing *the horse raced past the barn* have been obtained: the specification of the representation itself in both symbolic and connectionist forms; the characterization of its well-formedness in terms of a purely symbolic grammar, a harmonic grammar, and the weight matrix of a recurrent connectionist network; and the specification of the function from syntax to semantics as a recursive symbolic function and as the weight matrix of a feed-forward net. We now consider the mental processes resulting from the arrival of the final word of the sentence, *fell.* A step-by-step account is given in (25) and sketched in Figure 8.

(25) Illustration (Figure 8)

Parsing; dynamics computes optimal representation, given words so far.

① A new word arrives: *fell.*

② The existing parse (*a*) is inconsistent with the new word, so must change; the syntactic network must shift to a substantially different state to accommodate this word.

③ The recurrent syntactic network circulates activation for some time after the arrival of *fell*; the activation values of its units oscillate until a new equilibrium is established.

④ During this time the network is maximizing Harmony, the Harmony landscape having shifted with the arrival of the new word.

⑤ The time required to process this word, and the probability of failing to do so successfully, are determined by the Harmony maximization process: how quickly and accurately it optimizes.

⑥ Assuming a successful optimization, when activation settles down after processing *fell*, the network state will realize a different tree (*b*), one that incorporates the new word.

⑦ The new tree is grammatical, since the weights $\mathbf{W}_{\mathcal{G}}$ in the network are such that optimizing Harmony means satisfying the grammar $\mathcal{G}$ (see Figure 5).

❽ The overall transition can be described at the symbolic level as moving from one tree to another, but there is no algorithm operating on symbolic constituents that describes the actual state transitions of the system that mediate between the initial and final state. In other words, there is no symbolic algorithm whose internal structure can predict the time and the accuracy of processing; this can only be done with connectionist algorithms.

Figure 8. Processing the new word *fell*

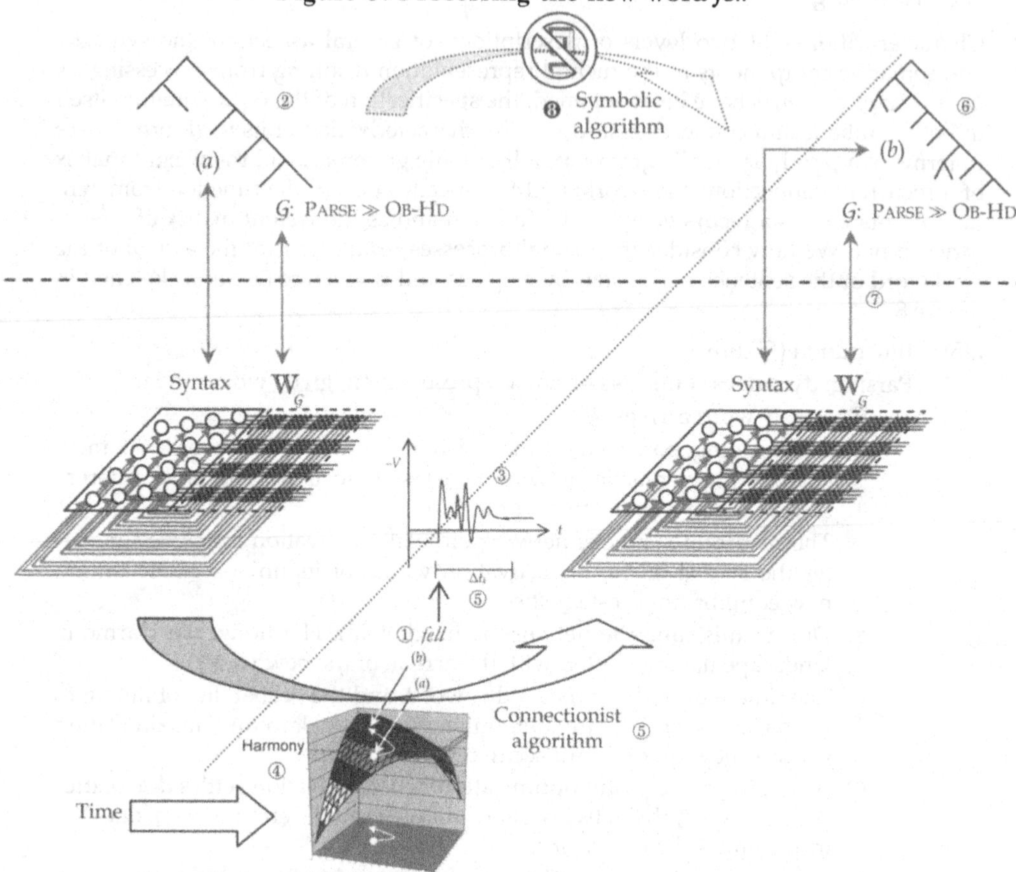

It is not yet possible to formulate a detailed model instantiating this account, but several results on this general problem (26) are reported in this book; they are summarized in (27). (28) mentions some key outstanding problems.

(26) General problem
Find a characterization of the outcome of connectionist activation processing, the resource requirements for the connectionist computation (time, number of units and connections, precision) required to produce an output, and the probabilities of different types of errors; relate all these characteristics to symbolic descriptions of the computation.

(27) Results
a. In harmonic networks, activation processing maximizes Harmony, in a

sense appropriate for the type of network (25.④) [Chapter 9].

b. The claim (25.❽) that there do not exist symbolic algorithms that accurately describe the computational processes at work in the network—that symbolic *representations*, but not symbolic *algorithms*, are "psychologically real"—is consistent with both symbolic explanation of the productivity of higher cognition and the computational reduction of symbolic cognition to neural computation [Chapter 23].

c. Example networks (using local representations)
Network for parsing context-free languages [Chapter 10]
CVNet for syllabifying consonant-vowel sequences [Chapter 21]
BrbrNet for syllabifying Berber words [Chapter 20]

(28) Open problems

a. Design comparable models using distributed rather than local representations.

b. Develop a general *theory* of processing ("settling") times Δt_k.

c. Develop a general theory of errors.

d. Find general characterizations of the sensitivity of network performance to representation structure and to damage.

e. Determine the extent to which *local* Harmony maxima impede the network's search for global Harmony maxima, the maxima relevant to optimization-based linguistic well-formedness ("competence").

8.6 Putting it all together

All the bits described above are brought together in Figure 9. This figure also explicitly characterizes the initial and final syntactic trees as those that are optimal according to OT: the tables at the top of the drawing are OT constraint tableaux in which the ranked constraints head successive columns, the leftmost being the most dominant (Chapter 4). Alternative syntactic parses of the input label the rows. A star indicates that a parse violates a constraint. The parse with the lowest-ranked violations is optimal (marked with a finger in the tableaux). When the unexpected final word *fell* arrives, the new optimal parse (*b*) differs substantially from the previous optimal parse (*a*). And this is what accounts for the high processing difficulty arising at this point in the sentence.

8.7 Learning

How does the language-processing system depicted in Figure 9 arise? A few results concerning the nativist hypothesis are presented in the book—although no commitment to (or endorsement of) this hypothesis is manifest in the research program. Three case studies are listed in (29): (29a) is experimental, (29c) is theoretical, and (29b) is an application of the theory to spontaneous child production data.

(29) Illustrations
  a. Infants' knowledge of universal phonological constraints [Chapter 17]
  b. Role of universal syntactic constraints in the earliest acquisition of clause structure [Chapter 18]
  c. Learning an OT syllabification grammar with genomically encoded constraints [Chapter 21]

Two central general learning problems of the theory are given in (30). Some results and open problems are listed in (30)–(32).

(30) General problems
  a. Given the universal elements of any OT grammar, find a learning procedure that determines the language-specific element: the ranking.
  b. Provide a mechanism for learning the universal elements of an OT grammar—representations, constraints (including the most abstract ones)—from experience, or provide an account of how these elements may be genetically encoded and how such a genome evolved.

(31) Results
  a. Language-particular ranking ↔ experience with positive data
     Constraint demotion algorithms can be defined; these adjust rankings so that optimal forms match observed forms [Chapter 12].
  b. Learnability ↔ initial state
     General learnability arguments entail properties of the initial grammar, if knowledge of universal constraints is innate [Chapter 17].
  c. Symbolic OT universal grammatical system ↔ HG ↔ abstract neural network architecture ↔ abstract genomic encoding
     A demonstration system addressing learning of basic syllabification, formally specified at four levels of description: (i) OT grammar, (ii) HG, (iii) abstract (localist) neural network, and (iv) abstract genome [Chapter 21]

(32) Open questions
  a. What types of OT constraints can be learned from experience, and how?
  b. How, in general, do symbolic OT learning algorithms relate to neural network learning?
  c. Can the demonstration system be adapted to distributed representations?

In closing, we hasten to reiterate that the above outline provides only a few of the most important open problems, ones that may fall near the limits of current results, rather than far beyond. No implication whatever is intended that other problems, large and small, have been solved. We would also like to repeat that the above outline is not expected to be understandable from start to finish on the basis of only Chapters 1 and 2: it is intended as a reference to be consulted as the necessary concepts are developed in the remaining chapters, hopefully making it easier to fill in the big picture that has been outlined here.

Figure 9. The big picture

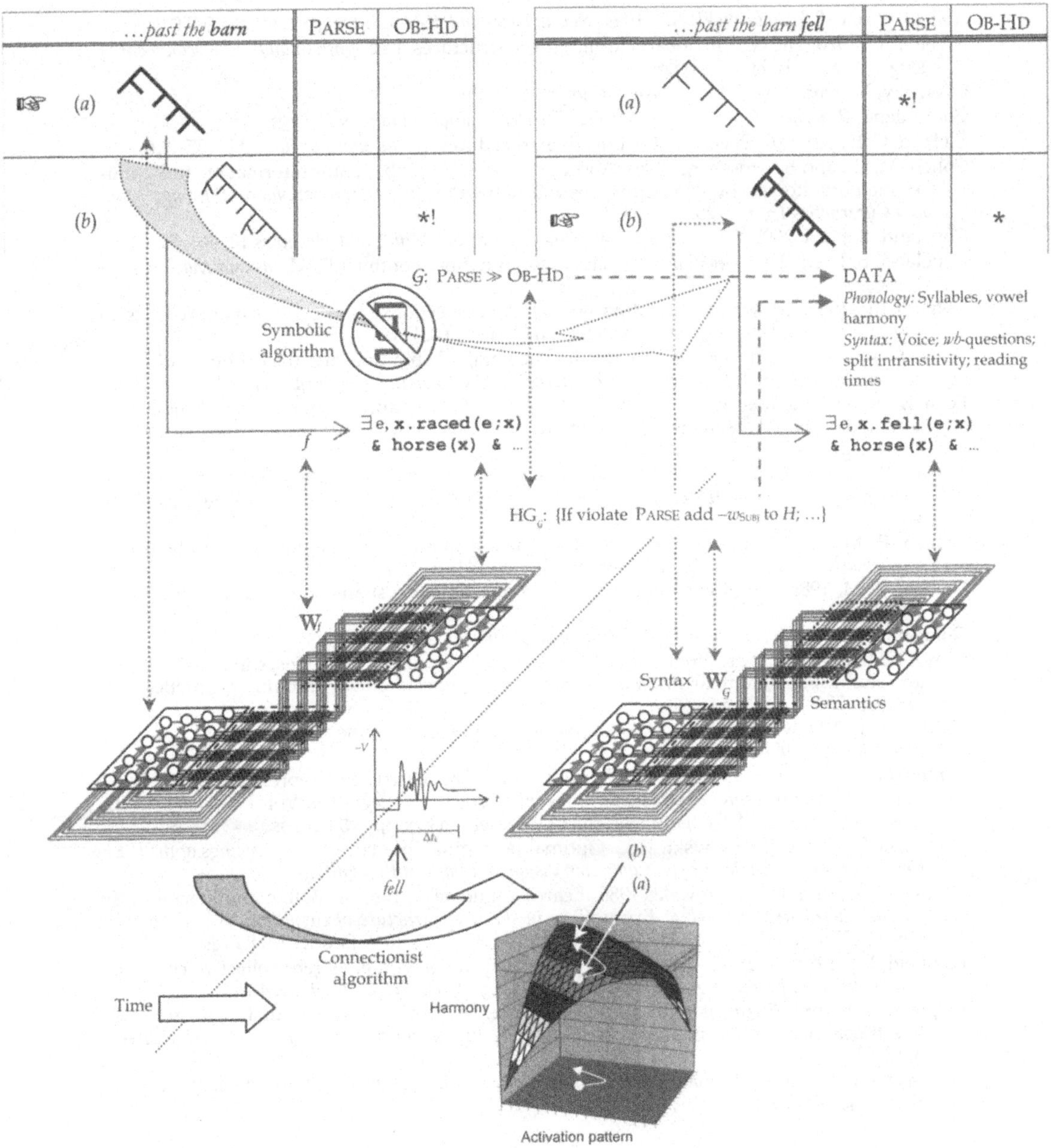

…past the **barn**	PARSE	OB-HD
☞ (*a*)		
(*b*)		*!

…past the barn ***fell***	PARSE	OB-HD
(*a*)	*!	
☞ (*b*)		*

G: PARSE ≫ OB-HD → DATA

Phonology: Syllables, vowel harmony

Syntax: Voice; *wh*-questions; split intransitivity; reading times

Symbolic algorithm

f

∃e, **x.raced(e;x) & horse(x) &** …

∃e, **x.fell(e;x) & horse(x) &** …

HG$_G$: {If violate PARSE add $-w_{\text{SUBJ}}$ to *H*; …}

$\mathbf{W}_f$

Syntax $\mathbf{W}_G$ Semantics

$-V$ t Δt_i

fell

Connectionist algorithm

Time

(*b*) (*a*)

Harmony

Activation pattern

References

ROA = Rutgers Optimality Archive, http://roa.rutgers.edu

Abbott, L., and T. J. Sejnowski, eds. 1999. *Neural codes and distributed representations*. MIT Press.

Bever, T. G. 1970. The cognitive basis for linguistic structures. In *Cognition and the development of language*, ed. J. R. Hayes. Wiley.

Chomsky, N. 1965. *Aspects of the theory of syntax*. MIT Press.

Churchland, P. S., and T. J. Sejnowski. 1992. *The computational brain*. MIT Press.

Cleland, C. E., ed. 2002. Special issue: Effective procedures. *Minds and Machines* 12, 157–326.

Cohen, M. A., and S. Grossberg. 1983. Absolute stability of global pattern formation and parallel memory storage by competitive neural networks. *IEEE Transactions on Systems, Man, and Cybernetics* 13, 815–25.

Copeland, B. J., ed. 2002. Special issue: Hypercomputation. *Minds and Machines* 12, 461–579.

Copeland, B. J., ed. 2003. Special issue: Hypercomputation (continued). *Minds and Machines* 13, 3–186.

Dolan, C. P. 1989. Tensor manipulation networks: Connectionist and symbolic approaches to comprehension, learning, and planning. Ph.D. diss., UCLA.

Dolan, C. P., and M. G. Dyer. 1987. Symbolic schemata, role binding, and the evolution of structure in connectionist memories. *IEEE International Conference on Neural Networks* 1, 287–98.

Eckhorn, R., H. J. Reitboeck, M. Arndt, and P. Dicke. 1990. Feature linking via synchronization among distributed assemblies: Simulations of results from cat visual cortex. *Neural Computation* 2, 293–307.

Geman, S., and D. Geman. 1984. Stochastic relaxation, Gibbs distributions, and the Bayesian restoration of images. *IEEE Transactions on Pattern Analysis and Machine Intelligence* 6, 721–41.

Golden, R. M. 1986. The "brain-state-in-a-box" neural model is a gradient descent algorithm. *Mathematical Psychology* 30–31, 73–80.

Golden, R. M. 1988. A unified framework for connectionist systems. *Biological Cybernetics* 59, 109–20.

Goldsmith, J. A. 1990. *Autosegmental and metrical phonology*. Blackwell.

Gray, C. M., P. Konig, A. K. Engel, and W. Singer. 1989. Oscillatory responses in cat visual cortex exhibit intercolumnar synchronization which reflects global stimulus properties. *Nature* 338, 334–7.

Hadley, R. F. 2000. Cognition and the computational power of connectionist networks. *Connection Science* 12, 95–110.

Hinton, G. E., J. L. McClelland, and D. E. Rumelhart. 1986. Distributed representation. In *Parallel distributed processing: Explorations in the microstructure of cognition*. Vol. 1, *Foundations*, D. E. Rumelhart, J. L. McClelland, and the PDP Research Group. MIT Press.

Hinton, G. E., and T. J. Sejnowski. 1983. Optimal perceptual inference. In *Proceedings of the IEEE Computer Society Conference on Computer Vision and Pattern Recognition*.

Hinton, G. E., and T. J. Sejnowski. 1986. Learning and relearning in Boltzmann machines. In *Parallel distributed processing: Explorations in the microstructure of cognition*. Vol. 1, *Foundations*, D. E. Rumelhart, J. L. McClelland, and the PDP Research Group. MIT Press.

Hopfield, J. J. 1982. Neural networks and physical systems with emergent collective computational abilities. *Proceedings of the National Academy of Sciences USA* 79, 2554–8.

Hopfield, J. J. 1984. Neurons with graded response have collective computational properties like those of two-state neurons. *Proceedings of the National Academy of Sciences USA* 81, 3088–92.

Hummel, J. E., and I. Biederman. 1992. Dynamic binding in a neural network for shape recognition. *Psychological Review* 99, 480–517.

Hummel, J. E., and K. J. Holyoak. 2003. A symbolic-connectionist theory of relational inference and generalization. *Psychological Review* 110, 220–64.

Lakoff, G. 1988. A suggestion for a linguistics with connectionist foundations. In *Proceedings of the Connectionist Models Summer School*, eds. D. S. Touretzky, G. E. Hinton, and T. J. Sejnowski. Morgan Kaufmann.

Legendre, G., Y. Miyata, and P. Smolensky. 1990a. Can connectionism contribute to syntax? Harmonic Grammar, with an application. In *Proceedings of the Chicago Linguistic Society 26*.

Legendre, G., Y. Miyata, and P. Smolensky. 1990b. Harmonic Grammar—a formal multi-level connectionist theory of linguistic well-formedness: An application. In *Proceedings of the Cognitive Science Society 12*.

Legendre, G., Y. Miyata, and P. Smolensky. 1990c. Harmonic Grammar—a formal multi-level connectionist theory of linguistic well-formedness: Theoretical foundations. In *Proceedings of the Cognitive Science Society 12*.

Marr, D., and T. Poggio. 1976. Cooperative computation of stereo disparity. *Science* 194, 283–7.

Plate, T. A. 1991. Holographic reduced representations: Convolution algebra for compositional distributed representations. In *Proceedings of the International Joint Conference on Artificial Intelligence 12*.

Plate, T. A. 1994. Distributed representations and nested compositional structure. Ph.D. diss., University of Toronto.

Pollack, J. 1988. Recursive auto-associative memory: Devising compositional distributed representations. In *Proceedings of the Cognitive Science Society 10*.

Pollack, J. 1990. Recursive distributed representations. *Artificial Intelligence* 46, 77–105.

Prince, A., and P. Smolensky. 1991. Notes on connectionism and Harmony Theory in linguistics. Technical report CU-CS-533-91, Computer Science Department, University of Colorado at Boulder.

Prince, A., and P. Smolensky. 1993/2004. *Optimality Theory: Constraint interaction in generative grammar*. Technical report, Rutgers University and University of Colorado at Boulder, 1993. ROA 537, 2002. Revised version published by Blackwell, 2004.

Shastri, L., and V. Ajjanagadde. 1993. From simple associations to systematic reasoning: A connectionist representation of rules, variables and dynamic bindings using temporal synchrony. *Behavioral and Brain Sciences* 16, 417–94.

Siegelmann, H. T. 1999. *Neural networks and analog computation: Beyond the Turing limit.* Birkhäuser.

Smolensky, P. 1983. Schema selection and stochastic inference in modular environments. In *Proceedings of the National Conference on Artificial Intelligence 3*.

Smolensky, P. 1986. Information processing in dynamical systems: Foundations of Harmony Theory. In *Parallel distributed processing: Explorations in the microstructure of cognition*. Vol. 1, *Foundations*, D. E. Rumelhart, J. L. McClelland, and the PDP Research Group. MIT Press.

Smolensky, P. 1987. On variable binding and the representation of symbolic structures in connectionist systems. Technical report CU-CS-355-87, Computer Science Department, University of Colorado at Boulder.

Smolensky, P. 1990. Tensor product variable binding and the representation of symbolic structures in connectionist networks. *Artificial Intelligence* 46, 159–216.

Smolensky, P., G. Legendre, and Y. Miyata. 1992. Principles for an integrated connectionist/symbolic theory of higher cognition. Technical report CU-CS-600-92, Computer Science Department, and 92–8, Institute of Cognitive Science, University of Colorado at Boulder.

Smolensky, P., M. C. Mozer, and D. E. Rumelhart, eds. 1996. *Mathematical perspectives on neural networks*. Erlbaum.

von der Malsburg, C., and W. Schneider. 1986. A neural cocktail-party processor. *Biological Cybernetics* 54, 29–40.

Wendelken, C., and L. Shastri. 2003. Acquisition of concepts and causal rules in SHRUTI. In *Proceedings of the Cognitive Science Society 25*.

3

Foundational Implications of the ICS Architecture: Unification in Cognitive Science

Paul Smolensky and Géraldine Legendre

The Integrated Connectionist/Symbolic Cognitive Architecture (ICS) is **split-level**: at the higher level, symbol structures allow specification of the form and content of the inputs and outputs of cognitive functions; at the lower level, units and connections allow specification of the processes by which these functions are computed. This unification of symbolic and connectionist computation enables ICS theory to break the stalemate between implementationalist and eliminativist explanations of cognition. More generally, we identify three types of integration that are important for progress in cognitive science: substantive integration, of the scientific content of different cognitive disciplines; methodological integration, of the diversity of research methods in different disciplines; and metatheoretic integration, of philosophies of science centered either on concrete model building or on formal principle development. Results reported in this book contribute to each of these types of integration.

Contents

Motivating the development of the Integrated Connectionist/Symbolic Cognitive Architecture (ICS) are the very basic, foundational considerations concerning neural and mental computation that were introduced in Chapter 1. Consequently, ICS gives rise to a number of foundational implications; they are introduced in this chapter and developed in Part IV.

Most importantly, relative to more familiar architectures that are either purely connectionist or purely symbolic, cognitive explanation within ICS theory is rather subtle. The division of explanatory labor between the symbolic and the connectionist levels of ICS is not easy to sort out; indeed, that analysis requires fairly elaborate argumentation, which consumes much of Chapter 23 and is summarized here in Section 1. This topic has been the subject of considerable debate in the literature.[1]

The design of ICS theory actually involves several quite different dimensions of integration, each central to the general enterprise of cognitive science. These dimensions are articulated and distinguished in Section 2. Section 3 continues this discussion by focusing on the integration of connectionist and symbolic approaches to the study of language. Finally, Section 4 identifies general thrusts of the research program presented in this book and considers the ways in which they attempt to address the various challenges of unification.

1 IMPLICATIONS FOR THE FOUNDATIONS OF COGNITIVE SCIENCE

The search for a coherent computational architecture for the mind/brain has led cognitive science into a major crisis. As discussed in Chapter 1, the computational architecture of the *brain* seems to be connectionist, while most successful explanation of the *mind* has depended on a very different architecture, symbolic computation. The ICS theory developed in this book aims to break the deadlock between the **eliminativists**—who claim that symbols have no place in a science of cognition—and the **implementationalists**—who maintain that symbolic computation provides all we need for a cognitive theory, with neural networks "merely implementing" symbolic theories (recall Box 1:8). ICS theory, we argue, takes us closer to a satisfactory computational characterization of a mind/brain, assigning both symbolic and connectionist computation essential roles that preserve the strength of the former for mental explanation, and the advantages of the latter for reducing cognition to neurally plausible elementary computations.

This argument is developed in detail in Chapter 23, which we only summarize here. As the argument is quite involved, the summary must skip quickly through claims that will ultimately require many pages to defend.

The foundation of the argument is an analysis of computational theories into

[1] See Smolensky 1987, 1988, 1990, 1991, 1994, 1995a, b; Fodor and Pylyshyn 1988; Fodor and McLaughlin 1990; Fodor 1991, 1997; Horgan and Tienson 1991; McLaughlin 1992, 1993; Smolensky, Legendre, and Miyata 1992; Aizawa 1997, 2003; and other papers cited in Chapter 23.

three levels based on but not identical to those of Marr (1982). At each level, it is important to relate the hypotheses of ICS and the **Purely Symbolic Architecture (PSA)**.

At the highest, **functional** level, ICS and PSA adopt the same type of symbolic description of higher cognition, exploiting the symbolic combinatorial strategy introduced in Section 1:3 to explain unbounded productivity and other important functional-level properties of cognition.

At the lowest, **physical** level, ICS and PSA (presumably) make equivalent assumptions about the structure of the brain at the level of neurons.

The key difference lies at the intermediate, **computational** level—the bridge between the functional and the physical levels. A computational-level theory takes high-level, abstract functions and breaks them down, successively and precisely, into smaller and smaller pieces, until finally reaching the elementary operations defining the computational architecture of that theory. The crisis in cognitive science arises because eliminativist connectionist theory has neurally appropriate small pieces, but lacks sufficiently powerful abstract functions, while just the reverse is true of symbolic theory.

Symbolic computation provides an effective means of formally defining abstract cognitive functions and formally decomposing these functions into the elementary operations of symbolic computation. This decomposition is satisfactory for implementing symbolic theory in conventional computers, or for studying whether abstract cognition is in principle possible within physical systems. The symbolic decomposition is not satisfactory, however, for demonstrating that abstract cognition is possible within *neural* systems; the primitives of symbolic theory do not come close to being plausibly within the capabilities of neural computation (see Box 1:6). To put it crudely, the problem is that the decomposition provided by symbolic computation has *symbols all the way down*: a neuron would have to behave like a symbol for this decomposition to reduce cognition to neural computation (Box 23:1).

At the computational level, ICS and PSA differ crucially. In ICS, there are two key decompositions and these do not align with one another; they correspond to analysis at two different sublevels within the overall computational level (see Box 1).

At a higher sublevel of the ICS computational level, representations are activity vectors, and these decompose into constituent vectors in a way parallel to the functional-level decomposition of complex symbol structures into their constituent symbol structures (Section 2:1). What makes ICS possible is the discovery that there is a formal equivalence or **isomorphism** between constituent decomposition in symbolic representations and in vectorial representations; this is the isomorphism codified in tensor product representations.

But at a lower sublevel of the ICS computational level, the decomposition is quite different. A representation—an activity pattern—is decomposed into the individual activation values of the network units over which the pattern is realized. Because ICS representations are distributed, this decomposition crosscuts the higher-level decomposition of a representation into its constituents: a single unit is part of the pattern for many different constituents, and the pattern for a single constituent is made up of many different unit activation values.

In ICS, therefore, a crucial transformation occurs between the higher and lower sublevels of the computational level: the higher sublevel aligns with symbolic constituents, the lower sublevel aligns with individual neurons. ICS provides a fully formal reduction, as required of a computational theory: it provides a formal mapping from symbol structures to activity vectors, another formal mapping from activity vectors to individual unit activity values, and finally (in principle) a formal mapping from unit activities to neural activities. Unlike PSA, ICS reduces abstract cognitive functions to elementary operations that fall within the computational capabilities of neural networks.

ICS is a **split-level** architecture. Only the higher computational sublevel provides **functionally relevant** structure; only the lower computational sublevel provides **physically relevant** structure. The higher-level decomposition into constituents is critical for identifying the functional significance of representations, including their compositional meanings. The lower-level decomposition into individual unit activities is essential for characterizing the *processes* that actually create representations. The computational resources required by cognitive processes are determined by the lower-level structure: the number of units required, the number of steps of activation spreading needed to produce a stable output, the consequences of imprecision or of error resulting from damage. A central obligation of a complete cognitive theory is to describe cognitive processes so as to predict relative processing times and other resource requirements; in ICS theory, this must be done in terms of processing algorithms defined at the lower computational sublevel: *connectionist* algorithms.

In contrast, a defining feature of the PSA architecture is that cognitive processes, including their resource requirements, are characterized by *symbolic* algorithms.[2]

However, as in PSA, in ICS mental *representations* have symbolic descriptions. In ICS theory, functions with symbolic inputs and outputs are computed—by processes that can be accurately described with connectionist but not symbolic algorithms.

At the functional level, ICS, like PSA, describes (higher) cognition in terms of symbolic functions. Thus, ICS theory provides symbolic explanations of functional-level phenomena, including the important problem of cognitive productivity (Chapter 1 (9)). In fact, quite a broad set of phenomena in cognitive science can be at least partially addressed at the functional level. It is tempting to say that ICS provides a symbolic "competence" theory but a connectionist "performance" theory. While there is some validity to this gloss, it is ultimately inadequate because many "performance" phenomena can in fact be addressed at the functional level, and these phenomena thus fall under the scope of symbolic explanations in ICS theory. This will be evident in Part III of the book where Optimality Theory—a central part of the

[2] As Cummins and Schwarz (1991, 64) put it: "the objects of semantic interpretation—the representations—are the objects of computation—the things manipulated by the algorithm."

higher, symbolic sublevel of ICS—is applied to a range of problems in the cognitive science of language that extends far beyond the boundaries of classical "competence" theories.

ICS differs crucially from the implementationalist approach because symbolic computation does not suffice for a theory of cognitive processes: connectionist computation is essential. And ICS theory departs critically from the eliminativist approach because connectionist computation does not suffice to explain functional-level phenomena, including those pertaining to the compositionality, systematicity, and semantics of mental representations, as well as the rich phenomena related to universal grammar.

The design of ICS attempts to take the implementationalist insight that symbolic computation is crucial for understanding the function of cognition and combine it with the eliminativist insight that the fundamentally connectionist character of cognitive computation is crucial for understanding cognitive processes. Unlike implementationalism, ICS theory provides a plausible reduction of cognition to neural computation; unlike eliminativism, ICS theory enables explanation of the functional properties that are central to human higher cognition. The hope is that ICS constitutes a step toward a comprehensive computational characterization of a mind/brain.

The integration that the ICS approach strives to achieve between connectionist and symbolic theory in general, and between connectionist and generative theories of language more specifically, actually involves several distinct dimensions of integration. Each of these is likely to prove critical for the ultimate success of a unified cognitive science. In the remainder of this chapter, these dimensions of unification are articulated and related to the ICS research program.

Box 1. The split-level architecture of ICS

The figure below shows the representations of simple trees discussed in Box 2:1. The top horizontal row shows a pattern of activity over 12 units realizing the tree **[$_X$A B]**. It can be decomposed into a sum of two other patterns, as shown by the dotted arrows labeled '+': one pattern is in the second row, a pattern over the last 8 units, which realizes **[A B]**; the other is in the bottom row, a pattern over the first 4 units, which realizes **X** at the tree root. The pattern realizing **[A B]** in the second row can itself be decomposed into a sum of two other patterns, as shown with the solid arrows labeled '+': one is the pattern for **B** in the right-child position (labeled '– **B**'), shown in the third row from the top; the other, shown in the next row down, is the pattern realizing **A** in the left-child position ('**A** –'). (Recall that white circles denote negative activation, so summing a white and a dark circle with the same area yields 0.)

This decomposition is an **intralevel** decomposition: it stays within the level of patterns of activity. The pattern realizing **[$_X$A B]** is decomposed into the patterns realizing its constituents. Thus, it is parallel to the decomposition of the symbol structure itself into its constituents; this is denoted '**[A B]** ⇝ {**A**, **B**}' in the figure. This de-

Box 1

composition is relevant to specifying **cognitive functions** and **semantic interpretation**, in both ICS and the Purely Symbolic Architecture (PSA): the combinatorial strategy builds the outputs of cognitive functions, and their meanings, from those of the constituents.

In PSA, this intralevel decomposition is also relevant for the description of mental **processes**: these are algorithms defined over symbolic constituents like **A** and **B**.

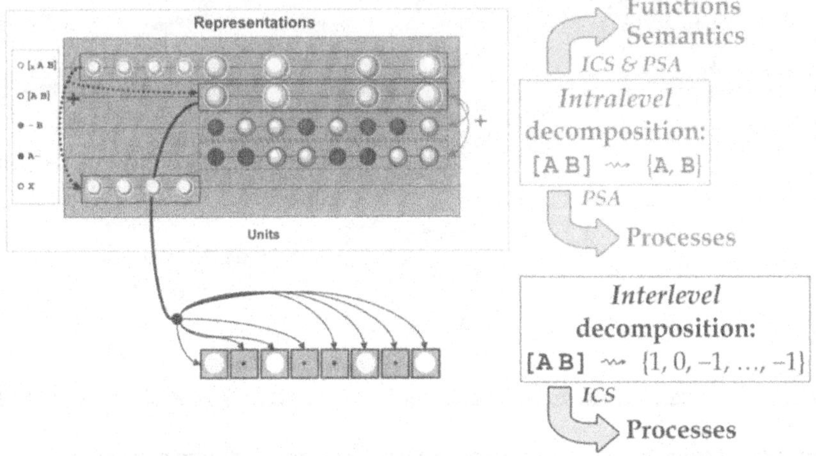

But in ICS theory, for describing mental processes it is not the intralevel decomposition that is relevant. What is relevant is another, **interlevel** decomposition: this decomposes, for example, the pattern for **[A B]** into its eight individual activation values. This is shown with the thick solid arrows taking the pattern in the second row (which realizes **[A B]**) and exploding it into the activities of eight separate units depicted as squares at the bottom of the figure. This interlevel decomposition is denoted '**[A B]** ⇝ {1, 0, −1, …, −1}' in the figure. In ICS theory, cognitive processes must be described by connectionist algorithms operating on individual activation values, the outcome of interlevel decomposition.

The preceding story for representations applies in corresponding fashion to rules or constraints. Under an *intra*level decomposition, the ICS weight matrix for the grammar $\mathcal{G}$ (Box 2:2) can be expressed as the sum of two other weight matrices, one for each rule of $\mathcal{G}$; this is shown in the figure below with the two arrows labeled '+'. This corresponds to the PSA decomposition of $\mathcal{G}$ into its constituent rules.

The *inter*level decomposition takes the total weight matrix for $\mathcal{G}$ and decomposes it into its individual weight values, as shown with the heavy solid arrows leading to the 12 squares at the bottom of the figure, which depict some of the 48 weights in the weight matrix for $\mathcal{G}$. Just as before, in PSA, the intralevel decomposition is relevant both to functions/semantics and to mental processes; but in ICS theory, the intralevel decomposition is relevant only to functions/semantics, and it is only the interlevel de-

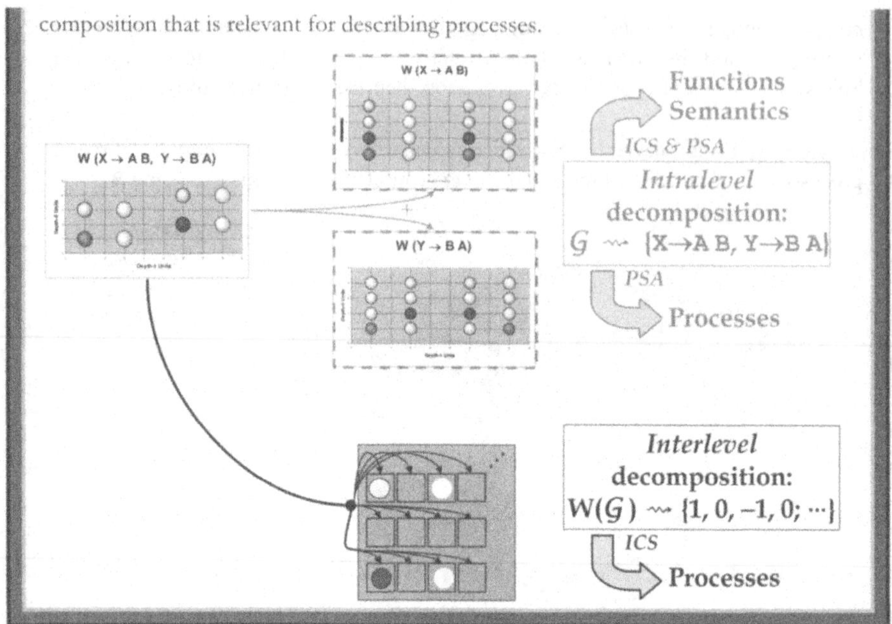

2 THE MULTIPLE CHALLENGES OF A UNIFIED COGNITIVE SCIENCE

Is cognitive science just a public relations gimmick, or is there something truly *new* about it as a field? After all, in each of the core cognitive disciplines —philosophy of mind, linguistics, cognitive psychology, artificial intelligence, and neuroscience—a great deal of research has been successfully conducted in isolation from the other fields—in some cases, for centuries. On our view, what is new about cognitive science as a field is the commitment to the proposition that the data and theories of these disciplines must be brought to bear directly on one another, and, ultimately, *integrated*. This is no small challenge, and in this section we distinguish several distinct types of integration and why we think them all important.

One of these dimensions, discussed in Section 2.3, concerns a somewhat subtle distinction in the philosophy of cognitive science between what we call **model-centered** and **principle-centered** research. While this distinction is certainly not entirely clear-cut, we find it useful for understanding the relations among a wide range of research methods growing out of quite different academic disciplines.

Of particular interest for the ICS approach is the role of connectionism in cognitive science: is it a source of division, or unity? This question is taken up in Section 3. Chapter 22 discusses at some length the relations between model- and principle-centered research, specifically in the case of connectionist approaches to language. It is argued that, despite the extremely important contributions of model-centered connectionist language research, there are compelling reasons for also conducting complementary research that is principle-centered; it is this type of research that is the focus of this book.

The challenges to unification that cognitive science faces weave together difficulties along many dimensions: conceptual incompatibilities, technical inadequacies, sociological differences, and divergent philosophies of science. In this section, we will attempt to articulate three general types of integration that we see as crucial goals for cognitive science, and that have shaped the research presented here.

2.1 Substantive integration and the central paradox of cognition

The first type of integration is the most straightforward.

(1) Substantive integration

A theory of cognition is **substantively integrated** if

a. it provides a satisfactory account of individual cognitive domains of both lower and higher cognition;

b. it **horizontally integrates** these domains by providing a coherent theory of the interrelation of cognition in these domains;

c. it **vertically integrates** accounts of cognition at the lower, neural level with abstract accounts of cognition at higher levels; and

d. it satisfactorily addresses the **central paradox** of cognitive architecture, providing a coherent account of the relation between the 'hard' and 'soft' aspects of cognition.

Substantive integration is clearly a highly demanding goal, itself encompassing several quite distinct dimensions.

In (1a), **higher cognition** refers to those rather abstract domains that are highly developed only in the human mind – for instance, problem solving, language, reasoning, and abstract planning. In these areas, most existing cognitive theory relies heavily on some sort of symbolic computation. These cognitive domains are to be contrasted with lower-level ones, already well developed in lower animals – for instance, pattern recognition, sensation, motor control, and simple types of memory. In these areas, symbolic computation has played a significantly less dominant role in cognitive theory. A horizontally integrated theory (1b) provides a coherent account of the interrelation of cognitive processes across the entire spectrum of domains, including both lower and higher cognition.

In contrast, vertical integration (1c) requires a coherent theory of the interrelation of the multiple levels of organization spanning from the neural level up to the highest mental levels (e.g., that of the theory of grammar). While horizontal integration has been a focus of cognitive architecture research from its early days (e.g., Newell 1990; Van Lehn 1991), the centrality of vertical integration for cognitive science has only become broadly recognized in the past decade or so (e.g., Churchland and Sejnowski 1992) – a result of connectionist theory as well as advances in neuroscience.

Two related but distinct 'higher/lower' axes are employed in the statement of substantive integration (1). The axis involved in horizontal integration—spanning from language and reasoning on the higher end to sensation and motor control on the lower end—is a scale of abstractness of the information relevant to a given domain of cognition. The axis relevant to vertical integration—ranging from symbol manipulation at the higher end to neurophysical interactions at the lower end—is a scale of abstractness of the level of analysis employed for scientifically characterizing the mind/brain. Clearly, these two axes are related; the more abstract information processing involved in language and reasoning has primarily been formalized using symbol manipulation, while accounts of sensation and motor control are quite naturally stated at a level much closer to the neurophysical.

In (1d), we attempt to isolate a fundamental aspect of the challenges of both horizontal and vertical integration. It concerns the vexing paradox at the heart of cognitive science first introduced in Chapter 1. On the one hand, formal theories of logical reasoning, grammar, and other higher mental faculties lead us to think of the *mind* as a machine for rule-based manipulation of highly structured arrays of symbols. Formal descriptions based in discrete mathematics, especially the theory of discrete computation, capture many of these 'hard' aspects of cognition, suggesting that the mind/brain is a discrete computer.

On the other hand, what we know of the *brain* compels us to think of human information processing in terms of the manipulation of a large unstructured set of numbers, the activation levels of interconnected neurons. Furthermore, the full richness and variation of human *performance*, both in everyday contexts and in the controlled environments of the psychological laboratory, seem to go beyond the limits of symbolic rule-based description, displaying strong sensitivity to subtle statistical factors in experience, in addition to structural properties of information. To capture these 'soft' aspects of cognition, it seems we must formally treat the mind/brain as a statistical, numerical computer.

To solve the central paradox of cognition is to resolve these contradictions—unifying the hard and soft aspects of cognition—by providing an integrated theory of the organization of the mind, the brain, behavior, and the environment.

A most tempting response to the central paradox, and substantive integration generally, is denial. The challenge of integration can always be evaded by simply denying the importance of one half of the material to be unified—denying the existence of one horn of the dilemma. For instance, adopting the view of eliminative connectionism (Box 1:8), one can evade any need for vertical integration by denying that higher-level human cognitive processes have in significant measure the character that symbolic theory attributes to them—qualitatively different from lower-level, nonsymbolic cognition. Language, say, might just be a kind of pattern recognition or signal processing; perhaps we 'recognize' the meaning of a sentence from a sound wave as we recognize the orientation of a surface from an image. But this sort of denial constitutes a huge step backward in our understanding of higher cognition and does not begin to do justice to the weight of evidence accrued by decades of symbolic cognitive research. Of particular relevance to the work in this book is the wealth of knowledge about language that depends crucially on structured symbolic descriptions. As difficult as it may be, integrating the hard, symbolic and the soft, numerical facets of cognition, in our view, is more promising than the prospect of building up, from low-level numerical operations alone, a theory of higher cognition with a degree of richness and empirical soundness that can begin to approach what we already have in symbolic theory.

The need for vertical integration can also be evaded by the opposite type of denial—denying the importance of the neural level to cognitive theory, as advocated for decades within cognitive science by the functionalist position. According to this position, the neural level is as irrelevant for the cognitive level of theorizing as are the details of machine language for writing programs in a high-level computer language. Such a perspective has been extremely productive, sanctioning important higher-level theorizing without prematurely imposing the straitjacket of neural realizability. But despite all its progress, the development of symbolic theory has not ultimately shed light on its neural realization (Box 23:1). Thus, it now seems appropriate that some significant portion of cognitive research adopt the working hypothesis, advocated by connectionists, that higher-level cognition is not so cleanly sealed off from its neural substrate and that we must explicitly incorporate knowledge of neural computation (as this knowledge accrues) if we are to develop a higher-level theory that correctly describes processing in the human brain.

Yet another type of denial rejects the importance of the soft facets of cognition—for example, by dismissing variability, gradedness, and statistical sensitivity in linguistic behavior as "mere performance noise" for which cognitive theory is not to be held responsible, except perhaps in some long-postponed future. This view evades the need for the substantive integration involved in resolving the central paradox. In our view, however, this move insulates cognitive theory from too much important data that can inform theory construction. The cognitive architecture we articulate in this book provides a deep connection between symbolic and numerical/statistical cognitive processing; it is our hope that this connection will enable future research developing detailed accounts of the precise relations between the discrete, structural and the continuous, numerical aspects of particular cognitive faculties.

Obviously, it is not our intent here to develop convincing arguments for the need for substantive integration, or for the other types of integration discussed below. We only wish to identify the kind of integrative goals toward which the research in this book is directed. In the end, our view amounts to this: understanding cognition is arguably the most difficult scientific challenge ever confronted, and we simply cannot afford to neglect any of the insight that has been gained by studying the abstract structure of higher cognition through symbolic theory, by studying the richness of behavior in both higher and lower cognition through experimental psychology, and by studying processing in the brain through cognitive and computational neuroscience. It is only by integrating the knowledge we have acquired through these multiple perspectives, only by squarely facing and resolving the central paradox of cognition, that we can hope to develop a truly successful science of cognition.

2.2 Methodological integration and sectarian warfare

The goal of substantive integration pertains to the *content* of cognitive theory. A second type of integration we believe to be important to cognitive science concerns its research *methods*.

(2) Methodological integration

A cognitive theory is **methodologically integrated** if

a. it incorporates the overall conceptualization of various cognitive domains that have been developed by individual cognitive disciplines;
b. its development effectively exploits the diverse research methods of these disciplines; and
c. its results constructively feed these disciplines and further their own particular goals.

As stated above, our integrative goals are motivated by the conviction that the mind/brain problem is of such difficulty that we must exploit every means available to us: this applies not just to the substantive insights that have been obtained, but also to the research tools that have been developed.

A still more compelling reason to pursue methodological integration is the risk of sectarian strife in a balkanized cognitive science containing predominantly segregated disciplines. The risks are easily seen. In the dominantly empiricist cultures of neuroscience and experimental psychology, it is not easy to appreciate the merit of abstract discussions of mind in which the objects of study cannot be directly measured; easy to dismiss the primary introspective data of generative linguistics as artifacts of linguists' own intuitions, and linguistic theory as a wildly implausible excess of abstraction. In the rationalist culture of formal linguistics, it is not easy to appreciate the need for painstaking experimentation; easy to dismiss experimental work as contributing little to the understanding of central theoretical issues. For cognitive scientists studying higher cognition, it is not easy to see the necessity, or even the value, of neuroscience. For neuroscientists, psychologists, and linguists, accustomed to strong empirical constraints on theory, it is not easy to appreciate the computationalists' culture in which formal, mathematical constraints play the dominant role in defining highly abstract problems and solutions; easy to dismiss computational models as too abstract or simplified to be relevant to the study of "real" cognition. And for all these cognitive scientists, it can be difficult to appreciate the contribution of philosophy, where questions are often so fundamental that even a clear formulation of a problem can be a major advance, and where the search for solutions spans centuries.

The risks of a divided cognitive science are all too real. Incompatibilities in the conception of what constitutes the key problems of cognition, the crucial data and sound research methods, the fundamental assumptions underlying cognitive theory—such inconsistency holds the potential for much destructive interference, always threatening to render cognitive science a whole that is much *less* than the sum of its parts.

The challenge of methodological integration is to confront head-on the inconsistencies across the divergent sciences of cognition, to forge a coherent, comprehensive theory that derives its strength from the diversity of perspectives that inform it. This is a challenge that increasing numbers of cognitive scientists are embracing, as new generations of scientists receive substantial interdisciplinary training during their academic critical period of graduate and postgraduate study. It is our hope that the work presented in this book will help further the case that constructive synergy can take the place of destructive interference between approaches to cognition traditionally seen as rivals. In particular, we see the work presented here as providing evidence that constructive interaction is indeed possible between symbolic theory and neural network theory, between generative grammar and connectionism. These approaches have in the past been separated, we believe, by a profound schism that goes even deeper than methodological divisions.

2.3 Metatheoretic integration: Model- versus principle-centered research

Cognitive science research seems to span a nonobvious but important fault line, a rift that, for example, divides much connectionist research from most work in symbolic theories like those of generative grammar. We do not believe this division to be a necessary one. At a metatheoretic level, one of this book's goals is to argue that connectionism can make a different kind of contribution than has been previously recognized; as a result, connectionism can exert a unifying rather than a divisive force within cognitive science.

To situate this potentially unifying role of connectionism, it is useful to regard research in cognitive science as divided very broadly into what we will call, lacking better terms, 'model-centered' and 'principle-centered' investigations. In both cases, research involves both more specific analyses and more general cognitive claims; the difference lies in their relative roles and prominence.

(3) Metatheoretic integration

A research paradigm is **metatheoretically integrated** if it supports both

a. **model-centered** research, by providing the technical resources for building precise, detailed accounts of empirical cognitive phenomena; and

b. **principle-centered** research, by providing cognitive principles of considerable generality that are precise enough to support formal analysis and that are supported by sound and fertile mathematical foundations.

Model-centered research focuses on specific analyses—prototypically in the form of implemented computational models—of particular behavioral phenomena—typically, effects measured in psychological experiments, or particular computational tasks that are abstracted from cognitive behavior. In model-centered research, the model is usually offered in the context of more general theoretical claims, but there is a marked asymmetry between these claims and the model. The theoretical claims are largely in the background, often because they are highly general and regarded as untestable in and of themselves: they need to be implemented in concrete models of particular facts before they can be tested. Major effort is directed toward implementing such models rather than toward formally articulating the principles per se and analyzing their logical consequences. As a result, the principles typically remain in a fairly imprecise form: alone, they do not allow any strong conclusions to follow. Instead, it is the model that is assigned the job of demonstrating the desired consequences; this is then taken as evidence in favor of the general claims.

In principle-centered research, the relative roles of specific accounts and general theoretical claims are reversed. Considerable effort is invested in clearly formulating the general claims, so they earn the title 'principles'. While general in scope, these principles must be sufficiently precise that one can actually deduce consequences from them. Furthermore, it must be possible to instantiate the general principles in specific accounts, in order to demonstrate their adequacy for explaining particular empirical phenomena. In the model-centered approach, the general background claims serve to motivate or enhance the appeal of the particular model in the spotlight; in the principle-centered approach, the specific accounts serve as a background for demonstrating the empirical adequacy of the general principles.

Chapter 22 elaborates in considerable detail the contrast between model- and principle-centered research, grounding the discussion in the case most relevant to the research presented in this book: connectionism as applied to language. The distinction is exemplified by two kinds of responses to the following situation. A fundamental connectionist hypothesis—say, that mental representations are distributed patterns of activity—is deemed extremely important, but, by itself, is simply too vague to enable more than loose predictions and questionable explanations. One response is to instantiate the hypothesis in very specific distributed representations for very specific cognitive tasks, and to use simulations of this specific instantiation to derive precise predictions. It is not the job of the hypothesis itself to directly enable predictions; that is the job of specific instantiations of the hypothesis. This is the model-centered approach.

A different response is to attempt to replace a vague hypothesis concerning distributed representations with a more formally precise hypothesis, but one that is still quite general. The resulting principle might assert that, generically for some broad domain like language or even higher cognition more generally, distributed representations are systems of vectors with precisely defined mathematical properties, from which can be deduced general consequences, which in turn can be instantiated and tested in specific situations. This is the principle-centered approach.

Both approaches, we believe, are essential for cognitive science; their complementary strengths and weaknesses are considered in Chapter 22. The model-centered approach is well developed within connectionist research, but the principle-centered approach is less so. The work reported in this book is largely directed toward the challenge of developing principle-centered approaches to a connectionist theory of higher cognition—especially, grammar.

In the remainder of this chapter, we offer a few brief remarks on the general role of connectionism in promoting integration within cognitive science.

3 Connectionism and Integration

Despite the history of divisiveness surrounding it, connectionism can in fact be a force for integration, offering cognitive science opportunities for overcoming substantive, methodological, and metatheoretic schisms.

Consider first the goal of substantive integration (1). In Chapter 23, it is argued that connectionism can promote vertical integration by providing a level of description intermediate between those of neurons and of symbols, and by exploiting this intermediate level as a bridge for bringing into contact theories of neural and mental computation. Furthermore, it is argued in Smolensky 1988 that connectionism provides a computational account of a unified cognitive architecture from which can emerge quite varied processes or **virtual machines** that serve the varying needs of diverse cognitive domains; this is a powerful means of achieving horizontal integration. Thus, the same fundamental connectionist computational mechanisms can be seen to underlie perceptual processes, memory, and certain higher-level processes; different principles of organization emerge as higher-level descriptions of different kinds of connectionist networks operating in different kinds of information-processing environments.

This conceptual integration notwithstanding, it proves technically quite difficult to relate connectionist computation to the symbolic computation dominating formal theories of higher-level cognition. Thus, connectionism in practice has not provided great progress on the important aspects of substantive integration involving higher cognition.

Indeed, connectionism has had a rather divisive influence with respect to higher cognition. The connectionist research devoted to higher cognition (and the rhetorical debate surrounding it) has tended toward one or the other extreme of eliminativism or implementationalism (Box 1:8). Eliminativist connectionist models are often used to argue that some concept from symbolic theory is misguided, crude, or superfluous. Implementationalist connectionist models are used to more or less directly implement symbolic concepts. The impact within cognitive science of both types of research seems to be a kind of polarization that is quite antithetical to the goal of methodological integration (2). Theorists of higher-level cognition tend to evaluate the eliminativist research as seriously missing the mark, in virtue of failing to address the target symbolic concepts with anything like the adequacy required to justify the conclusion that these concepts can be eliminated. Neither are these theorists generally impressed by the implementationalist research; they typically judge that the implementations do not do justice to the true symbolic concepts, nor do they find them very theoretically or computationally enlightening. We believe the net effect is that the majority of cognitive scientists studying higher-level cognition have at best become entrenched in their initial suspicion that connectionism has little to offer them in the pursuit of their scientific goals—at worst, they have concluded from strong eliminativist claims that connectionists are trying to seriously roll back the clock in the understanding of higher cognition.

Connectionism's influence with respect to metatheoretic integration (3) has also been rather divisive. That connectionism has proved itself an extremely fruitful vehicle within the model-centered approach is a well-attested—if not uncontroversial—view. Not surprisingly, examples are most common within the subdisciplines where model-centered research dominates: connectionism has been a significant impetus in promoting the success of theory (qua modeling) within neuroscience; connectionist modeling rapidly became a central part of theory (qua modeling) within cognitive psychology; and connectionist techniques in artificial intelligence and in computer applications enjoyed considerable success within a short time.

By contrast, with respect to principle-centered research, connectionism's contribution has been strikingly smaller. While suggestive glimpses of their inner workings are frequently achieved, connectionist models are sufficiently difficult to understand that it is usually quite mysterious why they fail, and—perhaps even more disturbing—just as mysterious why they succeed to the extent that they do. Such mysteries must give way to principled theory if connectionism is to become principle-centered—but this is an enormous technical challenge. Inadequacies of connectionist work construed as principle- rather than model-centered research were pointed out in a number of early critiques, from philosophical (Fodor and Pylyshyn 1988), linguistic (Lachter and Bever 1988; Pinker and Prince 1988), and psychological (McCloskey 1992) perspectives.

The purported fact—call it '*F*'—that connectionism is not effective as a vehicle for principle- as opposed to model-centered research has itself served as yet another source of divisiveness within cognitive science. Proponents of the principle-centered approach can use *F* to dismiss or deride connectionism. Proponents of connectionist modeling can recruit *F* for an argument against the viability of a principle-centered approach.[3] Agreeing on the validity of *F*, both connectionist modelers and anticonnectionists favoring principle-centered research can use it to drive a wedge into the rift separating them.

We aim to dissolve this conflict by arguing—with, among others, Stephen Grossberg (1982, 1988) and James McClelland (1991)— that *F* is in fact false, that connectionism *can* make important contributions to principle-centered research. Rather than further widening the schism between model- and principle-centered cognitive sci-

[3] A somewhat flamboyant articulation of the argument might be this: "Connectionist models have proven themselves as models of human behavior, and as our current best description of neural computation, so they are the best models of the mind/brain we have; but, clearly, connectionist models are *just too complicated* to admit the sort of precise, powerful, general principles presupposed by the principle-centered approach—therefore, such principles don't exist."

Box 1

ence, we hope to illustrate in this book how connectionism can actually help to integrate the two approaches, by providing both a powerful platform for modeling and new general principles that increase the scope of principle-centered research within cognitive science. In order to explore in more depth the unifying potential of connectionism, especially with respect to metatheoretic integration, in Chapter 22 we take a detailed look at this issue in the context of language.

This chapter concludes with a brief synopsis of the relation between the types of integration we have identified and the general research results presented in this book.

4 ILLUSTRATIVE RESULTS AND INTEGRATIVE GOALS

The contributions presented in this book are offered as evidence that the integrative goals (1)–(3) articulated in Section 2 can guide fruitful research in cognitive science. As an overview, we now briefly note how six general results bear on the integrative goals. These results are listed in (4); for each, references are given to relevant principles of ICS introduced in Chapter 2, or other relevant discussion above.

(4) Summary of selected general results

a. *Mental representation.* The mathematical formalism introduced in Chapter 5 and developed in Chapters 7–8 shows in precise terms how a mental representation can be simultaneously a fully distributed pattern of numerical activities at one level of analysis and the functional equivalent of a (possibly recursive) symbolic structure when analyzed at a higher level. [P_1: Chapter 2 (1), (2)]

b. *Mental processes.* In Chapter 8, it is shown in mathematical detail, and illustrated by computer simulation, how mental processing can be simultaneously a massively parallel process of spreading activation at one level of analysis and, at a higher level, a kind of parallel holistic manipulation of symbolic structures—even structures containing recursive embedding. A large class of functions computed via this symbol manipulation can be formally specified by symbolic programs. [P_2: Chapter 2 (3), (4)]

c. *Optimization of well-formedness.* In Chapter 9, it is demonstrated that the overall effects of spreading activation, in important classes of networks, can be analyzed at a higher level as a process of optimization, in which an output representation is constructed that maximizes a connectionist measure of well-formedness, Harmony. [P_3: Chapter 2 (5)]

d. *Harmonic Grammar* (HG). In Section 6:2, the preceding results are combined to define HG, which provides in Chapter 10 a new characterization of formal languages and which is employed in Chapter 11 to address a long-standing problem in natural language concerning the interface of syntax and semantics. This formalism constitutes a novel integration of connectionist and symbolic computation. [HG: Chapter 2 (6), (7)]

e. *Optimality Theory* (OT). In Chapter 12, HG is further developed to a new theory of the computational structure of universal grammar, OT. This theory is shown to enable precise characterizations of what it is that grammars of different languages share, and just how they differ, with respect to key aspects of phonology and syntax. It is also shown (in Part III) to provide new connections between grammatical theory and empirical studies of the acquisition and processing of language. [P_4: Chapter 2 (8); Chapter 4]
f. *Productivity*. Chapter 23 brings previous results to bear on a central problem in the foundations of cognitive science, allowing a novel explanation of how higher cognition can achieve, with finite and fixed resources, processing competence that displays a high degree of systematicity and productivity. [Section 1 of this chapter]

4.1 Relevance to integrative goals

The results summarized in (4) represent, we now suggest, a certain degree of progress in the achievement of the three integrative goals (1)-(3).

Consider first the imperative of substantive integration to face the challenges of higher cognition (1a). The cognitive problems of grammar and productivity addressed in (4d-f) are among the most central in higher cognition. Indeed, the results on language in (4e) bear directly on the universal theory of grammar, surely one of the bastions of higher cognitive theory. And—as emphasized in Fodor and Pylyshyn 1988, an influential critique of connectionist theory—the problem of productivity addressed in (4f) has a central role in understanding all of higher cognition.

Turning to the other imperative of the goal of substantive integration—to situate the theory of higher cognition in a theoretical context that is both vertically and horizontally integrated (1b-d)—we observe that results (4a-c) on representation, processing, and well-formedness provide the supporting pillars of a vertically integrated theory, built from general notions of connectionist computation that cut across many cognitive domains and so simultaneously provide the foundation for horizontal integration. In addition to its novel application to grammar developed in our research, the principle of optimal well-formedness has been applied in previous research to the perceptual problem of finding the optimal interpretation of an image, and to the problem of content-addressed memory, to find the optimal fit between stored items and a partial retrieval cue. The representations developed in (4a) apply not just to language, but to all domains of cognition where symbolic structure plays a role, whether the structure be discrete or continuous. Thus, the results (4) together constitute meaningful progress toward achieving the goal of substantive integration.

Progress toward the goal of methodological integration (2) is also represented. Results (4d-f) concerning grammar and productivity target problems that have been of central interest in two traditional cognitive disciplines: theoretical linguistics and the philosophy of mind. The formulations of these problems that are adopted here are those that have been developed by the practitioners of these fields. The data addressed are also those recognized in those fields. The theoretical constructs of those disciplines play a major role. And the established methods of those disciplines—generative-linguistic and philosophical analysis—are being incorporated into the multidisciplinary methodology under development in the ICS research program. In each case, collaboration or published dialogue involving linguists or philosophers has ensured that the work is part of a vigorous two-way interaction between a new interdisciplinary cognitive science perspective and established perspectives of the relevant individual disciplines.

Finally, the results presented in this book also address the goal of metatheoretic integration (3), to support both model- and principle-centered cognitive research. That connectionism can effectively support model-centered research is well established; our contribution is to show how connectionism can also support principle-centered research. While it does not develop "connectionist models" in the traditional sense, the ICS research program does include model-centered research, developing formal techniques for constructing concrete, detailed accounts of specific empirical phenomena. The grammar formalisms of HG and OT enable very specific accounts of empirical phenomena including the argument structure of intransitive verbs in French (Chapter 11), universal syllable structure (Chapter 13), vowel harmony systems (Chapter 14), simple clause structure (Chapter 15) and *wh*-questions (Chapter 16), aspects of the initial and final state of the phonological grammar of English learners (Chapter 17), the development of children's first sentences in French (Chapter 18), the online processing of sentences in English (Chapter 19), universals of auxiliary verb selection (Chapter 20), and the unusual syllabification system of a Berber dialect (Chapter 20). Addressing computational rather than empirical problems, the research program also develops in detail precise accounts of the distributed connectionist realization of the recursive binary-tree data structure (Chapter 8), the specification of formal languages by harmonic grammars (Chapter 10), the acquisition of grammars from positive examples and the computation of grammatical parses of inputs (synopsized in Chapter 12), and the encoding of a small universal grammar fragment in an abstract genome (Chapter 21).

With respect to the metatheoretic goal of supporting principle-centered research (3b), we note that each of the results summarized in (4) takes the form of precise yet general cognitive principles, centered on novel concepts for understanding cognition that arise from viewing a connectionist computational model and a symbolic computational model as two descriptions, at different levels of analysis, of one and the same cognitive system. The connectionist technical innovations of the research presented here—including, with others, the technical components of the results summarized in (4)—contribute to the soundness and power of the general mathematical framework supporting a connectionist theory of higher cognition. Original symbolic technical contributions have also provided innovations in grammar formalism, especially within OT. Key to the results presented in this book are mathematical bridges between the continuous, numerical model of computation underlying connectionism and the discrete, symbolic computation of virtual machines that emerge as higher-level descriptions of appropriately constructed connectionist systems. These mathematical foundations provide the kind of technical support needed to make progress on the central paradox of cognition.

4.2 Caveats

Given the inherent difficulty and ambition of the integrative goals identified here, the contributions in this book constitute only a tiny step on the road to meeting those goals. Concerning the claims for the results presented in this book, a number of major caveats are in order; two general ones will be taken up here.

First, while considerable effort has been put into the formulation and analysis of the principles we present, beginning in Chapter 5, it is clear that these are all merely working hypotheses that will undergo major refinement, revision, and perhaps rejection in the course of subsequent research. While rather precise formulation of the principles is necessary for much of the research we discuss, this level of precision should not be mistaken as implying that we believe the principles are now ready to be etched in stone. Ultimately more important than the exact formulation of the principles is the general theoretical approach to cognition they embody and *the kind of research they make it possible to do.* We intend the principles given here to be taken as representative of a class of principles, largely unexplored, that embody the same general approach and that allow the same kind of research. (Chapter 7 explicitly considers a number of variants of the first principle P_1, Chapter 2 (1)–(2), and identifies concretely the sense in which P_1 is a pure representative of the whole class of more elaborate variants.)

Second, the computational principles presented are quite general and therefore *potentially* applicable to a wide variety of problems in higher cognition. But of course the extent of their actual validity in various cognitive domains remains for the most part to be put to the empirical test. The adequacy of the principles as judged by certain computational, linguistic, and foundational criteria is addressed in Parts II, III, and IV, but this of course constitutes a tiny fraction of the tests to which such general principles must ultimately be subjected. In particular, crucial empirical directions for future work are investigation of the biological underpinnings of these principles and their embodiment in detailed psychological models. The near absence of empirical testing of the principles discussed below against the kind of data central to cognitive psychology and neuroscience is a regrettable deficiency in the current state of the research program—although early work addressing naturally occurring and experimental data from child language and online sentence processing is discussed in Chapters 17–19.[4] As implied by the general discussion in Section 2.3 of the model-

[4] It is unclear at this point how best to pursue the question of whether the principles have adequate support in empirical neuroscience. The right kind of question, of course, is not "How much detailed neural data can we explain with Harmony maximization?" but rather "Is there a higher level of

Box 1

versus principle-centered divide, our initial focus of research addressing issues central to the theory of computation, linguistics, and philosophy of mind, rather than those of neuroscience or cognitive psychology, may be understood as a consequence of differences among these fields in the prominence of principle-centered research, along with our high-level goal of demonstrating that connectionism can contribute to principle-centered and not just model-centered research in cognitive science. In order to do justice to the integrative goals set forth in this chapter, however, future research must more comprehensively bring to bear on each problem the wide range of empirical and theoretical perspectives that makes cognitive science such a rich discipline-in-formation.

analysis of biological neural computation where Harmony is maximized, to a reasonable approximation?" It is worth noting that while the primary motivations for introducing Harmony were psychological and computational rather than neural (Smolensky 1983, 1984, 1986), neural motivation was explicitly cited for the introduction of very closely related Lyapunov functions (Cohen and Grossberg 1983; Hopfield 1982, 1984). Thus, while the real question remains to be addressed, it is nonetheless historically accurate to say that principles virtually identical to that of Harmony maximization arose from the attempt to mathematically model biological neural networks. (Concerning the relation of ICS theory to neuroscience, see Box 1:6.)

References

Aizawa, K. 1997. Exhibiting vs. explaining systematicity: A reply to Hadley and Hayward. *Minds and Machines* 7, 39–55.

Aizawa, K. 2003. *The systematicity arguments*. Kluwer.

Churchland, P. S., and T. J. Sejnowski. 1992. *The computational brain*. MIT Press.

Cohen, M. A., and S. Grossberg. 1983. Absolute stability of global pattern formation and parallel memory storage by competitive neural networks. *IEEE Transactions on Systems, Man, and Cybernetics* 13, 815–25.

Cummins, R., and G. Schwarz. 1991. Connectionism, computation, and cognition. In *Connectionism and the philosophy of mind*, eds. T. E. Horgan and J. Tienson. Kluwer.

Fodor, J. A. 1991. Replies. In *Meaning in mind: Fodor and his critics*, eds. B. Loewer and G. Rey. Blackwell.

Fodor, J. A. 1997. Connectionism and the problem of systematicity (continued): Why Smolensky's solution still doesn't work. *Cognition* 62, 109–19.

Fodor, J. A., and B. P. McLaughlin. 1990. Connectionism and the problem of systematicity: Why Smolensky's solution doesn't work. *Cognition* 35, 183–204.

Fodor, J. A. , and Z. W. Pylyshyn. 1988. Connectionism and cognitive architecture: A critical analysis. *Cognition* 28, 3–71.

Grossberg, S. 1982. *Studies of mind and brain: Neural principles of learning, perception, development, cognition, and motor control*. Reidel.

Grossberg, S., ed. 1988. *Neural networks and natural intelligence*. MIT Press.

Hopfield, J. J. 1982. Neural networks and physical systems with emergent collective computational abilities. *Proceedings of the National Academy of Sciences USA* 79, 2554–8.

Hopfield, J. J. 1984. Neurons with graded response have collective computational properties like those of two-state neurons. *Proceedings of the National Academy of Sciences USA* 81, 3088–92.

Horgan, T. E., and J. Tienson. 1991. Structured representations in connectionist systems? In *Connectionism: Theory and practice*, ed. S. Davis. Oxford University Press.

Lachter, J., and T. G. Bever. 1988. The relation between linguistic structure and associative theories of language learning—a constructive critique of some connectionist learning models. *Cognition* 28, 195–247.

Marr, D. 1982. *Vision*. W. H. Freeman.

McClelland, J. L. 1991. Toward a theory of information processing in graded, random, interactive networks. Technical report PDP.CSN.91.1, Department of Psychology, Carnegie Mellon University.

McCloskey, M. 1992. Networks and theories: The place of connectionism in cognitive science. *Psychological Science* 2, 387–95.

McLaughlin, B. P. 1992. Systematicity, conceptual truth, and evolution. In *Philosophy and the cognitive sciences*, eds. C. Hookway and D. Peterson. Royal Institute of Philosophy, Supplement no. 34.

McLaughlin, B. P. 1993. The connectionism/classicism battle to win souls. *Philosophical Studies* 71, 163–90.

Newell, A. 1990. *Unified theories of cognition*. Harvard University Press.

Pinker, S., and A. Prince. 1988. On language and connectionism: Analysis of a parallel distributed processing model of language acquisition. *Cognition* 28, 73–193.

Smolensky, P. 1983. Schema selection and stochastic inference in modular environments. In *Proceedings of the National Conference on Artificial Intelligence 3*.

Smolensky, P. 1984. The mathematical role of self-consistency in parallel computation. In *Proceedings of the Cognitive Science Society 6*.

Smolensky, P. 1986. Information processing in dynamical systems: Foundations of Harmony Theory. In *Parallel distributed processing: Explorations in the microstructure of cognition*. Vol. 1, *Foundations*, D. E. Rumelhart, J. L. McClelland, and the PDP Research Group. MIT Press.

Smolensky, P. 1987. The constituent structure of connectionist mental states: A reply to Fodor and Pylyshyn. *Southern Journal of Philosophy* 26 (Supplement), 137–63.

Smolensky, P. 1988. On the proper treatment of connectionism. *Behavioral and Brain Sciences* 11, 1–74.

Smolensky, P. 1990. In defense of PTC: Reply to continuing commentary. *Behavioral and Brain Sciences* 13, 407–11.

Smolensky, P. 1991. Connectionism, constituency, and the language of thought. In *Meaning in mind: Fodor and his critics*, eds. B. Loewer and G. Rey. Blackwell.

Smolensky, P. 1994. Computational theories of mind. In *A companion to the philosophy of mind*, ed. S. Guttenplan. Blackwell.

Smolensky, P. 1995a. Constituent structure and explanation in an integrated connectionist/symbolic cognitive architecture. In *Connectionism: Debates on psychological explanation*. Vol. 2, eds. C. Macdonald and G. Macdonald. Blackwell.

Smolensky, P. 1995b. On the projectable predicates of connectionist psychology: A case for belief. In *Connectionism: Debates on psychological explanation*. Vol. 2, eds. C. Macdonald and G. Macdonald. Blackwell.

Smolensky, P., G. Legendre, and Y. Miyata. 1992. Principles for an integrated connectionist/symbolic theory of higher cognition. Technical report CU-CS-600-92, Computer Science Department, and 92-8, Institute of Cognitive Science, University of Colorado at Boulder.

VanLehn, K., ed. 1991. *Architectures for intelligence*. Erlbaum.

4

Optimality: From Neural Networks to Universal Grammar

Alan Prince and Paul Smolensky

A major component of the Integrated Connectionist/Symbolic Cognitive Architecture (ICS) research program is a grammatical architecture, Optimality Theory. This chapter provides a quick, self-contained introduction to this theory, its relation to connectionist networks, and its relevance to basic questions of language acquisition. A systematic exposition of the theory is presented in Chapter 12.

Can concepts from the theory of neural computation contribute to formal theories of the mind? The research presented here explores the implications of one principle of neural computation, optimization, for the theory of grammar. Optimization over symbolic linguistic structures provides the core of a new grammatical architecture, Optimality Theory. The proposition that grammaticality equals optimality sheds light on a wide range of phenomena, from the gulf between production and comprehension in child language, to language learnability, to the fundamental questions of linguistic theory: what is it that the grammars of all languages share, and how may they differ?

This chapter reprints an article by the same title published in *Science* 275, 1604–10 (1997). Some minimal overlap with material in previous chapters results from the autonomy of the original article. A few pointers to other chapters are inserted and a few typographical changes made for consistency with the present book. Numbered footnotes are from the original article.

Contents

It is evident that the sciences of the brain and those of the mind are separated by many gulfs, not the least of which lies between the formal methods appropriate for continuous dynamical systems and those for discrete symbol structures. Yet recent research provides evidence that integration of these sciences may hold significant rewards. Research on neural computation has identified optimization as an organizing principle of some generality, and current work is showing that optimization principles can be successfully adapted to a central domain within the theory of mind: the theory of grammar. In this chapter, we explore how a reconceptualization of linguistic theory through optimization principles provides a variety of insights into the structure of the language faculty, and we consider the relations between optimality in grammar and optimization in neural networks.

Some of the contributions of the optimization perspective on grammar are surprising. The distinction between linguistic knowledge in the abstract and the use of this knowledge in language processing has often been challenged by researchers adopting neural network approaches to language; yet we show here how an optimization architecture in fact strengthens and rationalizes this distinction. In turn, this leads to new formal methods by which grammar learners can cope with the demands of their difficult task, and new explanations for the gap in complexity between the language children produce and the language they can comprehend. Optimization also provides a fresh perspective on the nature of linguistic constraints, on what it is that grammars of different human languages share, and on how grammars may differ. And this turns out to provide considerable analytical leverage on central aspects of the long-standing problems in language acquisition.

1 Optimality Theory

Linguistic research seeks to characterize the range of structures available to human language and the relationships that may obtain between them, particularly as they figure in a competent speaker's internalized **grammar** or implicit knowledge of language. Languages appear to vary widely, but the same structural themes repeat themselves over and over again, in ways that are sometimes obvious and sometimes clear only upon detailed analysis. The challenge, then, is to discover an architecture for grammars that both allows variation and limits its range to what is actually possible in human language.

A primary observation is that grammars contain constraints on the well-formedness of linguistic structures, and these constraints are heavily in conflict, even within a single language. A few simple examples should bring out the flavor of this conflict. English operates under constraints entailing that its basic word order is subject-verb-object; yet in a sentence like *what did John see?* it is the object that stands first. This evidences the greater force of a constraint requiring question-words like *what* to appear sentence-initially. Yet even this constraint is not absolute: one must say *who saw what?* with the object question-word appearing in its canonical position; the potential alternative, *who what saw?*, with all question-words clumped at the front, which is indeed grammatical in some languages, runs afoul of another principle of clause structure that is, in English, yet stronger than the requirement of placing question-words first. Thus, *who saw what?* is the grammatical structure, satisfying the constraints of the grammar not perfectly, but **optimally**: no alternative does better, given the relative strength of the constraints in the grammar of English.

Similar conflicts abound at all levels of linguistic structure. In forming the past tense of *slip*, spelled *slipped* but pronounced *slipt*, a general phonological constraint on voicing in final consonant sequences favors the pronunciation *pt* over *pd*, conflicting with the requirement that the past tense marker be given its basic form *-d*; and the phonological constraint prevails.[1] In an English sentence like *it rains*, a constraint requiring all words to contribute to meaning (unlike the element *it* in this usage)[†] conflicts with a structural constraint requiring all sentences to have subjects; and the latter controls the outcome. Such examples indicate that a central element in the architecture of grammar is a formal means for managing the pervasive conflict between grammatical constraints.

The key observation is this: in a variety of clear cases where there is a strength asymmetry between two conflicting constraints, *no amount of success* on the weaker constraint can compensate for failure on the stronger one. Put another way: any degree of failure on the weaker constraint is tolerated, so long as it contributes to success on the stronger constraint. Extending this observation leads to the hypothesis that a grammar consists entirely of constraints arranged in a **strict domination hierarchy**, in which each constraint is strictly more important than—takes absolute priority over—all the constraints ranked lower in the hierarchy. With this type of constraint interaction, it is only the ranking of constraints in the hierarchy that matters for determining optimality: no particular numerical strengths, for example, are necessary. Strict domination thus limits drastically the range of possible strength-interactions between constraints to those representable with the algebra of total order.

Strict domination hierarchies composed of very simple well-formedness constraints can lead to surprisingly complex grammatical consequences. Furthermore, different rankings of the same set of constraints can give rise to strikingly different linguistic patterns. These properties show that strict domination, though a narrow mechanism, answers to the basic requirements on the theory of human language, which must allow grammars to be built from simple parts whose combination leads to specific kinds of complexity and diversity. **Optimality Theory** (OT), originally presented in 1991 (Prince and Smolensky 1991), offers a particularly strong version of a strict-domination-based approach to grammatical optimization.[2] OT hypothesizes

[1] Basic work on this phenomenon in neural network models, and critiques, includes Rumelhart and McClelland 1986 and Pinker and Mehler 1988.

[†] With weather verbs, *it* is a *dummy* pronoun: it has no referent in the world. Unlike many other languages, English does not permit subjectless declarative sentences.

[2] The basic sources are Prince and Smolensky 1993/2004, McCarthy and Prince 1993a, b. These primarily address phonology; the following early and basic works address syntax, including the topics mentioned in the text: Legendre, Raymond, and Smolensky 1993; Grimshaw 1997; Samek-Lodovici

that the set of well-formedness constraints is **universal**: not just universally available to be chosen from, but literally present in every language. A grammar for a particular language results from imposing a strict domination ranking on the entire universal constraint set. Also universal is the function that determines, for each input to the grammar, the set of candidate output structures that compete for optimality; every language considers exactly the same set of options for realizing an input. The observed force of a given constraint can vary from absolute (never violated) to nil (always violated), with many steps and stops along the way, depending on its position in the strict domination hierarchy for a given language, and depending on the membership in the output candidate set for a given input.

OT thus provides a direct answer to the classic questions of linguistic theory: what do the grammars of different languages have in common, and how may they differ? What they share are the universal constraints and the definition of which forms compete; they differ in how the constraints are ranked, and, therefore, in which constraints take priority when conflicts arise among them. For example, the two constraints in conflict in English *it rains* are ranked differently in Italian: the constraint against meaningless words outranks that against subjectless sentences, and the resulting grammatical sentence is simply *piove* (literally, 'rains'). [See discussion in Section 12:1.4.]

OT connects a number of lines of research that have occupied linguists in the last several decades: the articulation of universal formal principles of grammars (Chomsky 1965; Chomsky and Halle 1968) and substantive universals of process and product (Stampe 1979; Perlmutter 1983); the generalization of well-formedness constraints across the outputs of formally disparate mechanisms (Kisseberth 1970; Chomsky 1981); the descriptive use of informal notions of linguistic optimization (Goldsmith 1993; Archangeli and Pulleyblank 1994; Burzio 1994; Chomsky 1995); and output-oriented analysis (Perlmutter 1971; Bybee and Slobin 1982; McCarthy and Prince 1986/1996). Such a unification is made possible by the basic notion that grammaticality means optimally satisfying the conflicting demands of violable constraints.

2 Markedness and Faithfulness Constraints

Within the universal constraint set, several subclasses have been distinguished. One class of universal constraints in OT formalizes the notion of structural complexity, or **markedness** (Jakobson 1962; Trubetzkoy 1939/1969; Chomsky and Halle 1968, Chap. 9). Grossly speaking, an element of linguistic structure is said to be marked if it is more complex than an alternative along some dimension; the relevant dimensions may sometimes correlate with comprehension, production, memory, or related physical and cognitive functions. The word-final consonant cluster *pd* is more marked than *pt*; sentences lacking subjects are more marked than those with subjects.

1996; Legendre, Smolensky, and Wilson 1998. These and many other OT papers may be accessed electronically on the Rutgers Optimality Archive; see Footnote 3.

Marked elements tend to be absent altogether in certain languages, restricted in their use in other languages, later-acquired by children, and in other ways avoided. This cluster of properties diagnostic of marked elements is given a uniform explanation in OT, which follows from their formal characterization: marked structures are those that violate structural constraints. We will call the set of all such constraints **MARKEDNESS**.‡

Phonological markedness constraints often induce context-dependent alteration of pronunciations. For example, the markedness of *pd* relative to *pt* is responsible for the alteration of the past tense suffix *d* to *t* in 'slipped': this is a context in which the more marked cluster is avoided. A more dramatic alteration is common in French, driven by syllabic markedness constraints. (Our presentation simplifies somewhat for ease of exposition; for details, see Tranel 1994 [and Section 22:4.2].) One such constraint, NOCODA, is violated by any syllable ending with a consonant—a **closed** syllable; the syllable-closing consonant is called a **coda**. Closed syllables are marked relative to syllables ending with a vowel. Another constraint, ONSET, is violated by syllables that begin with a vowel.

In French, the masculine form of the word for 'small', written *petit*, is pronounced with or without the final *t*, depending on the context. Spelling, though often merely conventional, in this case accurately represents the abstract sound-sequence that a speaker internalizes when the word is learned: we write this sequence /pɛtit/. When the following word is vowel-initial, the final *t* is pronounced, beginning a syllable: *pɛ.ti.t øf* 'little egg'. Elsewhere—when the following word begins with a consonant, or when there is no following word—/pɛtit/ is pronounced *pɛ.ti*, with loss of the final lexical *t*: *pɛ.ti.pa* 'little step'. (Adjacent syllables are separated by a period in the examples.) The phonological grammar of French determines how 'small' is pronounced in a given context, that is, which grammatical **output** (pronunciation) corresponds to an **input** /pɛtit .../. The final *t* is not pronounced when so doing would violate NOCODA; the constraint ONSET determines that when the *t* precedes a vowel, it begins a syllable and is pronounced.

A second class of universal constraints in OT, **FAITHFULNESS**, is a direct consequence of the optimization perspective. (For significant extensions of FAITHFULNESS within OT, see McCarthy and Prince 1995; Benua 1995.) An optimal (grammatical) representation is one that optimally satisfies the constraint ranking among those representations containing a given input. The existence of many different optimal representations is due to the existence of many different inputs. The faithfulness constraints tie the success of an output candidate to the shape of the corresponding input; each faithfulness constraint asserts that an input and its output should be identical in a certain respect. For example, the constraint called PARSE asserts that every segment of the input must appear in the output: it penalizes deletion of material in the input-output mapping. (The French input-output pair (/pɛtit/, *pɛ.ti*) shows a violation of PARSE.) Another constraint, known as FILL, penalizes insertion of new mate-

‡ For consistency with the rest of the book, this chapter uses 'MARKEDNESS' in place of the term in the original article, 'STRUCTURE'.

rial that is not present in the input. Other constraints demand featural identity—one of these is violated when the English past tense suffix *d* is pronounced *t*. As with all constraints in the universal set, these constraints are violable, and much grammar turns on resolving the tension between markedness constraints, which favor simple structures, and the faithfulness constraints, which favor exact replication of the input, even at the cost of structural complexity.

As a general illustration of this relationship [developed in detail in Chapter 13], consider the confrontation between PARSE and NOCODA, which must play out in every language. These constraints are in conflict, because one way to avoid a closed syllable (thereby satisfying NOCODA) is to delete any consonant that would appear in syllable-final position (thereby violating PARSE, which forbids deletion). Consider first a grammar in which NOCODA dominates PARSE, which we will write as NOCODA ≫ PARSE. Syllabification is grammatically predictable and therefore need not be present in the input. Suppose a hypothetical unsyllabified input word /batak/ is submitted to this grammar for syllabification and pronunciation. A large range of syllabified candidate outputs (pronunciations) is to be evaluated, among which we find the faithful *ba.tak* and the progressively less faithful *ba.ta, bat, ba, b,* and *Ø* [silence], as well as *a.tak, tak, ak,* and many, many others. Observe that a very wide range of candidate output options is considered; it is the universal constraint set, ranked, that handles the bulk of the selection task.

Which of these candidates is optimal, by the hierarchy NOCODA ≫ PARSE? The faithful form *ba.tak,* which ends on a closed syllable, is ruled out by top-ranked NOCODA, because there are other competing output candidates that satisfy the constraint, lacking closed syllables. Among these, *ba.ta* is best—the most **harmonic**—because it involves the least violation of PARSE: a single deletion. It is therefore the optimal output for the given input: the grammar certifies the input-output pair (/batak/, *ba.ta*) as well formed: the final lexical *k* is unpronounced. The optimality computation just sketched can be represented conveniently in a **constraint tableau** as shown in Figure 1A. (For the sake of expositional simplicity, we are ignoring candidate outputs like *ba.ta.ki,* in which new material—the vowel *i*—appears at the end, resulting in a form that also avoids closed syllables successfully. Dealing with such forms involves ranking the anti-insertion constraint FILL with respect to PARSE; when FILL ≫ PARSE, deletion rather than insertion is optimal.) We conclude that in a language where NOCODA ≫ PARSE, all syllables must be open: for any output candidate with a closed syllable, there is always a better competitor that lacks it.

Consider now a grammar in which, contrariwise, we have PARSE ≫ NOCODA (see Figure 1B). Given the input /batak/, we have exactly the same set of output candidates to consider, since the candidate set is determined by universal principles. But now the one violation of PARSE in *ba.ta* is fatal; instead, its competitor *ba.tak,* which has no losses, will be optimal. (In the full analysis, we set FILL ≫ NOCODA as well, eliminating insertion as an option.) The dominance of the relevant faithfulness constraints ensures that the input will be faithfully reproduced, even at the cost of violating the markedness constraint NoCoda. This language is therefore one like English in which syllables will have codas, if warranted by the input.

Figure 1. Constraint tableaux in Optimality Theory

A

/batak/			NoCoda	Parse
a.		*ba.tak*	*!	
b.	☞	*ba.ta*		*
c.		*bat*	*!	* *
d.		*ba*		* *! *

B

/batak/			Parse	NoCoda
a.	☞	*ba.tak*		*
b.		*ba.ta*	*!	
c.		*bat*	*! *	*
d.		*ba*	*! **	

The table in A displays the optimality computation in graphic form. The input is listed at the head of the first column and (selected) output candidates occupy the cells below it. The constraints in the hierarchy are listed in domination order left to right across the first row. Other rows show the evaluation of a candidate with respect to the constraint hierarchy. The hand points to the optimal candidate. An asterisk indicates a constraint violation. The number of asterisks in a cell corresponds to the number of times the constraint is violated: for example, there are three asterisks in the Parse cell of row (d) because the input-output pair (/batak/, *ba*) involves three instances of nonparsing or deletion of segments. The exclamation point marks a fatal violation—one that ensures suboptimal status. Cells after the fatal violation are shaded, indicating that success or failure on the constraint heading that column is irrelevant to the optimality status of the candidate, which has already been determined by a higher-ranked constraint. In this example, which recapitulates the discussion of the minigrammar NoCoda ≫ Parse in the text, the interaction of just two constraints is depicted, and only a small sampling of the candidate set is shown. Given this ranking, the word /batak/ would be pronounced *bata*, as in the optimal candidate (b). Tableau B shows the effect of reranking: in a different language, in which Parse ≫ NoCoda, candidate (a) would be optimal; /batak/ would therefore be pronounced *batak*.

Domination is clearly **strict** in these examples: no matter how many consonant clusters appear in an input, and no matter how many consonants appear in any cluster, the first grammar will demand that they all be simplified by deletion (violating Parse as much as is required to eliminate the occasion for syllable codas) and the second grammar will demand that they all be syllabified (violating NoCoda as much as is necessary). No amount of failure on the violated constraints is rejected as excessive, as long as failure serves the cause of obtaining success on the dominating constraint.

Constraint interaction becomes far more intricate when crucial ranking goes to a depth of three or more; it is not unusual for optimal forms to contain violations of many constraints. OT research in syllable structure expands both the set of relevant markedness constraints and the set of faithfulness constraints that ban relevant disparities between input and output. The set of all possible rankings provides a restrictive typology of syllable structure patterns that closely matches the basic empirical findings in the area, and even refines prior classifications [Chapter 13]. Many other areas of phonology and syntax have been subject to detailed investigation under OT.[3] Here as elsewhere in cognitive science, progress has been accompanied by disputes at various levels, some technical, others concerning fundamental matters. The results obtained to date, however, provide considerable evidence that optimization ideas in general and OT in particular can lead to significant advances in resolving the central problems of linguistic theory.

3 Optimality Theory and Neural Network Theory

The principal empirical questions addressed by OT, as by other theories of universal grammar, concern the characterization of linguistic forms in and across languages. A quite different question is, can we explicate at least some of the properties of OT itself on the basis of more fundamental cognitive principles? A significant first step toward such an explanation, we will argue, derives from the theory of computation in neural networks.

Linguistic research employing OT does not, of course, involve explicit neural network modeling of language. The relationship we seek to identify between OT and neural computation must be of the type that holds between higher-level and lower-level systems of analysis in the physical sciences [Figure 1:2]. For example, statistical mechanics explains significant parts of thermodynamics from the hypothesis that matter is composed of molecules, but the concepts of thermodynamic theory, like temperature and entropy, involve no reference whatever to molecules. Like thermodynamics, OT is a self-contained higher-level theory; like statistical mechanics, we claim, neural computation ought to explain fundamental principles of the higher-level theory by deriving them as large-scale consequences of interactions at a much lower level. Just as probabilistic systems of point particles in statistical mechanics give rise to nonprobabilistic equations governing bulk continuous media in thermodynamics, so too should the numerical, continuous optimization in neural networks give rise to a qualitatively different formal system at a higher level of analysis: the

[3] Examples include segmental repertories, stress patterns, vowel harmony, tonology, reduplicative and templatic morphology, syntax-phonology and morphology-phonology relations, case and voice patterns, principles of question formation, interaction of syntactic movement and clause patterns, structure of verbal complexes, order and repertory of clitic elements, the interaction between focus and the placement and retention of pronominal elements, the interpretation of anaphoric relations, the nature of constraints like the Obligatory Contour Principle, and the compatibility of related grammatical processes. [See Part III.] Readers interested in pursuing any of these topics may consult the Rutgers Optimality Archive at http://roa.rutgers.edu/, which includes many papers and an extensive bibliography.

nonnumerical optimization over discrete symbolic representations—the markedness calculus—of OT.

To make contact with the abstract level at which mental organization like that of grammar resides, the relevant concepts of neural computation must capture rather high-level properties (Pinker and Prince 1988; Smolensky 1988; McCloskey 1992; Prince 1993). Because of the complexity and nonlinearity of general neural network models, such concepts are in short supply; one of the few available is the method of **Lyapunov functions.** A Lyapunov function assigns a number to each possible global state of the dynamical system in such a way that as the system changes state over time, the value of the function continually increases. Lyapunov functions have been identified for a variety of model neural networks and given various names, the term **energy function** being the most popular (Hopfield 1982, 1984; Cohen and Grossberg 1983; Hinton and Sejnowski 1983; Smolensky 1983; Golden 1988; for recent review articles, see Hirsch 1996, Smolensky 1996a [and Chapter 9]). We will use the term **Harmony function** since the work we discuss follows most directly along the path initiated in Harmony Theory (Smolensky 1986).

In the particular class of model neural networks admitting a Harmony function, the input to a network computation consists of an activation pattern held fixed over part of the network. Activation then flows through the net to construct a pattern of activity that maximizes—optimizes—Harmony, among all those patterns of activity that include the fixed input pattern [ICS principle P_3: HMax; Chapter 2 (5)]. The Harmony of a pattern of activation is a measure of its degree of conformity to the constraints implicit in the network's "synapses" or **connections.** As illustrated in Figure 2A–C, an inhibitory connection between two model "neurons" or **units,** modeled as a negative weight, embodies a constraint that when one of the units is active, the other should be inactive: this is the activation configuration that maximizes Harmony at that connection. An excitatory connection, modeled as a positive weight, embodies the constraint that when one of the units is active, the other should be active as well. In a complex, densely interconnected network of units, such constraints typically conflict; and connections with greater numerical magnitude embody constraints of greater importance to the outcome. A complete pattern of activation that maximizes Harmony is one that optimally balances the typically conflicting demands of all the constraints in the network.

An activity pattern can be understood as a representation of the information that it constitutes; the Harmony of any activity pattern measures the well-formedness of that representation with respect to the constraint system embodied in the connection weights. For a fixed input, a Harmony-maximizing network produces the output it does because that is the most well-formed representation containing the input. The knowledge contained in the network is the set of constraints embodied in its synaptic connections, or equivalently, the Harmony function these constraints define. This knowledge can be used in different ways during processing, by fixing input activity in different parts of the network and then letting activation flow to maximize Harmony: see Figure 2D.

Figure 1

Figure 2. Harmony maximization in a neural network

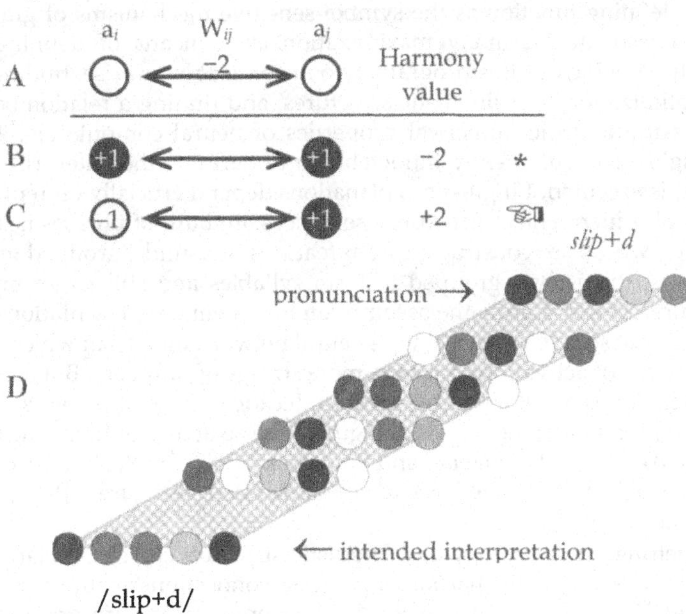

The basic Harmony function for a neural network is simply $H = \Sigma_{\alpha\beta}\, a_\alpha W_{\alpha\beta} a_\beta$, where a_α is the activation of unit (abstract neuron) α and $W_{\alpha\beta}$ is the strength or weight of the connection to unit α from unit β. In A, units α and β are connected with a weight of −2: this inhibitory connection constitutes a constraint that if one of these units is active, the other should be inactive. The microactivity pattern shown in B violates this constraint (marked '*'): both units have activity +1, and the constraint violation is registered in the negative Harmony $a_\alpha W_{\alpha\beta} a_\beta = (+1)(-2)(+1) = -2$. The activity pattern in C satisfies the constraint, with Harmony +2. Of these two micropatterns, the second maximizes Harmony, as indicated by the hand. In a network containing many units, the Harmony of a complete activity pattern is just the sum of all the micro-Harmonies computed from each pair of connected units.

In D, a hypothetical network is depicted for relating English phonological inputs and outputs. The topmost units contain a pattern for the pronunciation *slipt* 'slipped'; the units at the bottom host a pattern for the corresponding interpretation /slip+d/. In between, units support a pattern of activity representing the full linguistic structure, including syllables, stress feet, and so on. The connections in the network encode the constraints of English phonology. When the pattern for /slip+d/ is imposed on the lowest units, activation flows to maximize Harmony, giving rise to the pattern for *slipt* on the uppermost units: this is production-directed processing. In comprehension, the pattern for *slipt* is imposed on the uppermost units, and Harmony maximization fills in the rest of the total pattern, including the interpretation /slip+d/.

Because the Harmony function for a neural network performs the same well-formedness-defining function as the symbol-sensitive mechanisms of grammar, it is natural to investigate Harmony maximization as a means of defining linguistic grammars. In carrying out this program, two major problems arise: finding a suitable notion of optimization over linguistic structures, and finding a relation between this abstract measure and the numerical properties of neural computation. The second problem might seem sufficiently intractable to undermine the enterprise, no matter how the first is executed. Linguistic explanations depend crucially on representations that are complex hierarchical structures: sentences are built of phrases nested one inside the other; words are constructed from features of sounds, grouped to form phonetic segments, themselves grouped to form syllables and still larger units of prosodic structure. At first glance, the assumption that mental representations have such structure does not seem compatible with neural network models in which representations are patterns of activation—vectors, mere strings of numbers. But a family of interrelated techniques developed over the past decade show that patterns of activation can possess a precise mathematical analogue of the structure of linguistic representations (Pike 1984; Dolan 1989; Dolan and Smolensky 1989; Smolensky 1990; Plate 1994 [and Chapters 5, 7, and 8]): the basic idea is illustrated in Figure 3 [ICS principle P_1: Rep_{ICS}, Chapter 2 (1)–(2)].

In this setting, the Harmony of a linguistic structure is just the Harmony of the pattern of activity realizing that structure. The connections in the network define which linguistic structures have maximal Harmony—which are grammatical. This directly suggests the notion of **Harmonic Grammar**, in which a grammar is a set of 'soft' or violable constraints on combinations of linguistic elements, each constraint having a numerical strength (Legendre, Miyata, and Smolensky 1990a, b) [Chapter 2 (6); Chapters 6, 10, 11, and 20]. This strength is the quantity by which the Harmony of a linguistic representation is diminished when the constraint is violated. Through an activation-passing computation implementing maximization of the Harmony function, the strengths determine which constraints are respected, and to what degree, whenever there is conflict; a grammatical structure is then one that best satisfies the total set of constraints defining the grammar, that is, has maximal Harmony.

This conception is straightforward, but obviously incomplete, for it is far from true that every weighting of the set of linguistic constraints produces a possible human language. To delimit the optimizing function narrowly enough, the strength relation between constraints must be severely regimented [Chapter 20]. And this is exactly what strict domination provides: in OT, no amount of success on weaker constraints can compensate for failure on a stronger one. This corresponds to the numerical strength of a constraint being much greater than the strengths of those constraints ranked lower than it in the hierarchy; so much so that the combined force of all the lower-ranked constraints can never exceed the force of the higher-ranked constraint. But as we have seen, strict domination means constraint interaction in grammar is highly restricted: only the relative ranking of constraints, and not particular numerical strengths, can be grammatically relevant. The grammatical consequence is

Figure 2

that, in many cases studied to date, the set of all rankings delimits a narrow typology of possible linguistic patterns and relationships.

Figure 3. Realizing structured representations as patterns of activity in neural networks

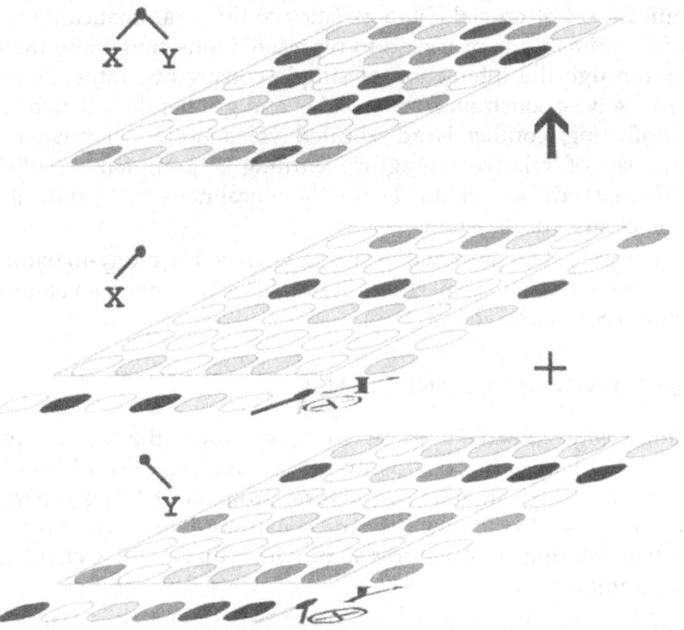

The top plane shows a pattern of activity **p** realizing the structure

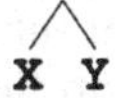

(e.g., a sentence in which **X** is the noun-phrase subject *big dogs* and **Y** a verb-phrase predicate *bite*); gray levels schematically indicate the activity levels of units in a neural network (circles). This pattern is produced by superimposing a pattern **x** realizing **X** in the left position (middle plane) on another pattern **y** realizing **Y** in the right position (bottom plane). Within the middle plane, the pattern **x** is a pattern **X** for **X** (right edge) times a pattern **r/** for 'left position' (bottom edge). The product operation here is the **tensor product** (⊗): in **x**, the activity level of the unit in row α and column β is just the activation of unit α in **X** times the activation of unit β in **r/**; and analogously for pattern **y**. Algebraically:

$$\mathbf{p} = \mathbf{x} + \mathbf{y};\ \mathbf{x} = \mathbf{X} \otimes \mathbf{r}/;\ \mathbf{y} = \mathbf{Y} \otimes \mathbf{r}\backslash;\ [\mathbf{x}]_{\alpha\beta} = [\mathbf{X}]_{\alpha}[\mathbf{r}/]_{\beta};\ [\mathbf{y}]_{\alpha\beta} = [\mathbf{Y}]_{\alpha}[\mathbf{r}\backslash]_{\beta}.$$

Since tensor products may be nested one inside the other, patterns may realize structures embedded in other structures. Through simple neural network operations, massively parallel structure manipulation may be performed on such patterns.

That strict domination governs grammatical constraint interaction is not currently explained by principles of neural computation; nor do these principles explain the universality of constraints that is central to OT and related approaches. These are stimulating challenges for fully integrating OT with a neural foundation. But the hypothesis that grammar is realized in a Harmony-maximizing neural network rationalizes a significant set of crucial characteristics of OT: grammaticality is optimality; competition for optimality is restricted to representations containing the input; complexity arises through the interaction of simple constraints, rather than within the constraints themselves; constraints are violable and gradiently satisfiable; constraints are highly conflicting; conflict is adjudicated via a notion of relative strength; a grammar is a set of relative strengths; learning a grammar is adjusting these strengths. OT's markedness calculus is exactly neural network optimization, specialized to the case of strict domination.

If the hypothesis that grammar is realized in a Harmony-maximizing neural network is correct, we would expect that it would lead to new developments in OT. We now turn to recent such work.

4 LINGUISTIC KNOWLEDGE AND ITS USE

Just as a numerically valued Harmony function orders the activity patterns in a model neural network from highest to lowest Harmony, so the ranking of constraints of an OT grammar orders linguistic structures from most to least harmonic: from those that best to those that least satisfy the constraint hierarchy. It is the constraint ranking and the ordering of structures it provides that is OT's characterization of knowledge of grammar.

Using this knowledge involves finding the structures that maximize Harmony, and this can be done in several ways (Tesar and Smolensky 1998a, b), directly following the lead of the corresponding neural network conception depicted in Figure 2. Use of grammatical knowledge for comprehending language involves taking the pronunciation of, say, a sentence and finding the maximum-Harmony linguistic structure with that pronunciation [Chapter 19]. This structure groups the given words into nested phrases and fills in implied connections between words, such as the possible interpretive link between *John* and *him* in *John hopes George admires him* (*him* = *John*), and the necessary antilink in *John admires him* (*him* ≠ *John*). The maximum-Harmony structure projected from the pronounced sentence by the grammar plays an important role in determining its meaning.

Producing a sentence is a different use of the very same grammatical knowledge. Now the competition is among structures that differ in pronunciation, but share a given interpretation. The ordering of structures from most to least harmonic constitutes grammatical knowledge that is separate from its use, via optimization, in comprehension and production; this is depicted schematically in Figure 4.

This view leads to a new perspective on a classic problem in child language. It is well known that, broadly speaking, young children's linguistic abilities in compre-

Figure 3

hension greatly exceed their abilities in production. Observe that this is a richer problem than many perception-action disparities—for example, we can recognize a violin without being able to play one—because real language comprehension requires sophisticated grammatical knowledge. In many cases, both the comprehension and production abilities can be captured by grammars, the "comprehension grammar" being closer to the adults' than is the "production grammar." Yet a grammar is usually seen as a characterization of linguistic competence independent of the cognitive factors involved in language use—so how can a child have two grammars, one for each type of use?

Figure 4. Knowledge versus use of grammar in Optimality Theory

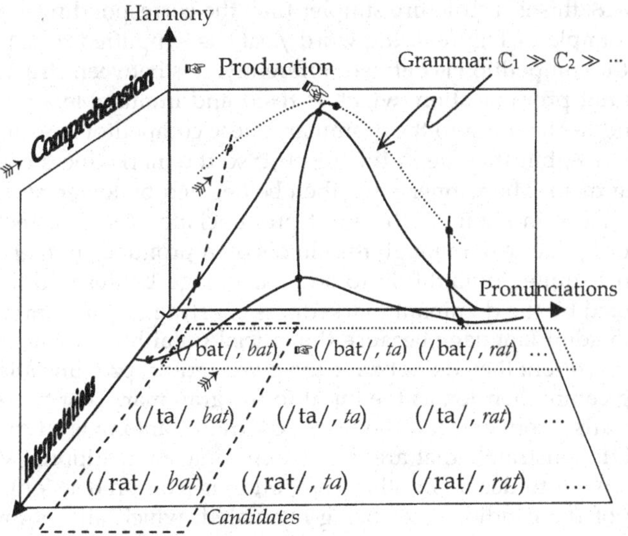

The pair (/bat/, *ta*) represents a structure in which the lexical item /bat/ is simplified and pronounced *ta.* The horizontal plane contains all such structures, and the vertical axis shows the relative Harmony of each structure, an ordinal rather than a numerical scale. This Harmony surface schematically depicts a young child's knowledge of grammar: MARKEDNESS dominates FAITHFULNESS. This knowledge can be used by optimization in two ways. In production of 'bat', the structures containing /bat/ compete (dotted box); the maximum-Harmony structure best satisfies top-ranked MARKEDNESS with the simplified pronunciation *ta* (peak of the dotted curve): this is marked ☞. In comprehension, the pronunciation *bat* is given, and competition is between the structures containing *bat* (dashed box). Since these are all pronounced *bat,* they tie with respect to MARKEDNESS; so lower-ranked FAITHFULNESS determines the maximum-Harmony structure to be (/bat/, *bat*), marked with ➳ (peak of the dashed curve). Correct comprehension results from the same grammar that gives incorrect—simplified—production.

OT provides a conceptual resolution of this dilemma (Smolensky 1996b). The child has only one grammar (constraint ranking) at a given time, a grammar that is evolving toward the adult grammar by reranking of constraints. Early child grammars have an interesting property: when used for production, only the simplest linguistic structures are produced. But when used for comprehension, the same grammar allows the child to cope rather well with structures much more complex than those she can produce.

The reason is essentially this. In early child grammars, markedness constraints outrank faithfulness constraints [Chapters 17 and 18]. In production, the input is an interpretation, and what competes are different pronunciations of the given interpretation. The winner is a structure that sacrifices faithfulness to the input in order to satisfy MARKEDNESS: this is a structure simpler than the corresponding adult pronunciation. (In the example of Figure 4, the word /bat/ is simplified to *ta*.) But during comprehension, the competition is defined differently: it is between structures that all *share* the given adult pronunciation, which is fixed and immutable, under the comprehension regime, as the input to the grammar. These competitors are all heavy violators of MARKEDNESS, but they tie in this respect; so the markedness constraints do not decide among them. The winner must then be decided by lower-ranked faithfulness constraints. (Thus, in Figure 4, the adult pronunciation *bat* is correctly comprehended as the word /bat/ even though the child's own pronunciation of /bat/ is *ta*.) Thus, production is quite "unfaithful" to adult language because faithfulness constraints are outvoted by the dominant markedness constraints. But comprehension is more "faithful" to adult language because the crucial unfaithful candidates are simply out of the competition: they do not have the given (adult) pronunciation, which is held fixed during comprehension as the input to the grammar. That two such different outcomes can arise from one and the same constraint ranking is a typical effect of optimization in OT: constraints that are decisive in some competitions (MARKEDNESS during production) fail to decide in other competitions (comprehension), depending on the character of the candidate set being evaluated, which allows lower-ranked constraints (FAITHFULNESS) to then determine the optimal structure.

This result resolves several related difficulties of two previous conceptions of child language. In the first, a grammar is a set of rules for sequentially transforming structures, ultimately producing the correct pronunciation of a given expression. This conception fails to adequately separate knowledge and use of grammar, so that a set of rules producing correct pronunciations is incapable of operating in the reverse direction, comprehension, transforming a pronunciation into an interpretation. (Even if the rule system could be inverted, children's "unfaithful production" and relatively "faithful comprehension" are simply not inverses of one another—the challenge is to provide a principled account for this divergence with a single grammar.) Furthermore, child grammars in this conception are typically considerably more complex than adult grammars, because many more transformations must be made in order to produce the "unfaithful" distortions characteristic of child productions.

In the second non-optimization-based conception, a grammar is a set of inviola-

Figure 4

ble constraints: a structure that violates any one of the constraints is ipso facto ungrammatical. Languages differ in the values of certain **parameters** that modify the content or applicability of constraints. Thus, the gap between child linguistic production and comprehension must be seen as resulting from two different sets of parameters, one for each type of use. Again, this fails to separate knowledge from use of grammar, and fails to provide any principled link between production and comprehension. By contrast, conceiving of grammar as optimization provides a natural distinction between use and knowledge of language, in such a way that a single grammar naturally provides relatively "faithful" comprehension at the same time as relatively "unfaithful" production.

The optimization perspective also offers a principled approach to a vexing fundamental problem in grammar learning. The constraints of a grammar refer to many hidden properties of linguistic structures, properties that are not directly observable in the data available for learning a language. For example, the way that words are grouped into nested syntactic phrases, or sounds grouped into prosodic constituents, is largely unobservable (or only ambiguously and inconsistently reflected in observables), and yet can differ from language to language. Learning a grammar requires access to this hidden linguistic structure, so that the grammar may be adjusted to conform to the configurations of hidden structure characteristic of the language being learned. But the hidden structure itself must be inferred from prior knowledge of the grammar: it cannot be directly observed.

Within OT, these coupled problems can be solved by successive approximation, as in related optimization problems outside grammar. The learner starts with an initial grammar (indeed, the early child grammar mentioned above). This grammar is used in the comprehension direction to impute hidden structure to the pronounced data of the target language. This hidden structure will initially be in error, because the grammar is not yet correct; but this structure can nonetheless be used to adjust the grammar so that, in the production direction, it outputs the inferred structures. With this revised grammar, the process continues with new learning data. As the grammar gets closer to the correct one, the hidden structure it assigns to learning data gets closer to the correct structure. While there are as yet no mathematical results demonstrating the success of this incremental learning method under general conditions, it has proved quite effective in related optimization problems such as speech recognition (Baum and Petrie 1966, Bahl, Jelinek, and Mercer 1983; for recent review articles, see Nádas and Mercer 1996, Smolensky 1996c); it has also performed quite successfully in preliminary computer simulation studies of OT grammar learning (Tesar 1997).

The central subproblem of this incremental learning strategy is this: given learning data including hidden structure (inferred on the basis of the current grammar), how can the grammar be improved? Here OT's optimization characterization of universal grammar provides considerable power. The grammars of human languages differ, according to the core hypothesis of OT, only in the way they rank the universal constraints. Thus, improving a grammar requires only reranking the constraints.

Given a grammatical structure from the language to be learned, there is a straightforward way to minimally rerank constraints to make that structure optimal, hence grammatical, in the revised grammar. And this procedure can be proved to efficiently converge on a correct grammar, when one exists. 'Efficient' here means that, even though there are $n!$ different constraint rankings of n universal constraints, no more than $n(n-1)$ informative learning examples are needed to converge on the correct ranking (Tesar and Smolensky 1993, 1998a). Corresponding results are not available within alternative general theories of how human grammars may differ: this is an indication of the learnability advantage arising from the highly structured nature of OT's optimization characterization of universal grammar [Chapter 12].

Will the connection between optimization in grammatical theory and optimization in neural networks lead to further progress at either level of cognitive theory? Will other theoretical connections between the sciences of the brain and of the mind prove fruitful? Of course, only time will tell. But we believe there is already in place a significant body of evidence that even a single high-level property of neural computation, properly treated, can yield a surprisingly rich set of new insights into even the most well-studied and abstract of symbol-processing cognitive sciences, the theory of grammar.[4]

[4] As indicated in the cited publications, much of the work discussed here is joint with our collaborators Géraldine Legendre, John McCarthy, and Bruce Tesar; we are most grateful to them and our colleagues Luigi Burzio, Robert Frank, Jane Grimshaw, and Colin Wilson for many stimulating conversations and invaluable contributions. For support of the work presented here, we acknowledge a Guggenheim Fellowship, the Johns Hopkins Center for Language and Speech Processing, and NSF grants BS-9209265 and IRI-9213894.

Figure 4

References

ROA = Rutgers Optimality Archive, http://roa.rutgers.edu

Archangeli, D., and D. Pulleyblank. 1994. *Grounded Phonology*. MIT Press.

Bahl, L. R., F. Jelinek, and R. L. Mercer. 1983. A maximum likelihood approach to continuous speech recognition. *IEEE Transactions on Pattern Analysis and Machine Intelligence* 5, 179–90.

Baum, L. E., and T. Petrie. 1966. Statistical inference for probabilistic functions of finite state Markov chains. *Annals of Mathematical Statistics* 37, 1559–63.

Benua, L. 1995. Output-output faithfulness. In *University of Massachusetts occasional papers in linguistics 18: Papers in Optimality Theory*, eds. J. Beckman, L. Walsh Dickey, and S. Urbanczyk. Graduate Linguistic Student Association, University of Massachusetts at Amherst. ROA 60.

Burzio, L. 1994. *Principles of English stress*. Cambridge University Press.

Bybee, J., and D. Slobin. 1982. Rules and schemas in the development and use of the English past tense. *Language* 58, 265–89.

Chomsky, N. 1965. *Aspects of the theory of syntax*. MIT Press.

Chomsky, N. 1981. *Lectures on government and binding*. Foris.

Chomsky, N. 1995. *The Minimalist Program*. MIT Press.

Chomsky, N., and M. Halle. 1968. *The sound pattern of English*. MIT Press.

Cohen, M. A., and S. Grossberg. 1983. Absolute stability of global pattern formation and parallel memory storage by competitive neural networks. *IEEE Transactions on Systems, Man, and Cybernetics* 13, 815–25.

Dolan, C. P. 1989. Tensor manipulation networks: Connectionist and symbolic approaches to comprehension, learning, and planning. Ph.D. diss., UCLA.

Dolan, C. P., and P. Smolensky. 1989. Tensor product production system: A modular architecture and representation. *Connection Science* 1, 53–68.

Golden, R. M. 1988. A unified framework for connectionist systems. *Biological Cybernetics* 59, 109–20.

Goldsmith, J. A. 1993. *The last phonological rule*. University of Chicago Press.

Grimshaw, J. 1997. Projection, heads, and optimality. *Linguistic Inquiry* 28, 373–422.

Hinton, G. E., and T. J. Sejnowski. 1983. Optimal perceptual inference. In *Proceedings of the IEEE Computer Society Conference on Computer Vision and Pattern Recognition*.

Hirsch, M. W. 1996. Dynamical systems. In *Mathematical perspectives on neural networks*, eds. P. Smolensky, M. C. Mozer, and D. E. Rumelhart. Erlbaum.

Hopfield, J. J. 1982. Neural networks and physical systems with emergent collective computational abilities. *Proceedings of the National Academy of Sciences USA* 79, 2554–8.

Hopfield, J. J. 1984. Neurons with graded response have collective computational properties like those of two-state neurons. *Proceedings of the National Academy of Sciences USA* 81, 3088–92.

Jakobson, R. 1962. *Selected writings I: Phonological studies*. Mouton.

Kisseberth, C. 1970. On the functional unity of phonological rules. *Linguistic Inquiry* 1, 291–306.

Legendre, G., Y. Miyata, and P. Smolensky. 1990a. Harmonic Grammar—a formal multi-level connectionist theory of linguistic well-formedness: An application. In *Proceedings of the Cognitive Science Society* 12.

Legendre, G., Y. Miyata, and P. Smolensky. 1990b. Harmonic Grammar—a formal multi-level connectionist theory of linguistic well-formedness: Theoretical foundations. In *Proceedings of the Cognitive Science Society* 12.

Legendre, G., W. Raymond, and P. Smolensky. 1993. An optimality-theoretic typology of case and grammatical voice systems. In *Proceedings of the Berkeley Linguistics Society 19*. ROA 3.

Legendre, G., P. Smolensky, and C. Wilson. 1998. When is less more? Faithfulness and minimal links in *wh*-chains. In *Is the best good enough? Optimality and competition in syntax,* eds. P. Barbosa, D. Fox, P. Hagstrom, M. McGinnis, and D. Pesetsky. MIT Press and MIT Working Papers in Linguistics. ROA 117.

McCarthy, J. J., and A. Prince. 1986/1996. Prosodic morphology 1986. Technical report RuCCS-TR-32, Rutgers Center for Cognitive Science, Rutgers University

McCarthy, J. J., and A. Prince. 1993a. Generalized alignment. In *Yearbook of morphology,* eds. G. Booij and J. van Marle. Kluwer.

McCarthy, J. J., and A. Prince. 1993b. Prosodic Morphology I: Constraint interaction and satisfaction. Technical report RuCCS-TR-3, Rutgers Center for Cognitive Science, Rutgers University, and University of Massachusetts at Amherst. ROA 482, 2001.

McCarthy, J. J., and A. Prince. 1995. Faithfulness and reduplicative identity. In *University of Massachusetts occasional papers in linguistics 18: Papers in Optimality Theory,* eds. J. Beckman, L. Walsh Dickey, and S. Urbanczyk. Graduate Linguistic Student Association, University of Massachusetts at Amherst. ROA 60.

McCloskey, M. 1992. Networks and theories: The place of connectionism in cognitive science. *Psychological Science* 2, 387–95.

Nádas, A., and R. L. Mercer. 1996. Hidden Markov models. In *Mathematical perspectives on neural networks,* eds. P. Smolensky, M. C. Mozer, and D. E. Rumelhart. Erlbaum.

Perlmutter, D. M. 1971. *Deep and surface structure constraints in syntax.* Holt, Rinehart and Winston.

Perlmutter, D. M., ed. 1983. *Studies in Relational Grammar 1.* University of Chicago Press.

Pike, R. 1984. Comparison of convolution and matrix distributed memory systems for associative recall and recognition. *Psychological Review* 91, 281–94.

Pinker, S., and J. Mehler, eds. 1988. *Connections and symbols.* MIT Press.

Pinker, S., and A. Prince. 1988. On language and connectionism: Analysis of a parallel distributed processing model of language acquisition. *Cognition* 28, 73–193.

Plate, T. A. 1994. Distributed representations and nested compositional structure. Ph.D. diss., University of Toronto.

Prince, A. 1993. In defense of the number *i*: Anatomy of a linear dynamic model of linguistic generalizations. Technical report RuCCS-TR-1, Rutgers Center for Cognitive Science, Rutgers University.

Prince, A., and P. Smolensky. 1991. Notes on connectionism and Harmony Theory in linguistics. Technical report CU-CS-533-91, Computer Science Department, University of Colorado at Boulder.

Prince, A., and P. Smolensky. 1993/2004. *Optimality Theory: Constraint interaction in generative grammar.* Technical report, Rutgers University and University of Colorado at Boulder, 1993. ROA 537, 2002. Revised version published by Blackwell, 2004.

Rumelhart, D. E., and J. L. McClelland. 1986. On learning the past tenses of English verbs. In *Parallel distributed processing: Explorations in the microstructure of cognition.* Vol. 2, *Psychological and biological models,* J. L. McClelland, D. E. Rumelhart, and the PDP Research Group. MIT Press.

Samek-Lodovici, V. 1996. Constraints on subjects: An optimality theoretic analysis. Ph.D. diss., Rutgers University. ROA 148.

Smolensky, P. 1983. Schema selection and stochastic inference in modular environments. In *Proceedings of the National Conference on Artificial Intelligence 3.*

Smolensky, P. 1986. Information processing in dynamical systems: Foundations of Harmony Theory. In *Parallel distributed processing: Explorations in the microstructure of cognition.* Vol. 1, *Foundations,* D. E. Rumelhart, J. L. McClelland, and the PDP Research Group. MIT Press.

Smolensky, P. 1988. On the proper treatment of connectionism. *Behavioral and Brain Sciences* 11, 1–74.

Smolensky, P. 1990. Tensor product variable binding and the representation of symbolic structures in connectionist networks. *Artificial Intelligence* 46, 159–216.

Smolensky, P. 1996a. Dynamical perspectives on neural networks. In *Mathematical perspectives on neural networks*, eds. P. Smolensky, M. C. Mozer, and D. E. Rumelhart. Erlbaum.

Smolensky, P. 1996b. On the comprehension/production dilemma in child language. *Linguistic Inquiry* 27, 720–31. ROA 118.

Smolensky, P. 1996c. Statistical perspectives on neural networks. In *Mathematical perspectives on neural networks*, eds. P. Smolensky, M. C. Mozer, and D. E. Rumelhart. Erlbaum.

Stampe, D. 1979. A dissertation in Natural Phonology. Ph.D. diss., University of Chicago.

Tesar, B. B. 1997. An iterative strategy for learning metrical stress in Optimality Theory. In *Proceedings of the Boston University Conference on Language Development 21*. ROA 177.

Tesar, B. B., and P. Smolensky. 1993. The learnability of Optimality Theory: An algorithm and some basic complexity results. Technical report CU-CS-678-93, Computer Science Department, University of Colorado at Boulder. ROA 2.

Tesar, B. B., and P. Smolensky. 1998a. Learnability in Optimality Theory. *Linguistic Inquiry* 29, 229–68.

Tesar, B. B., and P. Smolensky. 1998b. Learning optimality-theoretic grammars. *Lingua* 106, 161–96.

Tranel, B. 1994. French liaison and elision revisited: A unified account within Optimality Theory. ROA 15.

Trubetzkoy, N. 1939/1969. *Principles of phonology* (translation of *Grundzüge der Phonologie)*. University of California Press.

Part II

Principles of the Integrated Connectionist/Symbolic Cognitive Architecture

The Integrated Connectionist/Symbolic Cognitive Architecture is defined by four basic principles that were introduced and motivated in Part I. In Part II, we articulate these principles into formal hypotheses, deducing their general implications and applying them to theoretical and empirical problems in cognitive science. Chapters 5 and 6 develop the technical hypotheses informally and intuitively, and summarize the rest of Part II. Chapter 5 introduces principles P_1–P_2 concerning distributed representation and processing; Chapter 6 introduces P_3–P_4 concerning optimization. Chapters 7–12 provide more formal definitions and more detailed analysis of implications, as well as some extensions and applications. Each of Chapters 7–11 may be read independently of the others, but Chapters 6–8 presume Chapter 5 and Chapters 9–11 presume Chapter 6. Chapters 7 and 8 provide more formal analysis and extensions of tensor product networks (principles P_1–P_2). Chapter 9 provides the formal analysis of Harmony maximization in neural networks (principle P_3). Harmonic Grammar, derived in Chapter 6, is applied in Chapters 10 and 11 to problems in formal language theory and natural language syntax/semantics, respectively. This leads to a systematic presentation of Prince and Smolensky's Optimality Theory (principle P_4) in Chapter 12. Development of Optimality Theory to unify multiple facets of the cognitive science of language is the topic of Part III.

5 Formalizing the Principles I: Representation and Processing in the Mind / Brain

Paul Smolensky

This chapter develops the first two principles of the Integrated Connectionist/Symbolic Cognitive Architecture (ICS), which relate representations and processing at the connectionist and symbolic levels (P_1: Rep_{ICS} and P_2: Proc_{ICS}). The formal heart of these principles is a mathematical equivalence between the fundamental objects and operations of symbolic computation and those of specially structured connectionist networks. A symbol structure corresponds to a structured vector—a list of activation values, a pattern of activity. Manipulation of symbol structures corresponds to connectionist processing of vectors by structured matrices—arrays of weights, patterns of connections. The concepts introduced in this chapter are fundamental to all of Parts II and IV. Situated in the ICS map sketched in Chapter 2, the topics are centered on ③ in Figure 4 (Rep_{ICS}) and ⑧ in Figure 7 (Proc_{ICS}).

Contents

The development of the Integrated Connectionist/Symbolic Cognitive Architecture (ICS) focuses on the search for principles with the properties enumerated in (1) (see Chapter 3 (1c), (3b)).

(1) Goals for ICS principles

a. *Integration.* Principles that integrate the connectionist and symbolic architectures 'vertically'—that is, across lower and higher levels of description

b. *Generality.* Principles that are sufficiently general to apply quite widely within and across higher cognitive domains

c. *Precision.* Principles that are—despite their generality—sufficiently precisely specified to advance the explanation, via formal analysis, of central properties of higher cognition

The principles of ICS were given initial formulation in Chapter 2. These principles lay out an approach to vertical integration and are quite general—but, as formulated in Chapter 2, they are too imprecise to entail any consequences. As discussed in some detail in Chapter 22, a principle-centered research program must be founded on principles that are sufficiently formally articulated to yield a rich set of entailments.

This chapter and the next formalize the ICS principles that will underlie the theoretical and empirical analyses in Chapters 7–23. As in Chapter 2, the discussion itself will be more intuitive than formal—but the subject will be the proper formal treatment of the principles. The first two sections of this chapter respectively address the first and second principles, P_1: Rep_{ICS} and P_2: $Proc_{ICS}$, developed in Chapter 2; the remaining two principles (P_3: HMax and P_4: OT) are taken up in Chapter 6. The first principle relates the lower-level description of mental representations as activation levels to the higher-level description of these representations as symbolic structures. This principle supports all the others and will therefore be developed slowly and in considerable detail. The remaining three principles will be discussed much more briefly in this chapter and the next and will be developed in later chapters (primarily Chapters 7–9, 11–12; see Table 2:1).

As remarked in Section 3:4.2, the formalizations of the ICS principles developed in this book are sufficiently general and precise to logically entail interesting cognitive consequences, but there is no doubt that improvements and alternatives can be developed: the current formulations are merely initial working hypotheses. Indeed, Chapter 7 develops some important extensions, formally connecting the principles as stated here with other proposals in the literature.

The third and final section of this chapter addresses the multilevel descriptions of cognition sought within the ICS research program. The formal structure of mental representations and processes laid out in the first two sections makes it possible to illustrate quite precisely the form of the various levels of ICS description.

The relevant mathematics is presented as needed in the text. These bits are collected and organized in Box 1, a concise summary that is necessarily rather dense; it is intended for reference or review, and not for instruction. (For introductory exposition, see for example Jordan 1986.) Exemplification and explication of the concepts are provided where relevant in the text of this chapter. Some of the applications to connectionist networks of the constructs of Box 1 are identified in Box 2. *No familiarity with these concepts is assumed*: all are explained in the text at the appropriate points in the chapter.

Box 1. Vectors and matrices: Linear algebra

Pattern of activity is formalized as **activation vector.** Vectors are designated with bold-faced roman letters in the metalanguage used in this book. Figure 1 in Section 1.1 shows four useful ways of conceiving of the activation vector: as a list of n numbers or **components—activation values**; as a point or arrow in an n-dimensional **activation space**; as n circles representing n network units with different shading (or size) symbolizing different activation levels; and as a graph with n points—an activity wave or pattern.

An activation vector is **local** if only a single unit is active at a time: every component of the activation vector is 0, except the one corresponding to the single active unit, which is (conventionally) 1. An activation vector that is not local is **distributed.** If each member of a set of entities, S, is represented by a different local vector, we have a **local representation** of S. If more than one unit is active in a pattern representing an entity in S, and some units are active in the representation of more than one entity, then we have a **distributed representation.**

The basic category of analysis is the **vector space** V, a set of vectors with a crucial property: for any two vectors **a** and **b** in V and any real number (or **scalar**) c, the vectors $\mathbf{a} + \mathbf{b}$ and $c\mathbf{a}$ are also in V. The fundamental vector space operations of addition and scalar multiplication can be defined either **constructively** or **axiomatically**. The constructive approach is spelled out in (1).

(1) The n-dimensional real vector space $V \equiv \mathbb{R}^n$ is the set of all ***n*-tuples** of real numbers. Such an n-tuple is specified by n real numbers, each having a distinct address or tag—usually 1, 2, …, n, although it is sometimes convenient to choose a different tag set of n values. The real numbers constituting a vector are called its **components** or its **elements.** The component with tag k of a vector **a** is written $[\mathbf{a}]_k$ or a_k, and **a** is customarily written $(a_1, a_2, \ldots, a_n)$—simply a list of n real numbers. Suppose $\mathbf{a} = (a_1, a_2, \ldots, a_n)$ and $\mathbf{b} = (b_1, b_2, \ldots, b_n)$ are any two vectors in V, and c is any real number. Then define

a. $\mathbf{a} + \mathbf{b} \equiv (a_1 + b_1, a_2 + b_2, \ldots, a_n + b_n)$ **vector addition** (or **superposition**);

b. $c\mathbf{a} \equiv (ca_1, ca_2, \ldots, ca_n)$ **scalar-vector multiplication;**

c. $\mathbf{0} \equiv (0, 0, \ldots, 0)$ the **zero vector.**

From these definitions, it is easy to show that the properties in (2) hold.

(2) Let **a** and **b** be any vectors in V, and c any real number. Then the following expressions denote other vectors in V that satisfy the following equations:

a. $\mathbf{a}+\mathbf{b} = \mathbf{b}+\mathbf{a}$; $(\mathbf{a}+(\mathbf{b}+\mathbf{c})) = ((\mathbf{a}+\mathbf{b})+\mathbf{c})$;

b. $c(\mathbf{a}+\mathbf{b}) = c\mathbf{a}+c\mathbf{b}$; $(c+d)\,\mathbf{a} = c\mathbf{a}+d\mathbf{a}$; $c(d\mathbf{a}) = (cd)\mathbf{a}$; $1\mathbf{a} = \mathbf{a}$;

c. $\mathbf{a}+\mathbf{0} = \mathbf{a}$.

In the axiomatic (as opposed to the constructive) approach, a vector space is simply *defined* as any set V, with some operation denoted '+', some operation of scalar multiplication, and some element labeled '**0**', for which (2) holds. That is, the conditions in (2) constitute the axioms defining a vector space.

The n components of a vector can be represented in our metalanguage in many ways. It makes no difference whether their n addresses—n tag values—are denoted with a single subscript or multiple subscripts: in the latter case, the tag consists of multiple **indices**; each subscript denotes one index. Superscripts may be used in place of subscripts when convenient. It also does not matter whether the elements of a vector are displayed as a horizontal row or vertical column or two-dimensional array. In this book, the tags of vector components are often made up of multiple indices, and the components of a vector are sometimes arranged in more than one dimension. The components may be separated typographically by commas, semicolons, or just white space, as convenient for a given expression. So if $n = 4$, the four elements of a vector **a** would typically be written (a_1, a_2, a_3, a_4), but they might also be written $(a_{00}, a_{01}; a_{10}, a_{11})$ or

(3) $$\begin{pmatrix} a_{00} & a_{01} \\ a_{10} & a_{11} \end{pmatrix}.$$

In the latter two notations, the tag of the vector, which takes on four values, consists of two indices, each taking on two values; a general element would be denoted $a_\alpha = a_{\alpha_1\alpha_2}$ where the indices α_1 and α_2 each take values in $\{0, 1\}$ and the tag α takes the four values $\{00, 01, 10, 11\}$. Superscripts may be used in place of subscripts: **a** (3) may be alternatively written $(a^0{}_0\ a^0{}_1\ a^1{}_0\ a^1{}_1)$, with general element $a_\alpha = a^{\alpha_1}{}_{\alpha_2}$.

A vector **b** is a **linear combination** of vectors $\mathbf{a}_1, \mathbf{a}_2, \ldots, \mathbf{a}_N$ iff **b** can be expressed as a weighted sum of the $\mathbf{a}_i$s—that is, iff there is a set of real numbers $c_1, c_2, \ldots, c_N$ for which (4) holds. (**Iff** abbreviates 'if and only if'. A Σ-expression denotes the sum of a collection of terms that differ only in the value of a specified variable; here, the variable i, which takes the values $1, 2, \ldots, N$.)

(4) $$\mathbf{b} = c_1\mathbf{a}_1 + c_2\mathbf{a}_2 + \cdots + c_N\mathbf{a}_N \equiv \sum_{i=1}^{N} c_i\mathbf{a}_i\,.$$

A set of vectors $\{\mathbf{a}_1, \mathbf{a}_2, \ldots, \mathbf{a}_N\}$ is **linearly independent** iff none of them is a linear combination of the others. A vector space is ***n*-dimensional** iff there is a set of n linearly independent vectors, but no larger such set. (The vector space $\mathbb{R}^n$ of n-tuples of real numbers is n-dimensional in this sense.)

A collection $\mathcal{A} = \{\mathbf{a}_i\}$ of n linearly independent vectors in an n-dimensional vector space V is called a **basis** of V. Any vector **b** in V can be expressed in one and only one way as a linear combination of the basis vectors $\mathcal{A}$, as in (4). Each weight in this weighted sum—each c_i of (4)—is a **component of b with respect to** $\mathcal{A}$. The component c_1 depends not only on $\mathbf{a}_1$, but on all the other $\mathbf{a}_i$s as well.

It is often useful to define a notion of length in a vector space, as in (5).

(5) The **(Euclidean) length** or **(L_2) norm** or **magnitude** of a vector **a**, written $\|\mathbf{a}\|$

a. It is constructively defined as

$$\|\mathbf{a}\| \equiv \sqrt{(\mathrm{a}_1)^2 + (\mathrm{a}_2)^2 + \cdots + (\mathrm{a}_n)^2}\,.$$

b. Its properties are

$\|\mathbf{a}\| > 0$ if $\mathbf{a} \neq \mathbf{0}$; $\|c\mathbf{a}\| = |c|\,\|\mathbf{a}\|$; $\|\mathbf{a}+\mathbf{b}\| \leq \|\mathbf{a}\| + \|\mathbf{b}\|$.

(The last property is the **triangle inequality**.) These are the axioms for a vector space norm $\|\ \|$.

c. For any vector **a**, $\hat{\mathbf{a}} \equiv \mathbf{a}/\|\mathbf{a}\|$ has length 1; it is the **unit vector** defining the **direction** of **a**. A vector **a** is completely determined by the combination of its direction $\hat{\mathbf{a}}$ and its length $\|\mathbf{a}\|$: $\mathbf{a} = \|\mathbf{a}\|\,\hat{\mathbf{a}}$. A vector with length 1 is said to be **normalized**.

The **dot product** or **inner product** of two vectors **a** and **b**, $\mathbf{a}\cdot\mathbf{b}$, is constructively defined as in (6a). It is essentially the correlation between the two patterns defined by the vectors; it can be used to define the **similarity** of **a** and **b** as in (6b). If the vector components are all 0s and 1s, $\mathbf{a}\cdot\mathbf{b}$ is the number of units that are active in both patterns. Two vectors are **orthogonal** if they have zero similarity—zero correlation; geometrically, such vectors are perpendicular. With local representations, any two distinct representations are orthogonal.

(6) Dot or inner product of two vectors

a. $\mathbf{a}\cdot\mathbf{b} \equiv \mathrm{a}_1\mathrm{b}_1 + \mathrm{a}_2\mathrm{b}_2 + \cdots + \mathrm{a}_n\mathrm{b}_n \equiv \Sigma_\alpha\, \mathrm{a}_\alpha\, \mathrm{b}_\alpha$.

b. $sim(\mathbf{a}, \mathbf{b}) \equiv \mathbf{a}\cdot\mathbf{b}$.

c. $\mathbf{a}\cdot\mathbf{b} = \mathbf{b}\cdot\mathbf{a}$; $(c\mathbf{a})\cdot\mathbf{b} = c(\mathbf{a}\cdot\mathbf{b})$; $(\mathbf{a}_1+\mathbf{a}_2)\cdot\mathbf{b} = \mathbf{a}_1\cdot\mathbf{b} + \mathbf{a}_2\cdot\mathbf{b}$; $\mathbf{a}\cdot\mathbf{a} > 0$ iff $\mathbf{a}\neq\mathbf{0}$.

d. $\|\mathbf{a}\|^2 = \mathbf{a}\cdot\mathbf{a}$.

e. $\mathbf{b} = \mathbf{W}\cdot\mathbf{a}$ iff $\mathrm{b}_\alpha = \mathbf{w}_\alpha\cdot\mathbf{a}$ where $\mathbf{w}_\alpha$ is row α of matrix **W**.

f. $\mathbf{a}\cdot\mathbf{b} = \|\mathbf{a}\|\,[\|\mathbf{b}\|\cos\theta_{\mathbf{ab}}] = \|\mathbf{a}\|\,[\text{perpendicular projection of } \mathbf{b} \text{ onto } \mathbf{a}]$.

It is easy to verify that the dot product has the formal properties in (6c); these are the axioms defining the dot product in the axiomatic approach. And (6d–e) give useful connections among the dot product, vector length, and matrix-vector multiplication, defined shortly. (6f) gives the geometric interpretation of the dot product; $\theta_{\mathbf{ab}}$ is the angle between **a** and **b**; for illustrations, see Box 8:2.

The ith component of a vector **b** relative to a basis $\mathcal{A} \equiv \{\mathbf{a}_1, \ldots, \mathbf{a}_n\}$—the coefficient c_i in (4)—can be computed as the dot product of **b** with a vector $\mathbf{a}^+_i$:

(7) $c_i = \mathbf{b}\cdot\mathbf{a}^+_i$.

The set $\{\mathbf{a}^+_1, \ldots, \mathbf{a}^+_n\}$ is the basis **dual** to $\mathcal{A}$; its defining property is that

(8) $\mathbf{a}_j \cdot \mathbf{a}^+_k = \delta_{jk} \equiv [1 \text{ if } j = k, \text{ otherwise } 0]$.

The symbol δ is the **Kronecker δ**; it is frequently used and always has this definition. Like c_1, $\mathbf{a}^+_1$ depends on all $\mathbf{a}_i$, not just $\mathbf{a}_1$. Dual bases are extremely useful, thanks to (7).

An ***n*×*m* matrix W** is a set of real numbers labeled by a *pair* of tags, the first tag having *n* values, the second, *m* values. A matrix is usually displayed as a rectangular array of numbers, with *n* (horizontal) rows and *m* (vertical) columns; the number in the αth row and βth column is denoted $[\mathbf{W}]_{\alpha\beta}$ or $W_{\alpha\beta}$. But the elements of a matrix can also be depicted as a single list; the address of an element of this list consists of two tags. The two tags of a matrix may be separated by white space, by a delimiter like a comma or semicolon, or by nothing, according to typographical convenience. As with a vector, a tag of a matrix may consist of multiple indices; for example, if $n = 4$ and $m = 8$, the elements of the matrix might be written

$$[\mathbf{W}]_{\alpha_1\alpha_2,\,\beta_1\beta_2\beta_3}.$$

Here the first tag α consists of two indices $\alpha_1\alpha_2$, each having values 0 and 1, for a total of $n = 2^2 = 4$ values for α; β consists of three indices each with values in {0, 1}, yielding $m = 2^3 = 8$ values. **W** thus has 4 × 8 = 32 elements.

The **matrix-vector product** of an $n \times m$ matrix **W** and an *m*-dimensional vector **a** is the *n*-dimensional vector **b** defined in (9).

(9) $\mathbf{b} = \mathbf{W} \cdot \mathbf{a}$ iff, for all $\alpha = 1, 2, \ldots, n$,

$$[\mathbf{b}]_\alpha = [\mathbf{W}]_{\alpha 1}[\mathbf{a}]_1 + [\mathbf{W}]_{\alpha 2}[\mathbf{a}]_2 + \cdots + [\mathbf{W}]_{\alpha m}[\mathbf{a}]_m \equiv \sum_{\beta=1}^{m} [\mathbf{W}]_{\alpha\beta}[\mathbf{a}]_\beta .$$

The '·' explicitly marking this product (and the matrix-matrix product defined below) will sometimes be omitted, as is customary. If the tags of the vectors are multiple indices, the first and second tags of **W** must match the index structure of **a** and **b**, respectively. Note that if the vector $\mathbf{w}_\alpha$ is row α of **W**, (9) can be rewritten using the dot product, as stated in (6e):

(10) $b_\alpha = \mathbf{w}_\alpha \cdot \mathbf{a}$.

Matrix-vector multiplication obeys the following equations:

(11) $\mathbf{W} \cdot (\mathbf{a} + \mathbf{b}) = \mathbf{W} \cdot \mathbf{a} + \mathbf{W} \cdot \mathbf{b}$; $\mathbf{W} \cdot (c\mathbf{a}) = c\mathbf{W} \cdot \mathbf{a}$.

The function f defined by multiplication by **W** assigns to an input **a** the output $\mathbf{W} \cdot \mathbf{a}$. In virtue of (11), f meets the defining properties of a **linear transformation**:

(12) $f(\mathbf{a} + \mathbf{a}') = f(\mathbf{a}) + f(\mathbf{a}')$; $f(c\mathbf{a}) = c[f(\mathbf{a})]$.

The sum of two matrices **X** + **W**, multiplication of a matrix by a real number (scalar) *c*, and the zero matrix **0** are defined by (13a) so that (13b) holds.

(13) Addition and scalar multiplication of matrices; the zero matrix **0**

a. $[\mathbf{X} + \mathbf{W}]_{\alpha\beta} \equiv [\mathbf{X}]_{\alpha\beta} + [\mathbf{W}]_{\alpha\beta}$; $[c\mathbf{W}]_{\alpha\beta} \equiv c[\mathbf{W}]_{\alpha\beta}$; $[\mathbf{0}]_{\alpha\beta} \equiv 0$.

b. $[\mathbf{X}+\mathbf{W}]\cdot\mathbf{a}=\mathbf{X}\cdot\mathbf{a}+\mathbf{W}\cdot\mathbf{a};\ [c\mathbf{W}]\cdot\mathbf{a}=c[\mathbf{W}\cdot\mathbf{a}];\ \mathbf{W}+\mathbf{0}=\mathbf{W}.$

From the definitions (13a) it follows that the set of $n\times m$ matrices, $\mathcal{M}_{nm}$, has the properties defining a vector space (2): $\mathcal{M}_{nm}$ is itself a vector space (of dimension nm).

Multiplying any vector by the zero matrix gives the zero vector: $\mathbf{0}\cdot\mathbf{a}=\mathbf{0}$. There is also a matrix that acts like 1 under multiplication.

(14) Identity matrix $\mathbf{1}_n$ on an m-dimensional vector space V

a. Constructive definition: $[\mathbf{1}_m]_{\alpha\beta}\equiv\delta_{\alpha\beta};\ \ \alpha,\beta=1,2,\ldots,m.$

b. Axiom: $\mathbf{1}_m\cdot\mathbf{a}=\mathbf{a}$ for every $\mathbf{a}\in V$.

As always, δ in (14a) is the Kronecker δ (8).

The n-dimensional vector $\mathbf{b}=\mathbf{W}\cdot\mathbf{a}$ (where $\mathbf{W}$ is $n\times m$ and $\mathbf{a}$ is m-dimensional) can itself be multiplied by an $l\times n$ matrix $\mathbf{X}$. The result is the same as multiplying $\mathbf{a}$ by a single $l\times m$ matrix that is defined to be the **matrix product** $\mathbf{X}\cdot\mathbf{W}$. That is, the product of two matrices is defined as in (15a) in order to ensure (15b). (15c) also follows.

(15) Matrix multiplication

a. $$[\mathbf{X}\cdot\mathbf{W}]_{\alpha\beta}\equiv[\mathbf{X}]_{\alpha1}[\mathbf{W}]_{1\beta}+[\mathbf{X}]_{\alpha2}[\mathbf{W}]_{2\beta}+\cdots+[\mathbf{X}]_{\alpha m}[\mathbf{W}]_{m\beta}\equiv\sum_{\gamma=1}^{m}[\mathbf{X}]_{\alpha\gamma}[\mathbf{W}]_{\gamma\beta}.$$

b. $[\mathbf{X}\cdot\mathbf{W}]\cdot\mathbf{a}=\mathbf{X}\cdot[\mathbf{W}\cdot\mathbf{a}].$

c. $\mathbf{1}_n\cdot\mathbf{W}=\mathbf{W}=\mathbf{W}\cdot\mathbf{1}_m.$

In the matrix $\mathbf{X}\cdot\mathbf{W}$, the γth column is $\mathbf{X}\cdot\mathbf{w}_\gamma$, where $\mathbf{w}_\gamma$ is the γth column of $\mathbf{W}$. Equivalently, the element of $\mathbf{X}\cdot\mathbf{W}$ in row α and column γ is the dot product of row α of $\mathbf{X}$ with column γ of $\mathbf{W}$.

An $n\times1$ matrix $\mathbf{A}$ is traditionally called a **column vector** (although it is a matrix); it has the n components $[\mathbf{A}]_{\alpha1}$. Similarly, a $1\times m$ matrix is a **row vector**. For any vector $\mathbf{a}$, $\mathbf{A}$ will denote the corresponding column vector. If $\mathbf{W}\cdot\mathbf{a}=\mathbf{b}$ (matrix-vector multiplication (9)), then $\mathbf{W}\cdot\mathbf{A}=\mathbf{B}$ (matrix-matrix multiplication (15)). Thus, the distinction between $\mathbf{a}$ and $\mathbf{A}$ is customarily not marked typographically.

The **transpose** of a matrix is defined constructively as in (16a) in order to yield (16b). The definition implies the properties given in (16c–f).

(16) The transpose of a matrix $\mathbf{W}$, written $\mathbf{W}^{\mathrm{T}}$

a. Defined constructively by $[\mathbf{W}^{\mathrm{T}}]_{\alpha\beta}\equiv[\mathbf{W}]_{\beta\alpha}$; satisfies

b. $\mathbf{a}\cdot[\mathbf{W}\cdot\mathbf{b}]=[\mathbf{W}^{\mathrm{T}}\cdot\mathbf{a}]\cdot\mathbf{b}.$

c. $[\mathbf{W}\cdot\mathbf{X}]^{\mathrm{T}}=\mathbf{X}^{\mathrm{T}}\cdot\mathbf{W}^{\mathrm{T}};\ [\mathbf{W}+\mathbf{X}]^{\mathrm{T}}=\mathbf{W}^{\mathrm{T}}+\mathbf{X}^{\mathrm{T}};\ [c\mathbf{W}]^{\mathrm{T}}=c[\mathbf{W}^{\mathrm{T}}];\ [\mathbf{W}^{\mathrm{T}}]^{\mathrm{T}}=\mathbf{W}.$

d. If $\mathbf{U}$ is a column vector, then $\mathbf{U}^{\mathrm{T}}$ is the row vector with the same numerical components, and vice versa.

e. $\mathbf{a}\cdot\mathbf{b}=\mathbf{A}^{\mathrm{T}}\cdot\mathbf{B}$, where the left side is the dot product, the right side, the matrix-matrix product. (Recall that $\mathbf{A}$ and $\mathbf{B}$ are the column vectors—$n\times1$ matrices—with the same components as $\mathbf{a}$ and $\mathbf{b}$. This equation ignores the distinction between a single number, $\mathbf{a}\cdot\mathbf{b}$, and a 1×1 matrix, $\mathbf{A}^{\mathrm{T}}\cdot\mathbf{B}$.)

f. If $\mathbf{W} = \mathbf{B} \cdot \mathbf{A}^T$, then $\mathbf{W} \cdot \mathbf{x} = c\mathbf{b}$, where $c = \mathbf{A}^T \cdot \mathbf{X} = \mathbf{a} \cdot \mathbf{x} = sim(\mathbf{a}, \mathbf{x})$.

The result in (16f) shows that $\mathbf{W}_{\mathbf{ba}} = \mathbf{B} \cdot \mathbf{A}^T$ is something like a 'soft' analogue of the symbolic rewrite rule **a** → **b**: multiplying by $\mathbf{W}_{\mathbf{ba}}$ maps **a** into **b**, and maps a vector **x** similar to **a** into a vector with the same direction as **b**, but with length multiplied by the degree of similarity *sim*(**a**, **x**). If **x** is orthogonal (maximally dissimilar) to **a**, then $\mathbf{W}_{\mathbf{ba}}$ maps **x** to **0**. (A somewhat less 'soft' analogue for **a** → **b** uses $\mathbf{a}^+$ in place of **a**, where $\mathbf{a}^+$ is the dual vector of **a** (8) with respect to a basis of vectors realizing symbols {**a**, **b**, …}. With $\mathbf{a}^+$, a vector **x** realizing any symbol **x** different from **a** will be mapped to **0** even if **x** is not orthogonal to **a**.)

A primary purpose of this chapter is to develop the following concept and show its central role in integrating connectionist and symbolic computation.

(17) Tensor product of vectors

a. Suppose two vectors **a** and **b** have tags α and β, respectively. Their tensor product, written $\mathbf{a} \otimes \mathbf{b}$, is constructively defined as the vector **c** with a tag μ consisting of the concatenation of α and β, and with components

$$c_\mu \equiv a_\alpha b_\beta \text{ where } \mu = \alpha\beta; \;\; \mathbf{c} = \mathbf{a} \otimes \mathbf{b}.$$

For example., suppose $\alpha \in \{0, 1\}$ (**a** is in a two-dimensional vector space) and $\beta \in \{0, 1, 2\}$ (**b** is in a three-dimensional space). Then $\mathbf{c} = \mathbf{a} \otimes \mathbf{b}$ lies in a $2 \cdot 3$ = six-dimensional space; it has a tag $\mu \in \{00, 01, 02, 10, 11, 12\}$; and its components are $c_{00} = a_0 b_0$, $c_{01} = a_0 b_1$, and so on. If the tags of **a** and **b** themselves consist of multiple indices, these indices become indices of the tag of $\mathbf{a} \otimes \mathbf{b}$, as in (17d).

b. $\mathbf{c} = \mathbf{a} \otimes \mathbf{b}$ has the same numerical components as the **outer product matrix** $\mathbf{C} \equiv \mathbf{A} \cdot \mathbf{B}^T$ (where as always **A** and **B** are the *column* vectors corresponding to **a** and **b**). $\mathbf{C}^T = \mathbf{B} \cdot \mathbf{A}^T$ has the same components as $\mathbf{b} \otimes \mathbf{a}$. The element of matrix **C** labeled by a pair of indices α, β (e.g., α =1, β = 2) is numerically equal to the element of vector **c** labeled by the single tag μ = αβ (e.g., μ = 12); for example, $[\mathbf{C}]_{1,2} = [\mathbf{c}]_{12} = [\mathbf{a}]_1 [\mathbf{b}]_2$.

c. The tensor product operation ⊗ obeys

$$(\mathbf{a} + \mathbf{a}') \otimes \mathbf{b} = \mathbf{a} \otimes \mathbf{b} + \mathbf{a}' \otimes \mathbf{b}; \;\; \mathbf{a} \otimes (\mathbf{b} + \mathbf{b}') = \mathbf{a} \otimes \mathbf{b} + \mathbf{a} \otimes \mathbf{b}';$$
$$(c\mathbf{a}) \otimes \mathbf{b} = c(\mathbf{a} \otimes \mathbf{b}) = \mathbf{a} \otimes (c\mathbf{b}).$$

d. The constructive definition in (17a) and the properties in (17c)—but not the matrix correspondence in (17b)—generalize to higher-order tensor products; for example, $\mathbf{e} \equiv \mathbf{d} \otimes \mathbf{c} = \mathbf{d} \otimes (\mathbf{a} \otimes \mathbf{b})$. The tag of this vector has three indices: it is a **third-rank tensor.** Its components are

$$e_{\delta\alpha\beta} \equiv d_\delta c_{\alpha\beta} = d_\delta (a_\alpha b_\beta) = d_\delta a_\alpha b_\beta; \;\; \mathbf{e} \equiv \mathbf{d} \otimes \mathbf{c} = \mathbf{d} \otimes \mathbf{a} \otimes \mathbf{b}.$$

e. If V is an n-dimensional vector space and U is an m-dimensional vector space, then $V \otimes U$ is a vector space of dimension nm. This is the **tensor product space**, the vectors of which are **tensors of rank two.** The elements of such a tensor have a tag that is the concatenation of two indices, the first having values in the tag set of V, the second, in the tag set of U.

f. In general, for k vector spaces $V_1, V_2, \ldots, V_k$ of dimensions $n_1, n_2, \ldots, n_k$, the space of **kth-rank tensors** $S = V_1 \otimes V_2 \otimes \cdots \otimes V_k$ is a vector space of dimension $n_1 n_2 \ldots n_k$. A vector $\mathbf{s}$ in this space has components labeled with k indices: $[\mathbf{s}]_{\alpha_1 \alpha_2 \cdots \alpha_k}$, with α_1 ranging over the n_1 tag values of V_1, α_2 over the n_2 tag values of V_2, etc. Given a sequence of vectors $\mathbf{a}_1, \mathbf{a}_2, \ldots, \mathbf{a}_k$ from the spaces $V_1, V_2, \ldots, V_k$ (respectively), the **kth-order tensor product** of these vectors is the tensor $\mathbf{s} = \mathbf{a}_1 \otimes \mathbf{a}_2 \otimes \cdots \otimes \mathbf{a}_k$ with components

$$[\mathbf{s}]_{\alpha_1 \alpha_2 \cdots \alpha_k} \equiv [\mathbf{a}_1]_{\alpha_1} [\mathbf{a}_2]_{\alpha_2} \cdots [\mathbf{a}_k]_{\alpha_k}; \ \mathbf{s} = \mathbf{a}_1 \otimes \mathbf{a}_2 \otimes \cdots \otimes \mathbf{a}_k.$$

Matrices defined on tensor product spaces are often themselves tensor products.

(18) Tensor product of matrices

a. If $\mathbf{W}$ is an $n \times m$ matrix, and $\mathbf{W}'$ an $n' \times m'$ matrix, then $\mathbf{W} \otimes \mathbf{W}'$ is an $(nn') \times (mm')$ matrix. Each of its two tags has two indices. The components are constructively defined by

$$[\mathbf{W} \otimes \mathbf{W}']_{\alpha\alpha', \beta\beta'} \equiv [\mathbf{W}]_{\alpha, \beta} [\mathbf{W}']_{\alpha', \beta'}.$$

b. The defining axiom thus satisfied is

$$[\mathbf{W} \otimes \mathbf{W}'] \cdot (\mathbf{v} \otimes \mathbf{v}') \equiv (\mathbf{W} \cdot \mathbf{v}) \otimes (\mathbf{W}' \cdot \mathbf{v}').$$

If $\mathbf{W}$ maps vectors in an m-dimensional vector space V to vectors in an n-dimensional space U, and $\mathbf{W}'$ maps vectors in m'-dimensional V' to n'-dimensional U', then $\mathbf{W} \otimes \mathbf{W}'$ maps from (mm')-dimensional $V \otimes V'$ to (nn')-dimensional $U \otimes U'$.

One final vector space concept resolves a technical difficulty in the definition of recursive representations (Section 1.3).

(19) Direct sum

Given two vector spaces V and U, of dimensions d_V and d_U, a new vector space of dimension $d_V + d_U$, the **direct sum** $V \oplus U$, is defined constructively as follows.

a. $V \oplus U$ is the set of ordered pairs of vectors from V and U (i.e., the Cartesian product $V \times U$). Thus, if $\mathbf{v} \in V$ and $\mathbf{u} \in U$, $(\mathbf{v}, \mathbf{u}) \in V \oplus U$. This vector is also written $\mathbf{v} \oplus \mathbf{u}$.

b. Addition and scalar multiplication are defined as follows:

$$(\mathbf{v}_1, \mathbf{u}_1) + (\mathbf{v}_2, \mathbf{u}_2) \equiv (\mathbf{v}_1 + \mathbf{v}_2, \mathbf{u}_1 + \mathbf{u}_2); \ c(\mathbf{v}, \mathbf{u}) \equiv (c\mathbf{v}, c\mathbf{u}).$$

That is,

$$(\mathbf{v}_1 \oplus \mathbf{u}_1) + (\mathbf{v}_2 \oplus \mathbf{u}_2) \equiv (\mathbf{v}_1 + \mathbf{v}_2) \oplus (\mathbf{u}_1 + \mathbf{u}_2); \ c(\mathbf{v} \oplus \mathbf{u}) \equiv (c\mathbf{v}) \oplus (c\mathbf{u}).$$

c. The zero vector of $V \oplus U$ is $(\mathbf{0}_V, \mathbf{0}_U) = \mathbf{0}_V \oplus \mathbf{0}_U$, where $\mathbf{0}_V$ and $\mathbf{0}_U$ are the zero vectors of V and U. Both V and U are naturally embedded within $V \oplus U$: $\mathbf{v} \in V$ embeds as $\mathbf{v} \oplus \mathbf{0}_U$, and $\mathbf{u} \in U$ as $\mathbf{0}_V \oplus \mathbf{u}$. When the vector spaces of $\mathbf{v}$ and $\mathbf{u}$ are clear, we can deploy quotation marks for an informal notation: '$\mathbf{v}$' $\equiv \mathbf{v} \oplus \mathbf{0}_U$; '$\mathbf{u}$' $\equiv \mathbf{0}_V \oplus \mathbf{u}$.

The vector space $\mathbb{R}^d$ (1) is just $\mathbb{R} \oplus \mathbb{R} \oplus \cdots \oplus \mathbb{R}$ (d times).

Box 1

Box 2. Linear algebra of connectionist networks

A connectionist network consists of two interrelated collections of variables. One is a set of numerical variables $a_1, a_2, \ldots, a_n$ making up the **activation vector a** of the network; a_β is considered to be the activity (or activation value) of an abstract element, unit β. A subset of the units will generally be designated input units; another subset, output units. The other variables make up an $n \times n$ **weight matrix W** of real numbers; the entry $[\mathbf{W}]_{\beta\gamma} \equiv W_{\beta\gamma}$ is called 'the weight (or strength) of the connection to unit β from unit γ'. Each activation value a_β evolves in time according to some **activation equation**; this equation involves only the activation values of units γ with nonzero connection weights to unit β, and the value of the weights, $W_{\beta\gamma}$. Each weight $W_{\beta\gamma}$ evolves in time according to a **learning equation** (or algorithm) that refers only to a_β and a_γ, and sometimes (for **supervised learning**) to additional values t_β and t_γ that are **target values** for a_β and a_γ provided by a **teacher**. Almost universally, weights evolve over time much more slowly than do activations.

A multitude of activation and learning equations have been studied. Many of these fall into the category of **quasilinear** networks; these are analyzed in Chapter 9. In such a network, the activation equation for unit α involves only a_α itself and a single number, the **input** to unit α, defined as

(1) $\iota_\alpha \equiv [\mathbf{W}]_{\alpha 1}[\mathbf{a}]_1 + [\mathbf{W}]_{\alpha 2}[\mathbf{a}]_2 + \cdots + [\mathbf{W}]_{\alpha m}[\mathbf{a}]_m \equiv \sum_{\beta=1}^{m} \mathbf{W}_{\alpha\beta}[\mathbf{a}]_\beta$.

(ι is the Greek letter iota.) By Box 1 (9), this means that the vector $\boldsymbol{\iota}$ of inputs is simply the matrix-vector product of **W** and **a**:

(2) $\boldsymbol{\iota} = \mathbf{W} \cdot \mathbf{a}$.

If $\mathbf{w}_\alpha$ is row α of **W**—the vector of weights *into* unit α—then, as in Box 1 (10), we can write (1) above as

(3) $\iota_\alpha = \mathbf{a} \cdot \mathbf{w}_\alpha = sim(\mathbf{a}, \mathbf{w}_\alpha)$.

The vector $\mathbf{w}_\alpha$ is like a template that unit α matches against the activation vector **a**: the more similar **a** is to this template, the more input flows into unit α.

In a **linear** network, the activation value of unit γ is simply equal to the input ι_γ that it receives.

In many networks, the way in which activation patterns represent information can be understood as follows. The *direction* of the activation vector **a** determines its **content**, while the *magnitude* of **a** determines its **strength**. This is easily seen with local representations. Suppose an activation vector **a** represents the first letter of a word, and the first two units locally represent the letters **A** and **B**, respectively. If only the first unit is active, we have an unambiguous representation of **A**. The activation of this unit may build up in time from zero to some value large enough to send appreciable activation to subsequent units for further processing. As the activation builds in time, the strength—or perhaps the confidence level—of the representation grows. Now if the first two units have activation values 0.75 and 0.5, we can interpret this as a representational state in which the hypothesis that the first letter is **A** is attributed a confidence level 0.75, with 0.5 being the corresponding confidence level for **B**. For this local representation, the direction of the pattern representing **A** is just (1 0 0 ...), while the direction for **B** is (0 1 0 ...). These directions determine representational content. The magnitude of these vectors in the representation is just the activation value of the corresponding local unit; this encodes representational strength. For distributed representations, the directions for the representations of **A** and **B** would be patterns in which many units have nonzero activation—but the same interpretation of direction and magnitude of activation vectors applies, as illustrated in this chapter.

The units of a network are often partitioned into different groups or **layers**, with limited connectivity between the groups. Thus, there may be connections between group 1 and group 2, but not between group 1 and group 3. Absent connections can be encoded as weights in **W** with permanent value zero. In a given network, if $W_{\beta\gamma}$ is not permanently set to zero, let's say that there is a **bona fide** connection to unit β from unit γ. If a network has no closed loops of bona fide connections, it is a **feed-forward** network; otherwise, it is **recurrent**.

If **W** is the weight matrix of a network, then the transpose matrix $\mathbf{W}^{\mathrm{T}}$ (Box 1 (16)) is the matrix of the network that results from reversing the directions of all connections (without altering connection strengths).

In a feed-forward network with bona fide connections from one layer L_1 of m units to another layer L_2 of n units, the total weight matrix **W** is an $N \times N$ matrix, where $N \equiv m + n$ is the total number of units. But all these weights are permanently set to zero except for the bona fide connections to L_2 from L_1; the weights on these connections form an $n \times m$ submatrix **M** of **W**; often **M** is called "*the* weight matrix" for the network, the zero weights of non–bona fide connections in **W** simply being ignored. **M** will also be called a **feed-forward** weight matrix.

Suppose **M** is the $n \times m$ feed-forward weight matrix from a group of m input units to a group of n *linear* intermediate units, and **X** is the $l \times n$ feed-forward weight matrix from those intermediate units to a group of l output units. Then the mapping of activation from the input units to the output units achieved by this network is the same as the mapping of the network that results from removing the intermediate group of n units and directly connecting the m input units to the l output units with the $l \times m$ feed-forward weight matrix $\mathbf{X} \cdot \mathbf{M}$. Multiplying the weight matrices to form $\mathbf{X} \cdot \mathbf{M}$ corresponds to cascading the connections of **M** into the connections of **X**, via an intermediate group of linear units.

There are a great many learning algorithms in the connectionist literature. Several of the most central ones can be characterized using the outer product, defined in Box 1 (17b). Suppose the input units send activation to another group of units, G. Then Hebbian learning, the δ-rule, and back-propagation (defined in any text on neural networks, such as Rumelhart, McClelland, and the PDP Research Group 1986) all have the following form: when an input pattern **i** is presented, the weights from the input units change by

(4) $\Delta \mathbf{W}^{(i)} = \eta\, \mathbf{G} \cdot \mathbf{I}^{T}$; $\Delta W^{(i)}_{\alpha\beta} = \eta\, g_{\alpha}\, i_{\beta}$.

Here η is a constant learning rate, $\mathbf{G}$ and $\mathbf{I}$ are the column vectors corresponding to $\mathbf{g}$ and $\mathbf{i}$, and $\mathbf{g}$ is either the activation vector of group G (Hebbian learning), or the δ/error-vector of G (δ-rule or back-propagation learning). Thus, the transfer of learning from one input $\mathbf{i}$ to another $\mathbf{i}'$—the output of $\Delta \mathbf{W}^{(i)}$ on $\mathbf{i}'$—is $\Delta \mathbf{W}^{(i)} \cdot \mathbf{i}' = (\eta\, \mathbf{G} \cdot \mathbf{I}^{T}) \cdot \mathbf{i}' = \eta\, sim(\mathbf{i}, \mathbf{i}')\, \mathbf{g}$, by (16f); transfer (or interference) between inputs is proportional to their degree of similarity, which is zero for orthogonal (e.g., local) representations.

1 P₁: REPICS — SYMBOLIC STRUCTURES AS PATTERNS OF ACTIVITY

The first ICS principle concerns the integration of symbolic and connectionist formalizations of mental representations. It was stated in Chapter 2 (1) as follows:

(2) **P_1. Rep$_{ICS}$**: Cognitive representation in ICS

Information is represented in the mind/brain by widely distributed activity patterns—activation vectors—that, for central aspects of higher cognition, possess global structure describable through the discrete data structures of symbolic cognitive theory.

In this section, we will gradually articulate this principle, successively taking up increasingly more complex types of structure, as shown in Table 1.

Table 1. Types of representational structure

Sec.	Structuring operation	Symbolic formalization: Structures	Symbolic formalization: Example	Connectionist formalization
1.1	Combining	Sets	$\{\mathtt{c}_1, \mathtt{c}_2\}$	?
1.2	Filler/role binding	Strings, frames	**AB** = $\{\mathtt{A}/r_1, \mathtt{B}/r_2\}$	??
1.3	Recursive embedding	Trees	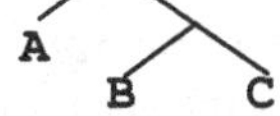	???

In Section 1, we start with the simple symbolic structure defined by sets: mere grouping or combining of elements. In Section 1.2, we consider more complex structures in which the combined elements fill different roles within the composite structure. And in Section 1.3, we consider recursive structures, in which the elements filling roles in a composite structure $\mathbf{s}$ are themselves structured in the same way as $\mathbf{s}$. Each of these types of structures has a familiar formalization within symbolic computation: these are listed and exemplified in Table 1. Each type of structure can be viewed as the result of a particular type of structuring operation: simple grouping of elements together (1.1); binding of structural roles to the atomic elements that fill them (1.2); binding of structural roles to elements that are themselves structured (1.3). The task at hand is to develop new formalizations of these structural operations appropriate for a parallel distributed processing (PDP) connectionist computational architecture. In these new principles, representations, at one level of analysis, are widely distributed patterns of activity, as stated in Rep_{ICS} (Abbott and Sejnowski 1999). More formally, the medium of representation is a space of **activation vectors** (see Box 2), and what we seek are operations on such a space that are suitable for formalizing the various structuring operations of Table 1. We will proceed by a series of leading questions.

1.1 Constituent combination by superposition

The most basic question about realizations of composite structures in distributed activation vectors was once colorfully posed as follows by Jerome Feldman (personal communication, 1983):

(3) The two-horse problem

If the representation of *one* horse fills up an entire network, how is it possible to represent *two* horses?

More prosaically: if the representation of a symbol **A** is distributed throughout a certain portion of a network, how can the representation of a second symbol **B** also be distributed throughout that same portion of the network—as is necessary for the distributed representation of even an extremely simple symbol structure like the set {**A**, **B**}?

Given that the representational medium we are working in is a space of activation vectors, to answer this question we turn to the fundamental operation used to combine elements in such spaces (Box 1 (1)).

(4) **The linear approximation**

With respect to central phenomena of higher cognition, the following approximation suffices for the analysis of the network realization of symbolic representations:

The Superposition Principle

The realization of the set {**A**, **B**} is the *superposition* or *vector sum* of the activation vectors realizing **A** and **B**.

The value of the Superposition Principle, or more generally of the linear approximation of which it is the fundamental assumption, is to be assessed here by how well it allows us to proceed with our task of developing connectionist structuring operations. We will see that it is rather successful in this regard, although future development of ICS theory will no doubt pursue nonlinear extensions of the methods developed here. The current linear analysis is intended as an initial approximation, as is standard in mathematical analysis in most scientific domains. For the most part, we will operate within the confines of the linear approximation in this book, without further comment (although see Chapters 7 and 9 for some discussion of representation and processing, respectively, in nonlinear networks). For tutorial introductions to the linear approximation in PDP networks, and some discussion of nonlinear extensions, see Jordan 1986 and Smolensky 1986 (see also van Gelder 1990).

The operation of vector addition—the essence of the Superposition Principle (4)—can be written and illustrated in many ways; several are shown in Figure 1. In the first row of this figure, we find our first element, symbolically denoted **A**, as shown in the leftmost column. The connectionist realization of **A** is a pattern of activity that is depicted in four ways. The most basic notation is the list of activation values defining this pattern of activity, say, (1.0, –1.0, 0.8), a simple pattern over three units. These three numbers can be seen as the coordinates of a point in **activation space**—in this simple case, a three-dimensional space, with one coordinate for each of the three activation values. It is conventional to denote this vector as an arrow from the origin to the point with the given coordinates, as shown in the column labeled 'arrow in activation space'.

Figure 1. Combination via vector addition

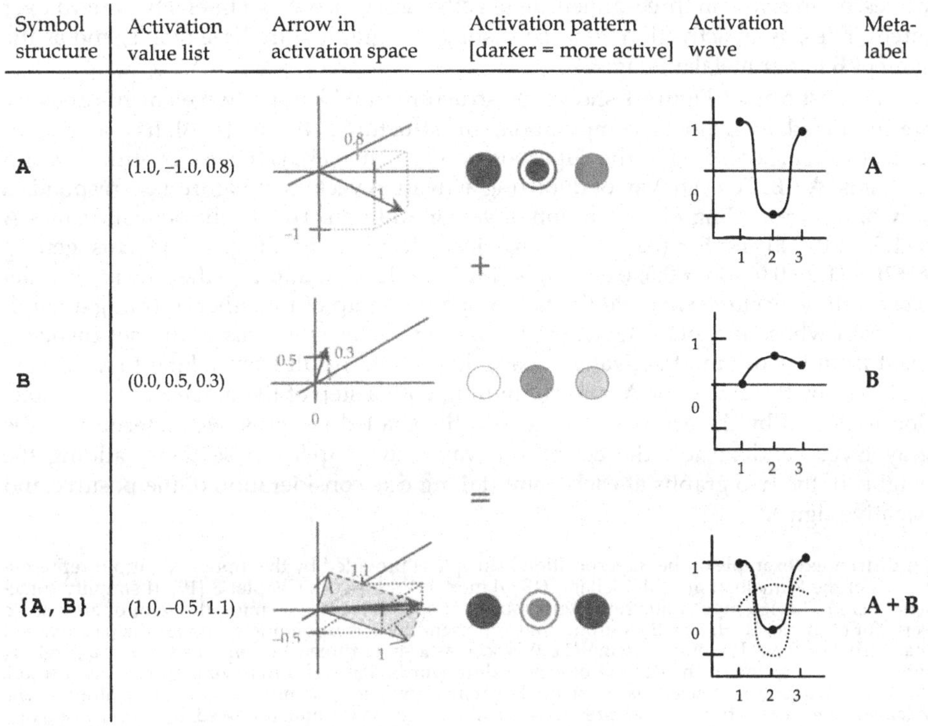

Symbol structure	Activation value list	Arrow in activation space	Activation pattern [darker = more active]	Activation wave	Meta-label
A	(1.0, –1.0, 0.8)	0.8, 1, –1		1, 0; 1 2 3	A
			+		
B	(0.0, 0.5, 0.3)	0.5, 0.3, 0		1, 0; 1 2 3	B
			=		
{A, B}	(1.0, –0.5, 1.1)	1.1, –0.5, 1		1, 0; 1 2 3	A + B

This vector can also be visualized as three circles, one for each unit, with the shade of gray of each circle indicating its activation value, darker shades denoting greater activity magnitude and a white border denoting negative activation levels. Often, activation levels are depicted by the area of the circles; white circles may be used to mark negative values, and black ones, positive values.

The next column of Figure 1 shows this same vector as an 'activation wave', a graph of the activation values of the three units. Only the three plotted points for one pattern are significant; the connecting curve serves only to group them together, and it could be replaced by straight lines or any other means of connection.

This vector will be denoted **A** in the metalanguage that constitutes our calculus of patterns of activity. The numbers (1.0, –1.0, 0.8) will be called the **components** or the **elements** of **A**; they may be separated by commas, semicolons, or white space, as typographical convenience dictates. The αth component of **A** will be written $[\mathbf{A}]_\alpha$ or A_α, where in this case the **tag** α may be 1, 2, or 3. $[\mathbf{A}]_\alpha$ is simply the activation level of unit number α in the activity pattern **A**.

In the second row of Figure 1 we find a second element, symbolically designated **B**, and its connectionist realization, a different pattern of activity over the same three units. This vector is also shown in five different notations: as a list of three activation values, as an arrow in three-dimensional activation space, as an intensity pattern over three circles, as an activation wave consisting of a graph with three points, and as the symbol **B** in our metalanguage.

The last row of Figure 1 shows the structure in which the two elements above it are combined. In symbolic computation, this structure is the set {**A**, **B**}. Its connectionist realization, according to the Superposition Principle (4), is the vector sum of **A** and **B**, that is, **A** + **B**. To each way of depicting activation vectors in Figure 1 corresponds a way of understanding this operation of vector addition. To add the activation lists **A** = (1.0, –1.0, 0.8) and **B** = (0.0, 0.5, 0.3), we just add corresponding components, getting **A** + **B** = (1.0 + 0.0, –1.0 + 0.5, 0.8 + 0.3) = (1.0, –0.5, 1.1). To add together the arrows depicting these vectors, we slide the tail of one to the tip of the other, forming a parallelogram whose diagonal depicts the resulting vector sum: this is the net displacement from the origin of activation space that would result from taking first the step indicated by the arrow for **A**, and continuing with a step of the magnitude and direction indicated by the arrow for **B**. To add the shaded patterns, we superimpose the gray levels; and to add the activation waves, we superimpose them, adding the heights of the two graphs at each point (taking due consideration of the positive and negative signs).[1]

[1] A distributed example of the Superposition Principle is provided by the input and output representations of the Rumelhart and McClelland (1986) model discussed in Chapter 8 (19). (I simplify somewhat here.) The 460 input units represent a string of speech sounds forming the stem of an English verb, for example, ⟨**lid**⟩ *lead*; the output units represent the corresponding string for the past tense of that verb, ⟨**lɛd**⟩ *led*. The output string ⟨**lɛd**⟩ is seen as a set of three 'Wickelphones', $\{_{\langle}\mathbf{l}_{\varepsilon}, {}_{l}\boldsymbol{\varepsilon}_{d}, {}_{\varepsilon}\mathbf{d}_{\rangle}\}$: $_{\langle}\mathbf{l}_{\varepsilon}$ represents an *l* sound in the context of a preceding word-edge and a following vowel *ε*, and so on. Each Wickelphone is viewed as a set of 'Wickelfeatures'; for example, one Wickelfeature in the Wickelphone $_{l}\boldsymbol{\varepsilon}_{d}$ is 'front-vowel preceded by liquid-consonant and followed by stop-consonant'. Each Wickelphone contains many such Wickelfeatures. Each of the 460 possible different output Wickelfeatures is represented by a single output unit. A single Wickelphone like $_{l}\boldsymbol{\varepsilon}_{d}$ is represented by

The example in Figure 1 illustrates a case of **distributed representation**: **A** and **B** are realized over the same units. It is not possible to localize the realization of **A** to one set of units and the realization of **B** to another, nonoverlapping, set of units. In the realization of the composite structure {**A**, **B**}, for example, the activity of the last unit, 1.1, is due partly to the presence of **A** (contributing activation 0.8) and partly to the presence of **B** (0.3). This raises the important question in (5).

(5) **The problem of inverting superposition**
Suppose a connectionist network contains an activation pattern in which distributed patterns representing multiple elements—parts—are superimposed to form the representation of the whole. In what sense does this single pattern *represent* those multiple elements? Can those individual elements be precisely identified by the theorist? How can the network process this representation in a way that is sensitive to the presence of the individual parts, given how they are all mixed together?

In the particular case illustrated in Figure 1, the question is, given the pattern for the structure as a whole, (1.0, –0.5, 1.1), how can the theorist identify the constituent parts precisely as (1.0, –1.0, 0.8) (= **A**) and (0.0, 0.5, 0.3) (= **B**), and how could a network processing this whole do so in a way that combines the appropriate processing for these two constituents, as required by the combinatorial strategy for explaining the productivity of cognition (Section 1:3)?

There are many facets to this question, not the least of which is the **semantic problem**, posed in Section 23:7.1.1.1: what exactly is required to justify the statement '*X* represents *Y*'? There is little consensus on the correct approach to answering this question among philosophers of cognitive science, despite (or perhaps because of) the considerable quantity of research that has been devoted to it. This is true even for would-be representations *X* in symbolic cognitive architectures—the answer for the relatively recent connectionist architecture is even less clear. This question will not be directly addressed in this book.

But we can make considerable progress by focusing on the technical core of the question. Given the pattern (1.0, –0.5, 1.1), can we assert that the constituents of this pattern are precisely the patterns **A** and **B**, rather than, say, **C**, **D**, and **E**, which, let us suppose, are the distributed patterns realizing three other symbols **C**, **D**, and **E**? The answer will be yes—as long as the vectors that realize symbols are *independent*: if the realizations are not independent, there is no such guarantee. This is hardly surprising: in any medium of representation, if the atoms of combination are not independent, there will be no unique way of decomposing a combination into its constituents. If a symbolic computational system is realized in a digital computer, for example, and the symbol **A** is realized as the bit pattern `00110101`, and the symbol **C** is real-

a pattern of activation over 460 units in which the units representing Wickelfeatures present in $_{l}\varepsilon_{d}$ have activation value 1, while all other units have activation 0. There is one such 460-dimensional vector for each of the three Wickelphones constituting ⟨**lɛd**⟩, and the pattern representing ⟨**lɛd**⟩ is just the vector obtained by adding together (i.e., superimposing) these three vectors. (Among the additional complexities of the actual model is the imposition of a maximal activation level of 1.)

ized as a bit pattern that is identical, then it will be impossible to distinguish the realization of any structure containing **A** from the corresponding structure containing **C** in its place. This is so obvious that it seems pointless to mention it. But this obviousness arises because in the digital medium, the condition of independence of realization is so trivial: the realizations of **A** and **C** are independent if they are nonidentical. In the representational medium of activation vectors, the condition of independence is less obvious, but it is in fact one of the most basic concepts of vector space theory.

A set of vectors is said to be **(linearly) independent** if no one of them is equal to a superposition of the others. More precisely:

(6) **Independence of vectors**

A set of vectors {**A**, **B**, **C**, ... } is (linearly) independent if no one of them is a weighted sum of the others—that is, if for every choice of numerical weights $w_{\mathbf{B}}, w_{\mathbf{C}}, \ldots$

$$\mathbf{A} \neq w_{\mathbf{B}}\mathbf{B} + w_{\mathbf{C}}\mathbf{C} + \cdots,$$

and similarly if **A** is exchanged with any other vector in the set.

The operation of multiplying a vector **B** by a number or 'scalar' w—**scalar multiplication**—consists simply in multiplying by w each of the components of **B**; for example, if $\mathbf{B} = (1.0, -0.8, 1.2)$ and $w = 0.5$, then $w\mathbf{B} = (0.5, -0.4, 0.6)$. Pictorially, this changes the size (or 'scale') of the arrow for **B** by a factor of w, while leaving its direction unchanged. (Multiplication by a negative scalar reverses the arrow's direction.)

Just as a digital realization of symbolic computation will fail if the bit patterns realizing different symbols are not independent, so a connectionist realization will fail if the activity patterns realizing different symbols are not independent, in the relevant—vector space—sense (6). But if these activity patterns *are* independent, we can be sure that combination by superposition can be correctly and precisely inverted. Returning to our earlier example, independence ensures that it is impossible for an activity pattern to be analyzable both as **A** + **B** and as **C** + **D** + **E**—impossible for a pattern of activity to be ambiguous between a realization of {**A**, **B**} and a realization of {**C**, **D**, **E**}. For ambiguity would mean that these two vector superpositions yield the same result:

(7) $$\mathbf{A} + \mathbf{B} \stackrel{?}{=} \mathbf{C} + \mathbf{D} + \mathbf{E}.$$

This is possible if and only if

(8) $$\mathbf{A} \stackrel{?}{=} -\mathbf{B} + \mathbf{C} + \mathbf{D} + \mathbf{E},$$

which is possible only if the vectors {**A**, **B**, **C**, **D**, **E**} are not linearly independent (6).

Thus, throughout the remainder of this book, except where explicitly stated otherwise, we will assume that (9) holds:

(9) **Independence assumption**

In a connectionist realization of symbolic computation, the activation vectors realizing the atomic symbols are (linearly) independent.

In a network with n units—defining an activation space of n dimensions—a randomly chosen set of up to n vectors will be independent, with probability 1; that is, *failure* of independence is the exceptional case, with probability 0. In such a network, however, it is not possible to have more than n independent vectors, so the number of units required for the realization of sets of symbols must be at least as great as the number of distinct symbols. In Chapter 8 we will see how, with distributed representations and large networks, the realizational capacity of a network can saturate 'gracefully' as the number of vectors exceeds n—precision degrades smoothly rather than catastrophically. We will also see that in the context of more complex structures, the independence assumption can be satisfied in the relevant sense even if the vectors realizing the elementary symbols **A**, **B**, ... are not independent (Chapter 8 (20) and Box 8:1)—this enables n units to represent far more than n symbols.

As we have seen, the independence assumption (9) ensures that given an activity pattern realizing a set of symbols, there is one and only one set of symbols realized by that pattern. Computational methods for actually computing which symbols these are require the further mathematical development in Chapter 8 (e.g., Boxes 1 and 2).

It remains to determine whether the constituents of a set are not only precisely defined and accessible to the theorist, but also accessible to computation in a connectionist network—accessible in the sense that processing of a composite representation is systematically related to processing of its parts, in the kinds of ways needed to instantiate the combinatorial strategy. We will return to this question in Section 2, which takes up processing; for now, we retain our focus on purely representational problems, and move on from the simple grouping structure exemplified by sets, to consider richer structures of the types crucial for higher cognition.

The results of this subsection can be summarized by filling in the first row of Table 1, yielding Table 2.

Table 2. Connectionist combination via vector addition (+)

	Structuring	Symbolic formalization		Connectionist formalization	
Sec.	operation	Structures	Example	Example	Vector operation
1.1	Combining	Sets	$\{\mathbf{c}_1, \mathbf{c}_2\}$	$\mathbf{c}_1 + \mathbf{c}_2$	Vector sum: +
1.2	Filler/role binding	Strings, frames	**AB** = $\{\mathbf{A}/r_1, \mathbf{B}/r_2\}$		?
1.3	Recursive embedding	Trees	A B C		??

1.2 Variable binding via the tensor product

A set is an unstructured collection of elements. Thus, for example, {**A**, **B**} and {**B**, **A**} denote the same set. When we move to true symbol *structures*, we must start to distinguish among the different **roles** in the overall structure played by different symbol tokens. A simple case is the symbol **sequence**, or **string**. And this brings us to our next problem:

(10) **The A + B = B + A problem**

Vector addition is commutative:

$$\mathbf{A} + \mathbf{B} = \mathbf{B} + \mathbf{A}.$$

So if simple vector addition is used to combine the activation vectors **A** and **B** that realize the two symbols **A** and **B**, then how can the distinction be made between the realizations of the two distinct strings **AB** and **BA**?

The solution to this problem must be that the contribution of **A** to the vector **AB** that realizes the string **AB** is distinguishable from its contribution to the vector **BA** that realizes **BA**.[2] The simplest example of such a difference is shown in the contrast between the first lines of panels A and A′ of Figure 2 (the rectangle enclosing two groups of five units each). These panels illustrate the **fully local** realization of the two symbol strings **AB** and **BA**, respectively. There are two horizontally separated groups of units, one hosting the realization of the first symbol in the string, the other, the second. In each group, there is a single unit dedicated to the realization of each type of symbol: the first for realizing **A**, the second for **B**, and so on.[3] In terms of activation *vectors*, the activity pattern over the first group of units is (1, 0, 0, 0, 0) = **A** for **A**, (0, 1, 0, 0, 0) = **B** for **B**, and so on. The total pattern of activation for **AB** is (**A** ; **B**); that is,

(11) $\mathbf{AB} = (\mathbf{A} ; \mathbf{B}) = (1, 0, 0, 0, 0 ; 0, 1, 0, 0, 0).$

(In (11), a semicolon has been used in lieu of a comma only to visually separate the activations of the two groups of units.) Now this vector can be expressed as the sum in (12):

(12)
$$\begin{aligned}
\mathbf{AB} &= (\quad \mathbf{A} \quad ; \quad \mathbf{B} \quad) \\
&= (1, 0, 0, 0, 0 ; 0, 1, 0, 0, 0) \\
&= (1, 0, 0, 0, 0 ; 0, 0, 0, 0, 0) \\
&\quad + (0, 0, 0, 0, 0 ; 0, 1, 0, 0, 0) \\
&= (\ \mathbf{A} \ ; \ \mathbf{0} \ ) \quad = \quad \mathbf{A}_1 \\
&\quad + (\ \mathbf{0} \ ; \ \mathbf{B} \ ) \quad\quad + \mathbf{B}_2
\end{aligned}$$

The vector $\mathbf{A}_1$ = (1 0 0 0 0 0 0 0 0 0) is the realization of **A** *in the role of first element of the*

[2] '**AB**' is to be read as a *single* metalanguage symbol. It denotes a vector realizing the string denoted '**AB**'; a more explicit notation of this might be '$\mathbf{a}_{AB}$'. '**AB**' consists typographically of an '**A**' preceding a '**B**', and *denotes* a symbol called '**A**' preceding a symbol called '**B**'. '**AB**' however does not, in general, denote a vector called '**A**' preceding a vector called '**B**'; the sense in which the single vector denoted '**AB**' (or '$\mathbf{a}_{AB}$') is "composed" of two other vectors called '**A**' and '**B**' (or '$\mathbf{a}_A$' and '$\mathbf{a}_B$') is exactly what is at issue in the text. In the simplest case—fully local realization—as in Figure 2A, $\mathbf{a}_{AB}$ *can* be presented as a vector $\mathbf{a}_A$ "preceding" (displayed left of) a vector $\mathbf{a}_B$ (11). This is just what makes this simple case special, and an easy starting point for deriving the general case, where the relation between $\mathbf{a}_A$ and $\mathbf{a}_B$ in $\mathbf{a}_{AB}$ is not "precedence."

[3] An example of this type of representation is the output encoding in the Plaut et al. (1996) model of Box 1:1. The output is a string of three sounds, the pronunciation of a monosyllabic English word. The output representation has three groups of units; the first contains one unit for each possible sound in the first syllable position, and similarly for the second and third positions.

string; $\mathbf{B}_2$ = (0 0 0 0 0 0 1 0 0 0) is the realization of **B** in the role of second element.

Figure 2. Fully local realization of symbol strings

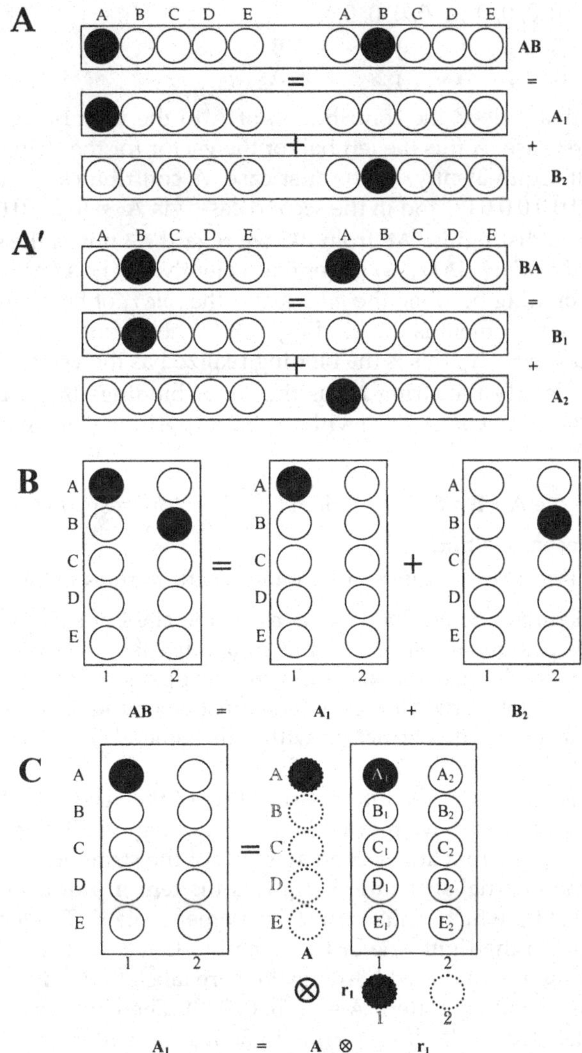

This pattern of activation **AB** realizing the string **AB** can be contrasted with the pattern **BA** realizing **BA** (shown in Figure 2A′). The decomposition of the new vector is shown in (13):

(13) $$\begin{aligned} \mathbf{BA} &= (\ \mathbf{B}\ ;\ \mathbf{A}\ ) \\ &= (0,1,0,0,0\,;1,0,0,0,0) \\ &= (0,1,0,0,0\,;0,0,0,0,0) \\ &\quad + (0,0,0,0,0\,;1,0,0,0,0) \\ &= (\ \mathbf{B}\ ;\ 0\ ) \quad = \mathbf{B}_1 \\ &\quad + (\ 0\ ;\ \mathbf{A}\ ) \quad\ \ + \mathbf{A}_2 \end{aligned}$$

And now we see that indeed the contribution of **A** to the vectors **AB** and **BA** is not the same: in the first case, **A** fills the left half of the vector for the string; in the second case, the right half. Equivalently, in the first case, **A** contributes via the constituent vector $\mathbf{A}_1$ = (1 0 0 0 0 0 0 0 0 0), and in the second case, via $\mathbf{A}_2$ = (0 0 0 0 0 1 0 0 0 0).

Thus, in order to distinguish **AB** from **BA**, we regard **AB** not as the simple set {**A**, **B**}, but as the set of *bindings* {**A**/r_1, **B**/r_2} (or equivalently, {**B**/r_2, **A**/r_1}): one element of this set, **A**/r_1, is a binding between the *filler* **A** and the *role* r_1 of being the first element of the string; the other element is the binding of **B** to the second-position role r_2. **A**/r_1 can be abbreviated simply $\mathbf{A}_1$; this is the binding realized as the vector $\mathbf{A}_1$.

To recap: we identify the string **AB** as the set of bindings {**A**/r_1, **B**/r_2} = {$\mathbf{A}_1$, $\mathbf{B}_2$} and then realize this set in compliance with the Superposition Principle (4):

(14) $\mathbf{AB} = \mathbf{A}_1 + \mathbf{B}_2$.

Our answer to the **A** + **B** = **B** + **A** problem (10) therefore rests on the following:

(15) **Filler/role decomposition**
A structure is a set of **bindings** of various structural **roles** to their **fillers**.

The class of a structure is determined by its roles; the class of strings is determined, for example, by the positional roles r_1, r_2, and so on, discussed above (although other types of roles may be defined for decomposing strings: see Section 8:2.3.1). These roles are variables, or slots, or attributes, which must be bound to particular values in order to individuate a particular structure within the general class (e.g., the particular string **AB**).

The next step is to identify the internal structure of the vector $\mathbf{A}_1$ that realizes the binding $\mathbf{A}_1$ = **A**/r_1. To this end, we redraw Figure 2A as Figure 2B, simply rotating the lines of units realizing the first and second symbols of the string **AB**. This allows us in Figure 2C to see the internal structure of $\mathbf{A}_1$: it is the **tensor product** of the vector **A** and the vector $\mathbf{r}_1$ = (1 0), which realizes the first-element role r_1. The tensor product is defined as follows. On the right side of the = sign in C is a vertical column of units shown as circles drawn with dotted borders; they are labeled 'A', 'B', … . These "dotted units" host the activation pattern **A** = (1, 0, 0, 0, 0). There is also a horizontal row of "dotted units" labeled '1', '2' (for r_1, r_2) with activation pattern $\mathbf{r}_1$ = (1, 0). The tensor product of these two "dotted vectors" is written $\mathbf{A} \otimes \mathbf{r}_1$; it is the pattern of activity in the box. There is one unit in the tensor product for each *pair* of dotted units, one from the column vector **A** and the other from the row vector $\mathbf{r}_1$. The activation value of each unit in the tensor product is the activation value of the dotted unit directly to its left multiplied by the activation value of the dotted unit directly below it; see Figure 3. In this simple local representation, all activation values are either 0 or 1; activation values of 1 have been shaded black in Figure 3 to show the relation to Figure 2C.

Figure 3. Simplest case of the tensor product (fully local)

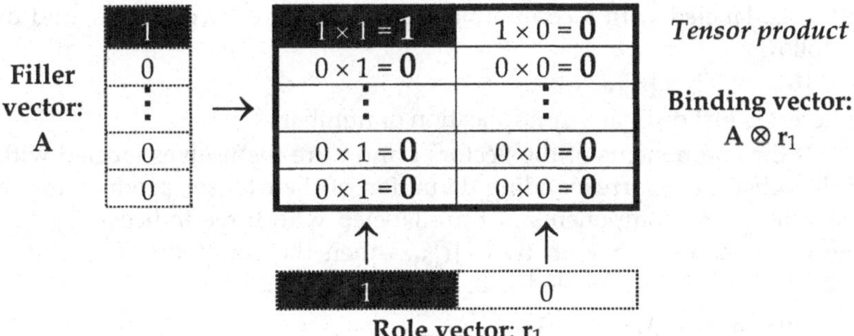

On the right side of the = sign in Figure 2C there are "solid units" within the box and "dotted units" to the left and below the box. It should be clear from the overall picture presented in Figure 2 that it is only the units within the box that constitute the realization of the binding $\mathtt{A}/r_1$; only these units are present in the vector $\mathbf{A}_1$. The dotted units outside the box are not part of $\mathbf{A}_1$ itself; rather, they constitute an *explication* of $\mathbf{A}_1$, showing how its structure is precisely that of the tensor product of a vector **A** realizing the filler and a vector $\mathbf{r}_1$ realizing the role. I will call $\mathbf{A}_1$ the **binding vector, A** the **filler vector**, and $\mathbf{r}_1$ the **role vector**.

In the vector **AB**—the realization of the symbol string **AB**—the binding vector $\mathbf{A}_1$ is present as one of the patterns superimposed to form the representation of the structure as a whole; the filler vector **A** and the role vector $\mathbf{r}_1$ do not themselves contribute *directly* to the superposition constituting **AB**; rather, they appear in it indirectly, as the factors that are multiplied together by the tensor product to form $\mathbf{A}_1$. I will also refer to the binding $\mathbf{A}_1$ as a **constituent** of **AB**, by which I mean *exactly this:* $\mathbf{A}_1$ is one of the symbol-realizing patterns superimposed to form **AB** (the other constituent being $\mathbf{B}_2$).

To formulate the preceding analysis in the general case:

(16) **Tensor product binding**

The binding $\mathtt{f}/r$ of a filler $\mathtt{f}$ to a role r is realized as a vector **f/r** that is the tensor product of a vector **f** realizing $\mathtt{f}$ with a vector **r** realizing r: $\mathbf{f/r} = \mathbf{f} \otimes \mathbf{r}$.[4]

A definition of the tensor product operation itself is spelled out in (17). This definition anticipates the need in Section 1.3 for *recursive* use of the tensor product operation, in which the units in activation patterns are labeled with multiple subscripts. It is this potential for recursive use that recommends the tensor product for building

[4] Again, as for '**AB**' in Footnote 2, '**f/r**' is a *single* metasymbol; see Footnote 2 for elaboration.

complex representations (this potential is lacking in the tensor product's simpler cousin in matrix algebra, the outer product: Box 1 (17b)).

(17) **Tensor product**

Let **f** be a vector with n components $[\mathbf{f}]_\alpha$ and **r** a vector with m components $[\mathbf{r}]_\beta$. Then the tensor product of these vectors, $\mathbf{b} = \mathbf{f} \otimes \mathbf{r}$, is a vector with $n \times m$ components, labeled with a compound tag consisting of two indices, and defined as follows:

$$[\mathbf{b}]_{\alpha\beta} = [\mathbf{f}]_\alpha \times [\mathbf{r}]_\beta,$$

where × is just ordinary multiplication of numbers.[5]

If the components of the vectors **f** and **r** are themselves labeled with multiple indices, the corresponding definition of their tensor product applies. For example, if the components of **f** are labeled with three indices—$[\mathbf{f}]_{\alpha\alpha'\alpha''}$—and the components of **r** with two—$[\mathbf{r}]_{\beta\beta'}$—then the components of their tensor product $\mathbf{b} = \mathbf{f} \otimes \mathbf{r}$ are labeled with five indices:

$$[\mathbf{b}]_{\alpha\alpha'\alpha''\beta\beta'} = [\mathbf{f}]_{\alpha\alpha'\alpha''} \times [\mathbf{r}]_{\beta\beta'}.$$

Thus, our solution to the **A + B = B + A** problem (10) combines the symbolic decomposition of structures into filler/role bindings (15) and the connectionist realization of these bindings via the tensor product (16).

1.2.1 From local to distributed representations of strings

So far, I have illustrated tensor product binding in only the simplest case, in which the vectors realizing both fillers and roles are completely localized patterns of activity: one unit in each vector has activation level 1, and all others have activation 0. Here, we see that tensor product binding can also provide distributed representations, including fully distributed representations in which every unit is part of the representation of every constituent. The mathematics we have in place is already adequate to the task: all we need do is move our example from fully localized patterns of activity to fully distributed ones. This we will do in two steps: first, we will consider distributed patterns for fillers, retaining local patterns for roles, and then we will take up the case in which both fillers and roles are realized with distributed patterns.

In Figure 4, the local patterns realizing the symbols **A** and **B** in Figure 2 have been replaced by distributed patterns.[6] In the top line of Figure 4A, the left half of the set of units hosts a distributed activity pattern **A** realizing **A**, while the right half hosts a dif-

[5] For example, suppose $n = 3$ and $\mathbf{f} = ([\mathbf{f}]_1, [\mathbf{f}]_2, [\mathbf{f}]_3) = (1, -3, 2)$. Suppose $m = 2$ and $\mathbf{r} = ([\mathbf{r}]_1, [\mathbf{r}]_2) = (0.1, -10)$. Then $\mathbf{f} \otimes \mathbf{r} = \mathbf{b}$ is a vector with six components: $\mathbf{b} = ([\mathbf{b}]_{11}, [\mathbf{b}]_{12}; [\mathbf{b}]_{21}, [\mathbf{b}]_{22}; [\mathbf{b}]_{31}, [\mathbf{b}]_{32}) = ([\mathbf{f}]_1 \times [\mathbf{r}]_1, [\mathbf{f}]_1 \times [\mathbf{r}]_2; [\mathbf{f}]_2 \times [\mathbf{r}]_1, \ldots) = (0.1, -10; -0.3, 30; 0.2, -20)$.

[6] McClelland and Rumelhart's (1981) classical model of the perception of letters in words uses this sort of representation in its input layer. For each of the letters in a four-letter word, there is a separate group of units. The distributed pattern of activity in the first of these four groups represents the first letter of the stimulus word. Different first letters correspond to different patterns over the same units. A letter's activation pattern is determined by the pattern of lines used to draw it, so letters with similar forms are represented by similar activation patterns.

ferent distributed pattern **B** realizing **B**. Just as before, this combined pattern **AB** realizes the string **AB**, and may be analyzed as the sum of two vectors, $\mathbf{A}_1$ (realizing **A** in the first position) and $\mathbf{B}_2$ (realizing **B** in the second position): equation (14) holds exactly here as well.

Figure 4. Semilocal realization of symbol strings

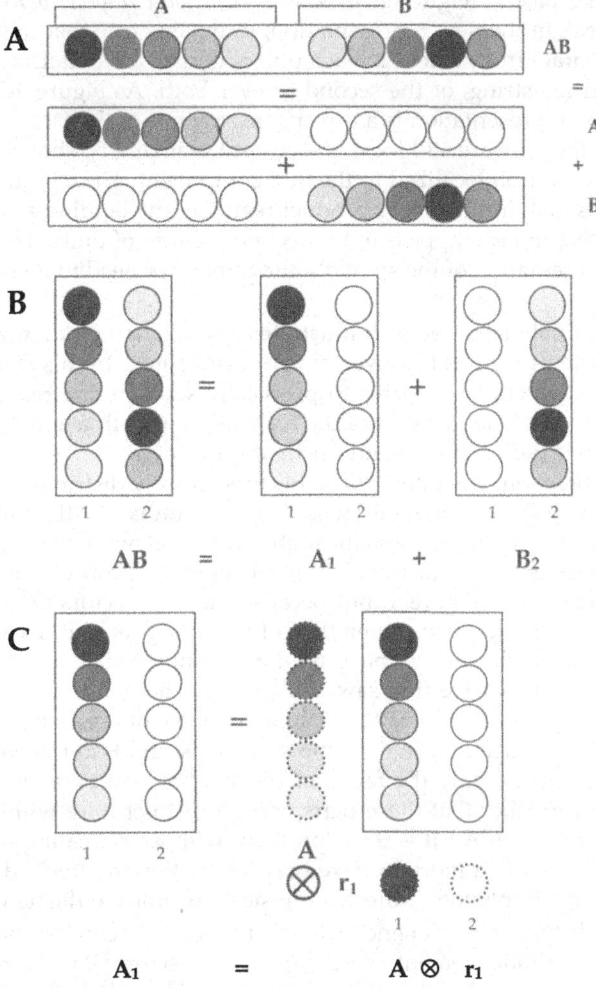

Figure 4B simply rotates the two subpatterns so that in Figure 4C we may readily see the internal tensor product structure of the constituent vector $\mathbf{A}_1$. As in the local case, it is simply the tensor product of the vector **A** (vertical, left of the box) with a vector

(1 0) = $\mathbf{r}_1$ realizing the role of 'first position' in the string (horizontal, below the box). The mathematical structure of Figure 4 is identical to that of Figure 2: only the activation patterns chosen for the illustration have changed. Under vector space analysis, the formal structure of the cases of local and distributed patterns realizing the symbols is exactly the same.

While the realization of **AB** shown in Figure 4 is clearly more distributed than its purely local counterpart in Figure 2, it is still local *with respect to realization of the roles*—it is **semilocal**. In the new representation, it remains true that the realization of **A** is physically separate from that of **B**; each unit is part of the pattern realizing either the first symbol in the string, or the second—never both. As Figure 4C makes clear, this property of the representation is a direct consequence of the fact that the activity patterns realizing the *roles* are still local: the pattern realizing r_1, shown in Figure 4C, is $\mathbf{r}_1$ = (1 0), with activation localized to the first component. The 0 in the second component of $\mathbf{r}_1$ means that, in the tensor product realizing the binding **A**/r_1 (the pattern in the box), no activation can appear in the second column of units. Thus, in order to delocalize the representation of the symbols altogether, we need to delocalize the role vectors.

Figure 5 is the final in our series. It illustrates a realization of **AB** in which the patterns chosen for role as well as filler vectors are distributed. In this **fully distributed representation**, it is no longer possible to physically separate the realizations of the two symbols: every unit is in fact part of the realization of both **A** and **B**. (Recall that a white-bordered circle indicates a negative activation value.)

In the next subsection, we will discuss this type of fully distributed realization of strings in more detail. For the moment, what is important is that the fully distributed case shares exactly the same mathematical structure that we have seen at work in more visibly transparent form in the fully local representation of Figure 2 and the semilocal representation of Figure 4. But because the role vectors are now nonlocal, the roles r_1 and r_2 (first and second members of the string) are not localized to separable parts of the network, and we have the kind of nontrivial superposition of the realizations of **A** and **B** that we first saw in Figure 1. There, two vectors realizing **A** and **B** were superimposed to realize {**A**, **B**}; here, two vectors realizing **A**/r_1 and **B**/r_2 are superimposed to realize **AB**. Binding the symbols **A** and **B** to role vectors is what allows us to represent not only the fact that the symbols are parts combined into a common whole, but further that these parts occupy distinct roles within that whole. This allows us to solve the $\mathbf{A}+\mathbf{B} = \mathbf{B}+\mathbf{A}$ problem without retreating from fully distributed representations to a more localized representation in which 'different structural roles' translates simply into 'different physical positions in the network'.

We must recall that the independence assumption (9) requires that the realizations of different symbolic elements be independent vectors. For the realizations of simple sets, this meant that the realizations of the atomic symbols **A** and **B** themselves had to be independent, for it was these patterns that were superimposed. Now it is the realizations of the bindings **A**/r_1 and **B**/r_2 that are superimposed, so it is these binding vectors that must be independent. The obvious extension of our earlier independence condition is given in (18).

Figure 5. Fully distributed realization of symbol strings

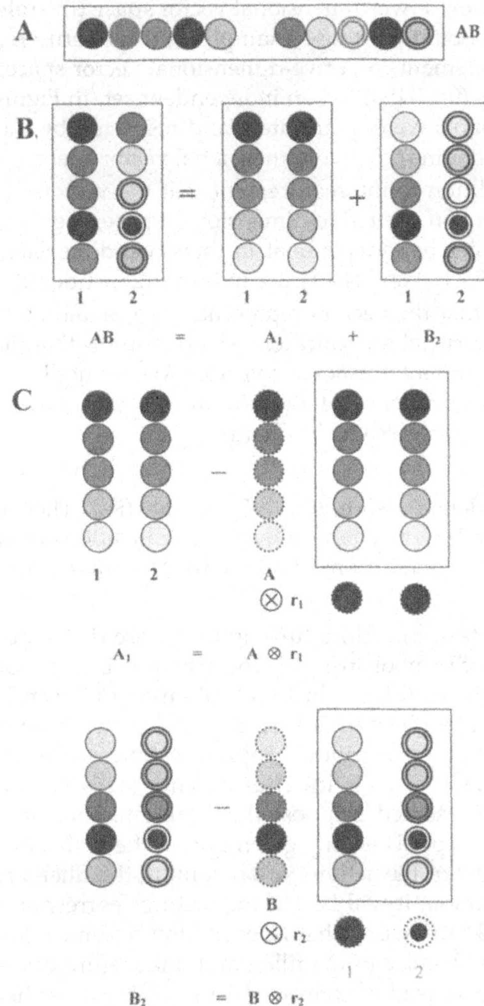

(18) **Independence assumption**

In a connectionist realization of symbolic computation, the activation vectors realizing the atomic symbols, and those realizing the role vectors, are (linearly) independent.

Here, it is understood that the patterns realizing the atomic symbols lie in one vector space and must be independent within that space, while the patterns realizing the roles lie in a different vector space and must be independent within that space. In the examples of Figure 2 and 4, the roles r_1 and r_2 were realized by the vectors (1 0) and (0 1), respectively: in their own two-dimensional vector space (the **role space**), these vectors are indeed independent. In those examples, the patterns realizing the atomic symbols **A**, **B**, ... were elements of a five-dimensional vector space; in Figure 2, these vectors were (1 0 0 0 0), (0 1 0 0 0), ..., an independent set. In Figure 4, the vectors realizing the atomic symbols were distributed, and restricted by the requirement that they must be independent in their five-dimensional vector space.

In Figure 5, in addition to the requirement that the vectors realizing the atomic symbols be independent in their five-dimensional space, we must require that the vectors realizing the roles be independent in their two-dimensional space. The role vectors used in Figure 5, (1 1) and (1 –1), are indeed independent.

We have required that the vectors representing roles and atomic symbols be independent, but what is crucial for realization of structure is that the patterns actually superimposed be independent: the *binding* vectors. We do not have to add a separate assumption for the independence of the binding vectors, however; the following theorem follows from results derived in Chapter 8:

(19) Proposition

Let the independence assumption (18) be satisfied. Then it follows that the binding vectors $\mathbf{f} \otimes \mathbf{r}$—as $\mathbf{f}$ ranges over the realizations of all the atomic symbols, and $\mathbf{r}$ over the realizations of all the roles—will form a linearly independent set.

The final issue we take up before turning to a more developed example of fully distributed realization of symbol strings is the semantic interpretation of the activity of individual units in the tensor product realization of a filler/role binding. A more precise formulation will be given in Section 8:2.2.2, but the intuition here is straightforward. A canonical type of distributed representation is one in which each unit's activity registers the presence (activity 1) or absence (activity 0) of some feature or property in the item represented. Suppose the representations of the atomic symbols and the roles are of this type. Then any given unit in the realization of a binding will be the numerical product of the activity of one unit in the filler's realization and one unit in the role's realization: it will be 1 if the features corresponding to those units are both present, and 0 otherwise. That is, each binding unit represents the *conjunction* of two features, one feature of the filler, and one feature of the role. Such representations have long been used in connectionist models under the name **conjunctive coding** (see, e.g., Hinton, McClelland, and Rumelhart 1986; McClelland and Kawamoto 1986).

As a simple example, consider *Josh fell.* The argument structure (Section 1:3.3) of the verb *to fall* has a role r for an undergoer, bound to the filler f, Josh. A distributed representation for such argument roles might employ a feature AFFECTED, which is present in (or true of) the role *r*. If this feature corresponds to the βth component of the role vector, then this component $[\mathbf{r}]_\beta = 1$. A distributed representation for fillers might involve a feature ANIMATE, which is certainly true of Josh. If the corresponding component of the filler vector is α, then $[\mathbf{f}]_\alpha = 1$. In the tensor product vector $\mathbf{f} \otimes \mathbf{r} = \mathbf{b}$ that represents the binding of Josh to the undergoer role, one of the units is labeled αβ; the activation value of this unit is $[\mathbf{b}]_{\alpha\beta} = [\mathbf{f}]_\alpha \times [\mathbf{r}]_\beta = 1$. This binding unit will be active if (and only if) the features corresponding to α and β are both present; it thus represents the conjunction ANIMATE & AFFECTED. This binding unit will also be active in the representation of *Josh grew*, but inactive in *the ball fell* and *Josh dropped the ball.*

Thus, tensor product binding is a descendant of the notion of conjunctive coding. Psychological models of memory for structured items (e.g., sequences) have for some time employed many of the same mathematical ideas (e.g., Murdock 1982; Pike 1984). Tensor product binding was first explicitly defined, analyzed, and employed in connectionist models in Dolan and Dyer 1987; Smolensky 1987, 1990; Dolan 1989; Dolan and Smolensky 1989; Legendre, Miyata, and Smolensky 1991.

1.2.2 Global structure illustrated

It is helpful to work out explicitly a very simple case of fully distributed representations of strings. In order to graphically display the example, it is necessary to severely restrict its scope.

As our alphabet of atomic symbols, we take {**A**, **B**, **C**, **D**}. We will consider only strings of length two, so the roles we employ are the ones introduced above, $\{r_1, r_2\}$: *element*$_1$ and *element*$_2$ of the string.

The vectors we choose for realizing the symbols and roles are as follows. The symbols will be realized in a two-dimensional vector space.

(20)

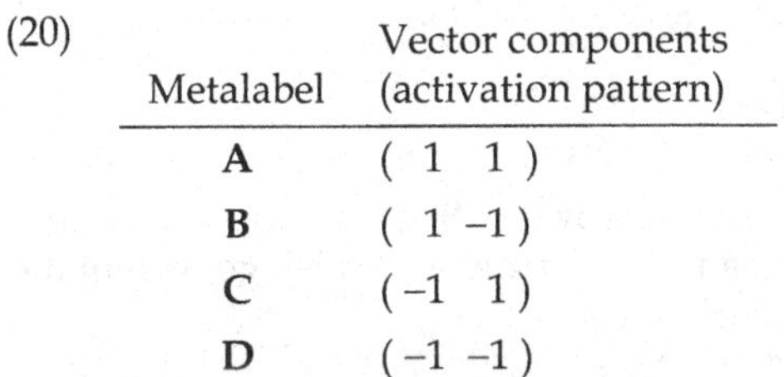

Metalabel	Vector components (activation pattern)
A	(1 1)
B	(1 –1)
C	(–1 1)
D	(–1 –1)

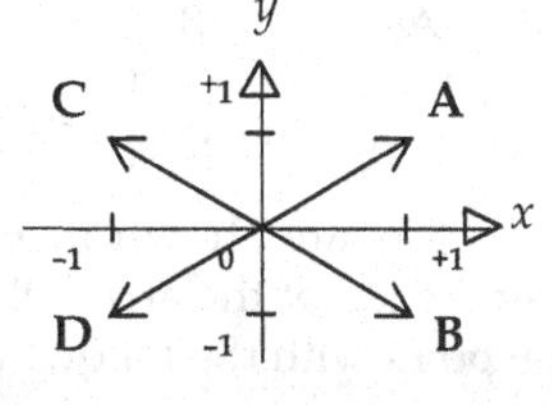

The roles will also be realized in a two-dimensional space.

(21)

Metalabel	Vector components (activation pattern)
$\mathbf{r}_1$	(1 1)
$\mathbf{r}_2$	(1 –1)

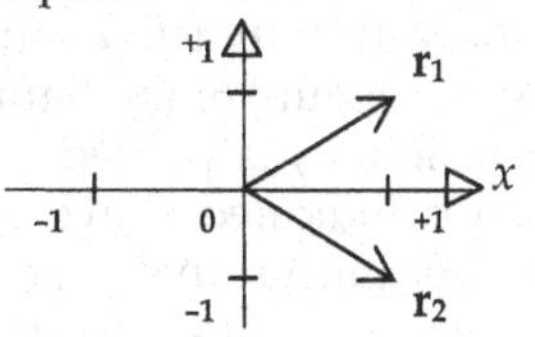

The filler vectors are not linearly independent (no more than two vectors can be independent in the two-dimensional filler space being employed in this simple illustration), so we are not guaranteed by the general mathematical analysis presented above that their identity will be preserved under superposition. Subsequent analysis in Chapter 8 (20) will show, however, that because the role vectors *are* independent, and each role is bound to at most one filler, no ambiguities can result in the distributed realizations of symbol strings: from the realization of a string, it can be uniquely determined which symbols appear in each position.

Computing the appropriate tensor products, we find the following patterns of activation realizing the possible bindings:

(22)

$$\begin{array}{r|ll}
\otimes & \mathbf{r}_1 = (1\ \ 1) & \mathbf{r}_2 = (1\ \ -1) \\
\hline
\mathbf{A} = \begin{pmatrix}1\\1\end{pmatrix} & \mathbf{A}_1 = \begin{pmatrix}1 & 1\\1 & 1\end{pmatrix} & \mathbf{A}_2 = \begin{pmatrix}1 & -1\\1 & -1\end{pmatrix} \\
\mathbf{B} = \begin{pmatrix}1\\-1\end{pmatrix} & \mathbf{B}_1 = \begin{pmatrix}1 & 1\\-1 & -1\end{pmatrix} & \mathbf{B}_2 = \begin{pmatrix}1 & -1\\-1 & 1\end{pmatrix} \\
\mathbf{C} = \begin{pmatrix}-1\\1\end{pmatrix} & \mathbf{C}_1 = \begin{pmatrix}-1 & -1\\1 & 1\end{pmatrix} & \mathbf{C}_2 = \begin{pmatrix}-1 & 1\\1 & -1\end{pmatrix} \\
\mathbf{D} = \begin{pmatrix}-1\\-1\end{pmatrix} & \mathbf{D}_1 = \begin{pmatrix}-1 & -1\\-1 & -1\end{pmatrix} & \mathbf{D}_2 = \begin{pmatrix}-1 & 1\\-1 & 1\end{pmatrix}
\end{array}$$

We can now readily compute the patterns realizing the two strings **AB** and **BA**.

(23)
$$\mathbf{AB} = \mathbf{A}_1 + \mathbf{B}_2 = \begin{pmatrix}1 & 1\\1 & 1\end{pmatrix} + \begin{pmatrix}1 & -1\\-1 & 1\end{pmatrix} = \begin{pmatrix}2 & 0\\0 & 2\end{pmatrix}$$

(24)
$$\mathbf{BA} = \mathbf{A}_2 + \mathbf{B}_1 = \begin{pmatrix}1 & -1\\1 & -1\end{pmatrix} + \begin{pmatrix}1 & 1\\-1 & -1\end{pmatrix} = \begin{pmatrix}2 & 0\\0 & -2\end{pmatrix}.$$

These two vectors are shown in Figure 6 using arrows; **AB** is the arrow resulting from placing the tail of the arrow $\mathbf{B}_2$ at the head of the arrow $\mathbf{A}_1$, which goes from the origin to the point with the following four coordinates:

(25)
$$\begin{pmatrix}w & x\\z & y\end{pmatrix} = \begin{pmatrix}2 & 0\\0 & 2\end{pmatrix}.$$

(25) shows how the four activation values of the binding units are paired with the coordinate axes in Figure 6; the figure shows how the x, y, and z axes are plotted. The fourth dimension, w, is plotted as follows. Each cube corresponds to a different w value, which is indicated above the cube; the values plotted are $w = -1, 0, 1, 2$. Of course, the two-dimensional page can't be used to unambiguously plot even a three-dimensional space, let alone the four-dimensional space we have here. But hopefully Figure 6 nonetheless helps to convey the relations among the binding vectors $\mathbf{A}_1$, $\mathbf{B}_1$,

$\mathbf{A}_2$, $\mathbf{B}_2$ and the vectors **AB**, **BA**.

Figure 6. String realizations in activation space

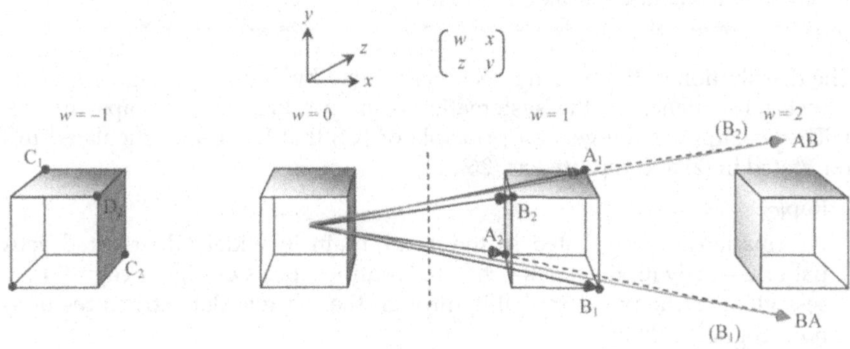

Figure 6 also plots the binding vectors involving the other symbols, **C** and **D**. This figure visually conveys some of the systematic relations linking these binding vectors that arise from their shared internal tensor product structure. For example, $\mathbf{A}_1$ and $\mathbf{A}_2$ are related by being respectively the product of $\mathbf{r}_1$ and $\mathbf{r}_2$ with a common vector: **A**. The visual manifestation of this relation in Figure 6 is that these vectors are at diagonally opposite corners of the back face of the cube; this same relation holds between $\mathbf{C}_1$ and $\mathbf{C}_2$, and on the front faces of their cubes, between the pairs $\mathbf{B}_1$, $\mathbf{B}_2$ and $\mathbf{D}_1$, $\mathbf{D}_2$ as well. Each binding with the first-position role r_1 is on the outer face of its cube (furthest from the origin) while its corresponding binding with the role r_2 is at the diagonally opposite corner of the inner face of its cube; see Demonstration 1.

Demonstration 1

Let $\mathbf{u} = (u_1, u_2)$ be the vector realizing one of the symbols {**A**, …, **D**}.[7] The relationship between $\mathbf{u}_1$ and $\mathbf{u}_2$ is captured by the difference vector

$$\Delta\mathbf{u} \equiv \mathbf{u}_1 - \mathbf{u}_2 = \mathbf{u}\otimes\mathbf{r}_1 - \mathbf{u}\otimes\mathbf{r}_2 = \mathbf{u}\otimes[\mathbf{r}_1 - \mathbf{r}_2] = \mathbf{u}\otimes[(1,1) - (1,-1)] = \mathbf{u}\otimes(0,2).$$

The components of this vector are

$$\begin{matrix} \otimes & \begin{bmatrix} 0 & 2 \end{bmatrix} \\ \begin{pmatrix} u_1 \\ u_2 \end{pmatrix} & \begin{pmatrix} 0 & 2u_1 \\ 0 & 2u_2 \end{pmatrix} \end{matrix} = \begin{pmatrix} \Delta w & \Delta x \\ \Delta z & \Delta y \end{pmatrix}.$$

This vector $\Delta\mathbf{u}$ extends from $\mathbf{u}_2$ to $\mathbf{u}_1$. Since its w-component Δw is zero, this vector lies within a single cube (points with a single w value); that is, $\mathbf{u}_2$ and $\mathbf{u}_1$ lie in the same w-cube whatever symbol **u** may denote. Similarly, since Δz is zero, $\mathbf{u}_2$ and $\mathbf{u}_1$ have the same value of z, that is, they lie on the same z-plane (relative to the z-axis directed "into" the paper, they have the same "depth"). Finally, $\mathbf{u}_2$ and $\mathbf{u}_1$ lie at opposite corners of the square with constant w and z value that they fall on. This is because, within

[7] u_1 is a single number, the first activation value in **u**. This should not be confused with $\mathbf{u}_1 \equiv \mathbf{u}\otimes\mathbf{r}_1$, a binding vector with four component numbers; $\mathbf{u}_1$ is the realization of the binding to role r_1 of the symbol realized by **u**.

that square, the vector $(\Delta x, \Delta y)$ is twice the vector (u_1, u_2), that is, in the same direction as **u**. All four vectors **u** realizing symbols are diagonally directed (20). They are also directed outward from the origin, so the vector from $\mathbf{u}_2$ to $\mathbf{u}_1$ is directed away from the origin; $\mathbf{u}_1$ is further from the origin than $\mathbf{u}_2$.

The distribution of the binding vectors revealed by Figure 6 is highly systematic —a direct consequence of the systematic tensor product relationships that relate them. This exemplifies the general principle of ICS that has been articulated in this section, stated in (2) and repeated as (26).

(26) Rep$_{\text{ICS}}$
Information is represented in the mind/brain in widely distributed activity patterns—activation vectors—that, for central aspects of higher cognition, possess global structure describable through the discrete data structures of symbolic cognitive theory.

The particular patterns that realize the role vectors will influence the exact geometric manifestation of the tensor product structure that relates the symbol bindings they define. What is crucially responsible for the systematic computational consequences of the systematic relations between bindings are the algebraic, tensor product relations only—their geometric counterparts are only an aid to the eye. These algebraic relations are guaranteed to hold by the principles of the theory we have been developing in this section.

Figure 7 expands on Figure 6 by plotting not only the vectors realizing strings involving **A** and **B**, but also a number of vectors realizing strings involving the remaining symbols. As before, Figure 7 shows the systematic relationships between individual bindings—like the relation between $\mathbf{C}_1$ and $\mathbf{C}_2$, which we can denote $\mathbf{C}_1 : \mathbf{C}_2$, where the filler is fixed while the role varies. In addition, Figure 7 shows the systematic relations between the vectors realizing related strings. For example, the pair **CA** : **CB** instantiates the same relation as the pair **AA** : **AB**—that is, **uA** : **uB**—and in Figure 7 this shared relation has the following geometric consequence: the **uA** vector is deeper and higher than the **uB** vector (deeper and higher by 2 units—that is, z- and y-coordinates differ by 2; Demonstration 2).

Demonstration 2
The vector from **uB** to **uA** is

$$\mathbf{uA} - \mathbf{uB} = [\mathbf{u} \otimes \mathbf{r}_1 + \mathbf{A} \otimes \mathbf{r}_2] - [\mathbf{u} \otimes \mathbf{r}_1 + \mathbf{B} \otimes \mathbf{r}_2] = \mathbf{A} \otimes \mathbf{r}_2 - \mathbf{B} \otimes \mathbf{r}_2 = [\mathbf{A} - \mathbf{B}] \otimes \mathbf{r}_2.$$

Since $\mathbf{A} - \mathbf{B} = (0, 2)$,

$$\begin{matrix} \otimes & \begin{bmatrix} 1 & -1 \end{bmatrix} \\ \begin{bmatrix} 0 \\ 2 \end{bmatrix} & \begin{pmatrix} 0 & 0 \\ 2 & -2 \end{pmatrix} \end{matrix} = \begin{pmatrix} \Delta w & \Delta x \\ \Delta z & \Delta y \end{pmatrix}.$$

Since $\Delta w = 0$, as in Demonstration 1 we know that **uA** and **uB** are in the same w-cube. Since $\Delta x = 0$, **uA** and **uB** must be on the same x-plane (the vertical planes going into the paper where x has a constant value). **uA** and **uB** differ only in their height (Δy = −2) and "depth" (Δz = 2); **uA** is 2 units lower and 2 units "deeper" than **uB**, whatever symbol **u** may realize.

Figure 7. Further string realizations in activation space

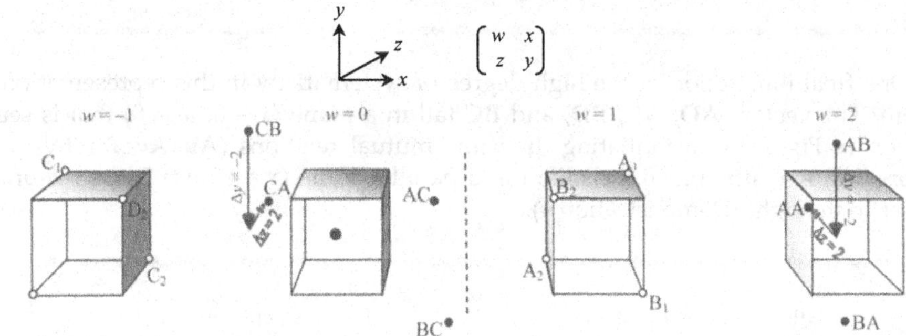

Other, higher-order, systematic relations among the vectors realizing related strings are illustrated in Figure 8. Emanating from the origin is a set of four arrows with dashed lines—something like a child's jack with four spokes; these are the realizations of the four symbols each bound to r_2. Now compare this four-way relationship with that connecting the four vectors **AA**, **AB**, **AC**, and **AD**: it is identical. The vectors realizing the four strings with **A** in first position emanate from the vector $\mathbf{A}_1$ in just the same way the dashed "jack" emanates from the origin. So do the vectors realizing the four strings with any other symbol in first position: the case of **B** is also shown in Figure 8, where now the hub of the spokes is $\mathbf{B}_1$ (Demonstration 3).

Figure 8. Systematicity of string realizations

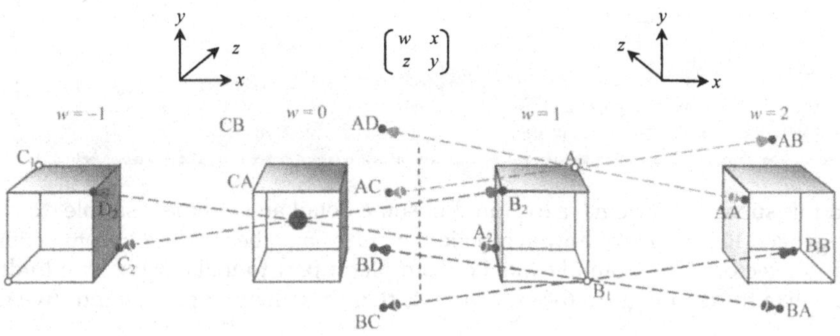

Demonstration 3
Since

$$\mathbf{uA} = \mathbf{u}_1 + \mathbf{A}_2, \quad \mathbf{uB} = \mathbf{u}_1 + \mathbf{B}_2, \quad \mathbf{uC} = \mathbf{u}_1 + \mathbf{C}_2, \quad \mathbf{uD} = \mathbf{u}_1 + \mathbf{D}_2,$$

the four string vectors **uA**, **uB**, **uC**, **uD** consist of the four binding vectors $\mathbf{A}_2$, $\mathbf{B}_2$, $\mathbf{C}_2$, $\mathbf{D}_2$ each displaced by $\mathbf{u}_1$. The four binding vectors $\mathbf{A}_1$, …, $\mathbf{D}_2$ make up the jack at the origin. Sliding the jack so that its center is located at $\mathbf{u}_1$ gives the four string vectors. This is true regardless of the symbol realized by **u**.

One final illustration of the high degree of systematicity in this representational system. The vectors **AD, AC, BD,** and **BC** fall in a plane ($x = 0$, $w = 0$) that is seen edge-on in Figure 8. Instantiating the same mutual relations (**Au** : **Av** : **Bu** : **Bv**), the vectors **AB, AA, BB,** and **BA** also fall in a parallel plane ($x = 0$, $w = 2$), two w-units further to the right (Demonstration 4).

Demonstration 4
The relations **Au** : **Av** : **Bu** : **Bv** are captured by the differences between these four vectors, given in the following table; each cell equals the vector labeling its column minus the vector labeling its row.

–	**Av**	**Bu**	**Bv**
Au	$\mathbf{v}_2 - \mathbf{u}_2$	$\mathbf{B}_1 - \mathbf{A}_1$	$(\mathbf{B}_1 - \mathbf{A}_1) + (\mathbf{v}_2 - \mathbf{u}_2)$
	Av	$(\mathbf{B}_1 - \mathbf{A}_1) - (\mathbf{v}_2 - \mathbf{u}_2)$	$\mathbf{B}_1 - \mathbf{A}_1$
		Bu	$\mathbf{v}_2 - \mathbf{u}_2$

All these differences are linear combinations of the vectors $\mathbf{B}_1 - \mathbf{A}_1$ and $\mathbf{v}_2 - \mathbf{u}_2$, where **u**, **v** is either **B**, **A** or **D**, **C**:

$$\mathbf{B}_1 - \mathbf{A}_1 = \begin{pmatrix} 1 & 1 \\ -1 & -1 \end{pmatrix} - \begin{pmatrix} 1 & 1 \\ 1 & 1 \end{pmatrix} = \begin{pmatrix} 0 & 0 \\ -2 & -2 \end{pmatrix} = \begin{pmatrix} \Delta w & \Delta x \\ \Delta z & \Delta y \end{pmatrix}$$

$$\mathbf{A}_2 - \mathbf{B}_2 = \begin{pmatrix} 1 & -1 \\ 1 & -1 \end{pmatrix} - \begin{pmatrix} 1 & -1 \\ -1 & 1 \end{pmatrix} = \begin{pmatrix} 0 & 0 \\ 2 & -2 \end{pmatrix} = \begin{pmatrix} \Delta w & \Delta x \\ \Delta z & \Delta y \end{pmatrix}$$

$$\mathbf{C}_2 - \mathbf{D}_2 = \begin{pmatrix} -1 & 1 \\ 1 & -1 \end{pmatrix} - \begin{pmatrix} -1 & 1 \\ -1 & 1 \end{pmatrix} = \begin{pmatrix} 0 & 0 \\ 2 & -2 \end{pmatrix} = \begin{pmatrix} \Delta w & \Delta x \\ \Delta z & \Delta y \end{pmatrix}$$

In every case, $\Delta w = 0 = \Delta x$, just as in Demonstration 2; thus, the four vectors in the relation **Au** : **Av** : **Bu** : **Bv** all lie in the same x-plane, with constant x and w values.

In this subsection, we have explored in some detail an extremely simple example of the general ICS theory of how symbolic structures may be realized in connectionist activation vectors. The example was kept simple in part to make it possible to draw pictures like those in Figures 6–8; the hope is that these help to give an intuitive feeling for the fundamental principle Rep$_{\text{ICS}}$ (26).[8] Even with only two units for realizing symbols and two for realizing roles, we already need to draw four-dimensional figures. Obviously, in any more interesting examples pictures will be of very limited help, and we will have to rely on algebraic notation. Fortunately, this notation is really quite simple; it is summarized in Table 3.

Table 3. Connectionist variable binding via the tensor product (⊗)

	Structuring	Symbolic formalization		Connectionist formalization	
Sec.	operation	Structures	Example	Example	Vector operation
1.1	Combining	Sets	$\{\mathbf{c}_1, \mathbf{c}_2\}$	$\mathbf{c}_1 + \mathbf{c}_2$	Vector sum: +
1.2	Filler/role binding	Strings, frames	AB = $\{$A$/r_1$, B$/r_2\}$	$\mathbf{A}\otimes\mathbf{r}_1 + \mathbf{B}\otimes\mathbf{r}_2$	Tensor product: ⊗
1.3	Recursive embedding	Trees	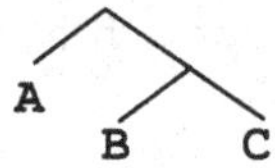 [tree: A, [B C]]		?

The final stage in the articulation of the first principle, Rep$_{\text{ICS}}$ (26), is to fill in the '?' in Table 3 regarding the realization of recursive embedding. Before moving on to this topic, let's consider the generality of the analysis developed in this subsection. In addition to its obvious applicability to strings of any length over an alphabet of any size, the analysis extends without modification from strings to any type of symbolic structure in which a fixed set of atomic elements may fill a fixed set of atomic roles: employing a term from Minsky 1975, I will call such structures 'frames'.

For example, consider a world under a description in which each possible state of the world is specified in terms of a fixed set of relationships that may hold among a fixed set of objects. A classic artificial intelligence 'blocks world' case (Winograd 1973) might involve a fixed set of locations L_i on a table and a fixed set of blocks B_j, a particular state of the world being specified by the fillers of a fixed set of roles such as r_j = B_j*'s-support*. That is, a state of this world is a set of filler/role bindings $\{\mathtt{f}_k/r_k\}$ in which $\mathtt{f}_k$ is the support of block B_k; this support is either one of the other blocks B_j or a location on the table L_i. The connectionist representation of such a world-state would be a vector **s** in the now-familiar form

(27) $\mathbf{s} = \Sigma_k\, \mathbf{f}_k \otimes \mathbf{r}_k.$

So if block B_3 supports block B_5, one constituent vector in the representation of the state is $\mathbf{c} = \mathbf{B}_3 \otimes \mathbf{r}_5$.

This example allows us to segue into the next subsection—the general problem of recursive embedding—because the roles it employs, $\{r_k$ = B_k*'s-support*$\}$, need not be viewed as atomic; they exhibit a very simple structure, consisting of the binding of a subfiller B_k to a subrole, r_{supp} = __*'s-support*. The tensor product may be used, recursively, to realize this binding in turn:

[8] The example explicitly instantiates the part of the ICS map depicted in Figure 2:4.

(28) $\mathbf{r}_k = \mathbf{B}_k \otimes \mathbf{r}_{supp}$.

For example, $\mathbf{r}_5 = \mathbf{B}_5 \otimes \mathbf{r}_{supp}$ because $\mathbf{r}_5$ is *B_5's-support*.

When these role vectors are substituted back into the equation for the world-state, we get

(29) $\mathbf{s} = \Sigma_k \mathbf{f}_k \otimes \mathbf{r}_k = \Sigma_k \mathbf{f}_k \otimes \mathbf{B}_k \otimes \mathbf{r}_{supp}$.

Because the original roles were further decomposed into subroles and subfillers, the overall representation involves the superposition of vectors each of which is the tensor product of *three* atomic vectors. So in our example,

(30) $\mathbf{c} = \mathbf{B}_3 \otimes \mathbf{B}_5 \otimes \mathbf{r}_{supp}$,

which is naturally interpreted as a tensor product realization of the binary relation **`supports(B₃, B₅)`**. (See Section 7:4 for further discussion of such **contextual roles**.) We now apply this same type of approach to the realization of recursive symbolic structures.

1.3 Embedding via recursively defined role vectors

The final problem concerning connectionist representation that we take up in this chapter concerns recursion.

(31) **The problem of embedding and recursion**

How can tensor product realization—where the vector **f/r** representing the binding of the filler **`f`** to the structural role *r* is $\mathbf{f} \otimes \mathbf{r}$—cope with embedded structure, where the filler is itself a complex structure, not an atomic symbol? Worse, how can it work when the embedding is unboundedly deep, as in recursive data structures?

The proposed approach to solving this problem has already been illustrated at the end of the previous subsection: we just recursively use tensor product realization for the complex fillers (or roles). The case we will examine is that of trees with binary branching. This type of recursive structure is of direct relevance to linguistic representations for the syntactic structure of sentences (e.g., Kayne 1984; Chomsky 1995); it is also a general-purpose recursive data structure, the basis, for example, of the structures processed by Lisp, the quintessential programming language for symbol manipulation (see Box 23:1). Here, we will assume that atomic symbols are placed only at the leaves of the tree; all internal tree nodes are unlabeled. The extension to the case of interior nodes labeled with atomic symbols is straightforward.

The recursive characterization of binary trees is simple: there are only two roles, r_0 = *left-subtree* and r_1 = *right-subtree* (in Lisp, the functions that extract these are respectively named **`car`** and **`cdr`**). A binary tree has each of these roles bound to a filler, which is itself either a binary tree or an atomic symbol.

The fundamental property essential to a connectionist realization of the structure of binary trees is given in (32).[9]

(32) **Recursive connectionist realization**

Let $\mathtt{s}$ be a binary tree with left and right subtrees $\mathtt{p}$ and $\mathtt{q}$; $\mathtt{s} = [\mathtt{p}\ \mathtt{q}]$, or, more graphically:

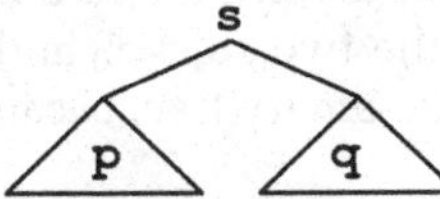

Given a connectionist realization of binary trees, let $\mathbf{s}$, $\mathbf{p}$, and $\mathbf{q}$ be the vectors realizing the trees $\mathtt{s}$, $\mathtt{p}$, and $\mathtt{q}$. Then the connectionist realization is **recursive** iff, for all trees $\mathtt{s}$,

$$\mathbf{s} = \mathbf{p} \otimes \mathbf{r}_0 + \mathbf{q} \otimes \mathbf{r}_1.$$

If either of the fillers $\mathtt{p}$ or $\mathtt{q}$ is an atomic symbol (e.g., $\mathtt{A}$), its realization is simply some vector $\mathbf{p}$ or $\mathbf{q}$ (e.g., $\mathbf{A}$) without further analyzable substructure. But if either of the fillers is itself a tree, then, given a recursive realization, the realization of that filler must also obey the fundamental equation, which, by the definition of a recursive realization, applies to the realization of all trees. If $\mathtt{q}$ is a tree rather than an atomic symbol, it can be expressed in terms of its left and right subtrees: $\mathtt{q} = [\mathtt{p}'\ \mathtt{q}']$. Then (32) entails

(33) $\mathbf{q} = \mathbf{p}' \otimes \mathbf{r}_0 + \mathbf{q}' \otimes \mathbf{r}_1$,

where $\mathbf{p}'$, $\mathbf{q}'$ are the realizations of the subtrees $\mathtt{p}'$ and $\mathtt{q}'$. This expansion of vectors realizing trees into the vectors realizing their subtrees may be recursively continued until the atomic symbols at the leaves of the tree have been reached.

Let's see how this works out in a simple case. Consider the structure $\mathtt{s} = [\mathtt{A}\ [\mathtt{B}\ \mathtt{C}]]$:

(34) $\mathtt{s}$ = A [B C] (tree: A; B C)

Here, $\mathtt{p}$ is the atomic symbol $\mathtt{A}$ while $\mathtt{q}$ is a subtree containing $\mathtt{B}$ and $\mathtt{C}$.

(35) $\mathtt{p} = \mathtt{A}$ $\quad \mathtt{q} = [\mathtt{B}\ \mathtt{C}]$ = B C

So in a recursive connectionist realization, the vectors $\mathbf{s}$, $\mathbf{p}$, and $\mathbf{q}$ realizing $\mathtt{s}$, $\mathtt{p}$, and $\mathtt{q}$ will obey (32),

(36) $\mathbf{s} = \mathbf{p} \otimes \mathbf{r}_0 + \mathbf{q} \otimes \mathbf{r}_1 = \mathbf{A} \otimes \mathbf{r}_0 + \mathbf{q} \otimes \mathbf{r}_1$,

and $\mathbf{q}$ will obey (33),

(37) $\mathbf{q} = \mathbf{B} \otimes \mathbf{r}_0 + \mathbf{C} \otimes \mathbf{r}_1$.

[9] As above, atomic symbols will be denoted by uppercase, typewriter-font characters such as '$\mathtt{A}$'; lowercase characters in the same font, such as '$\mathtt{a}$', will be variables denoting either an atomic symbol or a composite symbol structure.

Substituting (37) into (36) yields

(38) $$\begin{aligned} \mathbf{s} &= \mathbf{A} \otimes \mathbf{r}_0 + [\qquad\quad \mathbf{q} \qquad\quad] \otimes \mathbf{r}_1 \\ &= \mathbf{A} \otimes \mathbf{r}_0 + [\mathbf{B} \otimes \mathbf{r}_0 \quad + \mathbf{C} \otimes \mathbf{r}_1] \otimes \mathbf{r}_1 \\ &= \mathbf{A} \otimes \mathbf{r}_0 + \mathbf{B} \otimes [\mathbf{r}_0 \otimes \mathbf{r}_1] + \mathbf{C} \otimes [\mathbf{r}_1 \otimes \mathbf{r}_1]. \end{aligned}$$

This last form is the complete expression for the realization of the tree **s** in terms of the realization of the atomic symbols it contains and the two roles r_0 and r_1. These two roles are all that we need to specify the structure of a binary tree, because we can use them recursively.

This expression for **s** (38) has another interpretation, which makes direct contact with the end of the previous subsection. The equation gives **s** as the superposition of three vectors, each of which is a tensor product of a vector realizing an atomic symbol and another vector, delimited by square brackets. This is a familiar form: a sum of filler/role binding vectors, each the tensor product of a filler vector and a role vector. From this new perspective, the fillers are simply atomic symbols; in the original, recursive decomposition, the fillers were either atomic symbols or subtrees. From the new perspective, the filler vectors are not structured. But the role vectors are: they are recursively composed of tensor products of the atomic role vectors $\mathbf{r}_0$, $\mathbf{r}_1$, as in (39).

(39) $$\begin{aligned} \mathbf{s} &= \mathbf{A} \otimes \mathbf{r}_0 + \mathbf{B} \otimes [\mathbf{r}_0 \otimes \mathbf{r}_1] + \mathbf{C} \otimes [\mathbf{r}_1 \otimes \mathbf{r}_1] \\ &= \mathbf{A} \otimes \mathbf{r}_0 + \mathbf{B} \otimes [\ \mathbf{r}_{01}\ ] + \mathbf{C} \otimes [\ \mathbf{r}_{11}\ ]. \end{aligned}$$

In the new perspective, the symbol B is viewed as filling a role in the structure as a whole: 'the left child of the right child of the root', which, in keeping with our convention that 0 ~ left and 1 ~ right, we designate r_{01}; its realization is already derived in (39):

(40) $\mathbf{r}_{01} = \mathbf{r}_0 \otimes \mathbf{r}_1.$

Similarly, C is viewed as filling the role 'the right child of the right child of the root', r_{11}, realized as

(41) $\mathbf{r}_{11} = \mathbf{r}_1 \otimes \mathbf{r}_1.$

Equations (40) and (41) exemplify a general recursion relation between role vectors in this new perspective in which the roles (rather than the fillers) are analyzed as possessing recursive structure. Let x designate some position in the binary tree—for example, the left child of the right child of the left child of the left child of the root, which we will notate simply $x = 0100$. Now consider the two children of this node x. The left child of x, *left-child*(x), is 'the left child of …' where '…' is the verbal description of position x; in our binary notation, this means *left-child*(x) = $0x$, that is, 0 followed by the binary sequence specifying x. Similarly, the right child of x is just $1x$. The connectionist realizations of the roles r_x, r_{0x}, and r_{1x} are the vectors $\mathbf{r}_x$, $\mathbf{r}_{0x}$, and $\mathbf{r}_{1x}$, which in any recursive realization must be systematically related. Indeed, (40) and (41) exemplify such systematic relations, in the simple case of $x = 1$. The general recursion relations (42) are quite intuitive.

(42) **Recursive role vectors for binary trees**

$$\mathbf{r}_{\mathit{left\text{-}child}(x)} = \mathbf{r}_{0x} = \mathbf{r}_0 \otimes \mathbf{r}_x \qquad \mathbf{r}_{\mathit{right\text{-}child}(x)} = \mathbf{r}_{1x} = \mathbf{r}_1 \otimes \mathbf{r}_x$$

These are readily understood in terms of the new perspective's analysis of the roles as structured. Thus, the roles r_{0x} = 'filling location $0x$ in the tree' and r_{1x} = 'filling location $1x$ in the tree' are analyzed as the result of inserting the subfillers 0 and 1 into the subrole r_x = 'filling location __x in the tree'. That is, in terms of filler/role bindings, the analysis is

(43) $r_{0x} = 0/r_x$; $r_{1x} = 1/r_x$.

The realizations of the subfillers 0, 1 are the vectors $\mathbf{r}_0$, $\mathbf{r}_1$, and the realization of the subrole is $\mathbf{r}_x$. By the general tensor product binding theory, the realizations are thus related exactly by equation (42).

We began this subsection with the question, how can filler/role decomposition cope with recursive structure? The answer is, by using itself recursively. This has been spelled out in the important case of binary trees. Chapter 8 develops this proposal further. The general analysis shows that if role vectors are defined recursively, as in (42), it follows that the realization is recursive, as defined in (32); we have also seen this in one particular example, (38).

A final question we will take up here is the meaning of '+' in such equations as (39), repeated in (44):

(44) $\mathbf{s} = \mathbf{A} \otimes \mathbf{r}_0 + (\mathbf{B} \otimes [\mathbf{r}_0 \otimes \mathbf{r}_1] + \mathbf{C} \otimes [\mathbf{r}_1 \otimes \mathbf{r}_1])$.

In what vector space is this addition performed? This question arises because, under the simplest interpretation, the first term $\mathbf{A} \otimes \mathbf{r}_0$ and the second term $\mathbf{B} \otimes [\mathbf{r}_0 \otimes \mathbf{r}_1]$ are vectors in different vector spaces. Because the latter vector involves one additional tensor product with a fundamental role vector ($\mathbf{r}_1$), the number of numerical components in the vector is greater, by a factor equal to the number of numerical components of the fundamental role vectors (which must be at least two, so that $\mathbf{r}_0$ and $\mathbf{r}_1$ may be independent). In connectionist terms, the number of activation values (units) needed to realize the B-binding is greater than the number needed to realize the A-binding, because the former involves a deeper tree position. Indeed, just like the total number of roles, the number of units over which bindings are realized increases geometrically with tree depth; it equals AR^d, where A is the number of units used to realize atomic symbols, and R the number used to realize the fundamental role vectors $\mathbf{r}_0$ and $\mathbf{r}_1$ (two, in the Section 1.2.2 example and the construction in Chapter 8).[10]

From the perspective of vector space theory, the natural interpretation of (44) involves the **direct sum** of vector spaces. To set up this sum, let $V_{(1)}$ be the vector space including the first term in (44), $\mathbf{A} \otimes \mathbf{r}_0$; the vectors composing $V_{(1)}$ are all the linear combinations of vectors of the form $\mathbf{a} \otimes \mathbf{r}_i$, where $\mathbf{a}$ is the vector realizing an atomic

[10] The number of units required for cognitively relevant structures is actually quite modest. Realizing trees with depth up to 6 (maximum of $2^6 = 64$ terminal symbols) with an alphabet of symbols realized by 16-bit vectors (65,536 symbols) requires $16(2^{6+1} - 1) = 2{,}032$ units. The size of tensor product representations is often greatly exaggerated; for example, the case claimed by Marcus (2001, 106) to require $24{,}300{,}000 = (10 \cdot 3)^5$ nodes actually requires $7{,}280 = 10(3^{5+1} - 1)$.

symbol and $\mathbf{r}_i$ is $\mathbf{r}_0$ or $\mathbf{r}_1$. These vectors have AR numerical components and realize symbols at depth 1 in the tree. Similarly, let $V_{(2)}$ be the vector space including the second (and third) term of (44), $\mathbf{B}\otimes[\mathbf{r}_0\otimes\mathbf{r}_1]$. These are all the linear combinations of vectors of the form $\mathbf{a}\otimes\mathbf{r}_i\otimes\mathbf{r}_j$, with AR^2 components, realizing symbols at depth 2. In general, let $V_{(d)}$ be the AR^d-dimensional vector space formed from vectors of the form $\mathbf{a}\otimes\mathbf{r}_i\otimes\mathbf{r}_j\otimes\cdots\otimes\mathbf{r}_k$ with d role vectors; these realize symbols at depth d. $V_{(0)}$ is just the vector space of linear combinations of the vectors $\mathbf{a}$ realizing symbols (or, equivalently, symbols located at depth 0, the tree root).

A vector space containing all the vectors in $V_{(d)}$ for all d is the direct sum in (45):[11]

(45) $V^* \equiv V_{(0)} \oplus V_{(1)} \oplus V_{(2)} \oplus \cdots .$

A vector $\mathbf{s}$ in this space is a sequence of vectors $(\mathbf{s}_{(0)}; \mathbf{s}_{(1)}; \mathbf{s}_{(2)}; \cdots)$ where each $\mathbf{s}_{(d)}$ is a vector in $V_{(d)}$. $\mathbf{s}$ is also written $\mathbf{s}_{(0)}\oplus\mathbf{s}_{(1)}\oplus\mathbf{s}_{(2)}\oplus\cdots$. So (44) can be interpreted as

(46) $\mathbf{s} = (\mathbf{A}\otimes\mathbf{r}_0) \oplus (\mathbf{B}\otimes[\mathbf{r}_0\otimes\mathbf{r}_1] + \mathbf{C}\otimes[\mathbf{r}_1\otimes\mathbf{r}_1]).$

Alternatively, it is natural to view each $\mathbf{s}_{(d)}$ as embedded in V^*; calling the embedded vector '$\mathbf{s}_{(d)}$' (quotation marks included), we have

(47) $`\mathbf{s}_{(d)}' \equiv \mathbf{0}_{(0)} \oplus \mathbf{0}_{(1)} \oplus \cdots \oplus \mathbf{0}_{(d-1)} \oplus \mathbf{s}_{(d)} \oplus \mathbf{0}_{(d+1)} \oplus \cdots ,$

where $\mathbf{0}_{(k)}$ is the zero vector of $V_{(k)}$. That is, '$\mathbf{s}_{(d)}$' is the element of V^* with $\mathbf{s}_{(d)}$ in the sequence position appropriate for its space $V_{(d)}$, and zero everywhere else. Then (44) can be interpreted as

(48) $\mathbf{s} = `\mathbf{A}\otimes\mathbf{r}_0' + `(\mathbf{B}\otimes[\mathbf{r}_0\otimes\mathbf{r}_1] + \mathbf{C}\otimes[\mathbf{r}_1\otimes\mathbf{r}_1])'.$

Writing this equation out explicitly in terms of sequences of vectors gives (49).

(49)
$$
\begin{array}{rrcllll}
 & & & (\,\mathbf{s}_{(0)}; & \mathbf{s}_{(1)}; & \mathbf{s}_{(2)}; & \mathbf{s}_{(3)}; \;\cdots) \\
 & `\mathbf{A}\otimes\mathbf{r}_0' & = & (\,\mathbf{0}_{(0)}; & \mathbf{A}\otimes\mathbf{r}_0; & \mathbf{0}_{(2)}; & \mathbf{0}_{(3)}; \;\cdots) \\
+ & `\mathbf{B}\otimes[\mathbf{r}_0\otimes\mathbf{r}_1]' & = & (\,\mathbf{0}_{(0)}; & \mathbf{0}_{(1)}; & \mathbf{B}\otimes[\mathbf{r}_0\otimes\mathbf{r}_1]; & \mathbf{0}_{(3)}; \;\cdots) \\
+ & `\mathbf{C}\otimes[\mathbf{r}_1\otimes\mathbf{r}_1]' & = & (\,\mathbf{0}_{(0)}; & \mathbf{0}_{(1)}; & \mathbf{C}\otimes[\mathbf{r}_1\otimes\mathbf{r}_1]; & \mathbf{0}_{(3)}; \;\cdots) \\
\hline
 & \mathbf{s} & = & (\,\mathbf{0}_{(0)}; & \mathbf{A}\otimes\mathbf{r}_0; & \mathbf{B}\otimes\mathbf{r}_0\otimes\mathbf{r}_1+\mathbf{C}\otimes\mathbf{r}_1\otimes\mathbf{r}_1; & \mathbf{0}_{(3)}; \;\cdots)
\end{array}
$$

Thus interpreted, the only type of vector sum we need employ is the ordinary operation: add corresponding numerical components.

In terms of connectionist networks, the direct sum approach amounts to the assumption that the network has a group of units for realizing symbols at depth 0 in the tree (simple atoms), a distinct and larger group of units for symbols at depth 1, and so on down to deeper depths. The patterns of activity realizing the symbols at any given depth are all superimposed upon one another, but different tree depths are

[11] This direct sum construction corresponds exactly to the standard construction in particle physics of Fock space, the vector space of states of systems of indeterminate numbers of particles; $V^{(k)}$ is the subspace of states containing k particles (e.g., Messiah 1961). Indeed, furthering the isomorphism, the state of a particle within the atom is a tensor product: the vector representing the internal state of the particle (e.g., its spin orientation) times the vector representing its orbital (the role it fills in the atom's structure).

separately localized: this is the **stratified realization** of binary trees. For our running example (49), the units realizing atoms at depth 1 host the vector $\mathbf{A}\otimes\mathbf{r}_0$, the units realizing atoms at depth 2 host a superposition of two patterns, $\mathbf{B}\otimes\mathbf{r}_0\otimes\mathbf{r}_1 + \mathbf{C}\otimes\mathbf{r}_1\otimes\mathbf{r}_1$, and all other units have activation zero.

While the direct sum approach yielding the stratified representation is the simplest and perhaps the most natural, another approach is proposed in Section 8:4.4. This approach yields fully distributed representations, in which symbols at different tree depths superimpose upon one another. The mathematics is more complex, but of basically the same character as the direct sum approach presented above.

A word about the '…' in (49). If tree depth is unbounded, then the number of units in the network realizing them, or the number of components in the vectors, must be unbounded as well. Algebraically, this is no problem; nothing in our mathematical analysis will depend on the vectors being of finite length. Of course, in a computer simulation, a finite cutoff to the depth of trees, or lengths of vectors, may be convenient. But with respect to foundational questions about the capabilities of connectionist computation to realize symbolic computation, since it is standard to adopt the idealization of no resource limitations in the symbolic case, it is appropriate to do the same in the connectionist case. In place of an unbounded or infinite Turing machine tape or von Neumann machine stack (Box 6:1), we have an unbounded or infinite set of units.

In the context of the theory of human cognition, as opposed to idealized computational analysis, it must be remembered that the vectors we are discussing specify the cognitive system at a single moment. The material in a tree being realized as a single vector here corresponds to the information that may be processed in parallel, at one time. Thus, whatever the status of the idealization that there is no limit to the length of sentences that may be understood or generated, there is no question that the quantity of information that can be processed in parallel by the human cognitive system is limited. In the ICS approach, the size of the network that is appropriate to model a human cognitive system must be empirically determined from the quantity of information that speakers can access and process at one time (Townsend and Bever 2001). At this time, we must leave analysis of such resource limitations of various human cognitive capacities as a topic for future research. (But see Section 2.2 for finite specification of unbounded networks, Section 8:3.2 for abstract analysis of the graceful saturation of the representation as capacity limits are exceeded, and Chapter 19 for another ICS approach to modeling the relative difficulty of different inputs to the human sentence processor.)

1.4 The principle Rep$_{\text{ICS}}$ formalized

The results of Section 1.3 complete our summary table (see Table 4).

In this section, we have been developing the most fundamental of the principles defining ICS, the principle relating connectionist representations—activation vectors—to symbolic representations—symbol structures. Having originally stated it rather vaguely as Rep_{ICS} (2), we can now articulate it somewhat more formally, as it pertains to higher cognitive (HC) domains where symbolic representations are implicated.

Table 4. Connectionist embedding via recursive role vectors

Sec.	Structuring operation	Symbolic formalization: Structures	Symbolic formalization: Example	Connectionist formalization: Example	Connectionist formalization: Vector operation
1.1	Combining	Sets	$\{\mathbf{c}_1, \mathbf{c}_2\}$	$\mathbf{c}_1 + \mathbf{c}_2$	Vector sum: +
1.2	Filler/role binding	Strings, frames	**AB** = $\{\mathtt{A}/r_1, \mathtt{B}/r_2\}$	$\mathbf{A}\otimes\mathbf{r}_1 + \mathbf{B}\otimes\mathbf{r}_2$	Tensor product: ⊗
1.3	Recursive embedding	Trees	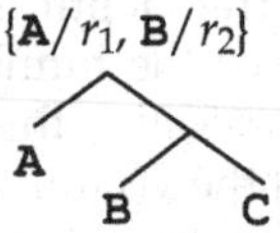	$\mathbf{A}\otimes\mathbf{r}_0 + [\mathbf{B}\otimes\mathbf{r}_0 + \mathbf{C}\otimes\mathbf{r}_1]\otimes\mathbf{r}_1$	Recursive role vectors: $\mathbf{r}_{\textit{left-/right-child}(x)} = \mathbf{r}_{0/1}\otimes\mathbf{r}_x$

(50) **Rep$_{\text{ICS}}$(HC)**: Integrated representation in higher cognition

a. In all cognitive domains, when analyzed at a lower level, mental representations are defined by the activation values of connectionist units. When analyzed at a higher level, these representations are distributed patterns of activity—activation vectors. For central aspects of higher cognitive domains, these vectors realize symbolic structures.

b. Such a symbolic structure $\mathbf{s}$ is defined by a collection of structural roles $\{r_i\}$ each of which may be occupied by a filler $\mathbf{f}_i$; $\mathbf{s}$ is a set of constituents, each a filler/role binding $\mathbf{f}_i/r_i$.

c. The connectionist realization of $\mathbf{s}$ is an activation vector

$$\mathbf{s} = \Sigma_i\, \mathbf{f}_i \otimes \mathbf{r}_i$$

that is the sum of vectors realizing the filler/role bindings. In these tensor product representations, the pattern realizing the structure as a whole is the superposition of patterns realizing all its constituents.[12] And the pattern realizing a constituent is the tensor product of a pattern realizing the filler and a pattern realizing the structural role it occupies.

d. In higher cognitive domains such as language and reasoning, mental representations are recursive: the fillers or roles of $\mathbf{s}$ have themselves the same type of internal structure as $\mathbf{s}$. And these structured fillers $\mathbf{f}$ or roles r in turn have the same type of tensor product realization as $\mathbf{s}$.

In this section, I have attempted to provide intuitive motivations for this particular approach to formalizing Rep_{ICS}. In conjunction with the other principles formalized below, this formulation of Rep_{ICS} (50), while surely preliminary, is sufficiently precise (and simple) to allow us to mathematically derive interesting consequences.

A number of important issues have not been treated here; some are taken up in

[12] For symbol structures realized in activation vectors, the whole is literally the sum of the parts.

the fuller development of Chapters 7 and 8, while others are pursued in published work cited there. Some foundational issues are taken up in Part IV, although the basic philosophical question—In virtue of what property does a connectionist representation represent?—must await future work.

The principle Rep_{ICS}(HC) (50) plays a central role in the research reported in the rest of this book, most of which falls into the category dubbed 'principle-centered' research in Chapter 3 (3): the general consequences of Rep_{ICS}(HC), when combined with other principles, are formally deduced. However, Rep_{ICS}(HC) also provides a valuable bridge from principle-centered to model-centered research. Tensor product representations, in the pure form discussed above, are simple enough to allow considerable formal analysis (see Chapter 8), but they also bear close relations to seemingly unrelated connectionist and similar models proposed in the literature, as discussed in Chapter 7. As already noted, preconnectionist 'vector' and 'matrix' psychological models of memory, developed to model experimental results on human memory for structured information, employ much the same mathematics (Murdock 1982; Pike 1984), and tensor product representations are a direct generalization of the conjunctive coding technique used in a number of early connectionist psychological models (e.g., McClelland and Kawamoto 1986; Rumelhart and McClelland 1986). Since their development, tensor product representations have themselves been explicitly used in cognitive models (e.g., Dolan and Dyer 1987; Dolan 1989; Humphreys, Bain, and Pike 1989; Wiles et al. 1990). And there are even intriguing suggestions that neural representations can have the general conjunctive character central to the tensor product (McNaughton and Smolensky 1991; Pouget and Sejnowski 1997a, b—see Chapter 7). Furthermore, as discussed in Chapter 8 and further in Smolensky 1990, a wide variety of specific representations employed in connectionist models in the literature are rather straightforwardly analyzed as special cases of tensor product representations; thus, principle Rep_{ICS}(HC) (50) unifies and rationalizes much of this literature, as regards issues of representation. Chapter 7 extends this result, showing that a number of different proposals for connectionist realization of structure—for example, the Recursive Auto-Associative Memory (RAAM) model (Pollack 1990; Callan and Palmer-Brown 1997; Melnik, Levy, and Pollack 2000), temporal firing-synchrony models (von der Malsburg and Schneider 1986; Gray et al. 1989; Eckhorn et al. 1990; Hummel and Biederman 1992; Shastri and Ajjanagadde 1993; Maass and Bishop 1999; Devnich, Stevens, and Hummel 2003; Hummel and Holyoak 2003; Wendelken and Shastri 2003), and Holographic Reduced Representations (Plate 1991a, b, 1995, 2003)—should not been seen as essentially different from the tensor product proposal, for they can in fact all be usefully analyzed as novel special cases, or direct extensions, of it.

As discussed in Box 1:2, there are good reasons to posit distributed representations. And indeed, generic tensor product representations are fully distributed. But as we saw in Section 1.2, special cases reduce to fully or semilocal representations. Thus, the principle Rep_{ICS}(HC) (50) contains no commitment to entirely distributed mental representations, with no localization whatever; rather, it provides a single formalism in which various degrees of distribution can be uniformly analyzed, from fully distributed to hyperlocal.[13] Furthermore, the vectorial analysis illuminates the relationship between local and distributed representations, showing them to be related as two coordinate systems in the activation vector space "rotated" with respect to one another: see Smolensky 1986 for an extended discussion (and Section 11:3.1.2).[14]

The equivalence between local and distributed representations is only partial. For a single, intact linear network using local representations there is an equivalent single, intact linear network using linearly independent distributed representations, the two systems being related by a linear transformation (very loosely, a generalized "rotation") of the coordinates in activation space. This equivalence means that the weight matrix in the local network can be transformed to produce a weight matrix for the distributed network; if an input to the local network is transformed to its distributed counterpart and processed by the transformed weight matrix, the output will be exactly the distributed transform of the output of the local network. This equivalence works both ways: if we start with a linear network using linearly independent distributed representations, we can transform it to an equivalent linear network using local representations. Any function that can be computed by one type of network can also be computed by the other.

But this equivalence breaks down when we depart from the core case of the single, intact linear network. There are several important respects in which local and distributed networks can differ.

(51) Nonequivalences between local and distributed networks

a. *Nonlinearity.* Units with nonlinear activation functions cannot be transformed exactly. (However, transformations of the input and output representations alone can be performed, leaving unchanged the activations of any internal nonlinear processing layers.)[15]

[13] Thus, even those who believe with Feldman (1989) that neural representations are not highly distributed should not see this as any objection to the use of the tensor product scheme as a connectionist means of realizing mental representations. If desired, special cases of the tensor product representation can be designed with any desired degree of locality, up to and including representations that dedicate a single node to an entire structure (e.g., a proposition: Ballard and Hayes 1984; Fodor and Pylyshyn 1988).

[14] In brief: The numerical components of activation vectors are normally defined as the activation values of individual units. The vector (1 0 0 0 ...) denotes a pattern in which the first unit is active, and all others are inactive: this is the first **basis vector** for the **unit** (or "neural") **basis** (see Box 1, after (4)). There is one such basis vector for each unit. These vectors point along the coordinate axes of the usual coordinate system. But the distributed patterns realizing symbols or other elements can also be used to form a basis – the **pattern** (or "conceptual") **basis** (assuming these patterns to be linearly independent, in accord with (9)). These basis vectors form the axes of a new coordinate system. With respect to these new coordinates, the components of an activation state directly specify the strength of each symbol in the state, rather than the degree of activation of each unit. Then a new network can be defined with one unit per symbol; to each state of the original network corresponds a state of the new network in which the activity of each new unit is the strength of its corresponding symbol in the first network's state. This new network employs local representations of the symbols.

[15] Suppose we are given an arbitrary (potentially nonlinear) network $\mathcal{N}$ with distinct input and output layers I, O hosting local representations; assume input to $\mathcal{N}$ consists of a clamped activation vector in I (i.e., there are no dynamics in I). Form a new network $\mathcal{N}'$, including $\mathcal{N}$ as a subpart, by adding new input and output layers I', O' that are connected to $\mathcal{N}$ via feed-forward connections: O feeds

b. *Local damage.* The effect of local damage is different, since activity that is localized in a local representation is not localized in a distributed representation, and vice versa.

c. *Learning time.* Local input representations have no similarity to one another; no unit is active in two different representations. The representing vectors are *mutually orthogonal* and hence learning on one input does not transfer to, or interfere with, learning on another (see Box 2 (4)). But distributed representations can be nonorthogonal: one input pattern can be quite similar to another, and if the function being learned requires that such similar inputs be mapped to dissimilar outputs, it can take many learning steps to eliminate the interference between the two similar distributed input patterns. Inversely, if the function being learned requires that similar inputs be mapped to similar outputs, the transfer of learning between similar distributed inputs can *reduce* learning time.

d. *Generalization.* During learning, the generalizations a network will make from training data to unseen data depend on the representation. Training on one input x will transfer to a novel input y under a distributed representation in which x and y are realized by similar vectors, but not in a local representation (which by definition entails that all distinct representations are orthogonal).

e. *Capacity.* A layer of n units can support only n local representations; the representational capacity is saturated entirely by n items. With distributed representations, more than n patterns can be used to encode more than n items; necessarily, these will not be linearly independent, but with large n the similarity between patterns can be small when n is exceeded by a relatively small amount; little similarity means near-orthogonality of patterns, which means only a small degree of confusion between items. Thus, for large n, with distributed representations the capacity limit of n items can be soft: exactness of representation degrades gracefully as n is exceeded. (Graceful saturation of distributed tensor product representations is analyzed in Section 8:3.2.)

In the remainder of this chapter, we take up the second principle of ICS that was introduced in Chapter 2; the final two principles are developed in Chapter 6. The three principles that remain will be given only high-level summaries; the substantive development of these principles will be left to the following chapters. Rep$_{\text{ICS}}$ has been

activation to O', which consists of linear units, and I' feeds to I, which we now take to consist of linear units (rather than having no dynamics and hosting only clamped patterns, as in $\mathcal{N}$). The weight matrix $\mathbb{W}_I$ from I' to I is a linear transformation that maps a linearly independent distributed representation in I' to the same local representation in I that is used in $\mathcal{N}$. The weight matrix $\mathbb{W}_O$ from O to O' takes the local representation of O in $\mathcal{N}$ to a linearly independent distributed representation in O'. Now $\mathcal{N}$ and $\mathcal{N}'$ are equivalent networks, the former using local and the latter distributed input/output representations. (Note that any hidden representations in $\mathcal{N}$ will be identically present in $\mathcal{N}'$.) The same transformation can be achieved in the reverse direction also, so long as the distributed representations used in the initial network are linearly independent. See Smolensky 1986 for an explanation of how to construct the matrices $\mathbb{W}_I$ and $\mathbb{W}_O$, and why linear independence is crucial.

singled out for lengthy discussion because most of the subsequent chapters depend on it—if not at a formal level, then at least as an existence proof that an architecture that is simultaneously PDP-connectionist on a lower level and symbolic on a higher level can indeed cope with some of the fundamental computational challenges of higher cognition.

2 P2: PROCICS—SYMBOLIC OPERATIONS AS PATTERNS OF CONNECTIONS

In Section 1, we formalized the first principle of ICS, Rep_{ICS}, developing a formal parallelism—a mathematical isomorphism—between symbolic structuring relations and relations among vectors denoting patterns of activation. We have thus established a precise sense in which unit activities can provide lower-level realizations of symbolic mental representations. Such representations are only of use, however, if connectionist mechanisms can effectively *process* them, providing a lower-level means of computing cognitive operations that may at a higher level be viewed as symbolic functions. This is the concern of the second principle of ICS, stated in Chapter 2 (3) and repeated here as (52).

(52) **P_2. Proc_{ICS}**: Cognitive processing in ICS

Information is processed in the mind/brain by widely distributed connection patterns—weight matrices—that, for central aspects of higher cognition, possess global structure describable through symbolic expressions for recursive functions of the type employed in symbolic cognitive theory.

In this section, we elaborate this principle formally, asserting rather than deriving results; demonstrations demand a level of mathematical development that is best deferred to Chapter 8.

Information is encoded in connectionist networks by activation vectors; vector space theory therefore provides the basis for the formalization of connectionist computation. Information processing in PDP networks is the spread of activation; as we will now see, the process employs the central operation of vector space theory—matrix-vector multiplication—by applying the matrix of connection weights to the vector of activations. In most networks, matrix multiplication is the core of the processing, around which more complicated operations may take place. Indeed, in its purest form, parallel distributed processing simply *is* matrix multiplication. We now pause to spell out exactly what this means. (Box 2 and Section 1:2 provide reviews.)

2.1 Linear processing in neural networks

The purest PDP connectionist network is the **linear associator** (see Figure 9). A linear associator contains a set of m input units on which resides an activation vector **i** encoding some input. There is a set of n output units that will host another activation vector **o** encoding the output associated with **i**, after activation has spread directly from the input units to the output units via a set of connections, each with its own strength or weight. If some input unit has activation value i and its connection to a particular output unit has weight W, then that output unit receives from that input unit an amount of activation equal to Wi (the numerical product of W and i). The output unit receives such activation from all the input units, and it simply adds up all these contributions to determine its own activation value o.

Figure 9. Linear associator

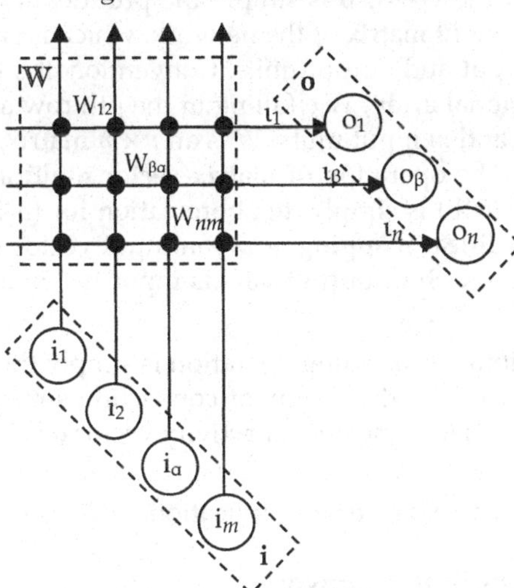

To write this out explicitly, let the input units be labeled 1, 2, ...; we will use the variable α to denote any one of these input unit labels. The activity of input unit α will be denoted i_α. The total set of input activation values, the input vector, is then **i** = $(i_1, i_2, \ldots, i_\alpha, \ldots, i_m)$. Using the variable β to denote the labels of the output units, and o_β to denote the activity of output unit β, we also have the corresponding output vector **o** = $(o_1, o_2, \ldots, o_\beta, \ldots, o_n)$. The weight of the connection *to* output unit β *from* input unit α is written $W_{\beta\alpha}$. The amount of activation that output unit β receives from input unit α is then $W_{\beta\alpha}\, i_\alpha$. The input received by output unit β, denoted ι_β (ι = iota), is just the sum of all such contributions:

(53) $\iota_\beta = W_{\beta 1} i_1 + W_{\beta 2} i_2 + \cdots + W_{\beta\alpha} i_\alpha + \cdots \equiv \Sigma_\alpha W_{\beta\alpha} i_\alpha.$

The last expression denotes the sum over all values of $\alpha = 1, 2, \ldots, m$ (Σ_α) of the weight to output unit β from input unit α ($W_{\beta\alpha}$) times the activity of input unit α (i_α). This expression for the total input received by a unit is common to the vast majority of connectionist networks; ι_β is said to be a **linear** function of **i**. What is special about a linear unit β is that its activation value a_β – the value determining how much activation it would send to other units – simply *is* ι_β. (In nonlinear units, a_β is typically a nonlinear function of ι_β.) Thus, (53) is also the equation for a_β. In the linear associator architecture, β is an output unit, so its activation value is also written o_β; thus, equation (53) becomes (54a). Collecting all $o_\beta = \iota_\beta$ values ($\beta = 1, 2, \ldots, n$) into the output vector **o**, (54a) is compactly expressed as (54b):

(54) Linear associator

a. $o_\beta = \Sigma_\alpha W_{\beta\alpha} i_\alpha \equiv W_{\beta 1} i_1 + W_{\beta 2} i_2 + \cdots;$

b. $\mathbf{o} = \mathbf{W} \cdot \mathbf{i}.$

Equation (54b) says that the vector **o** is simply the product of the matrix **W** and the vector **i**. Here **W** is the **weight matrix** of the network, which is simply the set of all the weights $W_{\beta\alpha}$ between input and output units. Conventionally, these numbers are arranged in a two-dimensional array, $W_{\beta\alpha}$ falling in the βth row and αth column. Since there are n output units and m input units, **W** is an $n \times m$ matrix, that is, a matrix with n rows and m columns. The operation **of matrix-vector multiplication**, here denoted by '·', is defined so that (54b) is simply an abbreviation for (54a). Equation (54) provides the definition of a **linear mapping** between input vector **i** and output vector **o** (for a single output, the graph of output versus input is a straight line through the origin). In sum:

(55) The core connectionist processing operation is simply the multiplication of the input activity vector **i** by the matrix of connection strengths **W**. In the purest case, the linear associator, the output activity vector **o** is

$$\mathbf{o} = \mathbf{W} \cdot \mathbf{i},$$

where '·' denotes matrix-vector multiplication, defined in (54).

2.2 Symbolic operations in ICS networks

An essential result concerning the tensor product representations developed in Section 1 is this: the mathematical isomorphism between symbolic structure and vector structure that is exploited by these representations extends to the basic *operations* of symbolic computation. The most fundamental operations on binary tree structures, for example, are those of extracting the left subtree (what we will call $\mathbf{ex}_0$), extracting the right subtree ($\mathbf{ex}_1$), and constructing a new tree by embedding two given trees as the left and right subtrees of the new tree (**cons**). With tensor product representations, these operations can be realized as the simplest type of connectionist operation, multiplication by a weight matrix; that is, they can be computed by the simplest type of connectionist network, the linear associator. These facts and some of the important results that follow from them are previewed in the remainder of this subsection; the results are derived in Chapter 8.

First, as just stated, extracting the left or right subtree of a tree is a matrix operation. That is, let **s** be the vector realizing `s = [x y]`, with **x** and **y** the vectors realizing `s`'s left and right subtrees `x` = $\mathbf{ex}_0$`(s)` and `y` = $\mathbf{ex}_1$`(s)`. (In general, `x` and `y` are complex trees in their own right.) Then there exist two matrices $\mathbf{W}_{ex0}$ and $\mathbf{W}_{ex1}$ obeying (56b):

(56) Extracting constituents of **s**, the realization of $\mathbf{s} = [\mathbf{x}\ \mathbf{y}]$

a. $\mathbf{x} = \mathbf{ex}_0(\mathbf{s})$ and $\mathbf{y} = \mathbf{ex}_1(\mathbf{s})$

b. $\mathbf{x} = \mathbf{W}_{ex0} \cdot \mathbf{s}$ and $\mathbf{y} = \mathbf{W}_{ex1} \cdot \mathbf{s}$

Consider now successively performing a sequence of two extraction operations—for example, first extracting the right child of **s**, getting **y**, then extracting the left child of **y**, getting a structure we'll call **z**. It then follows directly from (56b) that this produces the same ultimate result as successively multiplying **s** by a sequence of matrices: (57).

(57) $\mathbf{y} = \mathbf{ex}_1(\mathbf{s});\ \mathbf{z} = \mathbf{ex}_0(\mathbf{y}) = \mathbf{ex}_0(\mathbf{ex}_1(\mathbf{s}))$

$\mathbf{y} = \mathbf{W}_{ex1} \cdot \mathbf{s}$

$\mathbf{z} = \mathbf{W}_{ex0} \cdot \mathbf{y} = \mathbf{W}_{ex0} \cdot (\mathbf{W}_{ex1} \cdot \mathbf{s})$

Now as spelled out in Box 1 (15), two successive matrix products are equivalent to a single matrix product:

$$\mathbf{W} \cdot (\mathbf{W}' \cdot \mathbf{s}) = (\mathbf{W} \cdot \mathbf{W}') \cdot \mathbf{s},$$

where $\mathbf{W} \cdot \mathbf{W}'$ is the matrix product of **W** and **W′**. Thus, we have (58):

(58) Sequencing extraction operations

Suppose **z** is the left constituent of the right constituent of **s**. Then the vector **z** realizing **z** can be computed from the vector **s** realizing **s** as follows:

$$\mathbf{z} = \mathbf{W}_{ex01} \cdot \mathbf{s},$$

where the matrix $\mathbf{W}_{ex01}$ is simply defined as the matrix product,

$$\mathbf{W}_{ex01} = \mathbf{W}_{ex0} \cdot \mathbf{W}_{ex1}.$$

This can be recursively repeated to any depth. Thus, the extraction of any subconstituent, no matter how deep in the tree, is achieved by multiplication of a single appropriate matrix, a matrix that crucially has a special structure: that of a product of instances of the fundamental matrices $\mathbf{W}_{ex0}$ and $\mathbf{W}_{ex1}$.

It will be shown in Chapter 8 that, like *extracting* constituents from an existing tree, *constructing* new trees from existing constituents can be performed by linear operations—simple matrix multiplications and additions—based on two fundamental matrices, $\mathbf{W}_{cons0}$ and $\mathbf{W}_{cons1}$.

(59) Construction of trees from constituents

If **x** and **y** are the vectors realizing trees **x** and **y**, then the vector realizing the composed tree $\mathbf{s} = [\mathbf{x}\ \mathbf{y}]$ is

$$\mathbf{s} = \mathbf{W}_{cons0} \cdot \mathbf{x} + \mathbf{W}_{cons1} \cdot \mathbf{y}.$$

This equation is actually equivalent to (32), which defined a recursive connectionist realization; it is repeated as (60):

(60) $\mathbf{s} = \mathbf{x} \otimes \mathbf{r}_0 + \mathbf{y} \otimes \mathbf{r}_1.$

This is because the matrices $\mathbf{W}_{cons0}$ and $\mathbf{W}_{cons1}$ are defined so that taking their matrix product with a vector **v**—as in (59)—achieves the same result as taking the tensor product of **v** with $\mathbf{r}_0$ and $\mathbf{r}_1$, respectively—as in (60). And like extraction, *sequences* of construction operations can be combined into a single matrix operation; and indeed, sequences of interleaved extraction and construction operations can also be so combined into a single composite matrix **W**.

This sort of matrix **W** is illustrated in Figure 10, which shows a linear associator called **PassiveNet**. This is actually a subpart of a larger network called **Active/PassiveNet** discussed in Section 8:4.3 (Legendre, Miyata, and Smolensky 1991). An input to PassiveNet is a vector **s** that realizes an arbitrarily complex tree **s** (the network can be extended to arbitrarily large size). The connections in PassiveNet perform the matrix multiplication $\mathbf{W} \cdot \mathbf{s}$ (55), producing an output vector **t** that realizes another complex tree **t**. Such a network realizes a complex, structure-sensitive function ***f*** that takes an input tree **s** to its corresponding output tree **t**. This recursive function ***f*** is given a symbolic description in (61a).

(61) Connectionist realization of a symbol-manipulating function

a. $f(\mathtt{s}) = \mathtt{cons(ex_1(ex_0(ex_1(s))),}$
$\qquad\qquad \mathtt{cons(ex_1(ex_1(ex_1(s))),\ ex_0(s)))}.$

b. $$\mathbf{W} = \mathbf{W}_{\text{cons0}}\left[\mathbf{W}_{\text{ex1}}\mathbf{W}_{\text{ex0}}\mathbf{W}_{\text{ex1}}\right] + \mathbf{W}_{\text{cons1}}\left[\mathbf{W}_{\text{cons0}}(\mathbf{W}_{\text{ex1}}\mathbf{W}_{\text{ex1}}\mathbf{W}_{\text{ex1}}) + \mathbf{W}_{\text{cons1}}(\mathbf{W}_{\text{ex0}})\right].$$

f takes as input the tree structure of an English sentence in the passive voice and produces as output a tree structure encoding a predicate calculus form of the "semantic interpretation" of the input sentence. In place of the extremely deep trees current in Chomskyan syntax, the tree structures here are simplified and distorted to minimize tree depth—linguistic fidelity is completely irrelevant to the point of this example. Input "passive" sentences are encoded in trees of the form

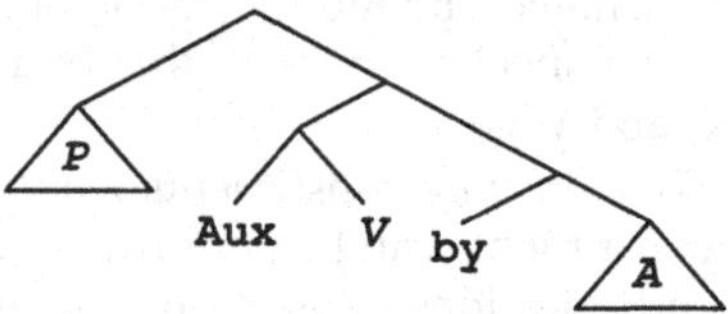

(where '*A*' denotes 'agent', '*V*' denotes 'verb', and '*P*' denotes 'patient': *P is V-ed by A*). Such an input tree is mapped by ***f*** into an output tree encoding *V*(*A*, *P*), namely,

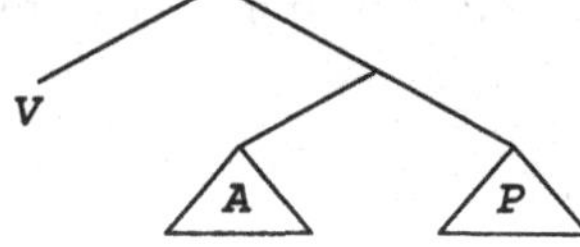

Here, the agent *A* and patient *P* arguments of the verb *V* are both arbitrarily complex noun phrase trees. (The function actually handles arbitrarily complex *V*s as well. **Aux** is the auxiliary verb, taken here as the marker of passive, such as *are* in *are admired*.) For example, for an input sentence $\mathtt{s} \equiv$ **[[X Y] [[Aux V] [by Z]]]**—(as in *few leaders are*

admired by George)—the function $\boldsymbol{f}$ produces the output **t** ≡ [**V** [**Z** [**X Y**]]] (*admire(George, few leaders)*).

Figure 10. Massively parallel symbolic computation in ICS: PassiveNet

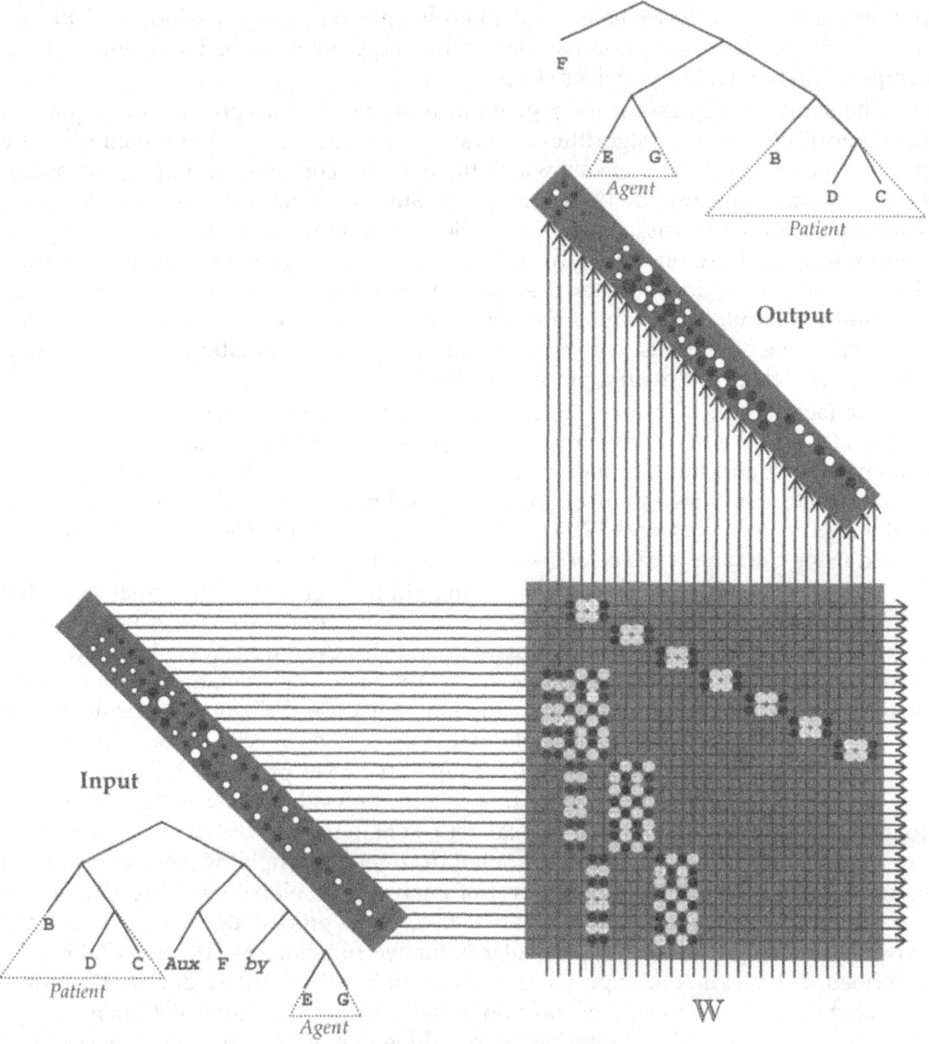

Figure 10 shows PassiveNet processing this particular example, the input and output trees being realized through the stratified recursive tensor product representations developed earlier in this chapter. The symbols **Aux**, **X**, **Y**, and so on, have arbitrarily chosen distributed realizations, and $\mathbf{r}_0$ and $\mathbf{r}_1$ are just the two-dimensional vectors used in the example of Section 1.2.2 above. The area of a square in the input or output layer encodes the activation level of the corresponding unit; black denotes positive and white negative values.

Obviously, this network is not offered as a contribution to natural language processing research! PassiveNet is of interest only because it performs all the required symbol manipulation in parallel, and handles entire embedded subtrees (e.g., complex NPs) as readily as it does simple symbols.

The symbolic expression for $\boldsymbol{f}$ given in (61a) can be interpreted as a sequential Lisp algorithm $\mathscr{A}$. This algorithm accurately describes the function computed by PassiveNet—but not the *means* by which the network computes it. In fact, the operation of the network cannot be described by any symbolic algorithm operating on symbolic constituents. PassiveNet is a simple one-step process—input vector mapped directly to output vector: the equivalent of a complex set of extraction and construction operations on constituents that are all performed simultaneously. Symbolic computation provides no way of reducing the one-step operation of PassiveNet to a set of primitive operations: that requires connectionist computation. (Careful examination of this claim is a main topic of Chapter 23.)

The fact that the function $\boldsymbol{f}$ (61a) is correctly realized by PassiveNet is explained by the fact that the net's weight matrix $\mathbf{W}$ possesses certain global structure: it is a certain product and sum of fundamental matrices $\mathbf{W}_{\text{ex0}}$, $\mathbf{W}_{\text{ex1}}$, $\mathbf{W}_{\text{cons0}}$, and $\mathbf{W}_{\text{cons1}}$. This global structure is shown in (61b); the correspondence between the internal structure of the expressions for $\boldsymbol{f}$ and $\mathbf{W}$ is evident. In Figure 10, the elements of $\mathbf{W}$ are displayed using the same area/color coding as the activation values.

Thus, we have a means of constructing simple networks like PassiveNet that compute arbitrarily complex symbolic (recursive) functions: we can prove that they do indeed correctly compute such functions, and therefore we can explain with complete precision and certainty how they do so. Yet such an explanation is not possible by means of symbolic algorithms; explanations must use the connectionist algorithm of a linear associator (54), with a weight matrix possessing special global structure.

Thus, while lacking any linguistic value, PassiveNet provides a simple illustration of the ICS computational perspective: at a lower level of analysis, PassiveNet is a connectionist network in which mental representations are distributed over many processing units, and outputs are computed from inputs simply by massively parallel spreading activation.[16] At a higher level of analysis, the global structure inherent in the activation vectors, and the weight matrices that process them, entails that the network provably computes a particular recursive function, $\boldsymbol{f}$. This function can be described with a symbolic expression, as in (61a); but the network does not compute the function in the step-by-step fashion standardly used to interpret such expressions. Rather, all the symbol manipulation is done in one step, in a massively parallel

[16] Thus, PassiveNet gives a simple, concrete illustration of the part of the ICS map sketched in Figure 2:7.

and distributed fashion. The computational resources required by the processing correspond to the number of units and weights needed, the precision with which individual units must operate, and the number of steps of activation spreading required to compute the output (i.e., 1)—not the number of symbols used, or the number of symbolic operations performed in interpreting the symbolic expression (61a).

Furthermore, as we will see in Chapter 8, the matrices **W** that compute a large family of such recursive functions—and hence the networks they define—can be characterized with a very simple equation, (62):

(62) $\mathbf{W} = \mathbf{I} \otimes \underline{\mathbf{W}}$.

This property will be expressed as '**W** has **feed-forward recursive tensor product structure**'. Here, $\underline{\mathbf{W}}$ is a finite weight matrix that rearranges symbols within some finite tree depth; it encodes the particular behavior of a particular function in a finite number of weights (in fact, important recursive functions—including $\mathbf{ex}_0$ and $\mathbf{ex}_1$—involve $\underline{\mathbf{W}}$ matrices containing only two weights). The **feed-forward recursion matrix** **I** is a fixed unbounded matrix—the same for all functions—with an extremely simple form: all its elements are either 0 or 1 (it is simply the global identity matrix on the vector space containing all tree realizations; see Box 1 (14) and (18) for definitions of identity matrix and matrix tensor product). In (62), **I** takes the finite number of elements in $\underline{\mathbf{W}}$ that govern rearrangements near the tree root and "copies" them unboundedly to fill up **W**, creating a matrix that performs the same rearrangement at unbounded depths in the tree. The idealization to unboundedly deep trees realized in unbounded (or infinite) networks or **W** matrices is immediate. The infinite behavior of recursive function evaluation is generated through the finite specification (or knowledge) $\underline{\mathbf{W}}$.

PassiveNet is representative of one important class of connectionist networks: feed-forward networks, where there are no closed loops of activation flow. The other class consists of the networks that do have such loops: **recurrent networks**. And an important subclass of these networks is the **harmonic networks**, which perform optimization: these are discussed in Chapter 6. Harmonic networks can realize important kinds of symbolic functions (including those determined by grammars). Like the weight matrices of feed-forward networks, the weight matrices of recurrent networks that compute an important class of recursive functions have a special structure—structure quite similar to that of their feed-forward counterparts: (62). In place of the feed-forward recursion matrix **I** is the **recurrent recursion matrix** **R**; its definition is best postponed until Chapter 8. The relevant structure for both feed-forward and recurrent networks is summarized in the principle (63), which characterizes the weight matrices defining ICS algorithms relevant to higher cognition.

(63) **Alg_{ICS}(HC,W)**: Recursive processing

Central aspects of many higher cognitive domains, including language, are realized in weight matrices with recursive structure. That is, feed-forward networks and recurrent networks realizing various cognitive functions have weight matrices with the respective forms

Feed-forward: $\mathbf{W} = \mathbf{I} \otimes \underline{\mathbf{W}}$; Recurrent: $\mathbf{W} = \underline{\mathbf{W}} \otimes \mathbf{R}$.

In either case, $\underline{\mathbf{W}}$ is a finite matrix of weights that specifies the particular cognitive function. **I** and **R** are the recursion matrices for feed-forward and recurrent networks: these are simply defined unbounded matrices that are fixed—the same for all cognitive functions.

This principle is the subject of extensive discussion in Chapter 8 (Section 4.1 for the feed-forward case, Section 4.2 for the recurrent case). The analysis shows how the special weight matrix structure specified in (63) entails the recursive properties of the functions these weights compute.

2.3 Summary

The goal of this section has been to formally elaborate the second ICS principle, Proc_{ICS} (52), repeated as (64).

(64) P_2. Proc_{ICS}: Cognitive processing in the ICS Architecture

Information is processed in the mind/brain by widely distributed connection patterns—weight matrices—which, for central aspects of higher cognition, possess global structure describable through symbolic expressions for recursive functions of the type employed in symbolic cognitive theory.

The first part of this principle states that in all domains, cognitive processing consists of spreading activation through widely distributed connection patterns; as (55) states, the core of such connectionist processing is the multiplication of activation vectors by weight matrices. The second part of Proc_{ICS} states that in central parts of higher cognitive domains, these weight matrices possess global structure describable through symbolic expressions for recursive functions. This is exemplified in (61), where the global structure of the matrix **W** (61b) is characterized by the isomorphic symbolic expression (61) for the recursive function ***f*** computed by the network. Another characterization of the global structure of **W** is given in Alg_{ICS}(HC,W), (63), which formally defines the kind of global structure enabling networks processing tensor product representations to achieve infinite competence with finite means, explaining how unboundedly productive behavior—correctly computing the values of various recursive functions over an unbounded set of possible inputs—can be specified by a finite store of knowledge. (At present, it is an open problem to completely characterize the set of recursive functions that can be computed by such networks; the claim is not that *all* recursive functions lie in this set. But Chapter 8 formally identifies a large family of functions that can be computed using these tensor networks.)

3 Multilevel Descriptions in ICS

ICS networks such as PassiveNet have multiple formal descriptions that differ along several dimensions. Most salient is the contrast between the atomic elements distinguishing the symbolic formalism (symbols) and the connectionist formalism (numbers). Also important is the distinction between lower-level, local descriptions of individual units and connections (numbers), on the one hand, and higher-level, global descriptions of entire patterns of activation (vectors) and patterns of connections (matrices), on the other. A more subtle contrast distinguishes descriptions that explicitly characterize the constituent structure of representations or processes from more unitary descriptions. Finally, there is the mundane distinction between general expressions using variables and specific expressions in which the variables have been assigned particular values.

Table 5. The space of descriptions of ICS systems

Level		Connectionist description: Representation	Connectionist description: Processing	Symbolic description: Function	Symbolic description: Representation
Higher (global)	a	$\mathbf{s}$	$f(\mathbf{s}) = \mathbf{W}\cdot\mathbf{s}$	$\mathtt{f}$	$\mathtt{s}$
	b	$\mathbf{s} = \Sigma_i \mathbf{c}_i = \Sigma_i \mathbf{f}_i \otimes \mathbf{r}_i$	$\mathbf{W}_{\mathcal{G}} = \Sigma_g \mathbf{W}^{(g)}$	$\mathtt{f}_{\mathcal{G}}[\{R_g\}]$	$\mathtt{s} = \{\mathtt{f}_i / r_i\}$
	c	$\mathbf{s} = \mathbf{p}\otimes\mathbf{r}_0 + \mathbf{q}\otimes\mathbf{r}_1$	$f(\mathbf{s}) = [\mathbf{I}\otimes\underline{\mathbf{W}}]\cdot\mathbf{s}$		$\mathtt{s} = [\mathtt{p\ q}]$
	d	$\mathbf{s} = \mathbf{A}\otimes\mathbf{r}_0 + \mathbf{B}\otimes\mathbf{r}_{01} + \mathbf{C}\otimes\mathbf{r}_{11}$	$f(\mathbf{s}) = [\mathbf{W}_{ex01}]\cdot\mathbf{s}$ $\mathbf{W}_{ex01} \equiv \mathbf{W}_{ex0}\mathbf{W}_{ex1}$	$\mathtt{f(s)} = \mathtt{ex}_0\mathtt{(ex}_1\mathtt{(s))}$	$\mathtt{s} = \mathtt{[A\ [B\ C]]}$ $= \{\mathtt{A}/r_0, \mathtt{B}/r_{01}, \mathtt{C}/r_{11}\}$
Lower (local)	a'	$[\mathbf{s}]_{\varphi\rho}$	$[f(\mathbf{s})]_\beta = \Sigma_\alpha W_{\beta\alpha}[\mathbf{s}]_\alpha$		
	b'	$[\mathbf{s}]_{\varphi\rho} = \Sigma_i [\mathbf{f}_i]_\varphi [\mathbf{r}_i]_\rho$	$[\mathbf{W}_{\mathcal{G}}]_{\alpha\beta,\alpha'\beta'} =$ $\Sigma_g [\mathbf{W}^{(g)}]_{\alpha\beta,\alpha'\beta'}$		
	c'	$[\mathbf{s}]_{\varphi\rho} = [\mathbf{p}]_\varphi[\mathbf{r}_0]_\rho +$ $[\mathbf{q}]_\varphi[\mathbf{r}_1]_\rho$	$[\mathbf{W}]_{\alpha\beta,\alpha'\beta'} =$ $[\mathbf{I}]_{\alpha,\alpha'}[\mathbf{W}]_{\beta,\beta'}$		
	d'	$\mathbf{s} = \{s^{(0)}_{\varphi}, s^{(0)}_{\varphi\rho_1}, s^{(0)}_{\varphi\rho_2\rho_1}, \ldots\}$ $[\mathbf{s}]^{(1)}{}_{\varphi\rho} = [\mathbf{A}]_\varphi[\mathbf{r}_0]_\rho$ $[\mathbf{s}]^{(2)}{}_{\varphi\rho'\rho} =$ $[\mathbf{B}]_\varphi[\mathbf{r}_0]_{\rho'}[\mathbf{r}_1]_\rho$ $+[\mathbf{C}]_\varphi[\mathbf{r}_1]_{\rho'}[\mathbf{r}_1]_\rho$	$[f(\mathbf{s})]_{\varphi\rho} =$ $\Sigma_{\rho'}[\mathbf{W}_{ex01}]_{\rho,\rho'}[\mathbf{s}]_{\varphi\rho'}$ $[\mathbf{W}_{ex01}]_{\rho,\rho'} =$ $\Sigma_{\rho''}[\mathbf{W}_{ex0}]_{\rho,\rho''} \times$ $[\mathbf{W}_{ex1}]_{\rho'',\rho'}$		
	d''	$[\mathbf{s}]^{(2)}{}_{321} = [1][1][1]$ $+ \cdots$	$[f(\mathbf{s})]_\beta = [\mathbf{s}]_{10\beta}$ $-[\mathbf{s}]_{01\beta}$		

Table 5 depicts the relations among many of the multiple descriptions occupying this multidimensional space. The concrete representation **s** = **[A [B C]]** is used for illustration, as is a simple symbolic function ***f*** that extracts the first subconstituent of the second constituent of its input. (Thus, ***f*****([A [BC]])** = **B**.) Connectionist descriptions are given in the left half, symbolic in the right half. Higher-level, global descriptions appear in the upper half; lower-level, local descriptions in the lower half. There are no symbolic descriptions at the lower level. Expressions are given at several levels of generality: the most general, using holistic variables (*a*); then, using variables for constituents (*b–c*); then, more specifically for a particular input and the particular function ***f*** (*d*); and finally, most specifically, for the case of the particular lower-level role and filler vectors employed in the particular example of Section 1.2.2 (*d*″).

Some of the detail in Table 5 anticipates formal developments of the ideas introduced in this chapter that are carried out in Chapters 8 and 10. Briefly, then, the descriptions in the table are as follows. In row *a*, the network realization of the symbolic function ***f*** operating on a representation **s** is identified as the linear operation of multiplying the vector **s** realizing **s** by a matrix **W** realizing ***f***. Row *b* shows the decomposition of **s** into constituents—filler/role bindings grouped into a set—and the corresponding decomposition of its realization **s** into constituents—tensor-product-binding vectors superimposed by vector addition. Analogously, a function $\boldsymbol{f}_{\mathcal{G}}$ is considered that is generated by a set of rules $\{R_g\}$ that are the 'constituents' of a grammar $\mathcal{G}$, and the corresponding connectionist realization of $\boldsymbol{f}_{\mathcal{G}}$ is defined by a weight matrix $\mathbf{W}_{\mathcal{G}}$ that is a superposition (sum) of weight matrices, each corresponding to a rule (Box 2:2). For the rest of the table, the simple ***f*** defined in the previous paragraph is used. In row *c*, a different decomposition of **s** identifies it as the binary tree with left and right subtrees **p** and **q**. The corresponding decomposition of **s** is also shown. A related decomposition of *f* identifies its recursive character by showing that it is generated via the recursion matrix **I**. In row *d*, our concrete simple function ***f*** is decomposed via the primitive functions $\mathbf{ex}_0$ and $\mathbf{ex}_1$, and the weight matrix realizing ***f*** is correspondingly decomposed into the basic matrices $\mathbf{W}_{\text{ex0}}$ and $\mathbf{W}_{\text{ex1}}$. Also given is our concrete example of a structure **s**, decomposed in both the ways shown in rows *b* and *c*. The vector **s** realizing this **s** is also shown, decomposed as in row *b*.

In the lower half of the table, the connectionist part of each of the rows in the upper half is expressed in terms of individual unit activations and connection strengths. The discussion in this chapter has derived the unit-level expressions for $[\mathbf{s}]_{\varphi\rho}$ in rows *a*′, *b*′, *c*′, and *d*′; these correspond directly to the vector-level expressions in rows *a*, *b*, *c*, and *d*, respectively. Finally, at the level of *d*′, it becomes possible to insert actual numbers for activations and weights; those shown in row *d*″ correspond to the particular numerical values of the example presented in Section 1.2.2. Turning to rows *a*′–*d*′ for *f*, these simply exhibit the component-level definitions of the expressions in rows *a–d*, employing the definition of matrix-vector product, matrix addition, matrix tensor product, and matrix-matrix product (all of which are summarized in Box 1). Row *d*″ explicitly employs some of the numerical components of $\mathbf{W}_{\text{ex01}}$, assuming the role vectors of Section 1.2.2; this level of detail requires the more advanced treatment developed in Chapter 8.

References

Abbott, L., and T. J. Sejnowski, eds. 1999. *Neural codes and distributed representations.* MIT Press.

Ballard, D. H., and P. J. Hayes. 1984. Parallel logical interference. In *Proceedings of the Cognitive Science Society 6.*

Callan, R. E., and D. Palmer-Brown. 1997. (S)RAAM: An analytical technique for fast and reliable derivation of connectionist symbol structure representations. *Connection Science* 9, 139–60.

Chomsky, N. 1995. *The Minimalist Program.* MIT Press.

Devnich, D., G. T. Stevens, and J. E. Hummel. 2003. Independent representation of abstract arguments and relations. In *Proceedings of the Cognitive Science Society 25.*

Dolan, C. P. 1989. Tensor manipulation networks: Connectionist and symbolic approaches to comprehension, learning, and planning. Ph.D. diss., UCLA.

Dolan, C. P., and M. G. Dyer. 1987. Symbolic schemata, role binding, and the evolution of structure in connectionist memories. *IEEE International Conference on Neural Networks* 1, 287–98.

Dolan, C. P., and P. Smolensky. 1989. Tensor product production system: A modular architecture and representation. *Connection Science* 1, 53–68.

Eckhorn, R., H. J. Reitboeck, M. Arndt, and P. Dicke. 1990. Feature linking via synchronization among distributed assemblies: Simulations of results from cat visual cortex. *Neural Computation* 2, 293–307.

Feldman, J. 1989. Neural representation of conceptual knowledge. In *Neural connections, mental computation,* eds. L. Nadel, L. A. Cooper, P. Culicover, and R. M. Harnish. MIT Press.

Fodor, J. A., and Z. W. Pylyshyn. 1988. Connectionism and cognitive architecture: A critical analysis. *Cognition* 28, 3–71.

Gray, C. M., P. Konig, A. K. Engel, and W. Singer. 1989. Oscillatory responses in cat visual cortex exhibit intercolumnar synchronization which reflects global stimulus properties. *Nature* 338, 334–7.

Hinton, G. E., J. L. McClelland, and D. E. Rumelhart. 1986. Distributed representation. In *Parallel distributed processing: Explorations in the microstructure of cognition.* Vol. 1, *Foundations,* D. E. Rumelhart, J. L. McClelland, and the PDP Research Group. MIT Press.

Hummel, J. E., and I. Biederman. 1992. Dynamic binding in a neural network for shape recognition. *Psychological Review* 99, 480–517.

Hummel, J. E., and K. J. Holyoak. 2003. A symbolic-connectionist theory of relational inference and generalization. *Psychological Review* 110, 220–64.

Humphreys, M. S., J. D. Bain, and R. Pike. 1989. Different ways to cue a coherent memory system: A theory for episodic, semantic and procedural tasks. *Psychological Review* 96, 208–33.

Jordan, M. I. 1986. An introduction to linear algebra in parallel distributed processing. In *Parallel distributed processing: Explorations in the microstructure of cognition.* Vol. 1, *Foundations,* D. E. Rumelhart, J. L. McClelland, and the PDP Research Group. MIT Press.

Kayne, R. S. 1984. *Connectedness and binary branching.* Foris .

Legendre, G., Y. Miyata, and P. Smolensky. 1991. Distributed recursive structure processing. In *Advances in neural information processing systems 3,* eds. R. P. Lippman, J. E. Moody, and D. S. Touretzky. Morgan Kaufmann.

Maass, W., and C. M. Bishop, eds. 1999. *Pulsed neural networks.* MIT Press.

Marcus, G. F. 2001. *The algebraic mind: Integrating connectionism and cognitive science.* MIT Press.

McClelland, J. L., and A. H. Kawamoto. 1986. Mechanisms of sentence processing: Assigning roles to constituents. In *Parallel distributed processing: Explorations in the microstructure of cognition.* Vol. 2, *Psychological and biological models,* J. L. McClelland, D. E. Rumelhart, and the PDP Research Group. MIT Press.

McClelland, J. L., and D. E. Rumelhart. 1981. An interactive activation model of context effects in letter perception: Part 1. An account of basic findings. *Psychological Review* 88, 375–407.

McNaughton, B. L., and P. Smolensky. 1991. Connectionist and neural modeling: Converging in the hippocampus. In *Perspectives on cognitive neuroscience,* eds. R. G. Lister and H. J. Weingartner. Oxford University Press.

Melnik, O., S. Levy, and J. Pollack. 2000. RAAM for infinite context-free languages. In *Proceedings of the International Joint Conference on Neural Networks.*

Messiah, A. 1961. *Quantum mechanics.* Elsevier Science. [Dover reprint, 2000.]

Minsky, M. 1975. A framework for representing knowledge. In *The psychology of computer vision,* ed. P. H. Winston. McGraw-Hill.

Murdock, B. B. J. 1982. A theory for storage and retrieval of item and associative information. *Psychological Review* 89, 316–38.

Pike, R. 1984. Comparison of convolution and matrix distributed memory systems for associative recall and recognition. *Psychological Review* 91, 281–94.

Plate, T. A. 1991a. Holographic reduced representations. Technical report CRG-TR-91-1, Computer Science Department, University of Toronto.

Plate, T. A. 1991b. Holographic reduced representations: Convolution algebra for compositional distributed representations. In *Proceedings of the International Joint Conference on Artificial Intelligence 12.*

Plate, T. A. 1995. Holographic reduced representations. *IEEE Transactions on Neural Networks* 6, 623–41.

Plate, T. A. 2003. *Holographic reduced representation: Distributed representation for cognitive structures.* CSLI Publications.

Plaut, D. C., J. L. McClelland, M. S. Seidenberg, and K. Patterson. 1996. Understanding normal and impaired word reading: Computational principles in quasi-regular domains. *Psychological Review* 103, 56–115.

Pollack, J. 1990. Recursive distributed representations. *Artificial Intelligence* 46, 77–105.

Pouget, A., and T. J. Sejnowski. 1997a. A new view of hemineglect based on the response properties of parietal neurones. *Philosophical Transactions of the Royal Society of London* B354, 1449–59.

Pouget, A., and T. J. Sejnowski. 1997b. Spatial transformations in the parietal cortex using basis functions. *Journal of Cognitive Neuroscience* 9, 222–37.

Rumelhart, D. E., and J. L. McClelland. 1986. On learning the past tenses of English verbs. In *Parallel distributed processing: Explorations in the microstructure of cognition.* Vol. 2, *Psychological and biological models,* J. L. McClelland, D. E. Rumelhart, and the PDP Research Group. MIT Press.

Rumelhart, D. E., J. L. McClelland, and the PDP Research Group. 1986. *Parallel distributed processing: Explorations in the microstructure of cognition.* Vol. 1, *Foundations.* MIT Press.

Shastri, L., and V. Ajjanagadde. 1993. From simple associations to systematic reasoning: A connectionist representation of rules, variables and dynamic bindings using temporal synchrony. *Behavioral and Brain Sciences* 16, 417–94.

Smolensky, P. 1986. Neural and conceptual interpretations of parallel distributed processing models. In *Parallel distributed processing: Explorations in the microstructure of cognition.* Vol. 2, *Psychological and biological models,* J. L. McClelland, D. E. Rumelhart, and the PDP Research Group. MIT Press.

Smolensky, P. 1987. On variable binding and the representation of symbolic structures in connectionist systems. Technical report CU-CS-355-87, Computer Science Department, University of Colorado at Boulder.

Smolensky, P. 1990. Tensor product variable binding and the representation of symbolic structures in connectionist networks. *Artificial Intelligence* 46, 159–216.

Townsend, D. J., and T. G. Bever. 2001. *Sentence comprehension.* MIT Press.

van Gelder, T. 1990. Compositionality: A connectionist variation on a classical theme. *Cognitive Science* 14, 355–84.

von der Malsburg, C., and W. Schneider. 1986. A neural cocktail-party processor. *Biological Cybernetics* 54, 29–40.

Wendelken, C., and L. Shastri. 2003. Acquisition of concepts and causal rules in SHRUTI. In *Proceedings of the Cognitive Science Society* 25.

Wiles, J., M. S. Humphreys, J. D. Bain, and S. Dennis. 1990. Control processes and cue combinations in a connectionist model of human memory. Technical report 186, Computer Science Department, University of Queensland.

Winograd, T. 1973. A procedural model of language understanding. In *Computer models of thought and language*, eds. R. Schank and K. Colby. W. H. Freeman.

6 Formalizing the Principles II: Optimization and Grammar

Paul Smolensky and Géraldine Legendre

This chapter develops the final two principles of the Integrated Connectionist/Symbolic Cognitive Architecture (ICS). These rest on a higher-level characterization of connectionist computation as a kind of optimization (P_3: HMax, formally developed in Chapter 9). Applying this optimization principle to language leads to two grammar formalisms: Harmonic Grammar (HG; Legendre, Miyata, and Smolensky 1990c) and Optimality Theory (P_4: OT; Prince and Smolensky 1993/2004). In this chapter, we formally derive HG by combining P_1: Rep_{ICS} and P_3: HMax. We explore the relation of higher-level HG analysis with lower-level connectionist description. We then summarize results of subsequent chapters showing that, despite its simplicity, HG is capable of characterizing arbitrarily complex formal languages (Chapter 10), and capable of capturing the strong interactions between syntactic and semantic constraints in a fragment of the grammar of French (Chapter 11). OT is presented in full in Chapter 12, and numerous OT applications are developed in Part III of the book. The topics are located within the ICS map in Figure 2:5.

Contents

The fundamental premise of the Integrated Connectionist/Symbolic Cognitive Architecture (ICS) is that the connectionist and symbolic frameworks for theories of cognition both contribute important computational principles of the mind/brain, but at different levels of analysis—the latter highly abstract, the former closer to the neural level. At the root of this conception is the idea that mental representations are instantiated in the activation values of connectionist units, and when analyzed at a higher level, as distributed patterns of activity, these same representations are seen as realizations of symbolic structures. But do the distributed patterns of activity defined in Chapter 5—tensor product representations—*really* have the kind of combinatorial syntactic structure needed to support symbolic computation? Can they really handle such structural complexities as embedding and recursion?

Affirmative answers to these questions were claimed in Chapter 5, based on arguments that, using simple connectionist operations, certain recursive functions can be computed over mental representations that are activation patterns possessing tensor product structure. In the present chapter, we pursue these questions further, focusing primarily on a particular computational arena in which recursive structure plays a crucial role: language.

Since recursive syntactic structure is present in very pure form in formal language theory (see Box 1), one of the sharpest ways to formulate the question of the adequacy of tensor product representations is as follows: Can such representations be used in parallel distributed processing (PDP) connectionist systems to capture formal languages? If so, to what level in the Chomsky hierarchy of formal languages? Can such systems capture the entire hierarchy, making them as powerful as Turing machines in the languages they define?

In this chapter, we describe formal results showing that the answer to the last question is *yes*. This requires that a theory of languages and grammars be formulated within ICS. The central concept in the ICS theory of language is that of relative well-formedness or **Harmony**. Well-formedness plays a central role in all of grammatical theory, of course; in the case of a formal language, an absolute notion of well-formedness is what distinguishes the symbol strings that belong to the language (those for which a well-formed parse, according to the grammatical rules, can be constructed). That a notion of well-formedness also plays a central role in connectionist theory is less obvious, but also true; and it is remarkable that by identifying connectionist well-formedness and linguistic well-formedness, a novel and quite powerful approach to grammar can be formulated.

We argue in this chapter that the computational principles of ICS are not merely *adequate* for supporting linguistic structure; in fact, they lead to significant advancements in grammatical theory. This marks a turning point in our presentation of research results. The first two principles of ICS, addressed in Chapter 5, concern how connectionist computation realizes symbolic computation; they constitute a contribution *to* the theory of connectionist computation *from* symbolic cognitive theory. The principles we take up in this chapter concern contributions in the reciprocal direction.

That connectionist principles lead to progress in symbolic theory argues against the implementationalist's claim (Box 1:8) that connectionist theory can merely fill in lower-level details without making contributions to theory at the *cognitive* level (see also Chapter 23).

Box 1. Formal languages and abstract automata: The Chomsky hierarchy, Turing machines, and all that

Formal language theory is a central topic within the classical theory of computation, a branch of pure mathematics (see, e.g., the textbook Hopcroft and Ullman 1979). It can be seen as a highly abstracted characterization of the combinatorial structure of natural languages, where the basic abstract symbols that are combined stand for words (syntax) or speech sounds (phonology). Formal language theory is however perhaps better regarded as simply one formalization of computation, of interest for the classes of computable functions it defines, and for its relations to other formalizations of computation, such as the abstract characterizations of the notion 'machine' provided by **automata theory**.

A **formal language** is a set $\mathcal{L}$ of strings (sequences) of symbols from an alphabet $\mathcal{A}$. For instance, $\mathcal{L}_1$ = {**b**, **ab**, **aab**, **aaab**, …} is a formal language over the alphabet $\mathcal{A}_1$ = {**a**, **b**}. A formal language may be specified by a **formal grammar**, which is a set $\mathcal{G}$ of **rewrite rules** such as $\mathcal{G}_1$ = {**S** → **aS**, **S** → **b**}; a string μ of symbols from $\mathcal{A}$ is in the language specified by $\mathcal{G}$ if and only if it can be produced by a sequence of rewrite operations in $\mathcal{G}$, starting with a special **start symbol S**. The rules in the grammar will typically involve not only the symbols in $\mathcal{A}$, the **terminal symbols**, but also a disjoint set of **nonterminal symbols**, including **S**. Nonterminal symbols label different types of constituents—substrings of symbols (they correspond to phrase types in natural language syntax, such as **NP** = Noun Phrase).

The following notational conventions will be used throughout this book:

lowercase Roman letter = terminal symbol (e.g., **a**)
uppercase Roman letter = nonterminal symbol (e.g., **S**)
lowercase Greek letter = string of terminal symbols (e.g., μ = **aab**)
uppercase Greek letter = string of symbols each of which may be either a terminal or a nonterminal (e.g., Γ = **aS**)

The language $\mathcal{L}_1$ defined above is the language specified by the above grammar $\mathcal{G}_1$: a string μ of symbols {**a**, **b**} is in $\mathcal{L}_1$ if and only if it can be created by starting with **S** and sequentially executing operations in which an **S** is replaced with either the substring **aS** (via the rule **S** → **aS**) or the symbol **b** (via the rule **S** → **b**). A sequence of applications of rules in $\mathcal{G}_1$ (a **derivation**) that generates a string such as **aab** gives rise to a **parse tree** for the string: (1).

In this tree, the substring **ab** at the right edge of the string **a<u>ab</u>** constitutes a **constituent** because it is grouped together in the tree. The substring **aa** at the left edge, by contrast, is not a constituent; the grouping represented by this tree is **a**[**ab**]. The constituent **ab** is in fact a constituent of type **S** that is **recursively embedded** within a larger constituent of type **S**. The tree (i) can be written more compactly as $[_{S}\mathbf{a}\ [_{S}\mathbf{a}\ [_{S}\mathbf{b}]]]$, where the recursive '**S** inside **S**' structure is evident.

(1)

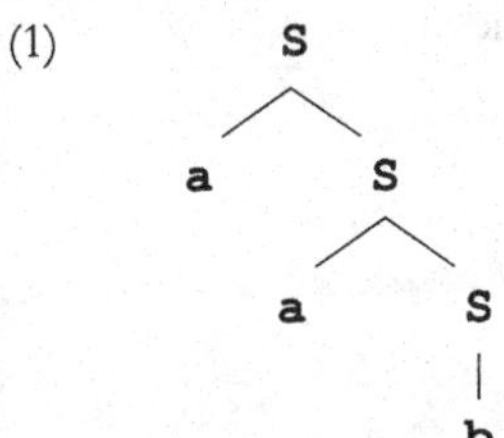

By restricting more and more tightly the set of allowed rewrite rules, a hierarchy of families of formal languages can be defined. At the top of this **Chomsky hierarchy** is the family of languages specified by **Type 0** or **unrestricted** grammars: rewrite rules $\Omega \to \Psi$ where, according to our convention, Ω and Ψ are each a substring of terminal and nonterminal symbols (Ω must be nonempty). Restricting to **Type 1** grammars, allowing only rewrite rules of the form $\Gamma\mathbf{A}\Delta \to \Gamma\Phi\Delta$ (i.e., "$\mathbf{A} \to \Phi$ in the context Γ—Δ"), gives a subfamily, the **context-sensitive** languages. Further restricting to **Type 2** grammars, allowing only rules of the form $\mathbf{A} \to \Phi$ (independent of context), yields the family of **context-free** languages. Most restricted is the set of **regular** languages, which (like $\mathcal{G}_1$ above) are specified by **Type 3** grammars in which all rules have the form $\mathbf{A} \to \mathbf{bC}$ or $\mathbf{A} \to \mathbf{d}$.

Each language family in the Chomsky hierarchy is generated (or recognized) by a corresponding family of abstract **machines** or **automata**; we discuss only the most general and most restricted cases here. The family of simplest automata, the **finite state machines**, can mimic the derivations of Type 3 languages: they are defined by a finite set of abstract **states**, and start in a special **start state** corresponding to **S**; they then repeatedly make transitions to new states, emitting a terminal symbol on each transition. Corresponding to the Type 3 grammar rule $\mathbf{A} \to \mathbf{bC}$ is the machine's transition from a state corresponding to **A** to a state corresponding to **C**, emitting the terminal symbol **b** in transit. (Corresponding to the rule $\mathbf{A} \to \mathbf{d}$ is the machine's emission of **d** in transit from the state corresponding to **A** to a special **terminal state**.)

At the opposite end of the machine hierarchy are the most powerful automata, **Turing machines**. These have an unlimited sequence of locations for storing symbols, and a finite-state-machine **controller** that repeatedly reads a symbol in the currently active storage location and, depending on the symbol read and the controller's current internal state, writes a new symbol in that location and moves left or right to the next location. In addition, we assume the Turing machine has a sequence of output stores with a first location containing the special symbol **#**. At any step, the controller can write a symbol from alphabet $\mathcal{A}$, or the symbol **#**, into the next output location. The language generated by this machine is the set of strings over $\mathcal{A}$ that are output between two end-markers **#**. The family of all languages over $\mathcal{A}$ that can be generated by some Turing machine—the **recursively enumerable** languages—is identical to the family of formal languages specified by Type 0 grammars over $\mathcal{A}$.

The Chomsky hierarchy of formal languages and corresponding hierarchy of automata can be depicted as follows (the names of the machines corresponding to Type 1 and Type 2 grammars have been given for completeness):

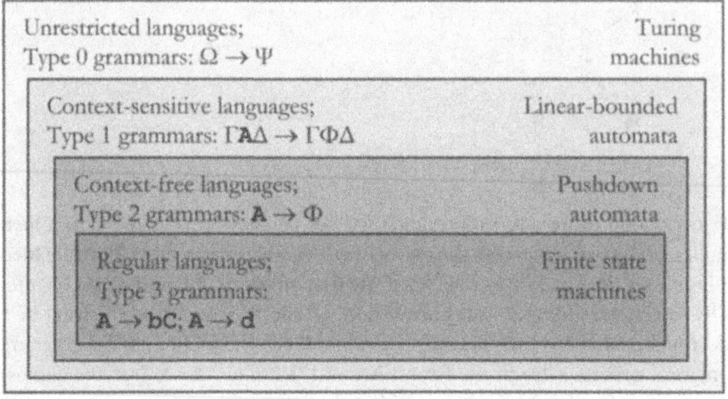

In Section 1, we introduce the ICS principle concerning Harmony maximization, or **optimization**, in neural computation—P_3: HMax, first introduced in Chapter 2 (5). This principle provides one answer to the question, what higher-level characterizations describe the computations performed in connectionist networks? This question is of central importance in ICS, since ICS identifies symbolic computation with higher-level formal descriptions of connectionist computation.

In Section 2, we show how P_3, together with the ICS principles P_1 and P_2 formulated in Chapter 5, leads to a general numerical-optimization-based grammar formalism, Harmonic Grammar. We discuss how this formalism can specify complex formal languages, despite its simplicity. We then turn to an application of Harmonic Grammar to a challenging problem in natural language, the interaction of syntactic and semantic constraints in a set of French sentence constructions.

In Section 3, we take up the final ICS principle, P_4, which characterizes the second optimization-based grammar formalism, Optimality Theory: this theory relies on nonnumerical optimization. The relation between the two grammar formalisms based on the optimization of Harmony, Harmonic Grammar and Optimality Theory, is a complex matter, discussed in Chapter 20 after both Harmonic Grammar and Optimality Theory have been further developed.

1 OPTIMIZATION IN NEURAL NETWORKS

To start the development of grammatical theory within ICS, we give an intuitive characterization of the connectionist notion of well-formedness: **Harmony**. The Harmony of an activation vector in a connectionist network is a numerical measure of the degree to which that vector respects the constraints encoded in the connection matrix: the degree to which the vector is well formed, according to the connections. Explaining this sentence will take most of this section.

1.1 Harmony of an activation vector

To begin at the beginning, consider a negative connection of weight, say, –0.8, from a unit α to a unit β (see Figure 1). This connection has the effect that if unit α is active, then unit β is inhibited by it: β receives negative activation from α. We can interpret this connection as enforcing a little constraint which says that if α *is* active, then β should *not* be active. This constraint has a strength, 0.8; if the connection weight were –8.0 instead, it would be implementing a constraint with the same content, but with ten times the strength.

Figure 1. Harmony of two micropatterns a and a′

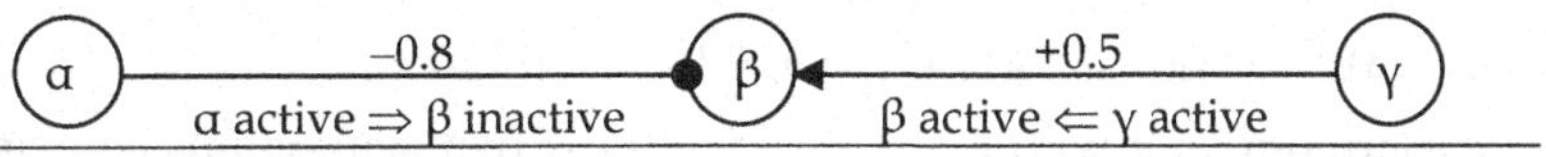

α —(–0.8)— β ◄—(+0.5)— γ

α active ⇒ β inactive   β active ⇐ γ active

a	$a_\alpha = +0.7$	$W_{\beta\alpha} = -0.8$	$\mathbf{a_\beta = +0.4}$	$W_{\beta\gamma} = +0.5$	$a_\gamma = +0.7$

$H_{\beta\alpha} = (+0.4)(-0.8)(+0.7) = -0.224$ $H_{\beta\gamma} = (+0.4)(+0.5)(+0.7) = +0.140$

$$H_{\beta\alpha}(\mathbf{a}) + H_{\beta\gamma}(\mathbf{a}) = \mathbf{-0.084}$$

a′	$a'_\alpha = +0.7$	$W_{\beta\alpha} = -0.8$	$\mathbf{a'_\beta = -0.4}$	$W_{\beta\gamma} = +0.5$	$a'_\gamma = +0.7$

$H_{\beta\alpha} = +0.224$ $H_{\beta\gamma} = -0.140$

$$H_{\beta\alpha}(\mathbf{a'}) + H_{\beta\gamma}(\mathbf{a'}) = \mathbf{+0.084}$$

Of course, unit β might also happen to have a *positive* connection from another unit γ—say, one of weight +0.5. This connection can be interpreted as implementing a constraint of opposite polarity: if unit γ is active, then unit β should be active too; this constraint has strength 0.5. If α and γ are both active, then β is subject to two conflicting constraints, and (assuming for simplicity that the activation levels of α and γ are equal) it is the stronger one that wins out: the negative activation received from the connection of weight –0.8 overcomes the positive activation received from the connection of weight +0.5, causing β to be inactive.

With respect to the single connection to β from α, all activity patterns can be assessed according to how well they respect the constraint corresponding to that connection. The constraint is violated by any activity pattern **a** in which both α and β are simultaneously active—for example, a pattern in which the activity of α is $a_\alpha = +0.7$ and that of β is $a_\beta = +0.4$. Because it is violated by **a**, this constraint therefore assesses **a** with negative Harmony; the numerical quantity, for reasons to be made clearer shortly, is computed as

(1) $H_{\beta\alpha}(\mathbf{a}) = a_\beta W_{\beta\alpha} a_\alpha = (+0.4)\ (-0.8)\ (+0.7) = -0.224.$

The Harmony of an activity pattern **a** with respect to a connection to β from α is simply the three-way product of the activation value of unit β (a_β) times the weight to β from α ($W_{\beta\alpha}$) times the activation value of α (a_α). If the weight is negative, and both activations are positive, the result is a negative number, indicating a violation of the constraint corresponding to that connection. The greater the weight of the connection (i.e., the strength of the constraint), and the greater the positive activations, the greater the significance of this violation, and the more negative is the assessed Harmony.

Now suppose further that in the pattern **a**, the activation value of unit γ is +0.7. Then the same pattern **a** *satisfies* the constraint corresponding to the connection (+0.5) to β from γ; the Harmony of **a** with respect to this constraint is positive:

(2) $H_{\beta\gamma}(\mathbf{a}) = a_\beta\ W_{\beta\gamma}\ a_\gamma = (+0.4)\ (+0.5)\ (+0.7) = +0.140.$

The *net* Harmony of **a** with respect to *both* these two connections combined is computed simply by adding together the individual Harmony values:

(3) $H_{\beta\alpha}(\mathbf{a}) + H_{\beta\gamma}(\mathbf{a}) = (-0.224) + (+0.14) = -0.084.$

This is negative: **a** satisfies the weaker constraint, but violates the stronger constraint, leading to a net violation indicated by a negative overall Harmony value.

Let us compare the pattern **a** with another pattern **a'**, identical to **a** except that the activation value of unit β is negative instead of positive: now, $a'_\beta = -0.4$, whereas before, $a_\beta = +0.4$. The new pattern **a'** now violates the weaker constraint (which says that γ is active so β should be too) while satisfying the stronger constraint (which says that α has positive activation so β should not). Reversing the sign of a_β to that of a'_β reverses the signs of all the Harmony values in the above equations, so now the value of $H(\mathbf{a'})$ with respect to these two connections is positive (+0.084). **a'** is more well formed than **a** with respect to these two connections: it conforms better to the set of two constraints. And indeed, as already discussed, the activation flow into β from both α and γ combined would have the net effect of inhibiting β, not exciting it, so activation flow will tend to generate pattern **a'** rather than pattern **a**.[1] The result of activation flow of course depends on the particular equations governing activation spread in the network; however, as we show momentarily, for an important class of networks, the result of spreading activation will be to create a pattern of activity that

[1] In some networks, activation values cannot be negative, but this should not obscure the point here. Instead of choosing $a'_\beta = -a_\beta$, let a'_β be *any* value less than a_β; then it will still follow that $H(\mathbf{a'}) > H(\mathbf{a})$. The lower the activation value of unit β, the more well formed the pattern. So the most Harmonic pattern will be the one with the lowest activation value for β that is possible in the particular network (which varies from network to network).

has maximum Harmony. This pattern is the one that **best satisfies** the pair of constraints corresponding to the pair of connections we have been considering. Thus, activation spread is a process of **parallel soft constraint satisfaction** (Hinton 1981; Feldman and Ballard 1982; Smolensky 1984; Ackley, Hinton, and Sejnowski 1985; Shastri 1985; Rumelhart et al. 1986; Stolcke 1989): the constraints are 'soft' in the sense that each may be overruled by other constraints and therefore violated in the final pattern—violation of a soft constraint in a licit representation is not impossible, in contrast to 'hard' constraints. A soft constraint may be violated, but at a cost: the Harmony is lowered, by amount depending on the strength of the violated constraint and the degree of violation.

In general, this account of activation spreading as parallel soft constraint satisfaction, or as a Harmony maximization process, applies not to a pair of connections, but to the complete set of connections in a network. The total Harmony of a pattern **a** in a network with connection weight matrix **W** is just the sum of the Harmony values of **a** with respect to all the individual connections. Thus, we have the following definition of well-formedness of an activity pattern in a PDP network:

(4) **Wf$_{\text{PDP}}$**

The Harmony of an activation vector **a** is defined to be

$$H(\mathbf{a}) = \Sigma_{\beta\alpha} H_{\beta\alpha} = \Sigma_{\beta\alpha}\, a_\beta W_{\beta\alpha} a_\alpha = \mathbf{a}^{\mathrm{T}} \cdot \mathbf{W} \cdot \mathbf{a}.$$

Here, $\Sigma_{\beta\alpha}$ means 'sum over all pairs of units β, α'. The last expression is simply a compact expression for this sum using matrix multiplication ('·'; see Chapter 5 (53) and Box 5:1); this way of producing a number, $H(\mathbf{a})$, from a vector **a** and a matrix **W** is fundamental to vector space theory. The symbol '^{T}' denotes the matrix **transpose** operation, which interchanges the rows and columns of a matrix: $[\mathbf{M}^{\mathrm{T}}]_{\alpha\beta} = [\mathbf{M}]_{\beta\alpha}$. For matrix algebra, the vector **a** can be taken to be a column vector, a matrix **A** with a single column: $[\mathbf{A}]_{\alpha 1} \equiv [\mathbf{a}]_\alpha$. The transpose of **A**, $\mathbf{A}^{\mathrm{T}}$, consists of a single row: $[\mathbf{A}^{\mathrm{T}}]_{1\beta} \equiv [\mathbf{a}]_\beta$. Then the double matrix product $\mathbf{A}^{\mathrm{T}} \cdot \mathbf{W} \cdot \mathbf{A}$ is a 1×1 matrix, a single number:

(5) $$[\mathbf{A}^{\mathrm{T}} \cdot \mathbf{W} \cdot \mathbf{A}]_{11} = \Sigma_\beta\, [\mathbf{A}^{\mathrm{T}}]_{1\beta}\, (\Sigma_\alpha [\mathbf{W}]_{\beta\alpha}\, [\mathbf{A}]_{\alpha 1}) = \Sigma_{\beta\alpha}\, a_\beta W_{\beta\alpha} a_\alpha = H(\mathbf{a}).$$

Equation (4) follows the usual convention in which **A**, $\mathbf{A}^{\mathrm{T}}$ are simply denoted **a**, $\mathbf{a}^{\mathrm{T}}$.

1.2 Harmony maximization

The reason for creating the concept of Harmony is that it figures into an important result from the theory of PDP connectionist computation: a theorem concerning Harmony maximization. To see intuitively the basis of this result, consider the contribution an individual activation value a_β makes to the Harmony in (4), which we now write as

(6) $$H(\mathbf{a}) = \Sigma_{\gamma\alpha}\, a_\gamma W_{\gamma\alpha} a_\alpha.$$

There are two types of terms containing a_β, ones with $\gamma = \beta$ and ones with $\alpha = \beta$:

(7) $$H_\beta \equiv \Sigma_\alpha a_\beta W_{\beta\alpha} a_\alpha + \Sigma_\gamma a_\gamma W_{\gamma\beta} a_\beta$$
$$= a_\beta [\Sigma_\alpha W_{\beta\alpha} a_\alpha] + \Sigma_\gamma a_\gamma W_{\gamma\beta} a_\beta$$
$$\equiv H_\beta^{\text{self}} + H_\beta^{\text{others}}.$$

(Here, we assume that units cannot send activation to themselves: $W_{\beta\beta} = 0$ for all units β.)[2] The quantity in square brackets is the input flowing into the unit β, which we call 'ι_β' (ι = iota; Chapter 5 (53)):[3]

(8) $$\iota_\beta \equiv \Sigma_\alpha W_{\beta\alpha} a_\alpha.$$

Thus, the first of the two terms in (7), which we will denote 'H_β^{self}', is just β's activation times its input: let us call this the **self-Harmony** of β. Focusing on just this term for the moment, we have

(9) $$H_\beta^{\text{self}} \equiv a_\beta [\Sigma_\alpha W_{\beta\alpha} a_\alpha] = a_\beta \iota_\beta.$$

What should the activation value of β do to maximize this? If the input to β is positive, $\iota_\beta > 0$, then a_β should be as large as possible. Thus, if β's activation function causes its activity to increase when it receives positive input ("excitation"), this will push the network toward maximum Harmony. If the input to β is negative, the reverse holds: to maximize *H*, β's activity should be as *small* as possible, and its activity will indeed decrease if its activation function converts negative input ("inhibition") into lower activation.

This is the essence of the **Harmony Maximization Theorem**—it is extremely simple. A number of complications must be taken into consideration, and these are mostly postponed until Chapter 9. But before leaving this basic analysis behind, we must return to the second term in the part of the Harmony dependent on β (7):

(10) $$H_\beta^{\text{others}} \equiv \Sigma_{\gamma\neq\beta} a_\gamma W_{\gamma\beta} a_\beta .$$

This may be thought of as the contribution β makes to the self-Harmony of the other units: it depends on the connections from β to other units γ, with weights $W_{\gamma\beta}$. When β's activity changes, the input it sends to other units changes also, which affects the self-Harmony of those other units. In general, this effect may be positive or negative; so, despite the arguments of the previous paragraph that β's *own* Harmony H_β^{self} will increase if it increases or decreases its activity in the face of positive or negative input (respectively), the *total* effect of this activity change might be to *lower* the network's Harmony, once account is taken of the additional effects β has on the self-Harmony of its neighbors.

There are special network architectures, however, that eliminate the possibility

[2] In general, self-connections introduce complications in Harmony maximization; see the recurring discussion of this issue in Chapter 9.

[3] To take a concrete example, suppose there are only three units and β = 1. Then

$$H \equiv (a_1W_{12}a_2 + a_1W_{13}a_3) + (a_2W_{21}a_1 + a_2W_{23}a_3) + (a_3W_{31}a_1 + a_3W_{32}a_2)$$
$$H_1 \equiv (a_1W_{12}a_2 + a_1W_{13}a_3) + a_2W_{21}a_1 + a_3W_{31}a_1$$
$$= a_1[W_{12}a_2 + W_{13}a_3] + a_2W_{21}a_1 + a_3W_{31}a_1$$
$$\equiv a_1[\iota_1] + (a_2W_{21}a_1 + a_3W_{31}a_1)$$
$$\equiv H_1^{\text{self}} + H_1^{\text{others}}.$$

that H will be lowered. One well-known case arises when the network is **symmetric**—meaning that the weight of the connection to any unit α from any other unit γ is the same as the weight of the connection between these same units going in the reverse direction: $W_{\alpha\gamma} = W_{\gamma\alpha}$. In this case, H_β^{others} is seen to be numerically equal to H_β^{self}, so that by changing β's activation to increase the latter, we are simultaneously increasing the former.[4]

Before stating a Harmony maximization result somewhat formally, we need to recall a high-level characterization of the kind of computation performed in PDP networks (Section 1:2). First, an input, encoded as an input vector **i**, is imposed (**clamped**) on a set of input units, where it remains unchanged throughout the computation.[5] Then activation flows from the input units to other units; each unit repeatedly **updates** its activation value in response to input from other units. Typically, this eventually **settles** and the overall activation vector of the entire network, **a**, no longer changes. The input vector **i** is a part of the total activation vector **a**, since the input units are a part of the total population of units in the network. We will phrase this as follows: the total vector **a** is a **completion** of the input vector **i**. Part of the total activation vector **a** is also the output vector **o**: this is the part of **a** that lists the activation values of the output units. Thus, as the network computes a completion **a** of an input **i**, part of what it's doing is mapping the input **i** to a corresponding output **o**; this mapping of **i** to **o** is the function f computed by the network.

In addition to the definition of Harmony, we need a definition that characterizes an important class of connectionist networks.

(11) Harmonic networks

A PDP network is **harmonic** if it possesses the following properties:

a. *Activation function.* If the total input to any unit is positive, its activation will increase (up to some limit, possibly); if negative, it will decrease (down to some limit, possibly).

b. *Connectivity.* The connectivity pattern is either feed-forward (no closed loops) or symmetric feedback ($W_{\beta\alpha} = W_{\alpha\beta}$: the connection weight to β from α equals that to α from β).

c. *Updating.* Units change their activation values one at a time, or they change their activity by a very small amount at each update (ideally, continuously in time).

Now we can state the theorem (based on work such as Hopfield 1982, 1984; Cohen and Grossberg 1983; Hinton and Sejnowski 1983b, 1986; Smolensky 1983, 1986; Geman and Geman 1984; Ackley, Hinton, and Sejnowski 1985; Golden 1986):[6]

[4] In the symmetric case, when $W_{\beta\gamma} = W_{\gamma\beta}$, the Harmony contribution of the connection *to* γ *from* β—$a_\gamma W_{\gamma\beta} a_\beta$—is equal to that of the connection *to* β *from* γ:

$$a_\beta W_{\beta\gamma} a_\gamma = a_\beta W_{\gamma\beta} a_\gamma = a_\gamma W_{\gamma\beta} a_\beta.$$

Thus, the corresponding terms in the sums defining H_γ^{others} and H_γ^{self} are equal.

[5] Clamping is not the only way of presenting an input to a network, but it is the one predominantly used, at least in cognitive modeling.

[6] The generality of this result emerged through the work of many people, as explained in the more

(12) Harmony Maximization Theorem

In harmonic networks, at each moment of processing, the Harmony of the total activation vector increases (or stays the same). Furthermore, for a very wide set of activation functions, the activation settles to a final vector that maximizes $H(\mathbf{a})$, among the vectors **a** that are completions of the input **i**.[7]

More precise formulations of (11) and (12) are presented in Section 9:3.3.

Harmony Maximization is fundamental to ICS because it makes it possible to reason at a level of analysis higher than that of individual units, connections, activation functions, updating procedures, and so on. Harmony Maximization enables most of this complexity to be encapsulated into a simple, yet powerful, principle that allows us to formulate a theory at a higher level.

We have now discussed the formal background to the third ICS principle introduced in Chapter 2 (5), where it was stated as follows:

(13) P_3. HMax (preliminary version)

a. (Harmony Maximization, general) In a number of cognitive domains, information processing in the mind/brain constructs an output for which the pair (input, output) is optimal: processing maximizes a connectionist well-formedness measure called Harmony. The Harmony function encapsulates knowledge as a set of conflicting soft constraints of varying strengths; the output achieves the optimal degree of simultaneous satisfaction of these constraints.

b. (Harmonic Grammar) Among the cognitive domains falling under Harmony Maximization are central aspects of knowledge of language—grammar. In this setting, the specification of the Harmony function is called a harmonic grammar. It defines a function that maps

input → output = parse(input).

We can now state a more articulated version of this principle, distinguishing the general character of PDP processing algorithms (Alg_{PDP}), the more specialized character of harmonic networks ($\text{Alg}_{\text{PDP}}(H)$), and resulting optimization characterization of the functions computed by these networks ($\text{Fun}_{\text{PDP}}(H)$): (14).

complete discussion in Chapter 9, which contains further references. Harmony Maximization is presumably just one of a whole family of principles waiting to be developed that allow higher-level analysis of various types of networks. Harmony Maximization represents one kind of behavior of dynamical systems like connectionist networks; dynamical systems theory characterizes a number of more exotic behaviors that are relevant to connectionist networks as well (e.g., Jordan 1986; Skarda and Freeman 1987; Cleeremans, Servan-Schreiber, and McClelland 1989; Pollack 1995; Hirsch 1996; Smolensky 1996; Blair and Pollack 1997; Rodriguez, Wiles, and Elman 1999; Rodriguez 2001).

[7] While (4) gives the core of the Harmony function needed in (12) for a large variety of networks, as shown in Chapter 9, it is often necessary to add a further term—the **unit harmony**—which is idiosyncratic to the particular activation function that units use to compute their activation. Generally, (4) is the part of the Harmony function that depends on the weights—the knowledge—in the network; the additional terms typically do not. For example, the simple case of a linear associator (Section 5:2.1) falls under theorem (12); the additional term one needs to add to (4) in that case is just $-\frac{1}{2}\,\Sigma_\alpha\, o_\alpha^2 \equiv -\frac{1}{2}\|\mathbf{o}\|^2$, where $\|\mathbf{o}\|$ is the Euclidean length of **o** (see Section 9:3.2.2.2).

(14) **P_3. HMax**

a. **Harmony Maximization**

Alg_{PDP}: In all cognitive domains, cognitive processes are spreading activation algorithms …

$Alg_{PDP}(H)$: … a core class of which are those operating in harmonic networks …

$Fun_{PDP}(H)$: … that perform parallel soft constraint satisfaction; that is, they complete input activation vectors to total activation vectors that maximize Harmony, optimally satisfying the soft constraints embodied in the network connections and encapsulated in the Harmony function defined in (4):

$$H(\mathbf{a}) = \mathbf{a}^{\mathrm{T}} \cdot \mathbf{W} \cdot \mathbf{a} \equiv \Sigma_{\beta\alpha}\, a_\beta W_{\beta\alpha} a_\alpha,$$

where **a** is the activation vector, **W** is the weight matrix, and the sum extends over all pairs of units α and β.

b. **Harmonic Grammar**

Knowledge of language — grammar — is realized in harmonic networks.

$Fun_{PDP}(H)$ is a logical consequence of $Alg_{PDP}(H)$ and not an independent hypothesis of the theory. Part (b) of the HMax principle states that grammar falls under principle $Alg_{PDP}(H)$ and therefore necessarily also under principle $Fun_{PDP}(H)$. Elaboration of the consequences of this principle for grammatical theory is the topic of the next section.

2 OPTIMIZATION IN GRAMMAR I: HARMONIC GRAMMAR

The importance of the processing assumption $Alg_{PDP}(H)$ is that it allows connectionist principles to inform analysis at a higher level. In higher cognitive domains, at such a level the representational assumption Rep_{ICS}(HC) (Chapter 5 (50)) applies: the vectors of interest have the form of tensor product representations. So what are the implications of having these two higher-level principles, Harmony maximization and tensor product representation, both in force? The analysis is undertaken in Section 2.1; for the moment, we simply state the result, which is remarkably simple:

(15) **Wf_{ICS}(HC)**: Harmonic Grammar Soft-Constraint Theorem

Suppose **a** is a tensor product vector realizing a symbolic structure **s** with constituents $\{\mathbf{c}_k\}$, according to Rep_{ICS}(HC).

a. The Harmony of this representation is

$$H(\mathbf{s}) \equiv H(\mathbf{a}) = \Sigma_{j \le k}\, H(\mathbf{c}_j, \mathbf{c}_k),$$

where $H(\mathbf{c}_j, \mathbf{c}_k)$ — the Harmony resulting from the co-occurrence of $\mathbf{c}_j$ and $\mathbf{c}_k$ in the same structure — is a constant for all **s**.[8]

[8] Restricting the sum to j, k pairs in which $j \le k$ ensures that each constituent pair is counted only once.

b. Equivalently, the $H(\mathbf{s})$ can be computed using the following rules:

R_{jk}: If **s** simultaneously contains the constituents $\mathbf{c}_j$ and $\mathbf{c}_k$, then add the numerical quantity $H(\mathbf{c}_j, \mathbf{c}_k)$ to H.

Each R_{jk} is called a **soft rule**, and the collection of soft rules defines a **harmonic grammar**. To determine the Harmony of a structure **s**, we simply find all rules R_{jk} that apply to **s** and add up all the corresponding Harmony contributions $H(\mathbf{c}_j, \mathbf{c}_k)$.

c. Soft rules can equivalently be recast as **soft constraints**. If $H(\mathbf{c}_j, \mathbf{c}_k)$ is a negative value $-w_{jk}$, then R_{jk} is interpreted as the following (negative) constraint, in which w_{jk} serves as a **weight** or **strength**:

C_{jk}: **s** does *not* simultaneously contain the constituents $\mathbf{c}_j$ and $\mathbf{c}_k$ (strength: w_{jk}).

If $H(\mathbf{c}_j, \mathbf{c}_k)$ is a positive value $+w_{jk}$, then R_{jk} corresponds to the following (positive) constraint:

C_{jk}: **s** *does* simultaneously contain the constituents $\mathbf{c}_j$ and $\mathbf{c}_k$ (strength: w_{jk}).

$H(\mathbf{s})$ is computed by adding the strengths of all the positive constraints that **s** satisfies and subtracting the strength of all the negative constraints that it violates.

d. With respect to the connectionist description, each Harmony contribution $H(\mathbf{c}_j, \mathbf{c}_k)$ can be calculated at the lower level in terms of the weight matrix **W** according to the formula

$$H(\mathbf{c}_j, \mathbf{c}_k) = H(\mathsf{c}_j, \mathsf{c}_k) = \Sigma_{\beta\alpha} [\mathsf{c}_j]_\beta (\mathrm{W}_{\beta\alpha} + \mathrm{W}_{\alpha\beta}) [\mathsf{c}_k]_\alpha = \mathsf{c}_j^{\mathrm{T}} \cdot (\mathbf{W} + \mathbf{W}^{\mathrm{T}}) \cdot \mathsf{c}_k,$$

where $[\mathsf{c}_k]_\beta$ is the activation value of unit β in the vector c_k that realizes $\mathbf{c}_k$.

e. $H(\mathbf{c}_j, \mathbf{c}_k)$ can be interpreted as the **interaction Harmony** of the pair $(\mathbf{c}_j, \mathbf{c}_k)$: the amount of Harmony contributed by $\mathbf{c}_j$ and $\mathbf{c}_k$ when they are present together, *beyond* the sum of the Harmonies of $\mathbf{c}_j$ and $\mathbf{c}_k$ in isolation.

This result is a simple kind of compositionality: the Harmony of a structure as a whole is the sum of the Harmonies contributed by all its constituents (considered pairwise).[9]

Let us illustrate soft constraints by discussing those that correspond to a conventional phrase structure rewrite-grammar rule, expressing a sentence (**S**) as a Noun Phrase (**NP**) followed by a Verb Phrase (**VP**).

(16) **S → NP VP**

This rule asserts the grammaticality of the local tree (17).

(17)

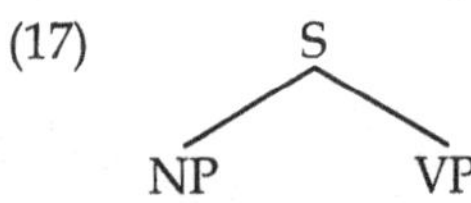

[9] This observation is due to Tom Wasow. Note that compositionality here is automatic, not stipulated.

Two corresponding soft constraints, informally stated, are:

(18) a. $R_{\mathbf{NP}/\mathbf{S}}$: If **s** contains a constituent labeled **S** and its left subconstituent is labeled **NP**, then add +2 to H.

b. $R_{\mathbf{S}\backslash\mathbf{VP}}$: If **s** contains a constituent labeled **S** and its right subconstituent is labeled **VP**, then add +2 to H.

That these rules instantiate the general soft rule schema for R_{jk} is fairly obvious. In (18a), for example, the constituent $\mathbf{c}_j$ is an **S** at some node in the parse tree, while the second constituent $\mathbf{c}_k$ is an **NP** at a node that is the left-child node of the **S**. The Harmony contribution from this pair, $H(\mathbf{c}_j, \mathbf{c}_k)$, is +2; that this quantity is positive means that this pair of constituents is well formed according to the grammar.[10]

The principle (15) Wf_{ICS}(HC) determines how the Harmony of a symbolic structure (e.g., a parse tree) **s** is computed in terms of its symbolic constituents. The computation is a simple one provided the quantities $H(\mathbf{c}_j, \mathbf{c}_k)$ are known. In that case, no reference to the connectionist description's activation vectors and weight matrices is required: the entire computation can be performed on the basis of the symbolic constituents alone. The numbers $H(\mathbf{c}_j, \mathbf{c}_k)$ encapsulate the details of the lower-level weights and activations into a form directly usable at the higher level. Thus, to apply the constraints $R_{\mathbf{NP}/\mathbf{S}}$ and $R_{\mathbf{S}\backslash\mathbf{VP}}$ (18), we need only know about the location of **S**, **NP**, and **VP** labels in a parse tree. We needn't know anything about the activation vectors used to realize these constituents, and the connections used to process them, except for what is encapsulated in (18): that the aggregate effect of all the relevant activations and weights is to assess a Harmony of +2 to the specified arrangements of constituents in a structure.

Given the ability to assess the Harmony of any symbol structure – provided by Wf_{ICS}(HC) – it is now (in principle) straightforward to determine the functioning of the grammar: apply principle $\text{Fun}_{\text{PDP}}(H)$, as follows. Imagine that the network receives a string of symbols, encoded as an input vector **i**, which it must parse according to its harmonic grammar. According to $\text{Fun}_{\text{PDP}}(H)$, the net effect of the processing in the network is to complete this input vector into a total pattern of activity **a** that has maximum Harmony; this normally involves adding constituents $\mathbf{c}_k$ to those already present in the input, for example, phrases that group together symbols in the input. The maximum-Harmony vector **a** is the parse of the input **i** according to the grammar encoded in the network's connections **W**.[11] That is, we have the following

[10] A few remarks should be made. First, in these soft rules, the two constituents referred to by $\mathbf{c}_j$, $\mathbf{c}_k$ can be the same; that is, a rule can refer to a single constituent, as in the rule (36) below. Second, in tensor product representations, a 'constituent' is a structure bound to some particular structural role, so it is perfectly legitimate to refer to roles such as 'left subconstituent', as in (18a). Finally, soft rules like (18) that correspond to rewrite rules like (16) must be **embedding invariant**: the Harmony of an **S**, **NP** pair must not depend on the level of its embedding in the tree. (This is an important part of the recursivity of the notion of well-formedness in formal languages.) Thanks to (15d), relating the Harmony of constituent pairs to the underlying weight matrix $\mathbb{W}$, it can be proven that the recurrent-network condition $\text{Alg}_{\text{ICS}}(\text{HC},\mathbb{W})$ defining the recursive tensor product structure of $\mathbb{W}$ (Chapter 5 (63)) entails embedding invariance; see Section 8:4.2.

[11] The bottom-up form of the logic here, then, is this: the weights **W** and representations $\{\mathbf{c}_k\}$ determine the set of $H(\mathbf{c}_j, \mathbf{c}_k)$'s by (15d); these pairwise Harmony values determine the soft rules R_{jk} by

symbolic version of $\text{Fun}_{\text{PDP}}(H)$:

(19) **$\text{Fun}_{\text{ICS}}(H,\text{HC})$**

Given an input symbolic structure *I*, the harmonic grammar assigns to *I* the output symbolic structure ('parse') **s** with maximal Harmony, among those which are completions of *I*. The higher the Harmony value of this parse structure **s**, the more well formed the grammar judges the input.

The input is always part of the parse structure. For phrase structure grammars (context-free grammars), the parse is a tree whose terminal symbols give the input string, and whose structure shows how the input symbols are grouped into constituent phrases. For formal grammars, we can arbitrarily impose a cutoff of acceptable Harmony for the parse in order for an input string to be judged sufficiently well formed by the grammar to be admitted into the language. For instance, we may choose a cutoff of 0: inputs assigned parses with negative Harmony are then not in the formal language, while those with nonnegative Harmony are.[12]

The remainder of this section consists of five subsections, each of which may be read independently of the others. The organization is as follows. Section 2.1 provides a formal derivation of the Harmonic Grammar formalism (15). Section 2.2 takes up a few formal issues concerning the relations between the lower- and higher-level characterizations of language processing implicit in Harmonic Grammar. Section 2.3 discusses the application of Harmonic Grammar to formal languages. Section 2.4 addresses an important optimization-based competence/performance distinction within ICS. Sections 2.1–2.4 all address computational issues. Section 2.5 turns to natural language, summarizing an application of Harmonic Grammar to a problem at the syntax-semantics interface.

2.1 Derivation of the Harmonic Grammar formalism

The purpose of this section is to derive the Harmonic Grammar formalism defined in (15). That is, we aim to show that HG follows mathematically from two ICS principles: P_2: $\text{Rep}_{\text{ICS}}(\text{HC})$ (Chapter 5 (50)), which states that representations subserving higher cognition, such as language, have tensor product structure, and P_3: HMax (14), which states that linguistic processing maximizes a Harmony function with a certain mathematical form. This section may be skipped as subsequent sections do not depend upon it.

According to HMax, the output of linguistic processing is an activation vector **a** that maximizes the following Harmony function:

(20) $$H(\mathbf{a}) = \mathbf{a}^{\mathrm{T}} \cdot \mathbf{W} \cdot \mathbf{a} \equiv \Sigma_{\beta\alpha}\, a_\beta\, W_{\beta\alpha}\, a_\alpha.$$

(15b); and these in turn determine which parse of an input has maximum Harmony and is therefore the correct parse, by (19).

[12] All inputs, even ungrammatical ones, are assigned a parse (structural description) by the grammar; this is a familiar notion in generative grammar. For a reinterpretation of Harmonic Grammar using an all-or-none definition of well-formedness, like that of Optimality Theory, see Sections 20:1.3–1.4.

According to $\text{Rep}_{\text{ICS}}(\text{HC})$, the vector **a** has the form

(21) $\mathbf{a} = \Sigma_i \, \mathbf{c}_i,$

where $\{\mathbf{c}_i\}$ are the vectors realizing the constituents $\{\mathsf{c}_i\}$ (filler/role bindings) of a symbol structure **s** realized by **a**. Inserting (21) into (20) gives

$$\begin{aligned}(22)\quad H(\mathbf{a}) &= \mathbf{a}^{\mathrm{T}} \cdot \mathbf{W} \cdot \mathbf{a} = (\Sigma_i \, \mathbf{c}_i)^{\mathrm{T}} \cdot \mathbf{W} \cdot (\Sigma_j \, \mathbf{c}_j) \\ &= \Sigma_k \, \mathbf{c}_k^{\mathrm{T}} \cdot \mathbf{W} \cdot \mathbf{c}_k + \Sigma_{i \neq j} \, \mathbf{c}_i^{\mathrm{T}} \cdot \mathbf{W} \cdot \mathbf{c}_j \\ &= \Sigma_k \, H(\mathsf{c}_k, \mathsf{c}_k) + \Sigma_{i \neq j} \, \mathbf{c}_i^{\mathrm{T}} \cdot \mathbf{W} \cdot \mathbf{c}_j,\end{aligned}$$

where c_k is the symbolic constituent realized by $\mathbf{c}_k$ and $H(\mathsf{c}_k, \mathsf{c}_k)$ is defined as follows:

(23) $H(\mathsf{c}_k, \mathsf{c}_k) \equiv \mathbf{c}_k^{\mathrm{T}} \cdot \mathbf{W} \cdot \mathbf{c}_k.$

$H(\mathsf{c}_k, \mathsf{c}_k)$ is exactly the Harmony of c_k in isolation. The second sum in (22) runs over all combinations of i and j, and thus counts each pair of constituents twice, once with $i < j$ and again with $i > j$ (e.g., the pair $\mathbf{c}_1$ and $\mathbf{c}_2$ is counted once with $i = 1, j = 2$, and again with $i = 2, j = 1$). We can reduce this to a sum with a single term for each pair (with, say, $i < j$) as follows. Using the fact[13] that

(24) $\mathbf{c}_i^{\mathrm{T}} \cdot \mathbf{W} \cdot \mathbf{c}_j = \mathbf{c}_j^{\mathrm{T}} \cdot \mathbf{W}^{\mathrm{T}} \cdot \mathbf{c}_i,$

we can rewrite the second sum in (22) as in (25),

$$\begin{aligned}(25)\quad \Sigma_{i \neq j} \, \mathbf{c}_i^{\mathrm{T}} \cdot \mathbf{W} \cdot \mathbf{c}_j &= \Sigma_{i<j} \mathbf{c}_i^{\mathrm{T}} \cdot \mathbf{W} \cdot \mathbf{c}_j + \Sigma_{i>j} \mathbf{c}_i^{\mathrm{T}} \cdot \mathbf{W} \cdot \mathbf{c}_j \\ &= \Sigma_{i<j} \mathbf{c}_i^{\mathrm{T}} \cdot \mathbf{W} \cdot \mathbf{c}_j + \Sigma_{i>j} \mathbf{c}_j^{\mathrm{T}} \cdot \mathbf{W}^{\mathrm{T}} \cdot \mathbf{c}_i \\ &= \Sigma_{i<j} \mathbf{c}_i^{\mathrm{T}} \cdot \mathbf{W} \cdot \mathbf{c}_j + \Sigma_{j>i} \mathbf{c}_i^{\mathrm{T}} \cdot \mathbf{W}^{\mathrm{T}} \cdot \mathbf{c}_j \\ &= \Sigma_{i<j} \mathbf{c}_i^{\mathrm{T}} \cdot (\mathbf{W} + \mathbf{W}^{\mathrm{T}}) \cdot \mathbf{c}_j \\ &= \Sigma_{i<j} H(\mathsf{c}_i, \mathsf{c}_j),\end{aligned}$$

where we have defined $H(\mathsf{c}_i, \mathsf{c}_j)$ as follows :

(26) $H(\mathsf{c}_i, \mathsf{c}_j) \equiv \mathbf{c}_i^{\mathrm{T}} \cdot (\mathbf{W} + \mathbf{W}^{\mathrm{T}}) \cdot \mathbf{c}_j.$

Now we can finally write the Harmony (22) in the desired form:

(27) $H(\mathsf{s}) \equiv H(\mathbf{a}) = \Sigma_k H(\mathsf{c}_k, \mathsf{c}_k) + \Sigma_{i<j} H(\mathsf{c}_i, \mathsf{c}_j) = \Sigma_{i \leq j} H(\mathsf{c}_i, \mathsf{c}_j).$

The Harmony of **a**, the realization of the structure **s** with constituents $\{\mathsf{c}_i\}$, is the sum of the Harmony resulting from all pairs of constituents, $H(\mathsf{c}_i, \mathsf{c}_j)$, including 'pairs' $(\mathsf{c}_i, \mathsf{c}_i)$ consisting of an element with itself. This establishes (15a) and (15d).

We turn now to the interpretation of (27). As noted previously in the discussion of (23), $H(\mathsf{c}_k, \mathsf{c}_k)$ is just $H(\mathsf{c}_k)$, the Harmony of c_k in isolation; this measures the degree to which the internal structure of the activation pattern $\mathbf{c}_k$ realizing the symbolic constituent c_k conforms to the soft constraints embodied in the network's connections. Now consider $H(\mathsf{c}_i, \mathsf{c}_j)$ when $i \neq j$; assume we've labeled the constituents so that $i < j$. Substituting $\mathbf{a} = \mathbf{c}_i + \mathbf{c}_j$ into equation (27) gives

[13] (24) can be seen by expanding out the matrix products; see (5):
$\mathbf{c}_i^{\mathrm{T}} \cdot \mathbf{W} \cdot \mathbf{c}_j \equiv \Sigma_{\beta\alpha} [\mathbf{c}_i]_\beta [\mathbf{W}]_{\beta\alpha} [\mathbf{c}_j]_\alpha = \Sigma_{\beta\alpha} [\mathbf{c}_i]_\beta [\mathbf{W}^{\mathrm{T}}]_{\alpha\beta} [\mathbf{c}_j]_\alpha = \Sigma_{\beta\alpha} [\mathbf{c}_j]_\alpha [\mathbf{W}^{\mathrm{T}}]_{\alpha\beta} [\mathbf{c}_i]_\beta \equiv \mathbf{c}_j^{\mathrm{T}} \cdot \mathbf{W}^{\mathrm{T}} \cdot \mathbf{c}_i.$

(28) $H(\mathbf{c}_i + \mathbf{c}_j) = \Sigma_{k \le l} H(\mathbf{c}_k, \mathbf{c}_l) = H(\mathbf{c}_i, \mathbf{c}_i) + H(\mathbf{c}_j, \mathbf{c}_j) + H(\mathbf{c}_i, \mathbf{c}_j)$.

This asserts that the Harmony of the pair $(\mathbf{c}_i, \mathbf{c}_j)$ in isolation is $H(\mathbf{c}_i, \mathbf{c}_i) + H(\mathbf{c}_j, \mathbf{c}_j)$—the sum of the Harmonies of the individual constituents in isolation—plus $H(\mathbf{c}_i, \mathbf{c}_j)$. So $H(\mathbf{c}_i, \mathbf{c}_j)$ can be interpreted as the interaction Harmony of $(\mathbf{c}_i, \mathbf{c}_j)$: the additional Harmony (positive or negative) arising from the co-presence of $\mathbf{c}_i$ and $\mathbf{c}_j$ beyond the sum of their individual Harmonies in isolation. This establishes (15e).

From (27), it is evident that computing the Harmony of a structure **s** can thus be achieved with the soft rules of (15b):

(29) R_{ij}: If **s** simultaneously contains the constituents $\mathbf{c}_i$ and $\mathbf{c}_j$, then add the numerical quantity $H(\mathbf{c}_i, \mathbf{c}_j)$ to H.

or the soft constraints of (15c):

(30) C_{ij}: *s* must/must *not* simultaneously contain the constituents $\mathbf{c}_i$ and $\mathbf{c}_j$ (strength: w_{ij}).

where the constraint reads 'must' if $H(\mathbf{c}_i, \mathbf{c}_j) > 0$, 'must not' if $H(\mathbf{c}_i, \mathbf{c}_j) < 0$, and where the strength w_{ij} is the magnitude $|H(\mathbf{c}_i, \mathbf{c}_j)|$. Each soft rule or constraint merely verbally describes one term in the sum (27). It must be remembered that in the rules/constraints, as in the sum, the cases where $i = j$ must be included. In such a case, R_{ii} requires that $H(\mathbf{c}_i, \mathbf{c}_i)$ be added to $H(\mathbf{s})$ whenever **s** contains the constituent $\mathbf{c}_i$, while C_{ii} asserts simply that **s** must/must not contain $\mathbf{c}_i$.

As a simple example relating to the exposition of tensor product representations in Chapter 5, if the string **s** = **abc** is decomposed using positional roles into the filler/role bindings $\{\mathbf{a}/r_1, \mathbf{c}/r_3, \mathbf{b}/r_2\}$, then

(31) $$H(\mathbf{abc}) = [H(\mathbf{a}/r_1, \mathbf{a}/r_1) + H(\mathbf{c}/r_3, \mathbf{c}/r_3) + H(\mathbf{b}/r_2, \mathbf{b}/r_2)] + [H(\mathbf{a}/r_1, \mathbf{b}/r_2) + H(\mathbf{a}/r_1, \mathbf{c}/r_3) + H(\mathbf{b}/r_2, \mathbf{c}/r_3)].$$

The first sum in square brackets is the first term $\Sigma_k H(\mathbf{c}_k, \mathbf{c}_k)$ of (27), the self-Harmonies of the individual constituents; the second sum in square brackets is the second term $\Sigma_{i<j} H(\mathbf{c}_i, \mathbf{c}_j)$ of (27), the interaction Harmonies of distinct constituent pairs.

2.2 Relations between lower and higher levels in Harmonic Grammar

According to the HG formalism (15), the Harmony of a structure is a sum of terms none of which depends on more than two constituents. This is significant because many dependencies in language and elsewhere are certainly higher than second order. For instance, even a simple phrase structure rule like **S → NP VP** expresses a *third*-order dependency, between a whole (**S**) and its two parts (**NP, VP**). This creates a challenge for capturing phrase structure with HG, a challenge requiring some rethinking of grammatical categories, as explained in Chapter 10.

That the Harmony of a structure is a sum of terms each depending on no more than two constituents is an instance of how in ICS lower-level structure percolates up and shapes the higher-level theory. A look at the derivation of the HG formalism in

Section 2.1 shows that the reason Harmony terms can depend on at most two constituents is that the expression for Harmony (4), $H(\mathbf{a}) = \mathbf{a}^{\mathrm{T}} \cdot \mathbf{W} \cdot \mathbf{a} = \Sigma_{\beta\alpha}\, a_\beta W_{\beta\alpha} a_\alpha$, has only two factors of **a**: it is second order or quadratic in the activation values **a**. This in turn is due to the fact that each connection in the underlying network directly connects only two units. A full demonstration of this claim requires the more elaborated methods of Section 9:2, but the basic reason is already visible in equation (9) above, which displays the essential structure, shown in (32):

(32) (Harmony at unit β) ~ (activation of β) × (input to β).

In the networks we consider, the input to β is a weighted sum of the activation values of its neighbors, which makes each term in the Harmony function second order in activation values: the activation of β times the activation of a neighbor.[14]

HG allows linguistic analysis to be conducted at two different levels. At the lower level, we can attempt to determine the individual connection strengths constituting the weight matrix **W**, and the individual activations constituting the vectors $\mathbf{c}_i$ realizing linguistic constituents; from this information we can directly compute the terms (26) determining the Harmony of structures:

(33) $H(\mathbf{c}_i, \mathbf{c}_j) \equiv \mathbf{c}_i^{\mathrm{T}} \cdot (\mathbf{W} + \mathbf{W}^{\mathrm{T}}) \cdot \mathbf{c}_j$.

Alternatively, we can take the quantities $H(\mathbf{c}_i, \mathbf{c}_j)$ *themselves* as our basic variables and attempt to determine them directly: this is higher-level analysis. In Chapter 11, we show how this can be done in a simple, but linguistically important, case (see Section 2.5 below for a summary). The problem is to find values $H(\mathbf{c}_i, \mathbf{c}_j)$ which together have the effect that certain given structures are grammatical, that is, of maximum Harmony. In Chapter 11, the data are an extensive set of acceptability judgments for sentences in which a large number of French intransitive verbs have been inserted into several special syntactic constructions. Values for the Harmony variables $H(\mathbf{c}_i, \mathbf{c}_j)$ are computed from the acceptability data using a new version of the back-propagation learning algorithm (Rumelhart, Hinton, and Williams 1986), adapted to a special network constructed to embody the *higher-level* structure of HG, in which the unknown variables $H(\mathbf{c}_i, \mathbf{c}_j)$ are treated formally as connection weights.

We have shown how it is possible to shift the primitive variables from the lower-level quantities—individual activations a_β and weights $W_{\beta\alpha}$—to the higher-level quantities—symbolic constituents $\mathbf{c}_i$ and their interaction Harmonies $H(\mathbf{c}_i, \mathbf{c}_j)$. This amounts to a **change of variables** in our formal description of the mind/brain, a change from "brain variables" to "mind variables," as it were. We close this section by briefly considering two of the questions that arise in such a change of variables.

(34) Changing from lower- to higher-level variables

a. As mentioned above, the higher-level variables $H(\mathbf{c}_i, \mathbf{c}_j)$ can sometimes be

[14] In more complex networks—rarely used in cognitive models—the input to β might depend on the *product* of activation values of several of its neighbors (e.g., the 'sigma-pi' networks of Rumelhart, Hinton, and McClelland 1986; Pollack 1995). If this product determining the input to β involves n neighbors, then, including the first factor in (32), the activation of β itself, the Harmony function becomes of order $n + 1$. In the standard case, $n = 1$, which is the case considered throughout this book.

computed by a numerical fit to data. When is this parameter-fitting exercise appropriately constrained? Since there is one variable $H(\mathbf{c}_i, \mathbf{c}_j)$ for each pair of constituents, the number of parameters $H(\mathbf{c}_i, \mathbf{c}_j)$ scales as C^2, where C is the number of possible constituents. The number of structures $\mathbf{s}$ that can be formed by combining N of these constituents scales roughly as C^N. Thus, as N grows beyond 2, achieving a good parameter fit to the Harmony of the composite structures rapidly becomes highly significant. In addition, in most linguistic situations there are invariances across roles; for example, in context-free formal languages, the well-formedness of a subtree is independent of where it is embedded in a larger tree. Then the number of free parameters drops enormously—essentially, from the square of the number of filler/role bindings to the square of the number of fillers, since Harmony is largely invariant under the change of a filler's role. (See Section 8:4.2 for a discussion of embedding invariance.)

b. Is it correct to treat the higher-level Harmony variables $H(\mathbf{c}_i, \mathbf{c}_j)$ as independent of one another? Is it possible that these variables are not independent because they all derive from the same lower-level weights and activity patterns (15d)? Roughly, the answer depends essentially on the relation between the number of independent units in the underlying network and the number of different constituents that may be realized in that network. Crudely speaking, if there are many more lower-level variables—connection weights and activation values—than higher-level variables—self- and interaction-Harmonies of constituents—then it is to be expected that any set of values for the higher-level variables $H(\mathbf{c}_i, \mathbf{c}_j)$ can be achieved by some choice of the lower-level variables, the activities in the constituent realization vectors $\mathbf{c}_i$, and the weights in $\mathbf{W}$. Then the fact that the higher-level variables $H(\mathbf{c}_i, \mathbf{c}_j)$ all derive from a common lower-level structure does not constrain these variables—they can independently be assigned any values. On the other hand, if it is possible to identify some strong constraints on the lower-level variables—for example, if a large number of different constituents were constrained to be represented as different activity patterns over a much smaller number of units—then, effectively, there might be fewer lower-level variables than higher-level ones, so that the space of possible values for the higher-level variables might be genuinely constrained by the fact that they are derived from the lower level.

2.3 Harmonic Grammar and formal languages

The utter simplicity of HG may give the impression that it is quite a weak formalism. Only pairs of constituents are examined. Each pair is crudely assigned a number, and these numbers are simply added up. Interactions would seem to be very limited. So it is reasonable to expect that this connectionist-derived linguistic formalism, HG, is too weak to handle "real syntax"—in the formal sense—like that of context-free phrase structure grammars. This expectation is, however, demonstrably false, as asserted by the following theorem:

(35) **Fun_{ICS}(CFL)**

Any context-free language can be specified by a harmonic grammar.

The proof of this theorem may be found in Section 10:1. The idea of the proof is rather simple: context-free rewrite rules like (16), **S** → **NP VP**, are replaced by HG soft rules like (18) '$R_{\text{NP/S}}$: If **s** contains a constituent labeled **S** and its left subconstituent is labeled **NP**, then add +2 to H'; such rules provide positive Harmony for legal dominations (constituent-subconstituent relations). At the same time, a carefully designed set of constraints like

(36) R_{S}: If **s** contains a constituent **S**, add –3 to H(**s**).

assess negative Harmony for all symbols (like **S**) that occur in the parse tree. The negative Harmony values in constraints like (36) are designed so that if the symbol has a legal parent in the tree, and the full number of required legal children, then its negative Harmony will be exactly canceled by the positive Harmony arising from all these legal dominations. The net result is that well-formed parse trees have zero Harmony while all other structures have negative Harmony—so the formal language is, as required, the set of those input symbol strings whose maximum-Harmony parse tree has the maximum-possible Harmony value: zero.

Extending theorem (35) from context-free grammars to unrestricted grammars is straightforward. The only complication is that parse structures are no longer simply trees, but more complex symbolic structures whose realization in tensor products has not yet been attempted explicitly; we know of no reason to expect any difficulties, however, given the utter generality of the tensor product technique for representing arbitrary symbolic structures. But as far as harmonic grammars at the symbolic level are concerned, there is no doubt: for any rewrite-rule grammar there is a corresponding harmonic grammar that generates the same formal language (see Section 10:1).

Unrestricted grammars are the formal-language equivalents of Turing machines: the former are the top of the Chomsky language hierarchy and the latter the top of the automaton hierarchy (recall Box 1). Thus, the power of the computational abstraction provided by ICS, HG, is as great as that of Turing machines. In this (very special) sense, at least, the goal of realizing the power of symbolic computation in PDP connectionist computation has been achieved, although implicit in this claim is an important competence/performance distinction to which we now turn.

2.4 A competence/performance distinction

The conclusion of the previous subsection was that harmonic grammars have computational power equivalent to that of Turing machines, as assessed by one key standard from theoretical computer science: the capacity for specifying formal languages.

To avoid misunderstanding of this claim, it is crucial to make what is usefully viewed as a competence/performance distinction for ICS—different in important respects from traditional competence/performance distinctions, but sharing enough central properties to justify the name. (See also Box 23:9.)

In this context, **competence** can be understood as an idealization of actual behavior—**performance**—in which we have removed the effects of limitations on computational resources: generally speaking, space, time, and precision. In symbolic computation, the competence idealization amounts essentially to assuming sufficient working memory, sufficient processing time, and complete accuracy of executing basic operations such as storing and retrieving items from particular memory locations, joining substructures to form larger structures, and so forth. In Harmony-maximizing PDP computation, however, the comparable competence idealization is accurate optimization, which requires, primarily, sufficient time.

The competence/performance distinction at issue in ICS turns critically on the difference between an input-output function and an algorithm for computing that function: this difference is explicitly marked on the labels for, on the one hand, $\text{Alg}_{\text{PDP}}(H)$ (14) and, on the other, $\text{Fun}_{\text{PDP}}(H)$ (14), and its special case for higher cognition, $\text{Fun}_{\text{ICS}}(H,\text{HC})$ (19).

A harmonic grammar specifies an input-output *function*, in terms of what is generally known as a constrained optimization formulation: the output is that completion of the input which maximizes (or optimizes) the Harmony function; the output specified by the grammar is in this sense optimal or most well formed.

How is this optimal output to be computed/constructed/found? This is the problem that a parsing *algorithm* must solve. It is not the job of grammars to compute: they merely specify functions, and their job is to abstractly determine, for any input, its correct output/parse/structural description. And this a harmonic grammar does, using a novel means of specification: optimization.

This means of specifying a function is derived from the underlying connectionist processing: $\text{Fun}_{\text{PDP}}(H)$ is a consequence of $\text{Alg}_{\text{PDP}}(H)$, via the Harmony Maximization Theorem (12). Thus, it should be possible to use the algorithms of harmonic networks (11) to compute the functions required by harmonic grammars. And, indeed, it is, although to date experience in doing so is extremely limited (see Chapter 20). But there is a gap between the connectionist algorithms of $\text{Alg}_{\text{PDP}}(H)$ and the HG functions of $\text{Fun}_{\text{PDP}}(H)$ that must now be examined.

Optimization theory distinguishes two kinds of optima: local and global. A **local** optimum is a solution that is better than any of its **neighbors**; this notion is relative to some concept of neighborhood in the space of possible solutions. In the PDP case, a local Harmony maximum is an activation vector **a** with the property that any small change in the activation of any of the units will lower the Harmony of the activity pattern. A **global** optimum is a solution that simply is better than *every* alternative. Thus, a local maximum **a** may not be a global maximum because it may be that a set of large changes to the activations in **a** would yield a higher Harmony pattern.

Computing the global maximum of Harmony functions is computationally intractable, and it is important to realize that neither connectionist networks nor any other known algorithm can exactly solve this problem efficiently, for arbitrary Harmony functions (i.e., arbitrary weight matrices or arbitrary sets of soft constraints in a harmonic grammar). There are two senses, then, in which the Harmony Maximization Theorem (12) holds. The first is that harmonic networks compute *local* Harmony maxima; this is true for a large variety of activation functions, as we will show in Chapter 9. For some special networks, a further result is true: there is a limit, which idealizes away from resource limitations, in which the *global* maximum is computed. For example, the spreading activation algorithm employed in Harmony Theory (Smolensky 1983, 1986) and the Boltzmann machine (Hinton and Sejnowski 1983a, 1986), sometimes called **simulated annealing** (Kirkpatrick and Gelatt 1983), is a probabilistic algorithm with the property that the probability of computing the global maximum approaches 100% as the amount of processing time is allowed to grow without bound (Geman and Geman 1984; see Section 9:4 for discussion).

The Harmony maximum employed in HG is the global maximum; at least as currently formulated, there is no notion of neighboring parses and no meaning therefore to 'local maximum'. The function specified by a harmonic grammar according to $\text{Fun}_{\text{ICS}}(H, \text{HC})$ constitutes a notion of grammatical competence. There is a gap between this and parsing algorithms governed by $\text{Alg}_{\text{PDP}}(H)$, which are potential models for linguistic performance. If rapid computation is required, the algorithms will compute local Harmony maxima rather than global maxima, leading to a kind of deviation from the competence theory that is as yet unexplored. On the other hand, there is an idealization of a perfect grammar-using network that is allowed unbounded time to compute the global maximum; in this limit, the PDP algorithm modeling performance exactly computes the function specifying competence.

A second kind of idealization appeared in the discussion of productivity in Section 5:2. The recursive tensor product representations used in ICS can achieve perfectly unambiguous realization of symbolic structure, but for this to occur, sufficiently large networks must be employed to cope with the size of symbol structures required. In the idealization of infinite productivity—unboundedly large trees being evaluated by recursive functions, unboundedly long sentences in a formal language, unboundedly deep recursion—unboundedly large networks are required. As already explained in Section 5:2.2, however, as in symbolic automata, this idealization is straightforwardly accommodated in ICS: these unboundedly large networks are unproblematically finitely specified.

2.5 An application to natural language syntax/semantics

A harmonic grammar is a set of soft constraints on the well-formedness of linguistic representations: weighted constraints determining which pairs of constituents are present (or absent) in well-formed representations. Such a conception of grammar has the potential to contribute to linguistic theory a formal means for computing well-formedness values from general tendencies rather than strict requirements. As an empirical test of HG, then, we can see whether formalizing tendencies and their interactions via HG soft constraints provides new insights into grammatical phenomena that have proved problematic for strict, hard-constraint formalisms.

We conducted such a test of HG in collaboration with Yoshiro Miyata in the early 1990s. This work is discussed in detail in Chapter 11; the linguistic details of the phenomenon and the relevant literature citations are best postponed until then. Here, we summarize the results at a general level.

In French, as in all languages, there are certain syntactic contexts in which only a subset of verbs can appear. Focusing on the simplest types of verbs—intransitive verbs, which by definition take only one noun phrase argument—we can say that each such syntactic context constitutes a **test** that only some intransitive verbs pass: these are the verbs that can be used in that context without producing ungrammaticality. An example is given in (37) (Legendre 1986).

(37) An unaccusativity test in French: Object raising (OR) with *faire*
  a. Une souris est facile à faire **mourir**.
     'A mouse is easy to make **die**.'
  b. *Une souris est facile à faire **courir**.
     'A mouse is easy to make **run**.'
  c. [singular noun phrase] est facile à faire ________
     '[singular noun phrase] is easy to make ________'
  d. [plural noun phrase] sont faciles à faire ________
     '[plural noun phrase] are easy to make ________'

The verb *mourir* 'die' passes this test (37a), while *courir* 'run' fails it, as indicated by the '*' marking (37b) as ungrammatical. The syntactic context defining this test is shown in (37c), with its plural variant shown in (37d). Depending on which verb is inserted into the slot at the end of the sentence, a semantically appropriate noun phrase argument is inserted at the beginning of the sentence. For reasons that will become clearer in Chapter 11, this sentence construction is called 'object raising with *faire*', which we'll abbreviate 'OR'. The intransitive verbs passing the OR test are called **unaccusative** verbs; they also pass a variety of other tests, defined by other syntactic constructions. These verbs are also characterized by certain semantic properties: change-of-state verbs like *die* are unaccusative, while activity verbs like *run* are not.

If all the statements in the previous paragraph were true, unaccusativity could be nicely described by hard constraints. However, they are only **tendencies**. The verbs passing different tests have a high degree of overlap, but they are not identical. The grammaticality of test sentences is usually determined by the inserted intransitive verb, but the noun phrase inserted into the sentence frame sometimes affects grammaticality too. Unaccusative verbs have a tendency to share certain semantic properties, but there are many exceptions: there is a degree of idiosyncrasy across verbs that semantics cannot eliminate (and that varies across languages). And acceptability judgments for these sentences are quite graded, to boot.

The semantic and syntactic tendencies characterizing the acceptability of test sentences can be formulated as a set of soft constraints in HG. For any given sentence, the grammar assigns a Harmony value: positive values indicate grammaticality, negative values indicate ungrammaticality, and values close to zero indicate a marginal level of grammaticality or ungrammaticality.

Such a grammar can achieve considerable descriptive success, as demonstrated in a series of increasingly comprehensive studies. The first looked at 4 syntactic tests (including OR) involving 143 verbs; the grammar correctly accounted for all but 2 of the corresponding 760 acceptability judgments (Legendre, Miyata, and Smolensky 1990a, b). In an expanded study examining these 143 verbs in 5 tests, the grammar correctly accounted for all but 3 of 885 judgments (Smolensky, Legendre, and Miyata 1992); and in the most comprehensive study, involving 183 intransitive verbs in 11 syntactic tests, it accounted for all but 14 of 3,608 judgments (Legendre, Miyata, and Smolensky 1991; Smolensky, Legendre, and Miyata 1992).

We take these studies to have shown that the insights into the phenomenon of unaccusativity provided by linguistic theory can in fact be taken to define a formal system of knowledge—a grammar—even though, descriptively, these insights appear on the surface to capture "mere tendencies" for certain syntactic and semantic factors to constrain one another. The constraints in these harmonic grammars are all simple, and all consonant with linguistic theory; once a formal means is provided for adjudicating the conflicts between them, they are sufficient to precisely account for a highly complex pattern of acceptability judgments. The means of adjudicating conflicts is encoded in the numerical strengths of the soft constraints.

At present, we see no prospects for predicting or explaining these strengths from more basic principles (but see Burzio 1997). The constraint strengths used in these studies of French unaccusativity were derived by a connectionist error-correcting learning algorithm; the somewhat involved analysis behind this algorithm is taken up in Chapter 11. As with any such parameter-fitting exercise, the significance of a good fit can only be determined by detailed examination of the problem; it must be ensured, for example, that the number of parameters does not exceed the number of independent data points being accounted for. Such analysis must be taken up in the context of a more detailed development of the actual harmonic grammars involved; see Chapter 11.

At a more substantive level, we believe these HG studies advance the theory of unaccusativity by showing how to formally integrate insights developed on both sides of the debate between syntax- and semantics-centered theories of unaccusativity. This is yet another respect in which the ICS research program described in this book contributes to integrating theoretical perspectives that have previously been taken as adversarial (see Chapter 3).

3 Optimization in Grammar II: Optimality Theory

In applying HG to phonology, Prince and Smolensky discovered that in a diverse set of phonological problems, the numerical strengths of soft constraints arrange themselves so that the constraints form **strict domination hierarchies**. In these hierarchies, when the soft constraints are ordered from weakest to strongest, each constraint turns out to be stronger than *all* the weaker constraints *combined*. Thus, any given constraint must be satisfied (if possible), regardless of whether that entails violating any number of weaker constraints—unless satisfying the constraint requires violating still stronger constraints that can otherwise be satisfied. In such situations, all the information carried by the numerical strengths of the soft constraints can be reexpressed nonnumerically as the ranking of the constraints in a domination hierarchy. In this more restricted case, the principle Wf_{ICS}(HC) (15) defining HG can be reformulated in nonnumerical terms.

Furthermore, Prince and Smolensky showed in a wide range of phonological domains how crosslinguistic variation can be explained through reranking of a common—**universal**—set of constraints. This led them to propose Optimality Theory (Prince and Smolensky 1991, 1993/2004), which was informally introduced in Chapter 4. OT will be systematically developed in Chapter 12; for present purposes, we simply reiterate the formulation of the fourth and final fundamental principle of the ICS cognitive architecture, P4: OT, from Chapter 2 (8).

(38) **P_4: OT (Optimality Theory)**

Grammar contains a core consisting of a set of universal violable constraints that apply in parallel to assess the well-formedness of linguistic structures. The conflicts between these constraints are resolved via language-specific strict domination hierarchies.

In Part III, this principle is applied to problems in both phonology and syntax through the perspectives of theoretical linguistics, computational linguistics, psycholinguistics (including processing and acquisition), and neurolinguistics (the neural and genetic encoding of grammatical knowledge). (For summaries, see Section 1:7.2.)

The remaining chapters of Part II provide the formal underpinnings of the four ICS principles P_1–P_4. Principles P_1–P_3 are applied to questions addressing the grammars of both formal and natural languages. Applications of P_4 are taken up in Part III.

References

ROA = Rutgers Optimality Archive, http://roa.rutgers.edu

Ackley, D. H., G. E. Hinton, and T. J. Sejnowski. 1985. A learning algorithm for Boltzmann machines. *Cognitive Science* 9, 147–69.

Blair, A., and J. Pollack. 1997. Analysis of dynamical recognizers. *Neural Computation* 9, 1127–42.

Burzio, L. 1997. Strength in numbers. In *University of Maryland Working Papers in Linguistics 5: Selected phonology papers from the Maryland Mayfest/Hopkins Optimality Theory Workshop 97,* eds. B. Moren and V. Miglio. Department of Linguistics, University of Maryland.

Cleeremans, A., D. Servan-Schreiber, and J. L. McClelland. 1989. Finite state automata and simple recurrent networks. *Neural Computation* 1, 372–81.

Cohen, M. A., and S. Grossberg. 1983. Absolute stability of global pattern formation and parallel memory storage by competitive neural networks. *IEEE Transactions on Systems, Man, and Cybernetics* 13, 815–25.

Feldman, J. A., and D. H. Ballard. 1982. Connectionist models and their properties. *Cognitive Science* 6, 205–54.

Geman, S., and D. Geman. 1984. Stochastic relaxation, Gibbs distributions, and the Bayesian restoration of images. *IEEE Transactions on Pattern Analysis and Machine Intelligence* 6, 721–41.

Golden, R. M. 1986. The "brain-state-in-a-box" neural model is a gradient descent algorithm. *Mathematical Psychology* 30–31, 73–80.

Hinton, G. E. 1981. A parallel computation that assigns canonical object-based frames of reference. *In Proceedings of the International Joint Conference on Artificial Intelligence 7.*

Hinton, G. E., and T. J. Sejnowski. 1983a. Analyzing cooperative computation. In *Proceedings of the Cognitive Science Society 5.*

Hinton, G. E., and T. J. Sejnowski. 1983b. Optimal perceptual inference. In *Proceedings of the IEEE Computer Society Conference on Computer Vision and Pattern Recognition.*

Hinton, G. E., and T. J. Sejnowski. 1986. Learning and relearning in Boltzmann machines. In *Parallel distributed processing: Explorations in the microstructure of cognition.* Vol. 1, *Foundations,* D. E. Rumelhart, J. L. McClelland, and the PDP Research Group. MIT Press.

Hirsch, M. W. 1996. Dynamical systems. In *Mathematical perspectives on neural networks,* eds. P. Smolensky, M. C. Mozer, and D. E. Rumelhart. Erlbaum.

Hopcroft, J. E., and J. D. Ullman. 1979. *Introduction to automata theory, languages, and computation.* Addison-Wesley.

Hopfield, J. J. 1982. Neural networks and physical systems with emergent collective computational abilities. *Proceedings of the National Academy of Sciences USA* 79, 2554–8.

Hopfield, J. J. 1984. Neurons with graded response have collective computational properties like those of two-state neurons. *Proceedings of the National Academy of Sciences USA* 81, 3088–92.

Jordan, M. I. 1986. Attractor dynamics and parallelism in a connectionist sequential machine. In *Proceedings of the Cognitive Science Society 8.*

Kirkpatrick, S., and C. D. Gelatt, Jr. 1983. Optimization by simulated annealing. *Science* 220, 671–80.

Legendre, G. 1986. Object raising in French: A unified account. *Natural Language and Linguistic Theory* 4, 137–84.

Legendre, G., Y. Miyata, and P. Smolensky. 1990a. Can connectionism contribute to syntax? Harmonic Grammar, with an application. In *Proceedings of the Chicago Linguistic Society 26.*

Legendre, G., Y. Miyata, and P. Smolensky. 1990b. Harmonic Grammar—a formal multi-level connectionist theory of linguistic well-formedness: An application. In *Proceedings of the Cognitive Science Society 12.*

Legendre, G., Y. Miyata, and P. Smolensky. 1990c. Harmonic Grammar—a formal multi-level connectionist theory of linguistic well-formedness: Theoretical foundations. In *Proceedings of the Cognitive Science Society 12*.

Legendre, G., Y. Miyata, and P. Smolensky. 1991. Unifying syntactic and semantic approaches to unaccusativity: A connectionist approach. In *Proceedings of the Berkeley Linguistics Society 7*.

Pollack, J. 1995. The induction of dynamical recognizers. In *Mind as motion: Explorations in the dynamics of cognition*, eds. R. F. Port and T. van Gelder. MIT Press.

Prince, A., and P. Smolensky. 1991. Notes on connectionism and Harmony Theory in linguistics. Technical report CU-CS-533-91, Computer Science Department, University of Colorado at Boulder.

Prince, A., and P. Smolensky. 1993/2004. *Optimality Theory: Constraint interaction in generative grammar*. Technical report, Rutgers University and University of Colorado at Boulder, 1993. ROA 537, 2002. Revised version published by Blackwell, 2004.

Rodriguez, P. 2001. Simple recurrent networks learn context-free and context-sensitive languages by counting. *Neural Computation* 13, 2093–118.

Rodriguez, P., J. Wiles, and J. L. Elman. 1999. A recurrent neural network that learns to count. *Connection Science* 11, 5–40.

Rumelhart, D. E., G. E. Hinton, and J. L. McClelland. 1986. A general framework for parallel distributed processing. In *Parallel distributed processing: Explorations in the microstructure of cognition*. Vol. 1, *Foundations*, D. E. Rumelhart, J. L. McClelland, and the PDP Research Group. MIT Press.

Rumelhart, D. E., G. E. Hinton, and R. J. Williams. 1986. Learning internal representations by error propagation. In *Parallel distributed processing: Explorations in the microstructure of cognition*. Vol. 1, *Foundations*, D. E. Rumelhart, J. L. McClelland, and the PDP Research Group. MIT Press.

Rumelhart, D. E., P. Smolensky, J. L. McClelland, and G. E. Hinton. 1986. Schemata and sequential thought processes in parallel distributed processing. In *Parallel distributed processing: Explorations in the microstructure of cognition*. Vol. 2, *Psychological and biological models*, J. L. McClelland, D. E. Rumelhart, and the PDP Research Group. MIT Press.

Shastri, L. 1985. Evidential reasoning in semantic networks: A formal theory and its parallel implementation. Technical report TR 166, Department of Cognitive Science, University of Rochester.

Skarda, C. A., and W. J. Freeman. 1987. How brains make chaos to make sense of the world. *Behavioral and Brain Sciences* 10, 161–95.

Smolensky, P. 1983. Schema selection and stochastic inference in modular environments. In *Proceedings of the National Conference on Artificial Intelligence 3*.

Smolensky, P. 1984. The mathematical role of self-consistency in parallel computation. In *Proceedings of the Cognitive Science Society 6*.

Smolensky, P. 1986. Information processing in dynamical systems: Foundations of Harmony Theory. In *Parallel distributed processing: Explorations in the microstructure of cognition*. Vol. 1, *Foundations*, D. E. Rumelhart, J. L. McClelland, and the PDP Research Group. MIT Press.

Smolensky, P. 1996. Dynamical perspectives on neural networks. In *Mathematical perspectives on neural networks*, eds. P. Smolensky, M. C. Mozer, and D. E. Rumelhart. Erlbaum.

Smolensky, P., G. Legendre, and Y. Miyata. 1992. Principles for an integrated connectionist/symbolic theory of higher cognition. Technical report CU-CS-600-92, Computer Science Department, and 92-8, Institute of Cognitive Science, University of Colorado at Boulder.

Stolcke, A. 1989. Unification as constraint satisfaction in structured connectionist networks. *Neural Computation* 1, 559–67.

7 Symbolic Computation with Activation Patterns

Paul Smolensky and Bruce Tesar

The heart of the integration of symbolic and connectionist computation in the Integrated Connectionist/Symbolic Cognitive Architecture (ICS) is P_1: Rep_{ICS}, a principle asserting that in higher cognitive domains, the mind/brain deploys tensor product representations. Chapters 7 and 8 respectively zoom out from and zoom in on this type of representation.

Chapter 7 shows that tensor product representations form the nucleus of an extended family of realizations of symbolic structure in patterns of activation. This family of generalized tensor product representations includes a wide range of proposals in the literature on connectionist, psychological, and neural modeling; five important examples are analyzed.

Chapter 8 formally defines tensor product representations and demonstrates that they possess a number of general properties making them suitable candidates as connectionist realizations of symbolic mental structures. Computations over tensor product representations are also analyzed.

Thus, Chapter 8 provides the formal foundations of the first two ICS principles, Rep_{ICS}—symbolic representations realized by activation vectors—and $Proc_{ICS}$—symbolic functions computed by weight matrices. Chapter 7 develops a more general formalization of Rep_{ICS}; its role in the big picture is indicated in (11b)–(12a) of the ICS map in Chapter 2.

Section 5 is a slightly modified version of Tesar and Smolensky 1994.

Contents

1 Realizing Symbolic Structure in Activation Vectors

Key to the vertical integration characteristic of the Integrated Connectionist/Symbolic Cognitive Architecture (ICS) (Chapter 3 (1c)) is the claim that symbolic computation can be realized in connectionist networks via patterns of activity. Chapter 5 (50) showed how tensor product representations substantiate that claim, providing a formal means of stating the most basic principle of ICS, Rep_{ICS}, as it pertains to higher cognition:

(1) Rep_{ICS}(HC): Integrated representation in higher cognition

a. In all cognitive domains, when analyzed at a lower level, mental representations are defined by the activation values of connectionist units. When analyzed at a higher level, these representations are distributed patterns of activity—activation vectors. For central aspects of higher cognitive domains, these vectors realize symbolic structures.

b. Such a symbolic structure **s** is defined by a collection of structural roles $\{r_i\}$ each of which may be occupied by a filler $\mathtt{f}_i$; **s** is a set of constituents, each a filler/role binding $\mathtt{f}_i/r_i$.

c. The connectionist realization of **s** is an activation vector

$$\mathbf{s} = \Sigma_i \, \mathbf{f}_i \otimes \mathbf{r}_i$$

that is the sum of vectors realizing the filler/role bindings. In these [**basic**] tensor product representations, the pattern realizing the structure as a whole is the superposition of patterns realizing all its constituents. And the pattern realizing a constituent is the tensor product of a pattern realizing the filler and a pattern realizing the structural role it occupies.

d. In higher cognitive domains such as language and reasoning, mental representations are recursive: the fillers or roles of **s** have themselves the same type of internal structure as **s**. And these structured fillers $\mathtt{f}$ or roles r in turn have the same type of tensor product realization as **s**.

As explained in Section 3:4.2, this is intended to be considered as only one particular formal instantiation among many possibilities worthy of study. It is important for the conceptual connection it provides between symbolic and connectionist computation, and for the precision it offers, enabling formal analysis (e.g., the derivation of Harmonic Grammar, Section 6:2.1). In this chapter, we explore the space of alternative formal instantiations of Rep_{ICS}, by examining other proposals in the literature concerning the realization of symbolic structures in numerical vectors. The somewhat surprising conclusion is that, despite compelling intuitions to the contrary, these alternatives are all closely related to tensor product representations—indeed, they are various special cases of a notion we develop in this chapter: generalized tensor product representations. This extended notion provides considerable insight into the space of possible vectorial representations of symbolic structures, yielding an explicit typology of representations differing along several dimensions.

How would ICS be affected by reformulating Rep_{ICS}, replacing the *basic* tensor product representations of (1) with the *generalized* tensor product representations to be defined below? Rep_{ICS} serves two central purposes in ICS. The first, and more important, is conceptual: it makes formally precise the idea introduced in Chapter 1 that connectionist and symbolic representations are two accounts of a single system, at different levels of analysis. This is crucial to the integrative character of ICS, discussed at length in Chapter 3. This role of Rep_{ICS} would not be affected at all by generalizing its formulation.

The second purpose of Rep_{ICS} was developed in Chapter 6, where it was shown that the particular formal structure of tensor product representations, when combined with the processing principle of Harmony Maximization, logically entails the particular formal structure of Harmonic Grammar (HG: Chapter 6 (15)). Some of the additional formal complexities introduced in generalizing the tensor product—for example, nonlinearity—would invalidate the derivation of HG in Section 6:2.1. It is currently an open question whether more sophisticated mathematical analysis allows a high-level grammar formalism like HG to be derived from these more complex connectionist representations. One possible outcome is that the more complex cases of generalized tensor product representations can be approximated by the simpler case of basic tensor product representations, under certain conditions—as nonlinear systems can often be approximated by linear ones, within a certain range of operation. Thus, extending Rep_{ICS} in the ways to be developed in this chapter may be a step toward going beyond the simplest version of ICS developed in this book, that governed by the linear approximation of Section 5:1.1.

In the terminology developed in Chapter 3, these two uses of tensor product representations constitute principle-centered research. But these representations can be used in model-centered research as well. In this chapter, we will mention some of this research, which provides empirical evidence for the validity of tensor product representations via experimental psychology and neuroscience. Some of this empirical evidence pertains to generalized tensor product representations and may ultimately bear on the question of which dimensions of generalization are psychologically or neurobiologically essential.

2 The Typology

In this chapter, we develop the typology shown in Table 1.[1] To explicate this typology, we must start with a definition of (basic) tensor product representations. A formal definition is given in Chapter 8, but the key ingredients are already implicit in the above statement of Rep_{ICS} (1). The first ingredient is the **filler/role decomposition** (1b): it breaks down symbol structures into a set of **bindings** of structural roles to the constituents that fill them. The second ingredient is the set of particular (activation)

[1] For a related typology, see Plate 1997.

vectors that realize individual roles and fillers. Once these are specified, the tensor product representation is fully determined: fillers are bound to roles via the tensor product, and filler/role bindings—constituents—are combined via superposition (vector addition): (1c).

Table 1. Typology of vectorial symbol structures

Typological Dimensions	Parietal cortex Sec. 3	Propositions Sec. 4	Synchrony Sec. 5	HRR Sec. 6	RAAM Sec. 7
a. Filler/role decomposition					
absolute positional	✓			✓	✓
versus contextual		✓			
versus formal			✓		
b. Realization vectors					
± distributed	+	+	–	+	+
c. Implementation					
± temporal	–	–	+	–	–
d. Binding					
± contracted	–	–	–	+	–
± squashed	–	–	–	–	+

So within the space of these (basic) tensor product representations, one dimension of variation is the filler/role decomposition: this is row *a* of Table 1. The second dimension is the pairing of vectors with fillers and roles: row *b*. Chapter 5 discussed the variation along this dimension between **local** and **distributed** (notated '±distributed' in Table 1): a local vector is one that has only a single nonzero element (all the activation is localized to a single unit). This dimension of variation was central in Chapter 5 but will not figure prominently in this chapter. Variation in filler/role decomposition type will be important, however. Chapter 5 considered primarily decompositions employing **absolute positional roles**, such as 'second position in a string' or 'left child of the tree root'. Here, and in Chapter 8, we will also discuss **contextual roles** like 'just after a vowel' or 'an argument of the verb *nosh*'. Finally, in Section 5.4 we introduce the notion of **formal roles** such as 'in the second binding'—when such a role is bound to both the filler **John** and the filler **agent**, we have a representation of John-as-agent.

In rendering a representation in a model more concrete, further dimensions of **implementation** arise: row *c* of Table 1. One of these, discussed at length in Section 5, concerns whether the elements of the vectors denote the activation of different units at a single time ('–temporal' in Table 1) or the activation of a single unit at different times ('+temporal'). Since it is the numbers themselves that define the representation per se, this distinction is outside the representation proper; rather, it is part of the implementation of the representation.

So far, we have remained within the space of basic tensor product representations. The dimensions of variation discussed above will be illustrated below with several models in the literature. The first, a model of spatial representations in parietal cortex (Pouget and Sejnowski 1997), illustrates a rather straightforward tensor product representation. The second, a model of propositional memory in analogical reasoning (Halford, Wilson, and Phillips 1998), illustrates contextual roles. The third is a scheme for binding roles and fillers via temporally synchronized firing of individual units (Shastri and Ajjanagadde 1993); it illustrates formal roles as well as implementation in temporally extended activation patterns. The corresponding columns in Table 1 characterize these models along the different typological dimensions, with boxes showing the most significant features for our expository purposes.

The first generalization of basic tensor product representations required to accommodate the remaining two examples involves the vectorial operation used to bind fillers to roles: this becomes a new dimension of variation among *generalized* tensor product representations (row *d* of Table 1). So far, the binding operation is the simple tensor product. The generalization involves following the tensor product operation with a subsequent operation: **tensor contraction**, which reduces the number of elements in the tensor. This operation, introduced in Section 6, reduces the size of a tensor (by reducing its rank—"dimension"—by two; that is, eliminating two of its indices or subscripts). This contraction of the tensor makes it possible to design representations in which vectors representing structures with different depths of embedding are the same size.

The other possible new operation, which follows the superposition of multiple bindings, is **squashing**: applying a nonlinear transformation to the sum of binding vectors for a given structure, thus squashing each element of the vector so that it remains between certain absolute minimum and maximum values. It is this operation that introduces nonlinearity into our representations for the first time.

It is appropriate to consider these more complex representations to be generalized tensor product representations because, even with these generalizations, the operation that literally binds fillers to roles is the simple tensor product. This tensor product may then be trimmed by contraction in the creation of a binding vector, but this postprocessing operation applies to the tensor product as a whole, with the filler already bound to its role. And the sum of bindings may be distorted by squashing, but again this postprocessing operation applies after the bindings have already been combined by superposition. So even after these generalizations, the binding per se of fillers to roles is achieved by the tensor product, and the combining per se of multiple bindings is achieved by superposition—exactly as in basic tensor product representations.

Table 1

Generalizing tensor product representations to allow postprocessing by contraction and/or squashing allows us to subsume under a single formalism all the representations discussed in this chapter, seeing each of them in its place in the typology of Table 1. We believe this provides useful insight into the multiple ways connectionist representations relate to one another and to symbolic representations. It also opens up a much wider space of representational possibilities, of which the examples explored in the literature to date are but a small sampling.[2]

3 Parietal Representation of Spatial Location

The first example we consider is a proposal by Alexandre Pouget and Terrence Sejnowski (1997) for the representation in parietal cortex of locations in the visual field to subserve sensorimotor transformations: mappings of visual inputs to motor responses. The representation they propose has a very interesting property: "the position of an object can be represented in multiple reference frames simultaneously, a property consistent with the behavior of hemineglect patients with lesions in the parietal cortex" (p. 222). That is, using a linear transformation implementable in a connectionist linear associator (Section 5:2), their representation can be readily transformed into one with either retinotopic or head-centered receptive fields (see below).

The basic problem here is that the spatial location of an object, relevant for motoric operations like grasping, is not directly accessible from the position of its image on the retina. Many factors are involved in, for example, determining the depth of the object; but even a simple fact—that the eyes can move—already raises interesting questions concerning the representation of spatial location. Is it relative to coordinates fixed on the retina—retinotopic coordinates? Or coordinates fixed relative to the head—head-centered coordinates? Or both, in different cortical regions? Or both, in one and the same cortical representation? This last possibility is what Pouget and Sejnowski propose with respect to parietal cortex.

Suppose a spot of light is presented on a screen. Computing the spot's spatial location requires combining the retinal location of its image with the current position of the eye. We might view the image of the spot at a given retinal position as a **filler** in the scene as a whole, the significance of which depends on the position of the eye, which might be seen as determining the **role** of that retinal position in constructing the scene. The contribution to the scene S made by the spot is the **filler/role binding** $\mathrm{r}_j/\mathrm{e}_k$, where r_j is the retinal position of the spot's image and e_k is the simultaneous eye position. The scene as a whole consists of a *set* of such bindings:

(2) $S = \{\mathrm{r}_{j(1)}/\mathrm{e}_{k(1)}, \mathrm{r}_{j(2)}/\mathrm{e}_{k(2)}, \cdots\}$,

where $\mathrm{r}_{j(1)}$ is the retinal position of the first spot, with simultaneous eye position $\mathrm{e}_{k(1)}$, $\mathrm{r}_{j(2)}$ and $\mathrm{e}_{k(2)}$ are their counterparts for the second spot, and so forth. (For consistency with Pouget and Sejnowski's figures, 'r' denotes the retinal position, even though

[2] There may well be proposals in the literature for vectorial realization of symbolic structure that fall outside the space of possibilities defined by our typology, but we do not know of any at this point.

here it is interpreted as a filler rather than a role.)

Figure 1. Network architecture
(From Pouget and Sejnowski 1997, Fig. 4.)

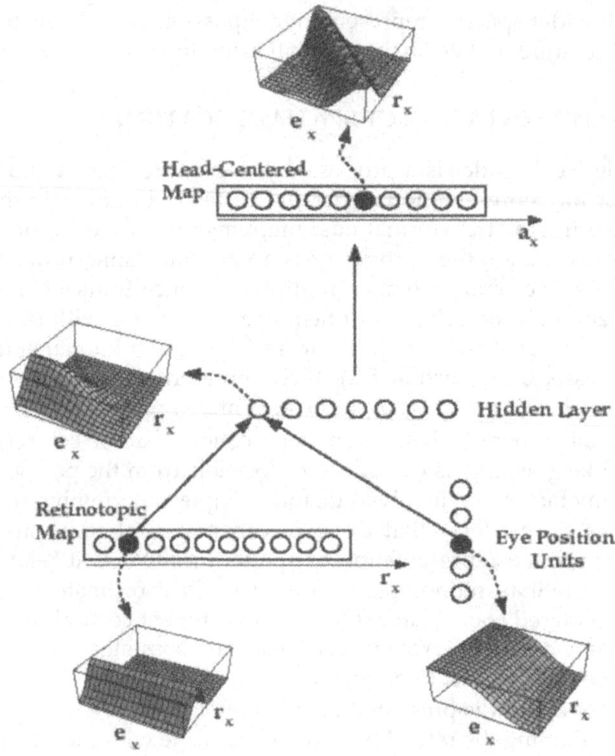

The tensor product representation of *S* would then be[3]

(3) $\mathbf{S} = \Sigma_i \, \mathbf{r}_{j(i)} \otimes \mathbf{e}_{k(i)}$.

Thus, the representation of a single spot (r, e) would be a pattern of activation in which the activity of the unit with indices α, β is

(4) $a_{\alpha,\beta}\,(r, e) = [\mathbf{r}]_\alpha[\mathbf{e}]_\beta$,

where the pattern of activity **r** represents the retinal position r and the pattern **e** represents the eye position e, and, as always, $[\mathbf{r}]_\alpha$ is the αth component of **r**.

[3] Using the *contextual* filler/role decomposition introduced in the next section, this situation can be more naturally interpreted as follows: *S* is a set of *pairs*, $S = \{(e_1, r_1), (e_2, r_2), \cdots\}$; the role filled by retinal position r_i is then the eye position e_i that defines its "context" (in the pair). The resulting tensor product representation would be identical to (3).

The retinal and eye positions r and e are actually two-dimensional; r = (r_x, r_y) and e = (e_x, e_y). But let us focus on just the x dimension, and understand 'r' to denote r_x and 'e' to denote e_x.

The network Pouget and Sejnowski propose is shown in Figure 1. The group of units in the lower left of this figure host a representation of the retinal position of a spot; those in the lower right, the simultaneous position of the eye. These send activation to the **hidden** group, which hosts the representation under study, the one proposed as a model of parietal cortex. From this hidden representation, it is possible to compute the position of the spot in head-centered coordinates, represented in the group of units at the top of the figure. The graphs show the responses of a unit in the corresponding group, responses as the retinal position r and eye position e vary; these response graphs will be discussed shortly.

Figure 2. A combined head- and retina-centered map (From Pouget and Sejnowski 1997, Fig. 5.)

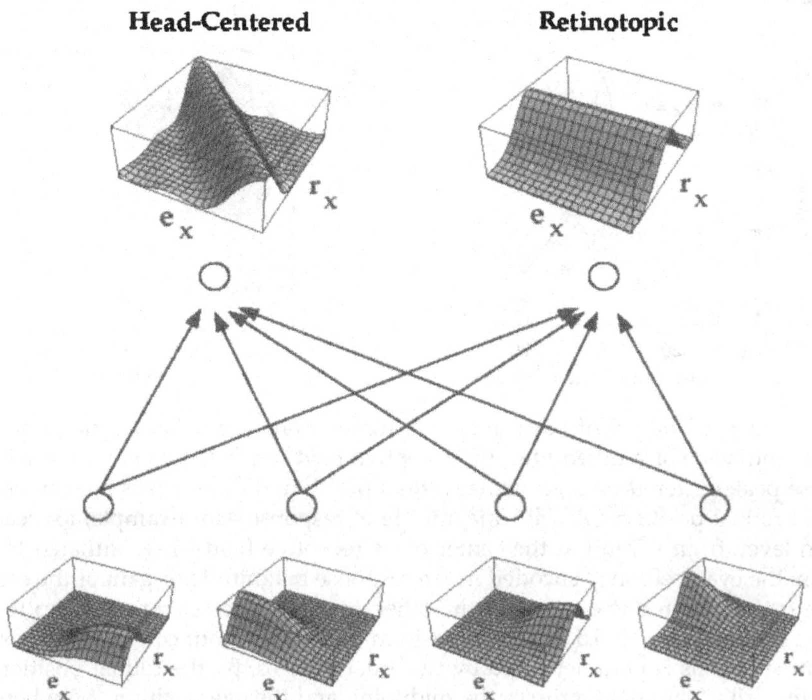

The uppermost portion of the network in Figure 1 is also shown in Figure 2; the units at the bottom of Figure 2 are the hidden units, and the upper-left unit is one from the head-centered representation. The upper-right unit is part of a retinotopic representation. The point is that from the hidden representation it is easy to compute both head- and retina-centered coordinates of a spot, so in this sense the hidden representation is a hybrid of the two.

Turning to the actual representation in parietal cortex, the response of cells to stimuli in different spatial positions—the receptive fields of parietal neurons—is shown in Figure 3. The variation in activity across retinal positions has the same peaked shape for different eye positions, and the peak remains at the same position as the eye position changes from 0 degrees (lower curve in Figure 3A) to 20 degrees (upper curve). But the overall magnitude of response is considerably greater at 20 degrees. Pouget and Sejnowski observe that these receptive fields can be mathematically modeled as a Gaussian function of r times a sigmoid function of e (Figure 4).

Figure 3. Response function of parietal neuron (From Pouget and Sejnowski 1997, Fig. 2.)

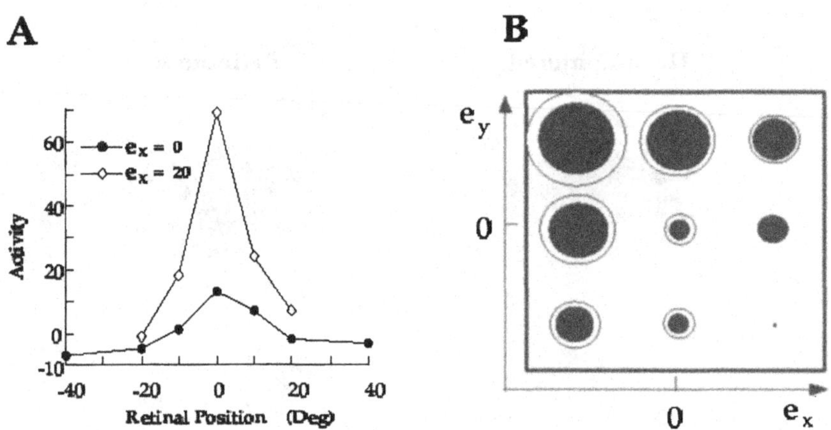

The proposed model of parietal spatial representation can be described qualitatively as follows. For a given unit, the receptive field is a bell-shaped curve with its response peak centered on a particular retinal position; different cells are centered at different retinal positions. A cell's magnitude of response—for example, its peak activation level, from stimuli at the center of its receptive field—is modulated by eye position: the eye position is encoded in the response magnitude or **gain** of the cell. As the eye sweeps from one extreme to the other, this gain grows from zero up to one, crossing the midpoint of 0.5 at an eye position that varies from cell to cell. Thus, the population of cells is parameterized by two quantities (α, β): the retinal position ($\hat{r}_\alpha$) where the cell's 'gain field' crosses the midpoint, and the eye position ($\hat{e}_\beta$) where the cell is most responsive. The two parameters α, β define a two-dimensional space of units we can consider to be laid out in a grid.

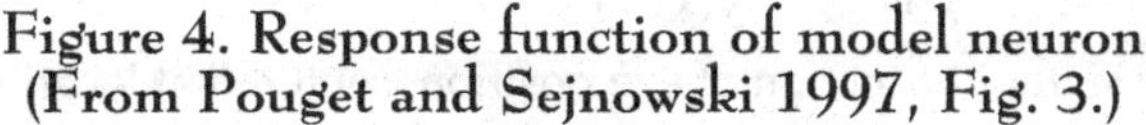
Figure 4. Response function of model neuron (From Pouget and Sejnowski 1997, Fig. 3.)

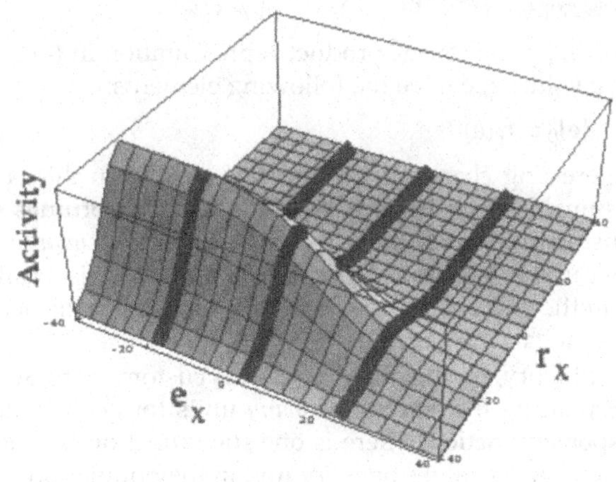

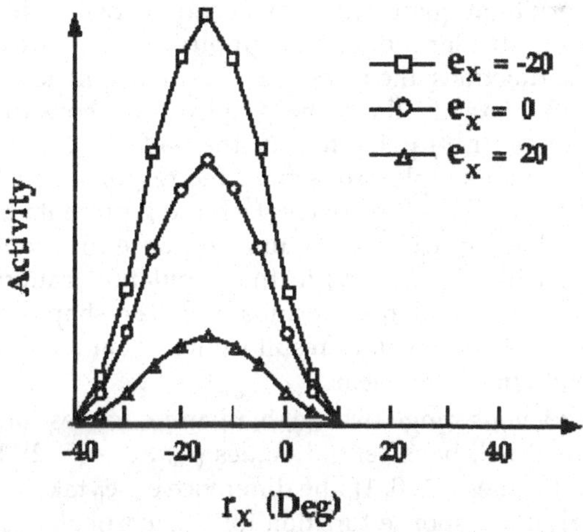

The quantitative analysis proceeds as follows. For a spot (r, e), the activation of the unit α, β is given by

(5) $a_{\alpha,\beta}(r, e) = g_{\alpha}(r) f_{\beta}(e)$,

where g_{α} is a Gaussian function of retinal position, centered at $\hat{r}_{\alpha}$,

(6) $g_\alpha(\mathrm{r}) = e^{-(\mathrm{r}-\hat{\mathrm{r}}_\alpha)^2/2\sigma^2} = g(\mathrm{r}-\hat{\mathrm{r}}_\alpha); \quad g(x) \equiv e^{-x^2/2\sigma^2},$

and f_β is a logistic sigmoid function of eye position, centered at location $\hat{\mathrm{e}}_\beta$:

(7) $f_\beta(\mathrm{e}) = \dfrac{1}{1+e^{-(\mathrm{e}-\hat{\mathrm{e}}_\beta)/T}} = f(\mathrm{e}-\hat{\mathrm{e}}_\beta); \quad f(x) = \dfrac{1}{1+e^{-x/T}}.$

Clearly, (5) is exactly the tensor product representation in (4), where the vectors **r**, **e** representing the values r, e have the following elements:

(8) $[\mathbf{r}]_\alpha \equiv g_\alpha(\mathrm{r}); \quad [\mathbf{e}]_\beta \equiv f_\beta(\mathrm{e}).$

There is an interesting change of perspective lurking in this equivalence (8). In neuroscience (presumably because early neural activity recordings measured only a single cell), it is customary to plot the activity of *one* cell for *many* stimuli (i.e., items represented). Let's call this the **unit response function**; there is a different such function for each unit in the population, and each function gives the activation values of one unit that represent varying stimuli.

In connectionist theory, on the other hand, it is customary to describe distributed representations by plotting the activity of *many* units for *one* stimulus; let's call this the **population response function**. There is one such function for each stimulus; each function gives the activation values of every unit in the population.

In both cases, however, we are ultimately interested in the activity of all units for all stimuli; so these two different ways of cutting the space serve the same end.

In fact, there is a very tight quantitative connection between the two types of response functions in this particular model. The graphs in the figures above (e.g., Figure 4) plot unit response functions: the response of a single unit across the range of (r, e) values represented. But exactly the same graphs also show the population response function for a single (r, e) pair—that is, the pattern of activity representing that pair. This follows from a simple property of the response functions (6) and (7): both f and g are functions of the *difference* between the represented values (r, e) and the α, β unit's central values ($\hat{\mathrm{r}}_\alpha$, $\hat{\mathrm{e}}_\beta$). For the unit response functions graphed in the figures, ($\hat{\mathrm{r}}_\alpha$, $\hat{\mathrm{e}}_\beta$) is fixed, while (r, e) vary; in the population pattern, (r, e) is fixed, while ($\hat{\mathrm{r}}_\alpha$, $\hat{\mathrm{e}}_\beta$) vary across the population of units α, β. The shapes of the graphs are the same because the same f and g values result from $\mathrm{r}-\hat{\mathrm{r}}_\alpha$ and $\mathrm{e}-\hat{\mathrm{e}}_\beta$ in both cases. A simplified example should make this clear.

Suppose first that r values range over {4, 5, 6} and e values range over {2, 4, 6}. One of the α, β units then will have central values ($\hat{\mathrm{r}}_\alpha$, $\hat{\mathrm{e}}_\beta$) = (5, 2). For this unit, the difference $\mathrm{r}-\hat{\mathrm{r}}_\alpha$ takes on values {–1, 0, 1}; the difference $\mathrm{e}-\hat{\mathrm{e}}_\beta$ takes on values {0, 2, 4}. So the two-dimensional unit response function for this particular unit plots the 3×3 array of values boxed in (9).

Now consider the population response function for (r, e) = (5, 6). This plots activity for α, β units where $\hat{\mathrm{r}}_\alpha$ varies over {4, 5, 6} and $\hat{\mathrm{e}}_\beta$ varies over {2, 4, 6}. The values of $\mathrm{r}-\hat{\mathrm{r}}_\alpha$ are then {1, 0, –1}, and the values of $\mathrm{e}-\hat{\mathrm{e}}_\beta$ are {4, 2, 0}. Thus, the activation values plotted in the population response are just the same as the 3×3 array in (9), although the sequence of values on each axis is reversed.

Figure 4 Table 1

(9) Values of unit response function with $(\hat{r}_\alpha, \hat{e}_\beta) = (5, 2)$

		2	4	6	e
r	$r - \hat{r}_\alpha$	0	2	4	$e - \hat{e}_\beta$
4	−1	$g(-1)f(0)$	$g(-1)f(2)$	$g(-1)f(4)$	
5	0	$g(0)f(0)$	$g(0)f(2)$	$g(0)f(4)$	
6	1	$g(1)f(0)$	$g(1)f(2)$	$g(1)f(4)$	

The generality of this result should be clear from the logic of the example. The same result obtains for any range of values of r and e, provided the values of r and e plotted in the unit response function are spaced like the centers of the units in the population. The unit and population response functions have the same shape.[4]

4 CONTEXTUAL ROLES: PROPOSITIONAL MEMORY

In Chapter 5, a letter-string such as **ABC** was decomposed with roles $position_1$, $position_2$, and so on—**absolute positional roles.** A sample binding is $\mathtt{B}/position_2$. Another way of viewing the string is to see **B** as filling a **contextual role**, for example, 'the letter preceding **C**' or r_{-C}. Such roles are discussed at some length in Chapter 8, so our consideration here will be brief.

The tensor product realization of such a contextual binding, $\mathtt{B}/r_{-C}$, is

(10) $\mathbf{B} \otimes \mathbf{r}_{-C}$.

Since the roles are in one-to-one correspondence with the atomic fillers here, one simple choice for $\mathbf{r}_{-C}$ is **C** itself; then the vector realizing $\mathtt{B}/r_{-C}$ is

(11) $\mathbf{B} \otimes \mathbf{C}$.

Thus, the total representation of ABC might be

(12) $\mathbf{ABC} = \mathbf{A} \otimes \mathbf{B} + \mathbf{B} \otimes \mathbf{C}$.

[4] A very different example of a connectionist realization that surprisingly turns out to be precisely a basic tensor product representation is the fractal representation of string sequences developed in Tabor 2000. Arbitrarily long strings from the alphabet {**a**, **b**, **c**} are represented as vectors in a two-dimensional space, as shown in the drawing to the left. Using the filler vectors **a**, **b**, **c**, and absolute-positional roles ($r_i \equiv$ 'ith symbol in the string'), this is exactly the tensor product representation arising from a recursively defined set of role vectors $\mathbf{r}_i = \mathbf{r}_{i-1} \otimes \mathbf{r}_1$ where the basic role vector $\mathbf{r}_1$ is just the *one-dimensional* vector (½). As in all the examples discussed in this chapter, an advantage to analyzing this as a tensor product representation is that it is then immediately clear how to make otherwise nonobvious extensions of the scheme to different dimensionality and to general distributed representations.

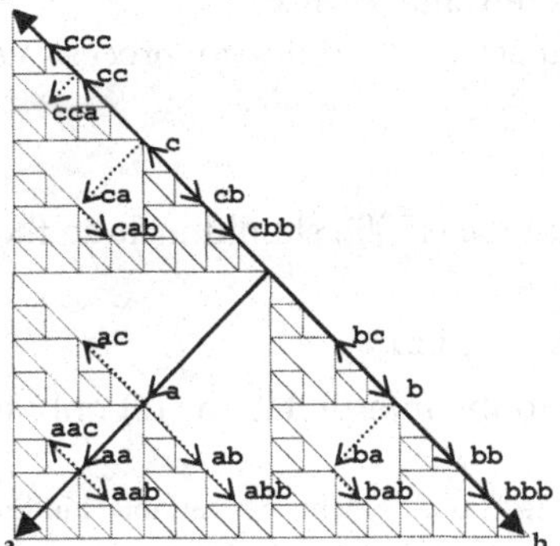

Contextual roles can consider a larger context than just a single neighbor. We might analyze **B** in **ABC** as filling the contextual role 'following **A** and preceding **C**', r_{A-C}. The above analysis can be extended to this case (see Chapter 8), resulting in realizing the role r_{A-C} as the vector $\mathbf{A} \otimes \mathbf{C}$; the representation of the filler $\mathbf{B}/r_{A-C}$ is

(13) $\mathbf{B} \otimes (\mathbf{A} \otimes \mathbf{C})$.

An equivalent representation that is more mnemonic exchanges the order of **B** and **A** (this rearranges the components of the tensors, but results in an equivalent representational system); then the vector realizing **ABC** is just

(14) $\mathbf{ABC} = \mathbf{A} \otimes \mathbf{B} \otimes \mathbf{C}$.

Such contextual role representations have been used in various models of how humans process propositional information (e.g., Wiles et al. 1992; Halford, Wilson, and McDonald 1995). Halford, Wilson, and Phillips (1998) use these representations as the foundation of their general theory of capacity limits for cognitive processing. On their theory, cognitive processes crucially involve **relations**; such a relation might be denoted symbolically as, say, `R(A,B,C)`, where `R` is a (third-order) relation and `A`, `B`, and `C` are the (three) arguments standing in this relation.[5] The vector realizing `R(A,B,C)` in working memory is then just the fourth-rank tensor

$$\mathbf{R}(\mathbf{A}, \mathbf{B}, \mathbf{C}) = \mathbf{R} \otimes \mathbf{A} \otimes \mathbf{B} \otimes \mathbf{C},$$

where **R**, **A**, **B**, **C** are the four activation vectors respectively realizing `R, A, B, C`. As relations become of higher order, the complexity of the network needed to realize them grows rapidly, in terms of both the number of units required and the intricacy of connection structure required to access the various dimensions. Thus, the highest order of the relations that can be represented and processed is a plausible metric of the processing capacity of such a system. Halford, Wilson, and Phillips (1998) argue that this metric of cognitive capacity sheds light on empirical data of several types: data from comparative psychology regarding the relative cognitive capacity of primate species; data from developmental psychology concerning the maturation of human children's cognitive capacity; data from cognitive psychology concerning adults' limits on processing highly complex information. (The tensor product representations involved are conjectured to reside in prefrontal cortex.)

As one example, consider the limited capacity of adults to process center-embedded sentences. In processing (15),

(15) *The boy the girl the man saw met slept.*

the result, according to Halford, Wilson, and Phillips (1998), should include the relations – or propositions – in (16).

(16) `slept(boy); met(girl, boy); saw(man, girl)`

The dependencies in the sentence (15) can lead to the interpretation (16) only by the

[5] Concerning relational processing and learning using temporal synchrony variable binding, see Hummel and Holyoak 2003 and Section 5.

satisfaction of constraints that interrelate all five arguments (one for **slept**, two each for **met**, **saw**; Halford, Wilson, and Phillips 1998, 830); this simultaneous-constraint-satisfaction problem requires an overall fifth-order representation, which is claimed to be "beyond the capacity of most adults" (p. 823). When participants judged the difficulty of a range of sentences (Andrews and Halford 1994), their ratings "strongly reflect[ed] the number of bindings that had to be processed in parallel" (Halford, Wilson, and Phillips 1998, 823; see also Phillips, Kamewari, and Hiraki 2003).[6] For other related applications of tensor product representations, see Wiles et al. 1992; Phillips 1994; Phillips, Halford, and Wilson 1995; Wilson and Halford 1998; Wilson, Marcus, and Halford 2001.

5 Patterns in Space-Time: Synchronous-Firing Variable Binding

Synchronous firing has been shown to be a rather robust property of certain types of model neural systems (e.g., Börgers and Kopell 2003; Hansel and Mato 2003). Such synchrony has been proposed as a way of solving the variable binding problem in neural networks (Gray et al. 1989; Eckhorn et al. 1990; Maass and Bishop 1999). Firing synchrony appears to be unrelated to earlier methods of variable binding, nearly all of which fall in the general category of tensor product representations, where vectors representing variables and values are bound together with the tensor product. In this section, we argue that, despite appearances, firing synchrony is also a case of tensor product representation. This analysis exposes two logically unrelated components of the synchronous firing idea. The most obvious is the idea of using time as a resource: spatiotemporal patterns of activation are used. This, we argue, is a purely implementational issue that does not bear on the complexity issues of variable binding. In contrast, the second idea does bear on genuinely representational issues, and is the source of most of the formal properties claimed for the synchrony scheme. Rather than being *explicitly* bound, a semantic role like **giver** is *implicitly* bound to a semantic filler like **John**—by explicitly binding each to a common **formal role**, via the tensor product. The analysis situates synchronous firing in a typology of alternative variable binding schemes and immediately yields novel, nonobvious extensions from local to distributed representations.

5.1 The variable binding problem reviewed

The variable binding problem is a classic challenge for connectionist networks processing structured data. One aspect of this problem is the binding of fillers to semantic roles, such as those distinguishing the arguments of a predicate. For example, the predicate **give(*x*, *y*, *z*)**—'***x*** gives ***z*** to ***y***'—has three semantic roles: **giver**, **recipient**, and **give-object**. (Here and throughout, we use the notation and terminology of Shastri and Ajjanagadde 1993.) A proposition such as **give(John, Mary,**

[6] The metric of sentence-processing difficulty developed in Gibson 1998, 2000 combines the number and the duration of unbound arguments; this metric may also be amenable to analysis as the complexity of the networks necessary to perform tensor product bindings.

book) may be understood as having three variable bindings: **giver = John**, **recipient = Mary**, and **give-object = book**.

5.2 Binding by synchronized firing

The new solution to the variable binding problem is inspired by phase synchronization of neurons, a biological mechanism of feature segmentation and linking suggested some time ago (von der Malsburg and Schneider 1986). Much of the motivating biological data and modeling has focused on perceptual modalities, especially vision (Gray et al. 1989; Eckhorn et al. 1990; Sejnowski 1999). Neurons functioning as feature detectors fire synchronously (or 'in phase') with other neurons responding to other features of the same entity, and out of phase with neurons responding to features of other entities.

Shastri and Ajjanagadde (1993) have proposed phase synchronization as a connectionist solution to the general dynamic variable binding problem, as have Hummel and Biederman (1992) (see also Hummel and Holyoak 2003 and references cited therein). These authors present their binding representation scheme as a more biologically plausible alternative to other kinds of connectionist variable binding schemes.

The representation system proposed by Shastri and Ajjanagadde (1993) uses single binary-valued nodes to represent roles and fillers. For the proposition **give(John, Mary, book)**, separate, single nodes represent each of **giver**, **recipient**, **give-object**, **John**, **Mary**, and **book** (see Figure 5).

Time is thought of as divided into cycles, each cycle having duration P (the period of the nodes). An active node fires once per cycle (inactive nodes don't fire at all). Two nodes are said to be **bound** together if they are both active, and their firings are synchronized; that is, they fire at the same time during each cycle.

Because each firing unit has a fixed pulse width W during which it is on, the number of independent sets of synchronized firings that can be represented within a cycle is P/W, which we will call N. A cycle may thus be viewed as a set of N **binding slots**, with each slot permitting the representation of the simultaneous binding of a set of nodes. An active node occupies exactly one of the binding slots by firing during the part of the cycle corresponding to that slot.

Thus, in the **give** example illustrated in Figure 5, the first slot is occupied by the **give-obj/book** binding, the second slot by **giver/John**, and so on. We will call the first slot the first **formal role**; this formal role is occupied by both **give-obj**, the **semantic role**, and by **book**, the **semantic filler**. These two elements occupying the first formal role constitute the **formal filler** of that role. The second formal role is occupied by the formal filler {**giver**, **John**}; one of these is a semantic role, the other a semantic filler. The crux of our analysis is displayed in Table 2.

Figure 5. Temporal synchrony variable binding

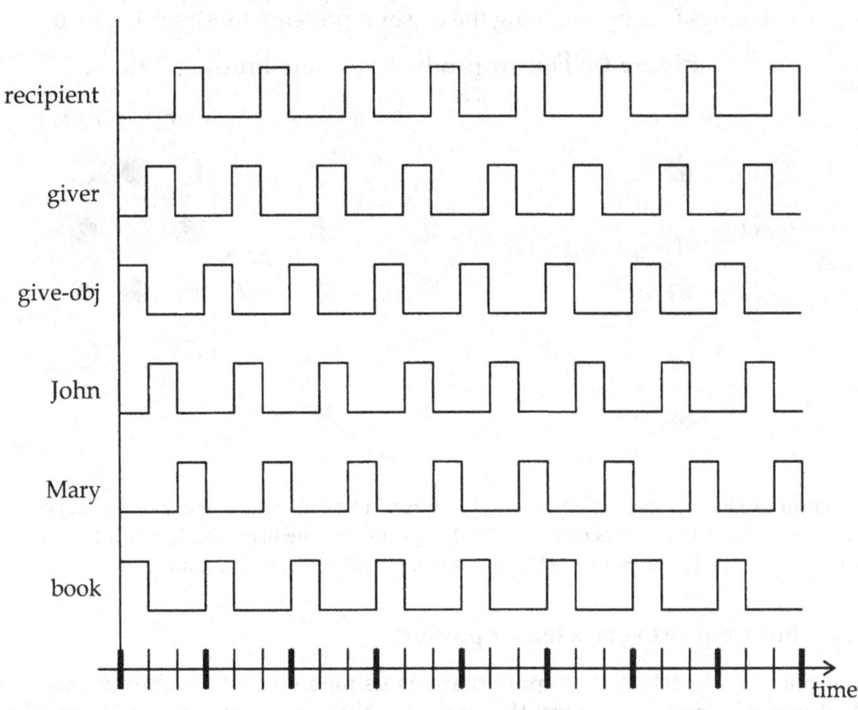

Temporal synchrony representation of **give(John, Mary, book)**, with $N = 3$ binding slots per cycle (after Shastri and Ajjanagadde 1993). Each label on the vertical axis denotes a single unit.

Table 2. Key to the analysis

formal role = 1 or 2 or ... or N *is occupied by*	e.g.: formal role = 1 *is occupied by*
formal filler = {a semantic role, its semantic filler }	formal filler = {**give-obj, book**}

5.3 Tensor product representations

On the face of it, phase synchrony binding seems a completely novel method of solving the variable binding problem, totally unrelated to other techniques. One of these techniques, of course, is tensor product representation. A tensor product representation binds a formal filler to a formal role by taking the tensor product of the tensor representing the filler and the tensor representing the role. Multiple bindings may be combined into one tensor representation by superimposing the representations of the individual bindings (i.e., by summing the tensor representations); see Figure 6.

Figure 6. Tensor product variable binding

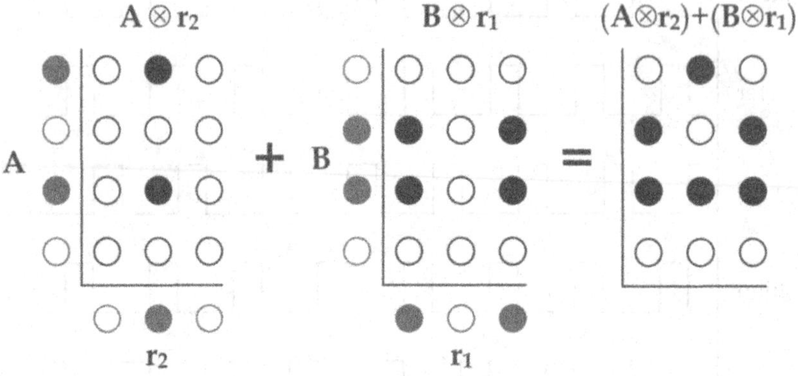

A tensor product representation of BA. The formal roles are r_1, r_2—first and second position—represented by the vectors $\mathbf{r}_1 = (1\ 0\ 1)$, $\mathbf{r}_2 = (0\ 1\ 0)$; the fillers are $\mathbf{A} = (1\ 0\ 1\ 0)$, $\mathbf{B} = (0\ 1\ 1\ 0)$. The representation of BA is $\mathbf{BA} = \mathbf{A} \otimes \mathbf{r}_2 + \mathbf{B} \otimes \mathbf{r}_1$, a rank-2 tensor.

5.4 Synchronized firing as a tensor product

Figures 5 and 6, depicting the representations using temporal synchrony and tensor product variable binding, suggest that the two schemes are entirely different. This is an illusion, however; dissolving this illusion is now our primary goal.

Figure 7A illustrates our analysis of temporal synchrony binding as a kind of tensor product representation. For each real unit—for example, **John**—in the temporal synchrony scheme, there is now an entire *row* of **virtual units**, each showing the activity of **John** during one time slot during one time cycle. We have simply replaced a bumpy activation trace with a row of virtual units showing the same activation values. Figure 7A is a **space-time diagram** of an activity pattern: the vertical axis is space, the horizontal axis time. A row of virtual units in Figure 7 shows the activity history over time of a single real unit in Figure 5; a column of units in Figure 7 shows the activity pattern over the whole Figure 5 network at a single moment of time.

Figure 7B shows one of the bindings in the full proposition **give(John, Mary, book)** shown in Figure 7A. This binding, **book/give-obj**, is the tensor product of the formal filler vector $\mathbf{f}_1$ shown along the right edge and the formal role vector $\mathbf{r}_1$ shown along the bottom. The formal role vector $\mathbf{r}_1$ has activation value 1 during the first slot of each time cycle. The formal filler vector $\mathbf{f}_1$ has activation value 1 in the locations corresponding to the units for **give-obj** and **book**; the subtlety is that the *formal* filler includes both the *semantic* filler (**book**) and the *semantic role* (**give-obj**). The *formal* role has no relation to the *semantic* role, which is part of the formal filler. Rather than using the tensor product to directly bind the semantic role and the semantic filler, these are implicitly bound together in virtue of both being explicitly bound (via the tensor product) to a common formal role, that is, time slot. In terms of equations: rather than $\mathbf{book} \otimes \mathbf{give\text{-}obj}$, we have $[\mathbf{book} + \mathbf{give\text{-}obj}] \otimes \mathbf{r}_1 = \mathbf{book} \otimes \mathbf{r}_1 + \mathbf{give\text{-}obj} \otimes \mathbf{r}_1$. The first alternative ($\mathbf{book} \otimes \mathbf{give\text{-}obj}$) instantiates the general tensor product binding scheme $\mathbf{formal\text{-}filler} \otimes \mathbf{formal\text{-}role}$ by setting the formal role = semantic role and the formal filler = semantic filler; this method, which we will dub the **formal = semantic approach,** is one way to use the tensor product technique to represent a proposition. Another way, illustrated in Figure 7, is to set the formal filler to be the superposition of a semantic role and its corresponding semantic filler, and set the formal role to be an arbitrary pattern, independent of the other formal roles used in the other bindings. We will call this the **formal ≠ semantic approach.**

Figure 7. Temporal synchrony as a tensor product

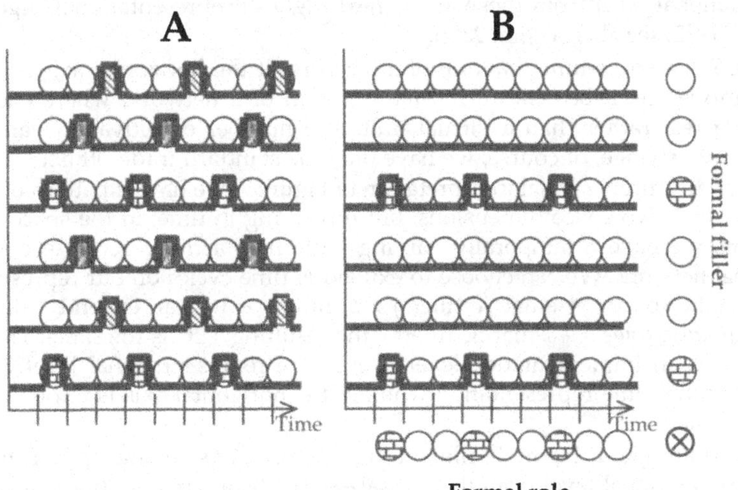

A: Temporal synchrony binding as a spatiotemporal tensor product representation. **B:** One of the three bindings that are superimposed in Panel A, **book/give-obj**, the tensor product of the indicated formal filler vector with the formal role vector.

Figure 7B shows only one of the three bindings present in Figure 7A; the other two are analogous. Just as prescribed by the general tensor product scheme, these three bindings are combined by superposition (i.e., summation); this yields exactly Figure 7A. In Figure 7A, we have distinguished the three bindings by using different shading patterns for their active units; in all cases, regardless of pattern, the shaded units have activation 1.

The real resource measure of a representation, we claim, is the number of activation values it requires; we call this **tensor element complexity** (TEC). The TECs of the formal = semantic and formal ≠ semantic representations differ. For the formal = semantic approach, the TEC is (#semantic roles)(#semantic fillers); for the other, it is N(#semantic roles + #semantic fillers). (Recall that N is the number of time slots in each cycle. We count only the activation values in a single cycle, since multiple cycles contain no more information.)

As Shastri and Ajjanagadde (1993) point out, temporal synchrony allows **`book`** to be bound to both **`give-obj`** and, say, **`own-obj`** in a single time slot; the tensor product analysis of this is simply $\mathbf{book} \otimes \mathbf{r}_1 + \mathbf{give\text{-}obj} \otimes \mathbf{r}_1 + \mathbf{own\text{-}obj} \otimes \mathbf{r}_1$.

5.5 A two-way formal/implementational representation typology

Viewing the synchronized firing model as a kind of tensor product has a number of advantages. Crucially, it allows us to clearly separate issues lying at Marr's lowest, implementational level from those at the next highest, representational/algorithmic level (Marr 1982; see also Section 23:2).

Figure 7 is a space-time diagram of a network. If the horizontal axis is changed from time to space, it becomes a normal diagram of a network, where each circle represents a real rather than a virtual unit. The number of activation values—the TEC—does not change, of course; we have only the standard trade-off between space and time. In the purely spatial interpretation of Figure 7, we have a pattern of activity distributed over two space dimensions, but unvarying in time; in the space-time interpretation, we have a temporally varying pattern of activity across a one-space-dimensional network. We can choose to expend N time cycles on our representation, and (#semantic roles + #semantic fillers) real units, or we can expend 1 time cycle and N(#semantic roles + #semantic fillers): the resulting TEC is the same. The choice here is clearly an implementation-level one: at the representational level, Figure 7 characterizes the same representation whether the horizontal axis is implemented in space or in time.

On the other hand, Figure 7, illustrating the formal ≠ semantic approach, differs at the representational level from the formal = semantic alternative (they have different TECs, for example). Thus, the temporal synchrony proposal combines two separate ideas residing at two different levels; these are shown along the two axes of the two-by-two minitypology of representations shown in Table 3 (in which 'f-' and 's-' abbreviate 'formal' and 'semantic', respectively). The TEC depends on the representational but not the implementational axis.

A larger and somewhat more general typology could be generated by considering additional representational and implementational issues, including those listed in Table 4. (The dimensions of typological variation considered here are, however, a subset of those included in the overarching typology of Table 1.)

Figure 7 *Table 2*

Table 3. A typology of representations

Typology: Complexity — *Representational axis*

Spatial semantic roles
time: 1
space: (#s-roles)(#s-fillers)
	Temporal semantic roles
	time: #s-roles
	space: #s-fillers
		formal = semantic
		#f-fillers = #s-fillers
		#f-roles = #s-roles
		TEC = (#s-roles)(#s-fillers)

Spatial "synchrony"
time: 1
space: N(#s-fillers + #s-roles)
	Temporal synchrony
	time: N
	space: #s-fillers + #s-roles
		formal ≠ semantic
		#f-fillers = #s-fillers + #s-roles
		#f-roles= N
		TEC = N(#s-fillers + #s-roles)

Spatial formal roles	**Temporal formal roles**	TEC = time-complexity × space-complexity

Implementational axis

Table 4. Representation- versus implementation-level issues

Representation-level issues
Distinction of formal and semantic roles and fillers
Local versus distributed representations
Dimensionality of the role and filler spaces (both semantic and formal)
Continuous versus discrete dimensional indexing
Range of tensor component values used (e.g., real, binary)
Separate versus overlapping subspaces for semantic roles and semantic fillers
Implementation-level issues
Complexity in space (number of neural units)
Complexity in time (intrinsic to neural units)
Complexity of units' activation (real versus binary, complex, 'label-passing')

5.6 Conclusion

The present analysis shows that temporal synchrony is not a new method of variable binding per se. Rather, it uses our familiar general method of variable binding, the tensor product. The temporal synchrony approach consists rather in two logically unrelated ideas at two different levels. The first is the implementation-level idea of using time as a representational dimension: in addition to using space as a resource for holding the activation values of a connectionist representation, we can also use time as such a resource. This is potentially quite useful for designing efficient artificial or biologically faithful networks.

The second, higher-level idea embodied in the temporal synchrony scheme is one that can barely be stated without the conceptual structure provided by tensor product representations. It is that a semantic filler/role pair like **`give-obj/book`** can be *implicitly* bound together by *explicitly* binding each of **`give-obj`** and **`book`** to a common formal role (using the tensor product). The tensor product analysis of temporal synchrony also offers a number of other contributions; for example, it makes the seemingly impossible generalization of the synchrony technique to distributed representations and overlapping firing patterns completely straightforward, and it allows direct formal analysis of inference over these representations, exploiting tensor calculus.

6 CONTRACTION: HOLOGRAPHIC REDUCED REPRESENTATIONS

All the representations discussed until now have been basic tensor product representations, conforming to the simple definition introduced in (1) and elaborated in Chapter 8. These representations share the property that as structures get more deeply embedded, the number of elements in the representing vectors grows rapidly. For example, the recursive representation of binary trees developed in Section 5:1.3 requires a number of units that grows exponentially in the depth of the trees represented. This is inevitable for *exact, general-purpose* representations: the number of trees that must be distinguished grows exponentially in tree depth, and these must be linearly independent if they are to enable arbitrary mappings via the usual connectionist operation of multiplication by a weight matrix, followed, perhaps, by a nonlinear squashing operation (the quasi-linear networks of Chapter 9).[7]

6.1 Tensor contraction

Inexact or special-purpose representations need not require as many units, however. One could simply discard a number of units in the tensor product representation: this was in fact done in the seminal model of the acquisition of the English past tense inflection by Rumelhart and McClelland (1986). This is discussed in Section 8:2.3.2.4.

[7] More precisely, suppose the vector realizing one structure S is not linearly independent of the vectors realizing a set of other structures $\{S_i\}$. Then (by definition) the realization of S is identical to a weighted mixture of the other structures: $\mathbf{S} = \Sigma_i c_i \mathbf{S}_i$. Then the weights processing these representations will treat S exactly as a weighted combination of their treatment of the S_i – once it is determined how these weights process the S_i, it is ipso facto determined how they process S. This representation is not general purpose in that the functions computed cannot treat S independently of the S_i. But for specific functions, it could be that S can in fact be treated identically to a mixture of the S_i– this could be the correct way of generalizing to S the knowledge the network has encoded for the S_i. For example, consider a completely compositional function $F(x, y) = (f(x), g(y))$. If (x, y) is represented by the sum of the representations of $(x, 0)$ and of $(0, y)$ – and thus is not linearly independent of them – $F \equiv F_1 + F_2$ can correctly generalize to (x, y) from the sub-functions $F_1(x, z) \equiv (f(x), 0)$ and $F_2(w, y) \equiv (0, g(y))$. In the special cases when such compositionality or modularity exists, special-purpose representations exploiting this modularity can escape the requirement of linear independence. If n values of x are represented by linearly independent patterns over n units, and m values of y similarly over m units, the combined network of $n + m$ units suffices for representing the $n \times m$ possible structures (x, y) – but only for the purposes of computing purely compositional functions such as F. Thus, compositional structure of cognitive functions enables a huge gain in representational efficiency.

Of concern now, however, is a more principled way of reducing the size of a tensor, an operation provided by tensor calculus: **contraction**. Recall that the individual numbers constituting a tensor are labeled by a set of *indices* (subscripts); the number of such indices is the *rank* ("dimensionality") of the tensor (Box 5:1). The contraction operation reduces the rank of a tensor by two, by selecting two indices of the tensor and "summing along the diagonal" defined by these two indices: the elements of the tensor with equal values of these two indices are added together, and all elements with unequal values of these two indices are ignored. In (17), this is illustrated with the contraction of a rank-3 tensor T to a rank-1 tensor S, written in several useful ways:

(17) $S = \mathbb{C}_{23}[T]$; $S_\alpha \equiv \Sigma_\beta T_{\alpha\beta\beta} = \Sigma_{\beta\lambda}\, \delta_{\beta\lambda} T_{\alpha\beta\lambda}$.

We will use '$\mathbb{C}$' to denote the contraction operator generally; the subscripts, when explicitly specified, identify which two indices are the target of contraction. In (17), it is the second and third indices of T we contract over. The first expression, $\Sigma_\beta T_{\alpha\beta\beta}$, explicitly shows we are setting these two indices to equal values—β—and summing. For a given value of α—say, 2—the elements $\{T_{2\beta\lambda}\}$ can be displayed like an ordinary two-index matrix; summing the diagonal elements of this matrix gives the αth element of the contraction S: S_2. (In matrix algebra, this is called the **trace** of the matrix.)

The final expression in (17), $\Sigma_{\beta\lambda}\, \delta_{\beta\lambda} T_{\alpha\beta\lambda}$, will be convenient below. For each element $T_{\alpha\beta\lambda}$ of T, we multiply by $\delta_{\beta\lambda}$, which is the **Kronecker $\boldsymbol{\delta}$** defined so that $\delta_{\beta\lambda} = 1$ if $\beta = \lambda$, and 0 otherwise. This wipes out all elements of T with unequal values of β and λ, while leaving unchanged the elements of T with equal values of β and λ. This enables us to sum over all *pairs* β and λ: the result will simply be S_α.

As an example of the use of tensor contraction, let us note its relation to matrix-vector multiplication. If $\mathbb{M}$ is a matrix and **v** a vector, their matrix-vector product is the vector

(18) $\mathbf{u} = \mathbb{M} \cdot \mathbf{v}$; $u_\alpha = \Sigma_\beta M_{\alpha\beta} v_\beta = \Sigma_{\beta\lambda}\, \delta_{\beta\lambda} M_{\alpha\beta} v_\lambda$.

Now $M_{\alpha\beta} v_\lambda$ is the $\alpha\beta\lambda$ element of the tensor product of $\mathbb{M}$ and **v**:

(19) $[\mathbb{M} \otimes \mathbf{v}]_{\alpha\beta\lambda} = M_{\alpha\beta} v_\lambda$.

Thus, comparing (18) with (17), we see that **u** is in fact the contraction (over the last two indices) of the tensor $\mathbb{M} \otimes \mathbf{v}$:

(20) $\mathbb{M} \cdot \mathbf{v} = \mathbb{C}_{23}[\mathbb{M} \otimes \mathbf{v}]$.

A second useful example of tensor contraction concerns the inner (or dot) product of two vectors. This is defined as

(21) $\mathbf{u} \cdot \mathbf{v} \equiv \Sigma_\beta\, u_\beta v_\beta$.

This is often used as a measure of the **similarity** of two vectors (see Box 5:1). Using the method of introducing δ, we have

(22) $\mathbf{u} \cdot \mathbf{v} \equiv \Sigma_\beta u_\beta v_\beta = \Sigma_{\beta\lambda}\, \delta_{\beta\lambda} u_\beta v_\lambda$.

But $u_\beta v_\lambda$ is just the $\beta\lambda$-element of the tensor product $\mathbf{u} \otimes \mathbf{v}$, so

(23) $\mathbf{u} \cdot \mathbf{v} = \Sigma_{\beta\lambda}\, \delta_{\beta\lambda} u_\beta v_\lambda = \Sigma_{\beta\lambda}\, \delta_{\beta\lambda}[\mathbf{u} \otimes \mathbf{v}]_{\beta\lambda} = \mathbb{C}[\mathbf{u} \otimes \mathbf{v}]$.

That is, the inner product of **u** and **v** is simply the contraction of their outer (tensor) product (over its only two indices).

It is worth noting that the operation of tensor contraction is **linear**—it preserves weighted summation. That is, suppose a tensor T is the weighted sum of two other tensors T′ and T″, with weights w' and w'':

(24) $T = w'\, T' + w''\, T''$.

For concreteness, suppose T is a rank-3 tensor, as in (17). Then (24) means that for all index values for α, β, and λ,

(25) $T_{\alpha\beta\lambda} = w'\, T'_{\alpha\beta\lambda} + w''\, T''_{\alpha\beta\lambda}$.

Thus, the contraction of T over its last two indices, S = $\mathbb{C}$[T], is, by (17),

(26) $$\begin{aligned} S_\alpha \equiv \Sigma_\beta\, T_{\alpha\beta\beta} &= \Sigma_\beta\, [w'\, T'_{\alpha\beta\beta} + w''\, T''_{\alpha\beta\beta}] \\ &= w'\, \Sigma_\beta\, T'_{\alpha\beta\beta} + w''\, \Sigma_\beta\, T''_{\alpha\beta\beta} \\ &= w'\, S'_\alpha + w''\, S''_\alpha, \end{aligned}$$

where S′ and S″ are the contractions of T′ and T″ over their last two indices. In other words:

(27) Linearity property of tensor contraction

$$T = w'\, T' + w''\, T'' \;\Rightarrow\; \mathbb{C}[T] = w'\, \mathbb{C}[T'] + w''\, \mathbb{C}[T'']$$

This expression holds generally, where T is a tensor of any rank, and $\mathbb{C}$ a contraction over any pair of indices (the same indices in each of its occurrences).

As we now see, the notion of tensor contraction can be used to relate tensor product representations to two interesting proposals in the literature for representing structure; we take up the first here, and the second in Section 7.

6.2 Holographic Reduced Representations

In an important series of papers, Tony Plate (Plate 1991a, b, 1993, 1994a, b, 1995, 1997, 1998a, b, 2000, 2003) developed the notion of **Holographic Reduced Representation**, or **HRR**. The key element is a proposal to achieve filler/role binding through the vector operation of **circular convolution**. This proposal derives from earlier work using the convolution operation, and its close relative, the correlation operation, in vector-based models of associative memory; since these operations are at the heart of optical holography, some of these models were dubbed 'holographic' (e.g., Willshaw 1981).

6.2.1 Circular convolution

Circular convolution is illustrated in (28) for two 3-element vectors, **x** and **y**.

(28) Circular convolution: $\mathbf{z} = \mathbf{x} \circledast \mathbf{y}$

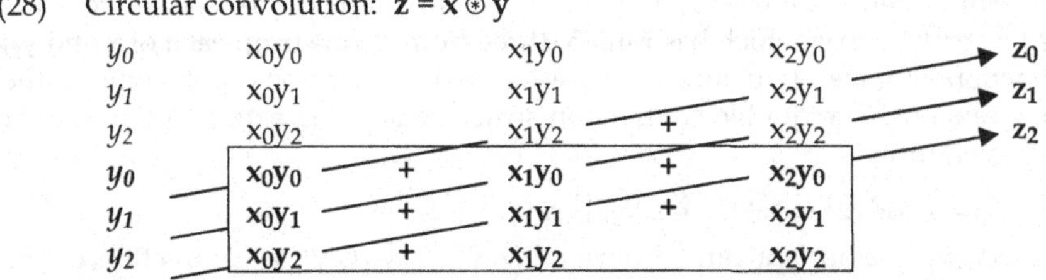

The box encloses the ordinary tensor product $\mathbf{y} \otimes \mathbf{x}$; for reasons soon to be apparent, it is convenient here to take 0 rather than 1 as the lowest index value. If we imagine the vertical axis to be closed into a circle, we would have $y_0\, y_1\, y_2\, y_0\, y_1\, y_2\, y_0 \cdots$; this is shown in (28) by displaying $\mathbf{y}$ a second time, in lighter type. Adding three elements from the tensor product along the indicated diagonals gives the three numbers z_0, z_1, z_2 constituting $\mathbf{z}$, the circular convolution of $\mathbf{x}$ and $\mathbf{y}$, written $\mathbf{x} \circledast \mathbf{y}$. The indices are determined by this condition: the three terms $x_\alpha y_\beta$ that are added together to form z_λ are exactly those for which λ is the value of $\alpha + \beta$ (mod 3). The value of $\alpha + \beta$ (mod 3) is just the remainder of $\alpha + \beta$ when it is divided by 3: either 0, 1, or 2. (Arithmetic modulo n is a kind of "circular" arithmetic—hence the name 'circular convolution'.) Thus, for example, when $\lambda = 1$, the three pairs (α, β) for which $\lambda = \alpha + \beta$ (mod 3) are $(0, 1)$, $(1, 0)$, and $(2, 2)$; thus, z_1 is the sum of the three $x_\alpha y_\beta$ terms $x_0 y_1$, $x_1 y_0$, and $x_2 y_2$.

In HRRs, circular convolution is used to bind filler vectors to role vectors. The key point is that *the binding vector has the same number of elements as the vectors being bound.* With basic tensor product binding, of course, this is not true: the binding vector has n^2 elements if each vector being bound has n elements.

Circular convolution is defined in general as follows. Let $\mathbf{x}$ and $\mathbf{y}$ be vectors each with n elements. Then $\mathbf{z} = \mathbf{x} \circledast \mathbf{y}$ is the vector with the following n elements:

(29) $z_\lambda = \Sigma_{\alpha\beta}\, T_{\lambda\alpha\beta} x_\alpha y_\beta$,

where

(30) $$T_{\lambda\alpha\beta} \equiv \delta^{(n)}_{\lambda,\alpha+\beta} = \begin{cases} 1 & \text{if } \lambda = \alpha + \beta \ (\text{mod } n) \\ 0 & \text{otherwise} \end{cases}.$$

For a given λ, multiplying each product $x_\alpha y_\beta$ by the corresponding $T_{\lambda\alpha\beta}$ wipes out all terms except those for which $\lambda = \alpha + \beta$ (mod n), so summing $T_{\lambda\alpha\beta} x_\alpha y_\beta$ over all α and β pulls out just those terms in the tensor product $\mathbf{x} \otimes \mathbf{y}$ that add together to form the component $\mathbf{z}_\lambda$ of the circular convolution vector $\mathbf{z} = \mathbf{x} \circledast \mathbf{y}$.

To see the contraction structure of circular convolution, we can rewrite (29):

(31) $z_\lambda = \Sigma_{\alpha\beta}\, T_{\lambda\alpha\beta} x_\alpha y_\beta = \Sigma_{\alpha\mu} \Sigma_{\beta\kappa} \delta_{\alpha\mu} \delta_{\beta\kappa} T_{\lambda\mu\kappa} x_\alpha y_\beta$.

In the final expression in (31), the indices α and β of T have been replaced by μ and κ, with Kronecker deltas $\delta_{\alpha\mu}$ and $\delta_{\beta\kappa}$ inserted so that the sums over μ and κ will pick out only those terms where both $\alpha = \mu$ and $\beta = \kappa$. The expression (31) is a *double* contraction of the tensor $\mathrm{T} \otimes \mathbf{x} \otimes \mathbf{y}$, which has rank 5 (three from T, one from each of **x** and **y**); each contraction removes two indices, so after two contractions, only one of the original five remains. The double contraction structure is made explicit by rewriting (31) in the nested form

(32) $z_\lambda = \Sigma_{\alpha\mu} \Sigma_{\beta\kappa} \delta_{\alpha\mu} \delta_{\beta\kappa} \mathrm{T}_{\lambda\mu\kappa} x_\alpha y_\beta = \Sigma_{\alpha\mu} \delta_{\alpha\mu} [\Sigma_{\beta\kappa} \delta_{\beta\kappa} \mathrm{T}_{\lambda\mu\kappa} x_\alpha y_\beta]$.

The bracketed expression is a rank-3 tensor $\mathrm{S} \equiv \mathbb{C}_{35}[\mathrm{T} \otimes \mathbf{x} \otimes \mathbf{y}]$, a contraction of the rank-5 tensor $\mathrm{T} \otimes \mathbf{x} \otimes \mathbf{y}$; then the outer sum is a contraction of S over its final two indices. Thus,

(33) $\mathbf{z} = \mathbf{x} \circledast \mathbf{y} = \mathbb{C}_{23}[\mathbb{C}_{35}[\mathbf{T} \otimes \mathbf{x} \otimes \mathbf{y}]]$.

We see, then, that the circular convolution of **x** and **y** is a double contraction of the tensor product of **x**, **y**, and a third tensor T that embodies the 'circular' structure (via its definition (30), which employs the circular arithmetic of addition modulo *n*).

To identify the relation of circular convolution to tensor product representations, we rewrite (31) as a nested sum, as in (32), but with the nesting reversed:

(34) $$\begin{aligned} z_\lambda &= \Sigma_{\alpha\mu} \Sigma_{\beta\kappa} \delta_{\alpha\mu} \delta_{\beta\kappa} \mathrm{T}_{\lambda\mu\kappa} x_\alpha y_\beta \\ &= \Sigma_{\beta\kappa} \delta_{\beta\kappa} [\Sigma_{\alpha\mu} \delta_{\alpha\mu} \mathrm{T}_{\lambda\mu\kappa} x_\alpha] y_\beta. \end{aligned}$$

Now define $\mathbf{x}^\dagger$ to be the rank-2 tensor in brackets in (34):

(35) $\mathbf{x}^\dagger \equiv \mathbb{C}_{24}[\mathbf{T} \otimes \mathbf{x}]$;

that is,

$$x^\dagger_{\lambda\kappa} = \Sigma_{\alpha\mu} \delta_{\alpha\mu} \mathrm{T}_{\lambda\mu\kappa} x_\alpha = \Sigma_\mu \mathrm{T}_{\lambda\mu\kappa} x_\mu = x_{\lambda-\kappa}.$$

($\lambda - \kappa$ is, like all subscript arithmetic here, modulo n.) For example, in the case $n = 3$,

(36) $$\mathbf{x}^\dagger = \begin{bmatrix} x_0 & x_2 & x_1 \\ x_1 & x_0 & x_2 \\ x_2 & x_1 & x_0 \end{bmatrix}.$$

We can now substitute $\mathbf{x}^\dagger$ for the bracketed expression in (34), giving

(37) $z_\lambda = \Sigma_{\beta\kappa} \delta_{\beta\kappa} [\Sigma_{\alpha\mu} \delta_{\alpha\mu} \mathrm{T}_{\lambda\mu\kappa} x_\alpha] y_\beta = \Sigma_{\beta\kappa} \delta_{\beta\kappa} x^\dagger_{\lambda\kappa} y_\beta$,

which is recognizable as another contraction:

(38) $\mathbf{z} = \mathbf{x} \circledast \mathbf{y} = \mathbb{C}_{23}[\mathbf{x}^\dagger \otimes \mathbf{y}]$.

A similar computation derives an alternate form of this expression:

(39) $\mathbf{z} = \mathbf{x} \circledast \mathbf{y} = \mathbb{C}_{13}[\mathbf{x} \otimes \mathbf{y}^\dagger]$.

6.2.2 Convolution variable binding and Holographic Reduced Representations

Like tensor product representations, HRRs are built from a filler/role decomposition of a set of symbol structures, a set *F* of vectors realizing fillers, and a set *R* of vectors realizing roles. The representation of a structure is the superposition (vector sum) of the representation of all the filler/role bindings making up the structure. The only difference between HRRs and tensor product representations is that the latter use the tensor product operator $\otimes$ to bind fillers to roles, while the former use the circular convolution operator $\circledast$. Corresponding to the tensor product representation schema

(40) $\mathbf{s}(\otimes, F, R) \equiv \Sigma_i\, \mathbf{f}_i \otimes \mathbf{r}_i$

is the HRR schema

(41) $\mathbf{s}(\circledast, F, R) \equiv \Sigma_i\, \mathbf{f}_i \circledast \mathbf{r}_i$.

Using the results of Section 6.2.1, it is simple to relate these two schemas.

Circular convolution is used in an HRR to bind a filler vector **f** to a role vector **r**, yielding a binding vector **b**:

(42) $\mathbf{b} = \mathbf{f} \circledast \mathbf{r}$.

Using (39) and (38), we can write this as

(43) $\mathbf{b} = \mathbf{f} \circledast \mathbf{r} = \mathbb{C}[\mathbf{f} \otimes \mathbf{r}^\dagger] = \mathbb{C}[\mathbf{f}^\dagger \otimes \mathbf{r}]$,

with $\mathbf{f}^\dagger$ and $\mathbf{r}^\dagger$ defined by **f** and **r** as in (35):

(44) $\mathbf{u}^\dagger \equiv \mathbb{C}[\mathbf{T} \otimes \mathbf{u}]$.

What (43) says is that binding **f** to the role vector **r** with circular convolution $\circledast$ is exactly equivalent to binding **f** to the related role vector $\mathbf{r}^\dagger$ using the tensor product $\otimes$, followed by contraction. Alternatively, this convolution binding is equivalent to binding the related filler vector $\mathbf{f}^\dagger$ to **r** via the tensor product, followed by contraction. By altering either the filler or the role vectors appropriately, convolution binding can be reproduced exactly by contracted tensor product binding.

This result motivates the following definition:

(45) Contracted tensor products

a. A **contracted tensor product binding** of two vectors **u** and **v** is

$$\mathbb{C}[\mathbf{u} \otimes \mathbf{v}],$$

where $\mathbb{C}$ is a tensor contraction.

b. A **contracted tensor product realization** of a symbol structure **s** is

$$\mathbb{C}[\Sigma_i \mathbf{f}_i \otimes \mathbf{r}_i],$$

where

$$\mathbf{s}(\otimes, F, R) \equiv \Sigma_i \mathbf{f}_i \otimes \mathbf{r}_i$$

is the standard tensor product realization of **s** with respect to a filler/role decomposition and sets F and R of filler and role vectors.

As we have just shown (43), binding by circular convolution is a kind of contracted tensor product binding. Thus, an HRR built by using circular convolution to bind fillers $\mathbf{f}_i$ to their (rank-1) role vectors $\mathbf{r}_i$ is a representation using contracted tensor product binding to bind the original (rank-1) fillers $\mathbf{f}_i$ to the modified (rank-2) role vectors $\mathbf{r}_i^\dagger$ (or, contracted tensor product binding of modified (rank-2) filler vectors $\mathbf{f}^\dagger_i$

with the original (rank-1) role vectors $\mathbf{r}_i$).

Not only are individual filler/role bindings in an HRR contracted tensor products—so too are representations of entire structures containing multiple bindings. This follows immediately from the fact that circular convolution is a contracted tensor product (43) and the linearity property of the contraction operator (27). Thus, the HRR for the structure (41) is

(46) $\mathsf{s}(\circledast, F, R) \equiv \Sigma_i \mathbf{f}_i \circledast \mathbf{r}_i = \Sigma_i \mathbb{C}[\mathbf{f}^\dagger_i \otimes \mathbf{r}_i] = \mathbb{C}[\Sigma_i \mathbf{f}^\dagger_i \otimes \mathbf{r}_i] = \mathbb{C}[\mathbf{s}(\otimes, F^\dagger, R)]$,

where $F^\dagger$ is the set of filler vectors F with each vector $\mathbf{f}$ replaced by $\mathbf{f}^\dagger$. Alternatively, we can retain the original filler vectors F and replace each role vector $\mathbf{r}$ in R by $\mathbf{r}^\dagger$, obtaining $R^\dagger$:

(47) $\mathsf{s}(\circledast, F, R) \equiv \Sigma_i \mathbf{f}_i \circledast \mathbf{r}_i = \Sigma_i \mathbb{C}[\mathbf{f}_i \otimes \mathbf{r}^\dagger_i] = \mathbb{C}[\Sigma_i \mathbf{f}_i \otimes \mathbf{r}^\dagger_i] = \mathbb{C}[\mathbf{s}(\otimes, F, R^\dagger)]$.

Thus, the representational *schema* provided by HRRs is a special case of the contracted tensor product schema; a particular HRR equals a particular contracted tensor product representation when either (but not both) the filler vectors or the role vectors of the HRR are modified by the † operator.

6.2.3 Models of human memory

Plate (1994a, Sec. 6.2) employs HRRs to model judgments of analogical similarity elicited in experiments by Gentner and Markman (1993). Participants were asked to judge the similarity of simple figures consisting of a pair of geometric shapes, where the similarity could be based on shared shapes or on shared relations between different shapes (relative size, relative position).

The vector **v** Plate employs to represent a small circle above a large square is given in (48):

(48) HRR representation of 'small circle above large square'

$$\mathbf{v} \equiv \langle \mathbf{smCircle} + \mathbf{lgSquare} \rangle + \langle \mathbf{vertical} + \mathbf{smCircle} \circledast \mathbf{above} + \mathbf{lgSquare} \circledast \mathbf{below} \rangle$$

$$\mathbf{smCircle} \equiv \langle \mathbf{small} + \mathbf{circle} \rangle$$

$$\mathbf{lgSquare} \equiv \langle \mathbf{large} + \mathbf{square} \rangle$$

$$\langle \mathbf{u} \rangle \equiv \mathbf{u} / \|\mathbf{u}\|.$$

This representation can be understood as follows.

In Chapter 5, we first introduced the idea of distributed superpositional representations with the simple case of sets, where {`A`, `B`} is realized by the superposition **A** + **B**. If 'small circle' is decomposed as a simple set of properties, {`small`, `circle`}, then its representation is simply **small** + **circle**.

The relation 'x above y' (where here, x = 'small circle' and y = 'large square') can be represented symbolically as `vertical`(x, y), which can be given the filler/role decomposition [*relation* = `vertical`; *above* = x, *below* = y]. Since x fills the role *above* and y the role *below*, these are realized using circular convolution binding as $\mathbf{x} \circledast \mathbf{above}$

and **y** ⊛ **below**. Now the symbol **`vertical`** fills the role *relation*. Suppose this role is realized by the vector $\mathbf{r}_0$. Then the binding for the relation is **vertical** ⊛ $\mathbf{r}_0$. Now unlike objects like **`smCircle`** that can fill various roles (*above*, *below*, etc.), **`vertical`** will always appear in this same role, *relation*. Thus, its contribution will always take the same form, **vertical** ⊛ $\mathbf{r}_0$; we may simply rename this binding vector itself **vertical**.

Superimposing these three binding vectors, for the particular values of x and y relevant here, produces the vector realizing **`vertical`**(**`smCircle`**, **`lgSquare`**):

(49) **vertical + smCircle ⊛ above + lgSquare ⊛ below.**

The figure as a whole is represented as a set of elements together with their relation, {x, y, **`vertical`**(x, y)}, so the vectorial representation of the particular figure in question superimposes the vector representing the relation, (49), and the representation of the two elements, **smCircle** and **lgSquare**. (The rationale for these representational choices, and for the technical device of normalizing vectors to unit length via the operator ⟨ ⟩, is rather technical and complex; see Plate 1994a.)

The primitive vectors used in the HRR model (here, **small, large, vertical, above, below, circle, square**) are randomly generated vectors with 512 elements; the statistical properties of the resulting relations are analyzed in Plate 1994a.

The similarity of two vectors is measured simply by their dot product, as is customary in connectionist modeling (see Box 5:1). Participants in the experiment were asked which of two displays was more similar to a given reference display, and Plate's model predicts they will prefer the display with greatest similarity, as measured by the dot product of the vectors representing the displays. This model correctly predicts the empirical preferences for the eight test cases used in the experiment.

This research continues a tradition within the cognitive psychology literature on memory for structured items (Metcalfe-Eich 1982 et seq.; Murdock 1982, 1984 et seq.; Pike 1984; Humphreys, Bain, and Pike 1989). The mathematical models proposed in this literature deploy vector operations similar to circular convolution, which are likewise cases of contracted tensor product representations. While it is clear that considerable future work remains to be done sorting out many details, the experimental evidence claimed as support for these models suggests that contracted tensor product representations of some kind may well be on the right track as accounts of how people actually represent structured information.

7 SQUASHING: RECURSIVE AUTO–ASSOCIATIVE MEMORIES

In the previous section, we showed that it may be useful to follow tensor product binding by a contraction operation that reduces the size of the binding vector. In this section, we consider an extension not to the binding operation, but to the operation of combining multiple bindings in the realization of a structure. This extension derives from Jordan Pollack's seminal work on **Recursive Auto-Associative Memories** or **RAAMs** (Pollack 1988, 1990 et seq.).

A concrete illustration of RAAM is provided by the realization of binary trees (see Section 5:1.3). The idea is illustrated in Figure 8.

Figure 8. A RAAM network

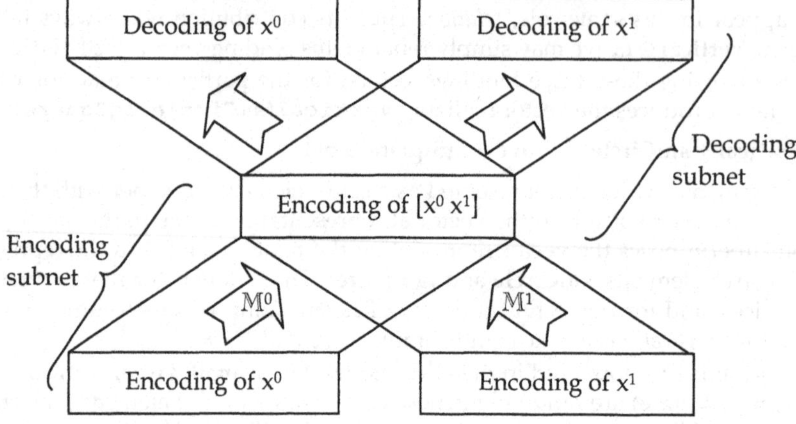

If patterns realizing **B** and **C** are placed in the two groups of input units at the bottom of the network in Figure 8, the result is a pattern at the middle layer that is taken to be the realization of the structure **[B C]**. This vector has the same number of elements as the vectors realizing **B** and **C**, so it may in turn be placed in the rightmost group of input units. If a pattern representing **A** is then placed in the leftmost group of input units, the resulting pattern in the middle layer is the representation of **[A [B C]]**: the constituent **[B C]** has been embedded inside a larger constituent that also includes **A**.

The top half of the network is used to *decode* trees. If the pattern we just constructed realizing **[A [B C]]** is placed in the middle layer, and the network has learned its task properly, the leftmost output units will host the vector realizing **A** and the rightmost the vector realizing **[B C]**. This latter vector can then be placed in the middle layer and the resulting patterns in the two halves of the output layer should be those for **B** and **C**.

The network is trained using back-propagation learning (Rumelhart, Hinton, and Williams 1986) so that the top half decodes what the bottom half encodes; when it is working correctly, the input should be reproduced on the output, despite the compression in between created by the middle layer. This network therefore is trained to perform **autoassociation**. Clearly, it is used recursively to encode and decode patterns for embedded structures.

While the *learning* in a RAAM is difficult to analyze, the *processing* is not. In Figure 8, we have labeled the weight matrix from the left half of the input layer to the middle layer '$\mathbb{M}^0$' and the matrix from the right half '$\mathbb{M}^1$'. These multiply their corresponding input vectors $\mathbf{x}^0$ and $\mathbf{x}^1$ to determine the input to the middle layer, and since these weights converge on the same set of middle units, these input vectors add:

(50) Input to middle RAAM layer, with input $(\mathbf{x}^0\ \mathbf{x}^1)$

a. From left half: $\boldsymbol{\iota}^0 = \mathbb{M}^0 \cdot \mathbf{x}^0$

b. From right half: $\boldsymbol{\iota}^1 = \mathbb{M}^1 \cdot \mathbf{x}^1$

c. Total input: $\boldsymbol{\iota} = \mathbb{M}^0 \cdot \mathbf{x}^0 + \mathbb{M}^1 \cdot \mathbf{x}^1$

Each unit at the middle layer computes its activation value by applying a nonlinear, sigmoidal function f to its input:

(51) Activation in the middle layer

a. Activation of the βth unit: $a_\beta = f(\iota_\beta) = \dfrac{1}{1+e^{-\iota_\beta}}$

b. Activation vector: $\mathbf{a} = \mathbf{F}[\boldsymbol{\iota}] = \mathbf{F}[\mathbb{M}^0 \cdot \mathbf{x}^0 + \mathbb{M}^1 \cdot \mathbf{x}^1]$
where $\mathbf{F}[\boldsymbol{\iota}] \equiv (f(\iota_1), f(\iota_2), \ldots)$

Now recall that matrix-vector multiplication is a kind of tensor contraction (20):

(52) $\mathbb{M} \cdot \mathbf{v} = \mathbb{C}[\mathbb{M} \otimes \mathbf{v}]$.

Then we can rewrite the activation vector at the middle layer as

(53) $\mathbf{a} = \mathbf{F}[\mathbb{M}^0 \cdot \mathbf{x}^0 + \mathbb{M}^1 \cdot \mathbf{x}^1] = \mathbf{F}[\mathbb{C}[\mathbb{M}^0 \otimes \mathbf{x}^0] + \mathbb{C}[\mathbb{M}^1 \otimes \mathbf{x}^1]]$.

Using the linearity of contraction (27), this can be expressed as

(54) $\mathbf{a} = \mathbf{F}[\mathbb{C}[\mathbb{M}^0 \otimes \mathbf{x}^0] + \mathbb{C}[\mathbb{M}^1 \otimes \mathbf{x}^1]] = \mathbf{F}[\mathbb{C}[\mathbb{M}^0 \otimes \mathbf{x}^0 + \mathbb{M}^1 \otimes \mathbf{x}^1]]$.

So we see that $\mathbf{x}^0$ and $\mathbf{x}^1$ are combined by the RAAM as follows:

(55) RAAM combination

a. Each of $\mathbf{x}^0$ and $\mathbf{x}^1$ is bound using the tensor product to its corresponding role (*left-child, right-child*), with $\mathbb{M}^0$ and $\mathbb{M}^1$ as role vectors, yielding $\mathbb{M}^0 \otimes \mathbf{x}^0$ and $\mathbb{M}^1 \otimes \mathbf{x}^1$.

b. These two bindings are superimposed, as in basic tensor product representations, yielding $[\mathbb{M}^0 \otimes \mathbf{x}^0 + \mathbb{M}^1 \otimes \mathbf{x}^1]$.

c. This is contracted, yielding $\mathbb{C}[\mathbb{M}^0 \otimes \mathbf{x}^0 + \mathbb{M}^1 \otimes \mathbf{x}^1]$—a contracted tensor product representation (45).

d. This vector is squashed element by element by the nonlinear function **F**, yielding the final result: $\mathbf{F}[\mathbb{C}[\mathbb{M}^0 \otimes \mathbf{x}^0 + \mathbb{M}^1 \otimes \mathbf{x}^1]]$.

Thus, RAAM perfectly exemplifies our target generalization of the basic notion of tensor product representations (1):

(56) A **generalized tensor product realization** of a structure **s** analyzed as a set of filler/role bindings $\{\mathbf{f}_i / r_i\}$ is

$\mathbf{s} = \mathbf{F}[\mathbb{C}[\Sigma_i\, \mathbf{f}_i \otimes \mathbf{r}_i]]$,

where $\mathbb{C}$ is a contraction over some set of tensor indices (possibly empty) and **F** is the element-by-element application of a function f (possibly the identity function):

$\mathbf{F}[\mathbf{v}] \equiv (f(v_1), f(v_2), \ldots)$.

When $\mathbb{C}$ is the trivial contraction (over no indices), and f is the identity function, this reduces to the basic tensor product realization defined in (1):

$\mathbf{s} = \Sigma_i\, \mathbf{f}_i \otimes \mathbf{r}_i$.

Since their introduction in Pollack 1988, RAAMs have been used in many interesting connectionist models (one rather recent example is Bodén and Niklasson 2000). RAAMs are often of interest because they *learn* which 'role vectors' $\mathbb{M}^0$ and $\mathbb{M}^1$ allow the relevant structures of the domain to be adequately encoded, despite the small size of the representation relative to a full (uncontracted) tensor product.

For example, Pollack (1990) trained a RAAM to encode a set of binary trees generated by a simple recursive context-free rewrite-rule grammar (recall Box 6:1). This grammar generated trees from the following 10 rules:

(57) **S → NP VP; S → NP V; VP → V NP; VP → V PP; PP → P NP;**
NP → D AP; NP → NP PP; NP → D N; AP → A AP; AP → A N.

These are parse trees for strings of five terminal symbols, including **V**(erb), **D**(eterminer), **A**(djective), **N**(oun), and **P**(reposition). Terminal symbols, but not nonterminal symbols such as **S**(entence) or **N**(oun)**P**(hrase), appeared as labels in these trees; the most complex tree in the training set, for example, was the **NP** [[**D** [**A N**]] [**V** [**P** [**D N**]]]].

Each of the five terminal symbols was realized by a single unit among a pool of 10 units (the extra 5 units being available for use by the network in designing its representations of trees). Thus, both the input and output layers of the RAAM contained two pools of 10 units each, and the hidden layer thus contained 10 units as well.

The RAAM was trained on 7 trees generated by the grammar, including the subtrees embedded within these complete trees; the RAAM saw 15 constituent trees. A cluster analysis of the patterns of activity over the 10 units that realized these trees showed them to be (roughly) clustered according to the type of constituent instantiated by the tree. For example, the activation vectors realizing the 2 trees in the training set that constituted **PP**s—[**P** [**D N**]] and [**P** [**D** [**A N**]]]—formed one cluster, as did the 3 trees instantiating **VP**s—[**V** [**D N**]], [**V** [**D** [**A N**]]], and [**V** [**P** [**D N**]]]. (The categories **S**, **NP**, and **AP** did not fall exactly into clusters.)

The RAAM trained on 15 trees was also able to successfully encode 31 other trees. (That is, when recursively encoded and then decoded by the RAAM, the vectors for these 31 trees were reconstructed within an activation error tolerance of 0.2 per unit, with activations ranging from 0 to 1.0.) Among these 31 new trees, there were 3 valid **NP**s, 4 valid **VP**s, and 12 valid **S**s; the remaining 12 trees were not legal according the grammar.

The procedures for encoding and decoding with a RAAM network are strictly sequential. But as shown in Chalmers 1990, RAAM representations can sometimes be employed for fully parallel structure processing: an input representation of a tree can be mapped to the output representation of a tree via a network that processes the input with massive parallelism, with no sequential construction or decomposition of trees. The computation studied in Chalmers 1990 is a tree manipulation analogous to the transformation that maps an English sentence in the active voice to its counterpart in the passive voice. This is clearly related to the fully parallel structure processing performable with standard tensor product representations (like the PassiveNet of Section 5:2 and Active/PassiveNet of Section 8:4.3); results of this sort concerning RAAM representations are based on computer simulation experiments, rather than the proof methods developed in Section 8:4 for analyzing parallel processing with standard tensor product representations.

References

Andrews, G., and G. S. Halford. 1994. Relational complexity and sentence processing. *Proceedings of the Annual Experimental Psychology Conference 21.*

Bodén, M., and L. Niklasson. 2000. Semantic systematicity and context in connectionist networks. *Connection Science* 12, 111–42.

Börgers, C., and N. Kopell. 2003. Synchronization in networks of excitatory and inhibitory neurons with sparse, random connectivity. *Neural Computation* 15, 509–38.

Chalmers, D. 1990. Syntactic transformations on distributed representations. *Connection Science* 2, 53–62.

Eckhorn, R., H. J. Reitboeck, M. Arndt, and P. Dicke. 1990. Feature linking via synchronization among distributed assemblies: Simulations of results from cat visual cortex. *Neural Computation* 2, 293–307.

Gentner, D., and A. M. Markman. 1993. Analogy—watershed or Waterloo? Structural alignment and the development of connectionist models of analogy. In *Advances in neural information processing systems* 5, eds. C. L. Giles, S. J. Hanson, J. D. Cowan. Morgan Kaufmann.

Gibson, E. 1998. Linguistic complexity: Locality of syntactic dependencies. *Cognition* 68, 1–76.

Gibson, E. 2000. The dependency locality theory: A distance-based theory of linguistic complexity. In *Image, language, brain,* eds. Y. Miyashita, A. Marantz, and W. O'Neil. MIT Press.

Gray, C. M., P. Konig, A. K. Engel, and W. Singer. 1989. Oscillatory responses in cat visual cortex exhibit intercolumnar synchronization which reflects global stimulus properties. *Nature* 338, 334–7.

Halford, G. S., W. H. Wilson, and M. McDonald. 1995. Complexity of structure mapping in human analogical reasoning: A PDP model. In *Proceedings of the Cognitive Science Society 17.*

Halford, G. S., W. H. Wilson, and S. Phillips. 1998. Processing capacity defined by relational complexity: Implications for comparative, developmental, and cognitive psychology. *Behavioral and Brain Sciences* 21, 803–64.

Hansel, D., and G. Mato. 2003. Asynchronous states and the emergence of synchrony in large networks of interacting excitatory and inhibitory neurons. *Neural Computation* 15, 1–56.

Hummel, J. E., and I. Biederman. 1992. Dynamic binding in a neural network for shape recognition. *Psychological Review* 99, 480–517.

Hummel, J. E., and K. J. Holyoak. 2003. A symbolic-connectionist theory of relational inference and generalization. *Psychological Review* 110, 220–64.

Humphreys, M. S., J. D. Bain, and R. Pike. 1989. Different ways to cue a coherent memory system: A theory for episodic, semantic and procedural tasks. *Psychological Review* 96, 208–33.

Maass, W., and C. M. Bishop, eds. 1999. *Pulsed neural networks.* MIT Press.

Marr, D. 1982. *Vision.* W. H. Freeman.

Metcalfe-Eich, J. 1982. A composite holographic associative recall model. *Psychological Review* 89, 627–61.

Murdock, B. B. J. 1982. A theory for storage and retrieval of item and associative information. *Psychological Review* 89, 316–38.

Murdock, B. B. J. 1984. A distributed memory model for serial-order information. *Psychological Review* 90, 316–38.

Phillips, S. 1994. Strong systematicity within connectionism: The tensor-recurrent network. In *Proceedings of the Cognitive Science Society 16.*

Phillips, S., G. S. Halford, and W. H. Wilson. 1995. The processing of associations versus the processing of relations and symbols: A systematic comparison. In *Proceedings of the Cognitive Science Society 17.*

Phillips, S., K. Kamewari, and K. Hiraki. 2003. Preliminary report on the link between relational complexity and visual attention. Talk presented at the Joint International Conference on Cognitive Science.

Pike, R. 1984. Comparison of convolution and matrix distributed memory systems for associative recall and recognition. *Psychological Review* 91, 281–94.

Plate, T. A. 1991a. Holographic reduced representations. Technical report CRG-TR-91-1, Department of Computer Science, University of Toronto.

Plate, T. A. 1991b. Holographic reduced representations: Convolution algebra for compositional distributed representations. *In Proceedings of the International Joint Conference on Artificial Intelligence.*

Plate, T. A. 1993. Holographic recurrent networks. In *Advances in neural information processing systems 5*, eds. C. L. Giles, S. J. Hanson, and J. D. Cowan. Morgan Kaufmann.

Plate, T. A. 1994a. Distributed representations and nested compositional structure. Ph.D. diss., University of Toronto.

Plate, T. A. 1994b. Estimating structural similarity by vector dot products of holographic reduced representations. In *Advances in neural information processing systems 6*, eds. J. D. Cowan, G. Tesauro, and J. Alspector. Morgan Kaufmann.

Plate, T. A. 1995. Holographic reduced representations. *IEEE Transactions on Neural Networks* 6, 623–41.

Plate, T. A. 1997. A common framework for distributed representation schemes for compositional structure. In *Connectionist systems for knowledge representation and deduction*, eds. F. Maire, R. Hayward, and J. Diederich. Queensland University of Technology.

Plate, T. A. 1998a. Chunks, bindings, star, and holographic reduced representations. *Behavioral and Brain Sciences* 21, 844–5.

Plate, T. A. 1998b. Structured operations with distributed vector representations. In *Advances in analogy research: Integration of theory and data from the cognitive, computational, and neural sciences*, eds. K. Holyoak, D. Gentner, and B. Kokinov. New Bulgarian University.

Plate, T. A. 2000. Analogy retrieval and processing with distributed vector representations. *Expert Systems* 17, 29–40.

Plate, T. A. 2003. *Holographic reduced representation: Distributed representation for cognitive structures.* CSLI Publications.

Pollack, J. 1988. Recursive auto-associative memory: Devising compositional distributed representations. In *Proceedings of the Cognitive Science Society 10.*

Pollack, J. 1990. Recursive distributed representations. *Artificial Intelligence* 46, 77–105.

Pouget, A., and T. J. Sejnowski. 1997. Spatial transformations in the parietal cortex using basis functions. *Journal of Cognitive Neuroscience* 9, 222–37.

Rumelhart, D. E., G. E. Hinton, and R. J. Williams. 1986. Learning internal representations by error propagation. In *Parallel distributed processing: Explorations in the microstructure of cognition*. Vol. 1, *Foundations*, D. E. Rumelhart, J. L. McClelland, and the PDP Research Group. MIT Press.

Rumelhart, D. E., and J. L. McClelland. 1986. On learning the past tenses of English verbs. In *Parallel distributed processing: Explorations in the microstructure of cognition*. Vol. 2, *Psychological and biological models*, J. L. McClelland, D. E. Rumelhart, and the PDP Research Group. MIT Press.

Sejnowski, T. J. 1999. Foreword: Neural pulse coding. In *Pulsed neural networks*, eds. W. Maass and C. M. Bishop. MIT Press.

Shastri, L., and V. Ajjanagadde. 1993. From simple associations to systematic reasoning: A connectionist representation of rules, variables and dynamic bindings using temporal synchrony. *Behavioral and Brain Sciences* 16, 417–94.

Tabor, W. 2000. Fractal encoding of context-free grammars in connectionist networks. *Expert Systems* 17, 41–56.

Tesar, B. B., and P. Smolensky. 1994. Synchronous-firing variable binding is spatio-temporal tensor product representation. In *Proceedings of the Cognitive Science Society 16.*

von der Malsburg, C., and W. Schneider. 1986. A neural cocktail-party processor. *Biological Cybernetics* 54, 29–40.

Wiles, J., G. S. Halford, J. E. M. Stewart, M. S. Humphreys, J. D. Bain, and W. H. Wilson. 1992. Tensor models: A creative basis for memory retrieval and analogical mapping. Technical report 218, Computer Science Department, University of Queensland.

Willshaw, D. 1981. Holography, associative memory, and inductive generalization. In *Parallel models of associative memory*, eds. G. E. Hinton and J. A. Anderson. Erlbaum.

Wilson, W. H., and G. S. Halford. 1998. Robustness of tensor product networks using distributed representations. In *Proceedings of the Australian Conference on Neural Networks* (ACNN'98).

Wilson, W. H., N. Marcus, and G. S. Halford. 2001. Access to relational knowledge: A comparison of two models. In *Proceedings of the Cognitive Science Society* 23.

8 Tensor Product Representations: Formal Foundations

Paul Smolensky

Tensor product representations, the formal cornerstone of the Integrated Connectionist/Symbolic Cognitive Architecture (ICS), are intuitively motivated at length in Chapter 5. In this chapter, these representations are formally defined and a number of their general properties are proven. A range of representations proposed in the connectionist cognitive modeling literature are analyzed as special cases of the general tensor product scheme. (A still wider range of representations is analyzed in Chapter 7.) Recursive tensor product representations are developed for the case of binary tree structures. A general analysis is provided of how simple connectionist networks can process such recursive representations to compute recursive functions and to realize formal grammars. The results fill in ③ of Figure 4, ⑦ of Figure 5, and ⑧ of Figure 7 in Chapter 2's ICS map. The material on grammar processing (Section 4.2) is closely connected to Chapter 10; it maybe helpful to read these together.

Sections 1–3 of this chapter are revised versions of a part of Smolensky 1990 (referred to here as 'TPAI'). The content has not been altered, but cross-references to other chapters in this book have been inserted, notation has been made consistent with this book, and additional explanation has been provided at some points. The literature cited predates 1990; for more recent relevant references, see Chapter 7. Much of the original content is omitted in this excerpt, and several sections have been abridged. Section 2.3.2 is greatly abbreviated; see TPAI and Smolensky 1987b for numerous examples of each type of representation. Sections 3.3–3.4 are numbered 3.8–3.9 in TPAI; the following sections have been omitted here:

3.3 Continuous structures and infinite-dimensional representations
3.4 Connectionist mechanisms for binding and unbinding
3.5 Binding-unit activities as connection weights
3.6 Values as variables
3.7 Representation of symbolic operations; recursive decompositions

Boxes 1–2 are based on the appendix of Smolensky 1995. The latter half of the chapter, Section 4, is a greatly extended treatment of ideas first set out in Smolensky, Legendre, and Miyata 1992, Sec. 3.2.1.

Contents

1 Introduction

1.1 The problem

The work reported here is part of an effort to extend the connectionist framework to naturally incorporate, without losing the virtues of connectionist computation, the ingredients essential to the power of symbolic computation (see also Smolensky 1986a, 1987a, 1988). This extended version of connectionist computation would integrate, in an intimate collaboration, the discrete mathematics of symbolic computation and the continuous mathematics of connectionist computation. This chapter offers an example of what such a collaboration might look like.

One domain where connectionist computation has much to gain by incorporating some of the power of symbolic computation is language. The problems here are extremely fundamental. Natural connectionist representation of a structured object like a phrase structure tree—or even a simple sequence of words or phonemes—poses serious conceptual difficulties, as I will shortly discuss. The problem can be traced back to difficulties with the elementary operation of binding a value to a variable. It is this basic problem that I address here.

I begin in Section 1.2 by discussing why natural connectionist representation of structured objects is a problem. I list several properties of the solution presented in this chapter.

First, though, it is worth commenting on where the research reported here fits into an overall scheme of connectionist theory. As in the symbolic approach, in the connectionist approach several components must be put together when constructing a model. Elements of the task domain must be represented, a network architecture must be designed, and a processing algorithm must be specified. If the knowledge in the model is to be provided by the designer, a set of connections must be designed to perform the task. If the model is to acquire its knowledge through learning, a learning algorithm for adapting the connections must be specified, and a training set must be designed (e.g., a set of input-output pairs). For most of these aspects of connectionist modeling, there exists considerable formal literature analyzing the problem and offering solutions. There is one glaring exception: the representation component. This is a crucial component, for a poor representation will often doom the model to failure, and an excessively generous representation may essentially solve the problem in advance. Representation is particularly critical to understanding the relation between connectionist and symbolic computation, for the representation often embodies most of the relation between a symbolically characterized problem (e.g., a linguistic task) and a connectionist solution.

Not only is the connectionist representation problem central, it is also amenable to formal analysis. In this chapter, the problem will be characterized as finding a **realization mapping** from a set of structured objects (e.g., trees) to a vector space, the set of states of the part of a connectionist network realizing those objects. The mélange of discrete and continuous mathematics that results is reminiscent of a related classical area of mathematics: the problem of representing an abstract group as a collection of linear operators on a vector space. The discrete aspects of group theory and the continuous aspects of vector space theory interact in a most constructive way. Group representation theory, with its application to quantum physics, in fact offers a useful analogy for the connectionist representation of symbolic structures. The world of elementary particles involves a discrete set of particle species whose properties exhibit many symmetries, both exact and approximate, that are described by group theory. Yet the underlying elementary particle state spaces are continuous vector spaces, in which the discrete structure is embedded. In the view that ultimately guides the research reported here, in human language processing, the discrete symbolic structures that describe linguistic objects are actually embedded in a continuous connectionist system that operates on them with flexible, robust processes that can only be approximated by discrete symbol manipulations.

One final note on terminology. In most of this chapter the structures being realized will be referred to as **symbolic structures**, because the principal cases of interest will be objects like strings and trees. Except when particular symbolic structures are considered, however, the analysis presented here applies to structured objects in general; it therefore applies equally well to objects like images and speech signals that are not typically considered 'symbolic structures'. With this understood, in general discussions I will indiscriminately refer to objects being realized as 'structures', 'structured objects', or 'symbolic structures'.

1.2 Distributed representation and connectionist variable binding

In this chapter, I propose a completely distributed representational scheme for variable binding: the **tensor product representation**. The tensor product of an n-dimensional vector $\mathbf{v}$ and an m-dimensional vector $\mathbf{w}$ is simply the nm-dimensional vector $\mathbf{v} \otimes \mathbf{w}$ whose elements are all possible products $v_i w_j$ of an element of $\mathbf{v}$ and an element of $\mathbf{w}$. This vector $\mathbf{v} \otimes \mathbf{w}$ is a **rank-2 tensor**: its elements are labeled by two **tags** i and j. A rank-1 tensor is simply an ordinary vector labeled by a single tag, and a rank-0 tensor is a simple number or **scalar**. Tensors of rank higher than two are created by taking tensor products of more than two ordinary vectors; if $\mathbf{w}$ is an l-dimensional vector, then $\mathbf{u} \otimes \mathbf{v} \otimes \mathbf{w}$ is a rank-3 tensor, the nml-dimensional vector consisting of all products $u_i v_j w_k$. The tensor product generalizes the matrix algebra concept of outer product to permit third- and higher-order products; the more general apparatus of tensor algebra is needed here because the recursive use of tensor product representations leads to rank-n tensors with $n > 2$.[1]

[1] For treatments of tensor algebra, see Nelson 1967; Loomis and Sternberg 1968, 305-320; Warner 1971, 54-62. For a short presentation directed to the current work, see Smolensky 1987b, App.; see also Box 5:1. While this chapter will not make extensive use of tensor calculus, setting the connectionist issues discussed here in the framework of tensor algebra provides a useful link to well-established mathematics. Certain virtues of the tensor calculus, such as the way it systematically manages the multiple

In the tensor product realization of the binding of a value to a variable, both the value and the variable can be arbitrarily nonlocal representations. Features of the tensor product representation, most of which distinguish it from previous representations, include those given in (1).

(1) General properties of tensor product representations

a. The representation rests on a principled and general analysis of structure: role decomposition (Section 2.2.1).
b. A fully distributed representation of a structured object is built systematically from distributed representations of both the structure's constituents and the structure's roles (Section 2.2.4).
c. Most previous connectionist representations of structured data, employing varying degrees of localization, are special cases (Section 2.3).
d. If a structure does not saturate the capacity of a connectionist network that represents it, the components of the structure can be extracted with complete accuracy (Section 3.1).
e. Structures of unbounded size can be represented in a fixed finite connectionist network, and the representation will saturate gracefully (Section 3.2).
f. The representation applies to continuous structures and to infinite networks as naturally as to the discrete and finite cases (Smolensky 1990 (TPAI), Sec. 3.3).
g. The binding mechanisms can be simply performed in a connectionist network (TPAI, Sec. 3.4).
h. The representation respects the independence of two aspects of parallelism in variable binding: generating versus maintaining bindings (TPAI, Sec. 3.4.1).
i. The components of structures can be simply extracted in a connectionist network (TPAI, Sec. 3.4.2).
j. A value bound to one variable can itself be used as a variable (TPAI, Sec. 3.6).
k. Connectionist representations of operations on symbolic structures, and recursive data types, can be naturally analyzed (Section 4; TPAI, Sec. 3.7).
l. Retrieval of representations of structured data stored in connectionist memories can be formally analyzed (Section 3.3).
m. A general sense of optimality for activity patterns representing roles in structures can be defined and analyzed (Section 3.4).
n. A connectionist 'recirculation' learning algorithm can be derived for finding these optimal representations (Section 3.4).

tags associated with higher-rank tensors, have proven important for actual connectionist systems built on tensor product representations: Dolan and Dyer 1987, 1988; Dolan and Smolensky 1988, 1989.

2 Connectionist representation and tensor product binding: Definition and examples

In this section, I first formally characterize the notion of a connectionist realization of a symbol system (which models a system of mental representations, in the case of primary interest here). Next, I reduce the problem of representing structured objects to three subproblems: decomposing the structures via roles, representing conjunctions, and representing value/variable bindings. In this regard, I discuss role decompositions and define the superpositional representation of conjunction and the tensor product representation for value/variable bindings. Finally, I show how various special cases of the tensor product representation yield previous connectionist representations of structured data.

2.1 Connectionist representation

The question of how to represent symbolic structures in connectionist systems will be treated formally as follows.

Connectionist representations are patterns of activity over connectionist networks; these patterns can extend over many processors in the network, as in distributed representations, or be localized to a single processor, as in a local representation. Such a pattern is a collection of activation values: a vector with one numerical component for every network processor. The space of representational states of a connectionist network thus lies in a vector space, with a dimension equal to the number of processors in the network. Each processor corresponds to an independent basis vector; this forms a **distinguished basis** for the space.[2] In many connectionist networks, the processor's values are restricted in some way; such restrictions are important when considering the dynamics of the network but are not central to the representational issues considered here, and they will be ignored. (For expositions of the application of vector space theory—linear algebra—to connectionist systems, see, for example, Jordan 1986, Smolensky 1986b, and Box 5:2.) In sum:

(2) *Definition.* The **activity states of a connectionist network** are the elements of a vector space V that has a distinguished basis $\{\hat{\mathbf{v}}_1, \hat{\mathbf{v}}_2, \ldots\}$.

Whenever I speak of a vector space representing the states of a connectionist network, a distinguished basis will be implicitly assumed. Rarely will it be necessary to deal explicitly with this basis. It will be useful to use the canonical **inner product** associated with the distinguished basis: the one in which the basis vectors are orthogonal and of unit norm. (Equivalently, this inner product of two vectors can be

[2] The numerical components of a vector in a vector space depend on the coordinate system or **basis** employed within the space (see Box 5:1). Normally, these numerical components denote the activation values of network processing units; this is the coordinate system provided by the distinguished basis. Other coordinate systems are sometimes useful, however, especially in analyzing distributed representations, where the activation values of individual units do not determine the semantic interpretation of a vector as directly as do the coordinates of vectors determined by axes directed along the distributed patterns (the **pattern basis** of Smolensky 1986b).

computed as the sum of the products of corresponding vector components with respect to the distinguished basis: Box 5:1 (6).) Whenever I speak of activity patterns being **orthogonal**, or of their **norm**, these concepts are taken to be defined with respect to this canonical inner product; the inner product of vectors **u** and **v** will be denoted $\mathbf{u} \cdot \mathbf{v}$.[3]

(3) *Definition.* A **connectionist realization** (or **representation**)[4] of the symbolic structures in a set S is a mapping ψ from S to a vector space V:

$$\psi : S \to V.$$

Of central interest are the images under the mapping ψ of the relations between symbolic structures and their constituents, and the images of the operations transforming symbolic structures into other structures. Also important are basic questions about the realization mapping ψ, such as whether distinguishable symbolic structures have distinguishable realizations:

(4) *Definition.* A connectionist realization ψ is **faithful** iff ψ maps no structure in S to the zero vector $\mathbf{0} \in V$ and ψ is one to one:[5]

$$\mathbf{s}_1 \neq \mathbf{s}_2 \Rightarrow \psi(\mathbf{s}_1) \neq \psi(\mathbf{s}_2).$$

2.2 Tensor product representation: Definition

The representation of structured objects explored in this chapter requires first that structures be viewed as possessing a number (possibly unbounded) of **roles** that, for particular instances of the given structural type, are individually bound to particular **fillers.** For example, a string may be viewed as possessing an infinite set of roles $\{r_1, r_2, \ldots\}$, where r_i is the role of the ith element in the string. A particular string of length n involves binding the first n roles to particular fillers. For example, the string **ABA** involves the bindings $\{\mathbf{A}/r_1, \mathbf{A}/r_3, \mathbf{B}/r_2\}$, using a notation in which $\mathbf{f}/r$ denotes the binding of filler $\mathbf{f}$ to role r; in this string, the roles r_i for $i > 3$ are all unbound. Now note that the structure has been characterized as the *conjunction* of an unordered set

[3] If the numerical components of two vectors **u** and **v** with respect to the distinguished basis are $(u_1, u_2, \ldots)$ and $(v_1, v_2, \ldots)$, then their inner or **dot** product is the number $\mathbf{u} \cdot \mathbf{v} \equiv u_1v_1 + u_2v_2 + \ldots \equiv \Sigma_\beta u_\beta v_\beta$.

[4] There is a central terminological awkwardness here (see also Footnote 2:2). In a symbolic cognitive theory, a symbol structure **s** *represents* some entity *e*, typically one external to the cognitive system. An activity vector **v** that *realizes* **s** ipso facto *represents e*. The vector **v** (and the system of which it is a part) is fundamentally of interest because of this representation relation to *e*; its realization relation to **s** is only indirectly of interest. In this sense, the system of vectors **v** is a representation first, and a realization second; thus, it is often most natural to speak of tensor product *representations* rather than tensor product *realizations*. But the set of represented entities *e* is not formalized in the present analysis; it is only the realization relation between **v** and **s** that is formalized. Thus, in this chapter it is usually most precise to speak of tensor product *realizations*. With this understanding of the exact relations involved throughout the chapter, I will take the liberty of using either 'representation' or 'realization' as seems most natural in a given context.

[5] Recall that a function f: $D \to R$ is **one-to-one**, or **injective**, if $x \neq y \Rightarrow f(x) \neq f(y)$. A one-to-one function need not be **surjective**, or **onto** its range R; that is, for some $z \in R$ there may be no $x \in D$ such that $f(x) = z$. If f is both injective and surjective, then it is **bijective** or a **one-to-one correspondence** between its domain D and its range R. Here, a connectionist realization ψ is never onto its range, the vector space V; almost all vectors $\mathbf{v} \in V$ are not the realization of any structure $\mathbf{s} \in S$.

of variable bindings. The problem of realizing the structure has been reduced to the problems of

1. representing the structure as a conjunction of filler/role bindings;
2. representing the conjunction operation;
3. representing the bindings in a connectionist network.

These problems are respectively considered in Sections 2.2.1 through 2.2.3 and brought together in Section 2.2.4.

2.2.1 Role decompositions of symbolic structures

As a formal definition of roles and fillers, let us take the following:

(5) *Definition.* Let S be a set of symbolic structures. A **role decomposition** F/R for S is a pair of sets (F, R), the sets of fillers and roles, respectively, and a mapping

$$\mu_{F/R} : F \times R \rightarrow Pred(S); \quad (\mathbf{f}, r) \mapsto \mathbf{f}/r.$$

For any pair $\mathbf{f} \in F$, $r \in R$, the predicate on S, $\mu_{F/R}(\mathbf{f}, r) = \mathbf{f}/r$, is expressed '**f fills role** r'.

The role decomposition has **single-valued roles** iff for any $\mathbf{s} \in S$ and $r \in R$, there is at most one $\mathbf{f} \in F$ such that $\mathbf{f}/r(\mathbf{s})$ holds (i.e., at most one filler).

The role decomposition is **recursive** iff $F = S$.

A role decomposition determines a mapping

$$\beta: S \rightarrow 2^{F \times R}; \quad \mathbf{s} \mapsto \{(\mathbf{f}, r) \mid \mathbf{f}/r\,(\mathbf{s})\}.$$

The set $\beta(\mathbf{s})$ will be called the **filler/role bindings in s**, and the mapping β will be called the **filler/role realization** of S induced by the role decomposition.

The role decomposition is **faithful** iff β is one-to-one (i.e., if distinct elements of S have nonidentical sets of bindings).

The role decomposition is **finite** iff for each $\mathbf{s} \in S$, the set of bindings in $\mathbf{s}$, $\beta(\mathbf{s})$, is finite.

Throughout this chapter, all role decompositions will be assumed to be finite, except where the infinite case is explicitly considered.

Recursive role decompositions are heavily used in the standard description of symbolic structures. For example, the description of a binary tree $\mathbf{s}$ as a structure whose left subtree and right subtree are both themselves binary trees is a recursive decomposition via the roles *left-subtree* and *right-subtree*. Extensive treatment of the recursive case appears in Section 4.

Faithful role decompositions are particularly useful because the filler/role realizations they induce allow us to identify each symbolic structure with a predicate having a simple conjunctive form:

(6) *Proposition.* Let F/R be a role decomposition of S. For each $\mathbf{s}_0 \in S$, define the predicate $\pi_{\mathbf{s}_0}$ by

$$\pi_{\mathbf{s}_0}(\mathbf{s}) = \bigwedge_{(\mathtt{f},r)\in\beta(\mathbf{s}_0)} \mathtt{f}/r(\mathbf{s}),$$

where $\wedge$ denotes conjunction. $\pi_{\mathbf{s}_0}(\mathbf{s})$ is true iff the structure $\mathbf{s}$ contains all the filler/role bindings in $\mathbf{s}_0$. Then if the role decomposition is faithful, the structure $\mathbf{s}_0$ can be recovered from the predicate $\pi_{\mathbf{s}_0}$. The structure thus recovered from a predicate π is denoted $\mathbf{s}[\pi]$.

Proof. This result follows immediately from the following lemma:

Lemma. The mapping β of a role decomposition maps elements of S into subsets of $F \times R$. These subsets possess a partial order, set inclusion $\subseteq$, which can be pulled back to S via β:

$\mathbf{s}_1 \leq \mathbf{s}_2$ iff $\beta(\mathbf{s}_1) \subseteq \beta(\mathbf{s}_2)$.

Suppose F/R is faithful. Then with respect to the partial order $\leq$, the set of elements of S for which the predicate $\pi_{\mathbf{s}_0}$ holds has a unique least element, which is $\mathbf{s}_0$. In this way, $\mathbf{s}_0$ can be recovered from its corresponding predicate $\pi_{\mathbf{s}_0}$.

Proof of lemma. Since $\beta(\mathbf{s})$ is the set of filler/role bindings in $\mathbf{s}$, $\mathbf{s}_1 \leq \mathbf{s}_2$ iff the bindings in $\mathbf{s}_1$ are a subset of those of $\mathbf{s}_2$:

$\mathbf{s}_1 \leq \mathbf{s}_2$ iff [for all $\mathtt{f} \in F$ and $r \in R$, $\mathtt{f}/r(\mathbf{s}_1) \Rightarrow \mathtt{f}/r(\mathbf{s}_2)$].

(So, for example, **AB** $\leq$ **ABC** with respect to the filler/role decomposition of strings introduced at the beginning of Section 2.2.) Now consider the set of elements $\mathbf{s}$ satisfying the predicate $\pi_{\mathbf{s}_0}$, denoted $S(\pi_{\mathbf{s}_0})$:

$$\begin{aligned} S(\pi_{\mathbf{s}_0}) &= \{\mathbf{s} \in S \mid \pi_{\mathbf{s}_0}(\mathbf{s})\} \\ &= \{\mathbf{s} \in S \mid \text{for all } \mathtt{f}/r \in \beta(\mathbf{s}_0),\ \mathtt{f}/r(\mathbf{s})\} \\ &= \{\mathbf{s} \in S \mid \text{for all } \mathtt{f} \in F \text{ and } r \in R,\ \mathtt{f}/r(\mathbf{s}_0) \Rightarrow \mathtt{f}/r(\mathbf{s})\} \\ &= \{\mathbf{s} \in S \mid \mathbf{s}_0 \leq \mathbf{s}\}. \end{aligned}$$

(So in the example, **ABC** $\in S(\pi_{\mathbf{AB}})$.) The set $S(\pi_{\mathbf{s}_0})$ contains $\mathbf{s}_0$, and $\mathbf{s}_0$ is a least element: $\mathbf{s}_0 \leq \mathbf{s}$ for every $\mathbf{s}$ in the set. It remains to show that there is no other least element. Consider any other element $\mathbf{s}_1 \in S(\pi_{\mathbf{s}_0})$. Since μ is faithful and $\mathbf{s}_1 \neq \mathbf{s}_0$, there is at least one binding $\mathtt{f}_1/r_1$ not shared by $\mathbf{s}_0$ and $\mathbf{s}_1$. Since $\mathbf{s}_1 \in S(\pi_{\mathbf{s}_0})$ and $\mathbf{s}_0$ is a least element of $S(\pi_{\mathbf{s}_0})$, we must have $\mathbf{s}_0 \leq \mathbf{s}_1$: all the bindings of $\mathbf{s}_0$ are also bindings of $\mathbf{s}_1$, so if these binding sets do not share $\mathtt{f}_1/r_1$, it must be that this binding is in $\beta(\mathbf{s}_1)$ but not in $\beta(\mathbf{s}_0)$: $\mathtt{f}_1/r_1(\mathbf{s}_1) \wedge \neg\mathtt{f}_1/r_1(\mathbf{s}_0)$, where '$\neg$' denotes 'not'. This implies $\neg(\mathbf{s}_1 \leq \mathbf{s}_0)$, so $\mathbf{s}_1$ cannot be a least element in $S(\pi_{\mathbf{s}_0})$.

2.2.2 Connectionist representation of conjunction

In connectionist models, the combination of representations is performed with pattern superposition, that is, vector addition (see Section 5:1.1). This method yields the following definition of a connectionist realization mapping ψ:

(7) *Definition.* Suppose S is a set of symbolic structures and F/R is a role decomposition of S with fillers F and roles R. Suppose further that ψ_b is a connectionist realization of the filler/role bindings:

$$\psi_b : \{\mathtt{f}/r \mid \mathtt{f} \in F, r \in R\} \to V,$$

where V is a vector space. Define a connectionist realization of S, $\psi_{F/R}$, by

$$\psi_{F/R}: S \rightarrow V; \quad \mathbf{s} \mapsto \sum_{(\mathbf{f},r)\in\beta(s)} \psi_b(\mathbf{f}/r).$$

(The realization of a structure is the sum or superposition of the realization of its bindings.) In this representation, if $\{b_i\}$ are the bindings in a structure s_0, we have

$$\psi\left(\mathbf{s}\left[\bigwedge_i b_i\right]\right) = \psi(\mathbf{s}_0) = \sum_i \psi_b(b_i).$$

Thus, $\psi_{F/R}$ is said to employ the **superpositional realization of conjunction.**[6] $\psi_{F/R}$ is called the **connectionist realization of S induced by** (i) the role decomposition F/R, (ii) the superpositional realization of conjunction, and (iii) the binding realization ψ_b.

The use of vector addition to realize conjunction has pervasive implications for the faithfulness of representations. If the realizations of $\mathbf{A} \wedge \mathbf{B}$ and $\mathbf{C} \wedge \mathbf{D}$ are to be distinguishable, then $\mathbf{A}+\mathbf{B}$ and $\mathbf{C}+\mathbf{D}$ must be different. This constrains the possible patterns **A**, **B**, **C**, and **D** that can realize **A**, **B**, **C**, and **D**. It will be guaranteed that $\mathbf{A}+\mathbf{B}$ and $\mathbf{C}+\mathbf{D}$ will be different if the vectors **A**, **B**, **C**, and **D** are all **linearly independent**: none of these vectors can be expressed as a weighted sum of the others (see Section 5:1.1). To guarantee the faithfulness of representations, it will typically be necessary to require that constituents be represented by linearly independent patterns. This restriction is an expensive one, however, since for n linearly independent patterns to exist, there must be at least n nodes in the network. And, as we will see in Section 3.3, some sets of structures contain so many shared bindings that they cannot be given linearly independent realizations, no matter how the bindings are realized; this is true, for example, of the set of strings {**AX**, **BX**, **AY**, **BY**}, when decomposed (as above) by the roles *first-position, second-position*.

The addition operation used for superposition in this chapter is arithmetic addition, in which $1 + 1 = 2$; in other words, the scalars for the vector spaces are real numbers under numerical addition. An important variation of this analysis would be to consider vector spaces over *Boolean* scalars {0, 1} under logical addition (OR), where $1 + 1 = 1$. This variation can still be regarded as tensor product representation, but with respect to a different set of scalars; the result would have quite a different character. Boolean tensor product representations are needed to exactly describe a number of existing connectionist models that use Boolean-valued units and correspondingly use Boolean rather than numerical superposition to realize conjunction. Comparing real-valued and Boolean tensor product representations in general is like comparing connectionist models with real-valued units to those with Boolean units: each type has a variety of strengths and weaknesses. To mention just two, threshold operations can often allow retrievals from lightly loaded Boolean systems to be exact

[6] Note that, like conjunction, vector addition is associative ($\mathbf{u}+[\mathbf{v}+\mathbf{w}] = [\mathbf{u}+\mathbf{v}]+\mathbf{w}$) and commutative ($\mathbf{u}+\mathbf{v} = \mathbf{v}+\mathbf{u}$). Were this not so, vector addition could not be used to realize conjunction.

(e.g., Willshaw 1981); but, on the whole, the mathematics of real scalars is simpler. For this reason, this book initiates the analysis of tensor product representations by considering only the real-valued case.

2.2.3 Connectionist representation of variable binding

It remains to consider the realization of filler/role bindings: the mapping ψ_b of (7). This section introduces the tensor product realization of variable binding.

The tensor product realization of a value/variable binding is quite simple to define (see Figure 1).

Figure 1. The tensor product realization of filler/role bindings

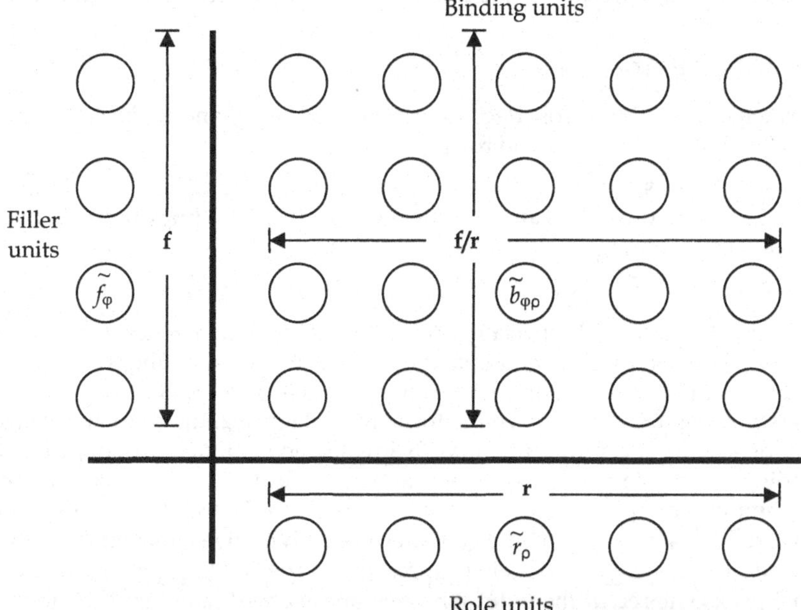

To bind a filler **f** to a role r, we first realize **f** as a pattern of activity **f** over a set of **filler units** $\{\tilde{f}_\varphi\}$ and realize r as a pattern of activity **r** over a set of **role units** $\{\tilde{r}_\rho\}$. The binding **f**/r is realized by a pattern of activity **f/r** over a set of **binding units** $\{\tilde{b}_{\varphi\rho}\}$: there is one binding unit for each *pair* of filler (φ) and role (ρ) units. The activity of the binding unit $\tilde{b}_{\varphi\rho}$ is simply the activity of the filler unit $\tilde{f}_\varphi$ in the pattern **f** times the activity of the role unit $\tilde{r}_\rho$ in the pattern **r**.

This procedure can readily be characterized in vector space terminology. The realization of the role r is a vector **r** in a vector space V_R. V_R is a real vector space with dimension equal to the number of role units $\tilde{r}_\rho$. The realization of the filler **f** is a vector **f** in a vector space V_F, a real vector space with dimension equal to the number of filler units $\tilde{f}_\varphi$. The realization of the binding $\mathtt{f}/r$ is the **tensor product** vector $\mathbf{f/r} = \mathbf{f} \otimes \mathbf{r}$ in the tensor product vector space $V_B = V_F \otimes V_R$ (Box 5:1 (17)).[7] V_B is a real vector space with dimension equal to the product of the dimensions of V_F and V_R. The components of the vector $\mathbf{f/r}$ are related to the components of **f** and **r** as follows. Each filler unit $\tilde{f}_\varphi$ corresponds to a vector $\hat{\mathbf{f}}_\varphi$ in V_F (the vector representing the pattern of activity in which that unit has activity 1 and all other units have activity 0). The complete set of vectors $\{\hat{\mathbf{f}}_\varphi\}$ forms the distinguished basis for V_F, and any vector **f** in V_F can be expressed in terms of this basis as a sequence of real numbers; these are the activities of all the units in the pattern corresponding to **f**. Exactly the same story holds for the roles. Then the tensor product space $V_B = V_F \otimes V_R$ has as a basis the set of vectors $\{\hat{\mathbf{b}}_{\varphi\rho} = \hat{\mathbf{f}}_\varphi \otimes \hat{\mathbf{r}}_\rho\}$. The $\varphi\rho$ component ($[\mathbf{b}]_{\varphi\rho} = [\mathbf{f/r}]_{\varphi\rho}$) of the vector $\mathbf{b} = \mathbf{f/r} = \mathbf{f} \otimes \mathbf{r}$ realizing the binding is the product of the φ component of **f** (f_φ) and the ρ component of **r** (r_ρ):

(8) $b_{\varphi\rho} = [\mathbf{f/r}]_{\varphi\rho} \equiv [\mathbf{f} \otimes \mathbf{r}]_{\varphi\rho} \equiv \mathrm{f}_\varphi \mathrm{r}_\rho.$

(9) *Definition.* Let F/R be a role decomposition of S. Let ψ_F and ψ_R be connectionist realizations of the fillers and roles:

$$\psi_F: F \to V_F; \quad \psi_R: R \to V_R.$$

Then the **tensor product realization** of the filler/role bindings induced by ψ_F and ψ_R is the mapping

$$\psi_b: \{\mathtt{f}/r \mid \mathtt{f} \in F, r \in R\} \to V_F \otimes V_R; \quad \mathtt{f}/r \mapsto \psi_F(\mathtt{f}) \otimes \psi_R(r).$$

Figure 2 shows an example specially chosen for visual transparency. Consider an application to speech processing, and imagine that we are representing the energy in a particular formant over time. For the roles here we take a series of time points and for the fillers the amount of energy in the formant. In Figure 2, the roles are realized as patterns of activity over five units, with greater activation levels depicted by darker shading. Each role r_ρ is a time point and is represented as a peaked pattern centered at unit number ρ; the figure shows the case $\rho = 4$. Each filler $\mathtt{f}$ is an energy level; in Figure 2, this is represented as a pattern of activity over four units: a single peak centered at the energy level being represented. The binding pattern is a two-dimensional peak centered at the point whose x- and y-coordinates are the time and energy values being bound together.

The example of Figure 2 is visually transparent because of the simple geometric structure of the patterns. Of course, there is nothing in the binding mechanism itself that requires this. The distributed representation of roles and fillers can be arbitrary patterns, and in general the tensor product of these patterns will be even more visually opaque than are the patterns for the roles and fillers; see Figure 3.

[7] '$\mathbf{f/r}$' is to be read as a *single* symbol denoting a single vector; see Footnotes 5:2, 4.

Figure 1

Figure 2. A visually transparent tensor product

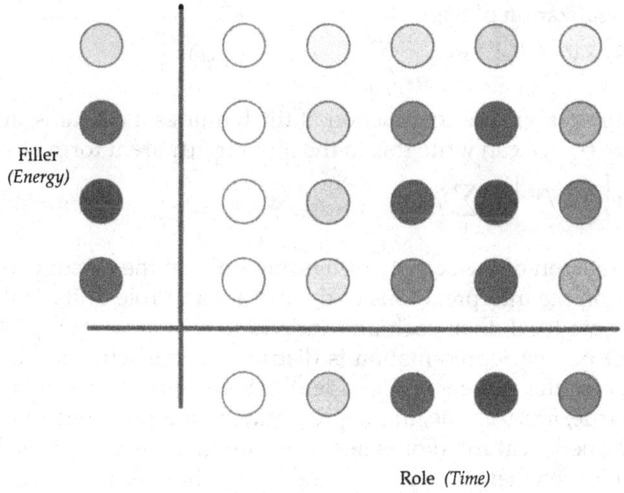

However, the mathematical simplicity of tensor product binding makes the general case, Figure 3, as easy to analyze as special cases like that of Figure 2.

Figure 3. A generic tensor product

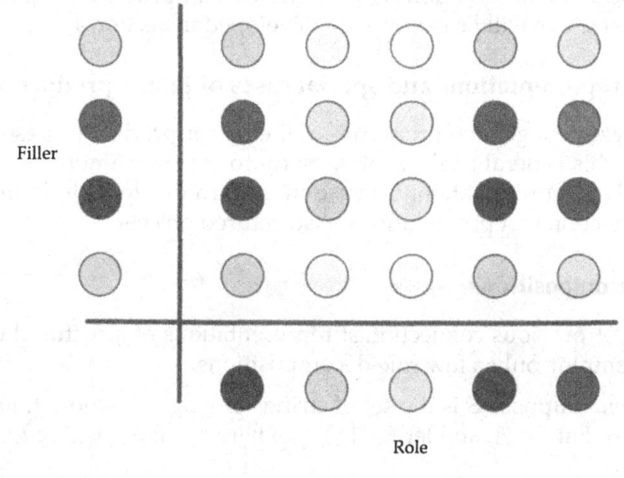

2.2.4 Tensor product representation

Putting together the previous representations, we have the following definition:

(10) *Definition.* Let F/R be a role decomposition of S, and let ψ_F and ψ_R be connectionist realizations of the fillers and roles. Then the corresponding **tensor product realization** of S is

$$\psi: S \to V_F \otimes V_R; \quad \mathbf{s} \mapsto \sum_{(\mathtt{f},r)\in\beta(s)} \psi_F(\mathtt{f}) \otimes \psi_R(r).$$

If we express $\mathbf{s}$ via the conjunction of the bindings it contains, and let $\mathbf{f} = \psi_F(\mathtt{f})$ and $\mathbf{r} = \psi_R(r)$, we can write this in the more transparent form

$$\psi\left(\mathbf{s}\left[\bigwedge_i \mathtt{f}_i / r_i\right]\right) = \sum_i \mathbf{f}_i \otimes \mathbf{r}_i.$$

The interpretation of the activity of binding units in the tensor product representation depends on the interpretations of the feature and role units. If the filler or role representations are local, then each unit individually represents a particular filler or role. If the filler or role representation is distributed, the activation of an individual node may indicate the presence of an identifiable feature in the entity being represented. This is true, for example, in a representation of a phoneme in which each unit represents a phonetic feature. (For expository simplicity, we can consider a local representation to be one where a given 'feature' is present in exactly one represented object, and a given object possesses exactly one 'feature'.) Then if the binding unit $\tilde{b}_{\varphi\rho}$ is active in the tensor product realization of a structure $\mathbf{s}$, the interpretation is that the feature represented by $\tilde{f}_\varphi$ is present in a filler of a role that possesses the feature $\tilde{r}_\rho$. In this sense, $\tilde{b}_{\varphi\rho}$ *represents the conjunction of the features represented by* $\tilde{f}_\varphi$ *and* $\tilde{r}_\rho$.[8] By using the tensor product representation recursively, we can produce conjunctions of more than two features; this will be extensively developed in Section 4.

2.3 Previous representations and special cases of tensor product realization

Section 3 analyzes the general properties of the tensor product representation. Before we proceed to this general analysis, it is useful to examine a number of special cases of tensor product representation, because these turn out to include most previously proposed connectionist representations of structured objects.

2.3.1 Role decompositions

The examples of previous connectionist representations of structured objects that we will consider employ only a few role decompositions.

(11) *Definition.* Suppose S is the set of strings of length no more than n from an alphabet A. Let $F = A$, and let $R = \{r_i\}_{i=1}^{n}$, where r_i is the role 'occupies the ith posi-

[8] For a more precise formulation, consider a simple case where the activity of unit $\tilde{f}_\varphi$ is 1 or 0 and indicates the truth value of the proposition 'there exists x among the represented objects such that the predicate $\tilde{f}_\varphi$ holds of x'; and suppose $\tilde{r}_\rho$ can be similarly interpreted. Then $\tilde{b}_{\varphi\rho}$ indicates the truth value of the proposition 'there exists x among the represented objects such that both predicates $\tilde{f}_\varphi$ and $\tilde{r}_\rho$ hold of x'. If this is true of n different values of x, in the superposition representing the structure as a whole, the value of $\tilde{b}_{\varphi\rho}$ will be n.

Figure 3

tion in the string'. Then F/R is the **positional role decomposition** of S.

This is the example given above in Section 2.2, in which the string **ABA** is represented by bindings $\{\mathbf{B}/r_2, \mathbf{A}/r_1, \mathbf{A}/r_3\}$. This decomposition is finite, has single-valued roles, and is faithful. This decomposition is the most obvious one, and the one most often used in previous connectionist systems.

The positional decomposition has an obvious extension to the case of finite strings of arbitrary length, where the set of roles becomes infinite; I will treat this as the case of the above definition with $n = \infty$. In the infinite case, the decomposition is still faithful, still has single-valued roles, and is still finite, since the strings are all of finite length. The infinite case will later be used to explore saturation of the tensor product representation.

There is a less obvious role decomposition of strings that was used to considerable advantage by Rumelhart and McClelland (1986), as we will soon see; it forms the basis of their 'Wickelfeature' representation. (The properties of this role decomposition are crucial to many of the criticisms of this model presented in Lachter and Bever 1988, Pinker and Prince 1988, Prince and Pinker 1988.)

(12) *Definition.* Suppose S is the set of strings of length no more than n from an alphabet A. Let $F = A \cup \{\langle, \rangle\}$, where $\langle$ and $\rangle$ are two new symbols meaning 'left string boundary' and 'right string boundary', respectively. Let $R = \{r_{x\_y} \mid x \in F, y \in F\}$, where r_{x_y} is the role 'is immediately preceded by x and immediately followed by y'. F/R is a role decomposition of S called the **1-neighbor context decomposition**.

Under this decomposition, the string **ABA** becomes the set of bindings $\{\mathbf{A}/r_{\langle\_\mathbf{B}}, \mathbf{B}/r_{\mathbf{A}\_\mathbf{A}}, \mathbf{A}/r_{\mathbf{B}\_\rangle}\}$. This decomposition does not have single-valued roles and is not faithful if $n \geq 4$ (the strings **AAA** $\equiv \mathbf{A}^3$ and $\mathbf{A}^4$ can't be distinguished). There is an obvious generalization to the k-neighbor context decomposition: it is faithful if $n < 2k + 2$.[9]

There are also obvious generalizations of the 1-neighbor context decomposition to differing size contexts on the left and right. A special case is the realization of pairs—say, strings with $n = 2$—where the roles are $R = \{r_{\_x} \mid x \in F\}$: the right-neighbor context. Omitting the unnecessary boundary symbols, the pair **AB** has the single binding $\mathbf{A}/r_{\_\mathbf{B}}$. This role decomposition, we will see in (18), is used in a powerful technique called 'conjunctive coding'.

While it is true that the positional role decomposition is more faithful than context decompositions for the realization of a *single* structure, it turns out that if multiple structures are to be simultaneously represented, the positional decomposition can be *less* faithful than the context decomposition. Suppose we are to realize the conjunction of **AB** and **CD** by superimposing the realization of the two pairs. What gets real-

[9] This decomposition gives the initial and final substrings of length up to $2k$, and all internal substrings up to length $2k+1$. These substrings uniquely determine strings of length no more than $2k+1$. But the strings $\mathbf{a}^{2k+1}$ and $\mathbf{a}^{2k+2}$ cannot be distinguished, so the decomposition is not faithful if $n > 2k+1$. If multiple occurrences of a binding are recognized, some ambiguities are resolved, but not all; for $k = 1$, **AACAABAA** and **AABAACAA** have the same bindings, with no repetitions. This example can be generalized to $k > 2$ by replacing '**AA**' with a sequence of $k+1$ **A**s. See also Prince and Pinker 1988.

ized is the union of the binding sets of the two structures. In the case of positional roles, this union is $\{\mathtt{A}/r_1, \mathtt{B}/r_2, \mathtt{C}/r_1, \mathtt{D}/r_2\}$; now it is impossible to distinguish what is being realized from the conjunction of **AD** and **CB**. However, with the right-neighbor context decomposition, the union of the binding sets is $\{\mathtt{A}/r_{\_\mathtt{B}}, \mathtt{B}/r_{\_\rangle}, \mathtt{C}/r_{\_\mathtt{D}}, \mathtt{D}/r_{\_\rangle}\}$, which can't at all be confused with the conjunction of **AD** and **CB**. With context decompositions, confusions can of course also result; these decompositions are not even faithful for realizing single structures.

An additional virtue of context decompositions is that they give rise to connectionist representations that give the network direct access to the kind of information needed to capture the regularities in many context-sensitive tasks; we will consider this below for the specific example of the Rumelhart and McClelland 1986 model.

2.3.2 Connectionist representations

Having looked at a few of the role decompositions that have been used in connectionist representations of structures, we can now consider examples of such representations. These are grouped according to the degree of locality in the representations of roles and fillers; we therefore start by distinguishing local and distributed connectionist representations in general, and then examine the degree of locality of various existing representations of structured objects. (The definitions in this section simply formalize the ideas informally developed in Section 5:1.2.1.)

2.3.2.1 Local and distributed representations

Local representations dedicate an individual processor to each item represented. In terms of the vector space of network states, these individual processors correspond to the members of the distinguished basis. Thus:

(13) *Definition.* Let ψ be a connectionist representation of a set X in a vector space V with distinguished basis $\{\hat{\mathbf{v}}_i\}$. ψ is a **local representation** iff it is a one-to-one mapping of the elements of X onto the set of basis vectors $\{\hat{\mathbf{v}}_i\}$. A connectionist representation that is not a local representation is a **distributed representation**.

2.3.2.2 Purely local realizations of symbolic structures

The first special case of the tensor product representation is the most local one (compare Figure 5:2):

(14) *Definition.* Let $\psi_{F/R}$ be the tensor product realization of S induced by a role decomposition F/R of S and two connectionist realizations ψ_F and ψ_R. Then $\psi_{F/R}$ is a **purely local tensor product representation** if ψ_F and ψ_R are both local representations.

Figure 3

2.3.2.3 Semilocal realizations of symbolic structures

The next most local special case is this (compare Figure 5:4):

(15) *Definition.* Let $\psi_{F/R}$ be the tensor product realization of S induced by a role decomposition F/R of S and two connectionist realizations ψ_F and ψ_R. If ψ_F is a distributed representation and ψ_R is a local representation, then $\psi_{F/R}$ is a **semilocal tensor product representation** or a **role register representation**.

2.3.2.4 Fully distributed realizations of symbolic structures

Now we come to the most distributed case (Figures 2–3; Figure 5:5):

(16) *Definition.* Let $\psi_{F/R}$ be the tensor product realization of S induced by a role decomposition F/R of S and two connectionist realizations ψ_F and ψ_R. If ψ_F and ψ_R are both distributed representations, then $\psi_{F/R}$ is a **fully distributed tensor product representation**.

Examples of fully distributed representations include the following:

(17) Coarse coding

A visually transparent example of a fully distributed tensor product representation using the positional role decomposition was given in Figure 3. The patterns representing roles here are examples of what have been called **coarse coding** representations (Hinton, McClelland, and Rumelhart 1986). It is traditional to focus on the numerous positions (roles) that activate a particular role unit (its **receptive field**); the formulation here focuses on the numerous role units activated by a particular positional role. These are merely two perspectives on the many-to-many relation between positions and units (see Section 7:3).

(18) Conjunctive coding

The McClelland and Kawamoto 1986 model (which learns to assign case roles to noun phrases in a clause frame) can be viewed as using a fully distributed representation of the output. Each output is a set of bindings of noun fillers to the case-frame slots of the verb. This output can be viewed as having roles like *loves-agent, loves-patient, eat-instrument, break-patient,* and so on; these roles can in turn be viewed as structured objects with two subroles: *verb* and *case-role.* The patterns representing the overall roles are the tensor product of a distributed pattern representing the verb (built from semantic verb features) and a local representation of the case-role. The representation of the overall roles is thus semilocal. The representation of the output as a whole is the tensor product of this distributed (albeit semilocal) representation of the roles and a distributed representation of the fillers (built of semantic features of nouns). This illustrates a kind of recursive tensor product representation developed in TPAI, Sec. 3.5 (and Chapter 5 (30)). Because of this nested structure, the output units in this model represent three-way conjunctions of features for nouns, verbs, and semantic roles: this has been termed **conjunctive coding**. (The "features" of semantic roles used in the model are of the local type mentioned in Section 2.2.4: they are in one-to-one correspondence with the semantic roles. A more distributed version of this model would employ real features of semantic roles, where each semantic role is a distributed pattern of features. Then the roles in the output as a whole would have fully distributed representations instead of semilocal ones.)

(19) Wickelfeatures

An example of a fully distributed representation employing the 1-neighbor context decomposition is the Rumelhart and McClelland 1986 model that learns to form the past tense of English verbs; see Figure 4. In this model, elements of S are strings of phonetic segments. The word *weed* corresponds to the string **wid**, which has the bindings $\{\mathbf{w}/r_{\langle\_\mathtt{i}},\ \mathbf{i}/r_{\mathtt{w\_d}},\ \mathbf{d}/r_{\mathtt{i}\_\rangle}\}$. The realization of this string is thus

$$\mathbf{w}\otimes\mathbf{r}_{\langle\_\mathtt{i}} + \mathbf{i}\otimes\mathbf{r}_{\mathtt{w\_d}} + \mathbf{d}\otimes\mathbf{r}_{\mathtt{i}\_\rangle}.$$

Figure 4. Rumelhart and McClelland 1986 representation of phonetic strings

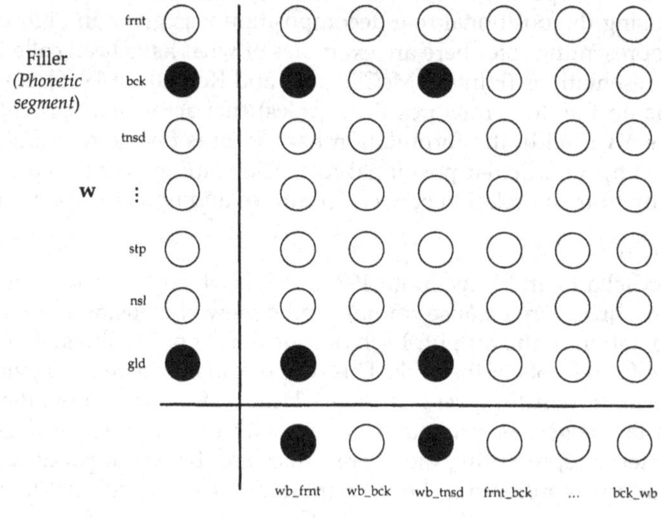

Role (*1-neighbor phonetic context*)

Feature abbreviations: wb = word_boundary, frnt = front, bck = back, tnsd = tensed, stp = stop, nsl = nasal, gld = glide

The filler vectors (e.g., **w**) are distributed patterns over a set of units representing phonetic features (e.g., *rounded, front, stop*). The role vectors (e.g., $\mathbf{r}_{\langle\_\mathtt{i}}$) are

Figure 4

patterns of activity over a set of units each of which represents the conjunction of a feature of the left neighbor (⟨) and a feature of the right neighbor (i). (In this model, both ⟨ and ⟩ possess the single feature *word_boundary*.) As in the previous example, since the roles are composite objects, they are in fact themselves further decomposed into subroles. The pair of phonetic segments defining the context is decomposed using the right-neighbor context decomposition, and the pattern representing the role r_{a_b} is the tensor product of patterns of phonetic features for **a** and **b**. To reduce the number of units in the network, many of the units arising in this further decomposition of the roles were in fact discarded. The overall structure of the representation of the roles can still be productively viewed as a tensor product from which some units have simply been thrown away.

2.4 Relations among purely local, semilocal, and fully distributed realizations

Purely local, semilocal, and fully distributed representations look quite different on the surface. Are they really as different as they seem? According to the definitions, the only difference lies in the relation between the representation vectors and the distinguished basis vectors indicating the individual processing units. Does this really matter?

The answer depends on the dynamics driving the connectionist network, and not solely on the representations themselves. If the dynamics is linear, so that the activity of every unit is exactly a weighted sum of the activity of its neighbors in the network, then networks using purely local, semilocal, and fully distributed representations will have exactly isomorphic behavior, subject to a few qualifications (Smolensky 1986b). Under the linear transformations that map these three cases into each other, locality is not preserved, so that local damage to the networks will have different effects, and what can be learned via the usual local connectionist learning procedures will be different. If the network contains nonlinear units, the isomorphism fails. Also, assuming finite networks, the local case accommodates only a fixed, finite set of fillers and roles; the semilocal case allows an unlimited number of fillers but only a finite set of roles. The fully distributed case, however, can accommodate an infinite set of fillers and roles in a finite network, as shown in Section 3.2. (For further discussion of differences between local and distributed representations, see Chapter 5 (51).)

3 Tensor Product Representation: Properties

In Section 2, I defined the tensor product representation and showed that several representations used in previous connectionist models are special cases of the tensor product representation. In this section, I will discuss a number of general properties of this representation. The case of interest is fully distributed representation; while most of the results apply also to the more localized special cases, in these cases they become rather trivial.

3.1 Unbinding

Until now, I have ignored a crucial and obvious question: if the realizations of all the variable bindings necessary for a particular structure are superimposed on top of each other in a single set of binding units, how can we be sure the binding information is all kept straight? (See Box 1 for exemplification.) In this section, we explore this question via the **unbinding** process: taking the tensor product realization for a complex structure and extracting from it the filler for a particular role (Box 2). Under what conditions can we perform this unbinding operation accurately?

(20) *Theorem.* Let $\psi_{F/R}$ be a tensor product realization induced by a role decomposition with single-valued roles. Suppose the vectors realizing the roles bound in a structure **s** are all linearly independent. Then each role can be unbound with complete accuracy: for each bound role r_i there is an operation that takes the vector $\psi_{F/R}(\mathbf{s})$ realizing **s** into the vector $\mathbf{f}_i$ realizing the filler $\mathtt{f}_i$ bound to r_i.

Proof. If the role vectors $\{\mathbf{r}_i\}$ being used are linearly independent, then they form a basis for the subspace of V_R that they span. To this basis there corresponds a **dual basis** $\{\mathbf{u}_i\}$ (= $\{\mathbf{r}^+_i\}$ in the notation of Box 5:1 (8)); these vectors by definition satisfy

$$\mathbf{r}_i \cdot \mathbf{u}_j = \delta_{ij} = \begin{cases} 1 & \text{if } i = j \\ 0 & \text{if } i \neq j \end{cases}.$$

That is, the inner (dot) product with $\mathbf{u}_i$ in V_R maps the single role vector $\mathbf{r}_i$ to 1 and all other role vectors to 0. Call $\{\mathbf{u}_i\}$ the **unbinding vectors** for roles $\{r_i\}$. (The matrix formed by combining all vectors $\{\mathbf{u}_i\}$ is just the inverse of the matrix formed from the vectors $\{\mathbf{r}_i\}$.) Now let **s** be the tensor product realization of a structure in which the roles $\{r_i\}$ are respectively bound to the fillers $\{\mathtt{f}_i\}$. Then we can extract $\mathtt{f}_i$ from **s**, or **unbind** r_i, by the **inner product in** V_R of **s** with the unbinding vector $\mathbf{u}_i$, defined as follows:

$$\mathbf{s} \cdot \mathbf{u}_i = \left(\sum_j \mathbf{f}_j \otimes \mathbf{r}_j\right) \cdot \mathbf{u}_i \equiv \sum_j \mathbf{f}_j (\mathbf{r}_j \cdot \mathbf{u}_i) = \sum_j \mathbf{f}_j \delta_{ji} = \mathbf{f}_i;$$

that is,

$$[\mathbf{s} \cdot \mathbf{u}_i]_\varphi = \sum_\rho \sum_j [\mathbf{f}_j]_\varphi [\mathbf{r}_j]_\rho [\mathbf{u}_i]_\rho \equiv \sum_j [\mathbf{f}_j]_\varphi (\mathbf{r}_j \cdot \mathbf{u}_i) = \sum_j [\mathbf{f}_j]_\varphi \delta_{ji} = [\mathbf{f}_i]_\varphi.$$

(21) *Definition.* The procedure defined in the preceding proof is the **exact unbinding procedure.**

Let unbinding of role r_i be performed as in the previous proof, but in place of the unbinding vector $\mathbf{u}_i$ use the role vector $\mathbf{r}_i$ itself. This is the **self-addressing unbinding procedure.**

Unlike the exact binding procedure, the self-addressing unbinding procedure is defined for any set of role vectors, even if they are not linearly independent (see Box 2).

(22) **Intrusion Theorem**

Suppose the self-addressing procedure is used to unbind roles. If the role vectors are all orthogonal, the correct filler pattern will be generated, apart from an overall magnitude factor. Otherwise, the pattern generated will be a weighted superposition of the pattern of the correct filler, $\mathbf{f}_i$, and all the other fillers, $\{\mathbf{f}_j\}_{j\neq i}$. In this superposition, the weight of each erroneous pattern $\mathbf{f}_j$ relative to the correct pattern $\mathbf{f}_i$, the **intrusion of role j into role i**, is

$$\frac{\mathbf{r}_i \cdot \mathbf{r}_j}{\|\mathbf{r}_i\|^2} = \cos\theta_{ji} \frac{\|\mathbf{r}_j\|}{\|\mathbf{r}_i\|},$$

where θ_{ji} is the angle between the vectors $\mathbf{r}_j$ and $\mathbf{r}_i$.

Proof. Repeating the computation of the previous proof with $\mathbf{r}_i$ replacing $\mathbf{u}_i$,

$$\mathbf{s} \cdot \mathbf{r}_i = \left(\sum_j \mathbf{f}_j \otimes \mathbf{r}_j\right) \cdot \mathbf{r}_i = \sum_j \mathbf{f}_j (\mathbf{r}_j \cdot \mathbf{r}_i) = (\mathbf{r}_i \cdot \mathbf{r}_i)\mathbf{f}_i + \sum_{j\neq i} (\mathbf{r}_j \cdot \mathbf{r}_i)\mathbf{f}_j.$$

In this weighted superposition, the ratio of the coefficient of each incorrect filler $\mathbf{f}_j$ to that of the correct filler $\mathbf{f}_i$ is

$$\frac{\mathbf{r}_j \cdot \mathbf{r}_i}{\mathbf{r}_i \cdot \mathbf{r}_i}.$$

The denominator is $\|\mathbf{r}_i\|^2$ and the numerator is $\cos\theta_{ji} \|\mathbf{r}_j\| \|\mathbf{r}_i\|$, giving the claimed result (see Box 5:1 (6)).

Since the tensor product binding realization is symmetric between role and filler, the unbinding procedures given above can also be used to retrieve a role pattern from the filler pattern to which it is bound. While there is no asymmetry between role and filler in the realization of a single binding, an asymmetry may result from the combination of many bindings in the realization of a structured object. For while role decompositions often involve single-valued roles, it is uncommon to encounter single-valued *fillers*. (For example, for strings, the role *first-element* has only one filler, but a filler **A** may fill many roles.) When multiple roles are bound to the same filler $\mathbf{f}_i$, unbinding as above but with the filler $\mathbf{f}_i$ replacing the role $\mathbf{r}_i$ (using the inner product in V_F rather than in V_R) will yield the superposition of all the role vectors bound to $\mathbf{f}_i$.

Box 1. Uniqueness of constituent decomposition exemplified

Consider the case of structures defined by two roles, r_0 and r_1 (e.g., binary trees, with the roles *left-subtree* and *right-subtree*). Assume that the vectors realizing these roles, $\mathbf{r}_0$ and $\mathbf{r}_1$, are linearly independent, and assume the realization of the fillers is faithful. (That is, since for the symbols **A** and **C**, **A** ≠ **C**, then for the vectors realizing them, **A** ≠ **C**. But the filler vectors {**A**, **B**, **C**, …} need not be linearly independent.) Suppose we are given a vector **v**; is it possible that this could be ambiguous between the realizations of two different structures? To begin with the simplest case, where the fillers of the roles are atomic symbols, this question becomes: is it possible that **v** could be ambiguous between the realization of a structure with bindings {**A**/r_0, **B**/r_1} (e.g., the tree **[A B]**) and that of a different structure with bindings {**C**/r_0, **D**/r_1} (e.g., the tree **[C D]**)?

Suppose (for the purpose of deriving a contradiction) that constituent decomposition *were* ambiguous, that is, that $\mathbf{v}$ could be written in two ways:

(1) $\mathbf{v} = \mathbf{A} \otimes \mathbf{r}_0 + \mathbf{B} \otimes \mathbf{r}_1$;

(2) $\mathbf{v} = \mathbf{C} \otimes \mathbf{r}_0 + \mathbf{D} \otimes \mathbf{r}_1$.

In order for this to constitute ambiguity, it would have to be that either $\mathbf{A} \neq \mathbf{C}$ or $\mathbf{B} \neq \mathbf{D}$. Suppose it were the case that $\mathbf{A} \neq \mathbf{C}$; exactly parallel reasoning would apply if $\mathbf{B} \neq \mathbf{D}$. With $\mathbf{A} \neq \mathbf{C}$, it would follow that $\mathbf{A} \neq \mathbf{C}$, since the realization of fillers is faithful. Now subtracting (2) from (1) would give

(3) $$\begin{aligned} \mathbf{0} &= [\mathbf{A} \otimes \mathbf{r}_0 - \mathbf{C} \otimes \mathbf{r}_0] + [\mathbf{B} \otimes \mathbf{r}_1 - \mathbf{D} \otimes \mathbf{r}_1] \\ &= [\mathbf{A} - \mathbf{C}] \otimes \mathbf{r}_0 + [\mathbf{B} - \mathbf{D}] \otimes \mathbf{r}_1, \end{aligned}$$

that is,

(4) $[\mathbf{A} - \mathbf{C}] \otimes \mathbf{r}_0 = [\mathbf{D} - \mathbf{B}] \otimes \mathbf{r}_1$.

Given the definition of the tensor product, in terms of components we would then have, for all φ and ϱ,

(5) $[\mathbf{A} - \mathbf{C}]_\varphi [\mathbf{r}_0]_\varrho = [\mathbf{D} - \mathbf{B}]_\varphi [\mathbf{r}_1]_\varrho$.

In order that $\mathbf{A} \neq \mathbf{C}$, it would have to be that these vectors differ in at least one component φ: call it φ^*; that is, $[\mathbf{A}]_{\varphi^*} \neq [\mathbf{C}]_{\varphi^*}$. Since $[\mathbf{A}]_{\varphi^*} - [\mathbf{C}]_{\varphi^*} \neq 0$, it would be possible to set $\varphi = \varphi^*$ in (5) and divide by $[\mathbf{A}]_{\varphi^*} - [\mathbf{C}]_{\varphi^*}$, resulting in

(6) $[\mathbf{r}_0]_\varrho = \left[([\mathbf{D}]_{\varphi^*} - [\mathbf{B}]_{\varphi^*})/([\mathbf{A}]_{\varphi^*} - [\mathbf{C}]_{\varphi^*})\right] [\mathbf{r}_1]_\varrho$.

Since this holds for all ϱ, it would then follow that

(7) $\mathbf{r}_0 = c\mathbf{r}_1$,

where the scalar $c \equiv ([\mathbf{D}]_{\varphi^*} - [\mathbf{B}]_{\varphi^*})/([\mathbf{A}]_{\varphi^*} - [\mathbf{C}]_{\varphi^*})$. This would contradict the assumption that the role vectors $\mathbf{r}_0$, $\mathbf{r}_1$ are independent. So it must not be possible for constituent decomposition of $\mathbf{v}$ to be ambiguous.

The preceding argument shows that constituent decomposition is unambiguous when the fillers are atoms. In the case of recursive structures such as binary trees, the lowest-level fillers in the tree are atoms, but higher fillers are themselves trees (subtrees of the full tree). In this case, the argument above can itself be applied recursively. Given $\mathbf{v}$, the argument shows that if $\mathbf{v}$ can be written in two ways,

(8) $\mathbf{v} = \mathbf{a} \otimes \mathbf{r}_0 + \mathbf{b} \otimes \mathbf{r}_1 = \mathbf{c} \otimes \mathbf{r}_0 + \mathbf{d} \otimes \mathbf{r}_1$,

then it must be that $\mathbf{a} = \mathbf{c}$ and that $\mathbf{b} = \mathbf{d}$. If $\mathbf{a}$ and $\mathbf{b}$ realize atoms, we are done: the above argument applies directly. If $\mathbf{a}$ realizes not an atom but a subtree, we just apply the same argument again, replacing $\mathbf{v}$ with $\mathbf{a}$, concluding that its constituent decomposition is unique. Either these are atoms, and we are done, or we are not, and we apply the argument once again to the nonatomic constituents. Eventually, the process must terminate by reaching atoms, by the definition of a tree.

Figure 4

Box 1

Box 2. Extraction of constituents exemplified

The process of constituent extraction can be illustrated with the help of a two-dimensional picture, if we take a simple enough case and break the problem into small enough pieces.

Consider the example discussed in Box 1, a vector **v** realizing the tree **[A B]**. To extract the left constituent is to compute **A** from the vector

(1) $\mathbf{v} = \mathbf{A} \otimes \mathbf{r}_0 + \mathbf{B} \otimes \mathbf{r}_1.$

Using the definition of the tensor product to rewrite this equation, the components of **v** are

(2) $v_{\varphi\varrho} = [\mathbf{A}]_\varphi [\mathbf{r}_0]_\varrho + [\mathbf{B}]_\varphi [\mathbf{r}_1]_\varrho.$

If we put together all the components with a fixed φ value φ^* and different ϱ values into a vector $\mathbf{v}^{(\varphi^*)}$ with components

(3) $[\mathbf{v}^{(\varphi^*)}]_\varrho \equiv v_{\varphi^*\varrho},$

then we get

(4) $\mathbf{v}^{(\varphi^*)} = A_{\varphi^*} \mathbf{r}_0 + B_{\varphi^*} \mathbf{r}_1.$

Our problem is to compute **A** from **v**, which we do by computing each component A_{φ^*} of **A** from the vector $\mathbf{v}^{(\varphi^*)}$. The method is shown in the following diagram:

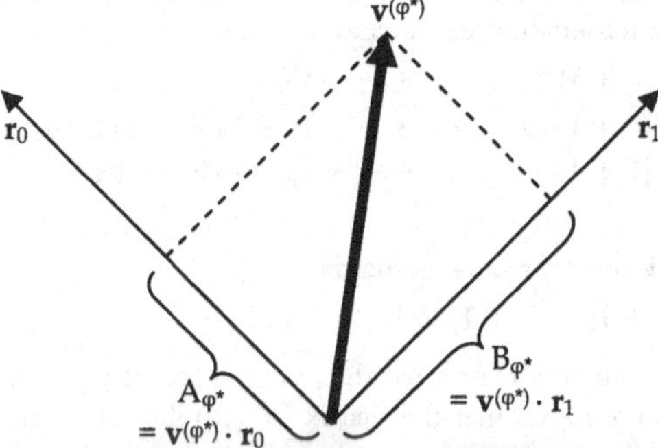

$\mathbf{v}^{(\varphi^*)}$ is a weighted combination of the vectors $\mathbf{r}_0$ and $\mathbf{r}_1$, and we need to determine the weight of $\mathbf{r}_0$, which is precisely the number A_{φ^*} we seek. But this can be done easily, using a basic vector operation: the dot product. The diagram illustrates the simplest case, when $\mathbf{r}_0$ and $\mathbf{r}_1$ are **orthonormal**: at right angles to each other and of length 1. In this case, we simply take the dot product of $\mathbf{v}^{(\varphi^*)}$ with $\mathbf{r}_0$, $\mathbf{v}^{(\varphi^*)} \cdot \mathbf{r}_0$, and the result is exactly what we want: A_{φ^*}. Geometrically, in this case, taking the dot product of $\mathbf{v}^{(\varphi^*)}$ with $\mathbf{r}_0$ amounts simply to determining the length of the perpendicular projection of $\mathbf{v}^{(\varphi^*)}$ onto an axis running through $\mathbf{r}_0$.

Algebraically, taking the dot product $\mathbf{v}^{(\varphi^*)} \cdot \mathbf{r}_0$ is performing the following computation:

(5) $A_{\varphi*} = \mathbf{v}^{(\varphi*)} \cdot \mathbf{r}_0 = \Sigma_\varrho [\mathbf{v}^{(\varphi*)}]_\varrho [\mathbf{r}_0]_\varrho = \Sigma_\varrho v_{\varphi*\varrho} [\mathbf{r}_0]_\varrho = \Sigma_{\varphi'\varrho} \delta_{\varphi*\varphi'} [\mathbf{r}_0]_\varrho v_{\varphi'\varrho} = [\mathbf{W}^{(0)} \cdot \mathbf{v}]_{\varphi*}.$

That is,

(6) $\mathbf{A} = \mathbf{W}^{(0)} \cdot \mathbf{v},$

where the symbol $\delta_{\varphi\varphi'}$—the Kronecker δ—denotes 1 if $\varphi = \varphi'$ and 0 if $\varphi \neq \varphi'$, and the matrix $\mathbf{W}^{(0)}$ has elements

(7) $[\mathbf{W}^{(0)}]_{\varphi,\varphi'\varrho} \equiv \delta_{\varphi\varphi'} [\mathbf{r}_0]_\varrho.$

$\mathbf{W}^{(0)}$ creates a rank-1 tensor **A** from a rank-2 tensor **v**, so its left matrix tag is a single index (φ) while its right tag is a pair of indices ($\varphi'\varrho$); the summation in the matrix multiplication '·' runs over this tag, that is, over all values of the pair of indices (recall Box 5:1 (3)).

Now the matrix of Kronecker δ values $\{\delta_{\varphi\varphi'}\}$ forms the **identity matrix** on the filler space V_F: $\mathbf{1}_F$. This means we can write $\mathbf{W}^{(0)}$ as follows:

(8) $\mathbf{W}^{(0)} = \mathbf{1}_F \otimes \mathbf{r}_0$; i.e., $[\mathbf{W}^{(0)}]_{\varphi,\varphi'\varrho} = [\mathbf{1}_F \otimes \mathbf{r}_0]_{\varphi,\varphi'\varrho} = [\mathbf{1}_F]_{\varphi\varphi'} [\mathbf{r}_0]_\varrho = \delta_{\varphi\varphi'} [\mathbf{r}_0]_\varrho.$

As we will see in Section 4, the full recursive function that extracts the left subtree of a tree must be realized by a matrix that maps tensor product vectors of rank $n+2$ (realizing trees of depth $n+1$) into tensor product vectors of rank $n+1$; **v** in our example here just involves the case of $n = 0$. For each n, it turns out we need

(9) $\mathbf{W}^{(n)} = \mathbf{1}_F \otimes \mathbf{1}_R \otimes \cdots \otimes \mathbf{1}_R \otimes \mathbf{r}_0$

with n factors of $\mathbf{1}_R$, the identity matrix on V_R. The matrix **W** that realizes the complete recursive extract-left-subtree function is

(10)
$$\begin{aligned} \mathbf{W} &= \mathbf{W}^{(0)} + \mathbf{W}^{(1)} + \cdots + \mathbf{W}^{(n)} + \cdots \\ &= \mathbf{1}_F \otimes \mathbf{r}_0 + \mathbf{1}_F \otimes \mathbf{1}_R \otimes \mathbf{r}_0 + \cdots + \mathbf{1}_F \otimes \mathbf{1}_R \otimes \cdots \otimes \mathbf{1}_R \otimes \mathbf{r}_0 + \cdots \\ &= \mathbf{1}_F \otimes [1 + \mathbf{1}_R + \cdots + \mathbf{1}_R \otimes \mathbf{1}_R \otimes \cdots \otimes \mathbf{1}_R + \cdots] \otimes \mathbf{r}_0 \\ &= \mathbf{I} \otimes \mathbf{r}_0, \end{aligned}$$

where **I** is the **feed-forward recursion matrix**

(11) $\mathbf{I} \equiv \mathbf{1}_F \otimes [1 + \mathbf{1}_R + \cdots + \mathbf{1}_R \otimes \mathbf{1}_R \otimes \cdots \otimes \mathbf{1}_R + \cdots].$

(This is simply the identity matrix for the entire space of representations of trees of all depths.) Section 4 shows that the matrix **W** (10) illustrates the general form of a large class of recursive functions:

(12) $\mathbf{W} = \mathbf{I} \otimes \underline{\mathbf{W}},$

where the finite matrix $\underline{\mathbf{W}}$ determining the function is simply the column vector $\mathbf{r}_0$.[10]

The preceding analysis of the case where $\{\mathbf{r}_0, \mathbf{r}_1\}$ are orthonormal vectors can be immediately generalized to the case where they are merely independent vectors; it suffices to replace $\mathbf{r}_0$, $\mathbf{r}_1$ in the previous equations with the unbinding vectors $\mathbf{u}_0$, $\mathbf{u}_1$. The following figure illustrates:

[10] In the more precise analysis of Section 4.1.4, we will see that in general, $\underline{\mathbf{W}} = \mathbf{u}_0^T$, where $\mathbf{u}_0$ is the unbinding vector corresponding to $\mathbf{r}_0$.

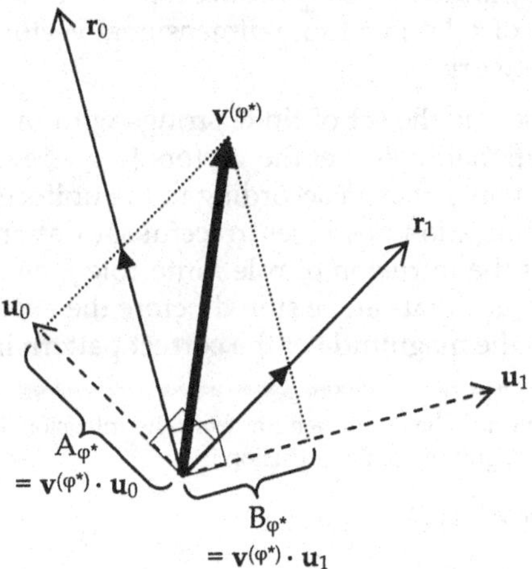

The unbinding vector $\mathbf{u}_0$ is orthogonal to $\mathbf{r}_1$; $\mathbf{u}_1$ is orthogonal to $\mathbf{r}_2$. The length of $\mathbf{u}_0$ is the inverse of the length of $\mathbf{r}_0$, while the length of $\mathbf{u}_1$ is the inverse of the length of $\mathbf{r}_1$. This entails that $\mathbf{u}_0 \cdot \mathbf{r}_1 = 0$ while $\mathbf{u}_0 \cdot \mathbf{r}_0 = 1$, and similarly with 1 and 0 interchanged.

3.2 Graceful saturation

Like a digital memory with n registers, a connectionist system that uses n pools of units to represent a structure with n roles has a discrete saturation point. Structures with n or fewer filled roles can be represented precisely, but for larger structures some information must be omitted entirely. The form of saturation characteristic of connectionist systems (e.g., connectionist memories) is less discrete than this; this is one aspect of the **graceful degradation** advertised for connectionist systems.

Aspects of graceful degradation can be formally characterized as follows:

(23) *Definition.* Let F/R be a role decomposition of S. A connectionist realization ψ of S has **unbounded sensitivity** with respect to F/R if for arbitrarily large n,

$$\psi\left(\bigwedge_{i=1}^{n} \mathbf{f}_i / r_i\right)$$

varies as $\mathbf{f}_i$ varies, for each $i = 1, 2, \dots, n$.

If for sufficiently large n the realization of structures containing n filler/role bindings is not faithful, then ψ **saturates**.

If ψ saturates and has unbounded sensitivity, then ψ possesses **graceful saturation.**

The tensor product representation, unlike local and role register representations, can exhibit graceful saturation. To see this, let us now consider an example that also illustrates how fully distributed tensor product representations can be used to represent an infinite number of roles in a finite-dimensional vector space corresponding to a finite connectionist network.

(24) *Theorem.* Suppose S is the set of finite strings with unbounded length, and let $\{r_i\}_{i=1}^{\infty}$ be the positional roles. Let the vectors $\{\mathbf{r}_i\}_{i=1}^{\infty}$ be unit vectors in N-dimensional space, randomly chosen according to the uniform distribution. Then this tensor product realization possesses graceful saturation. The expected value of the magnitude of the intrusion of role i into role j is proportional to $N^{-1/2}$. The number of bindings n that can be stored before the expected total magnitude of intrusions equals the magnitude of the correct pattern increases as $N^{1/2}$.

Proof. Since all role vectors have unit length, from the Intrusion Theorem (22), the expected value of the magnitude of the intrusion is

$$\mathrm{EI} = \frac{1}{V_{N-1}} \int_0^{\pi} |\cos\theta_{ji}|\, V(\theta_{ji})\, d\theta_{ji}\,.$$

Here V_{N-1} is the $(N-1)$-dimensional volume of the unit sphere in N-space, and $V(\theta_{ji})$ is the volume of the subset of the unit sphere in N-space consisting of all vectors having angle θ_{ji} with the vector $\mathbf{r}_i$. This subset is in fact a sphere in $(N-1)$-space with radius $\sin\theta_{ji}$. To see this, choose a Cartesian coordinate system in N-space in which the first coordinate direction lies along $\mathbf{r}_i$. Then the first coordinate x_1 of all points in the subset is $\cos\theta_{ji}$. Since all points lie on the unit sphere, we have

$$1 = \sum_{i=1}^{N} x_i^2 = \cos^2\theta_{ji} + \sum_{i=2}^{N} x_i^2,$$

which implies

$$\sum_{i=2}^{N} x_i^2 = 1 - \cos^2\theta_{ji} = \sin^2\theta_{ji}.$$

Thus, the subset is a sphere in $(N-1)$-space with radius $\sin\theta_{ji}$. Therefore,

$$V(\theta_{ji}) = V_{N-2}\sin^{N-2}\theta_{ji}\,.$$

Thus, the expected intrusion is

$$\mathrm{EI} = \frac{V_{N-2}}{V_{N-1}}\, 2 \int_0^{\pi/2} \sin^{N-2}\theta\cos\theta\, d\theta$$

$$= \frac{V_{N-2}}{V_{N-1}}\, 2 \int_0^{1} z^{N-2}\, dz = \frac{V_{N-2}}{V_{N-1}} \frac{2}{N-1}$$

(using the substitution $z = \sin\theta$, which implies $dz = \cos\theta\, d\theta$). The ratio of volumes of spheres of successive dimensions V_{N-2}/V_{N-1} is a complex expression taking different forms depending on whether N is odd or even (see the appendix of Smolensky 1987b). Since these details are quite irrelevant to the general behavior as N increases, we can look at the mean of two successive such ratios (using the geometric mean since the quantities are ratios); this is given by the simple expression[11]

[11] There is a rough calculation suggesting that, as the dimension N grows, the expected inner product of role vectors should decrease with the square root of N. Suppose for the first N role vectors we chose an orthonormal basis. For the next vector, suppose we choose one that is equidistant from all the others; an example is the vector whose components in the orthonormal basis are $C^{-1}(1, 1, ..., 1)$. In

$\sqrt{(N-1)/2\pi}$.

The result then is

$$\mathrm{EI} = \sqrt{\frac{2}{\pi(N-1)}}.$$

As claimed, the expected interference falls as $N^{-\frac{1}{2}}$.

For a structure involving n bindings, the expected total magnitude of intrusions of all $\{r_j\}_{j \neq i}$ into r_i is $(n-1)$EI. This equals unity at

$$n = \sqrt{\pi/2}(N-1)^{\frac{1}{2}} + 1,$$

which increases as the square root of N.

The estimate of interference given in the preceding theorem is extremely conservative, since it computes the expected sum of the *absolute values* of all intrusions. In fact, for any given component of the desired filler, the errors caused by intrusions will typically be of both signs, producing a net error potentially much smaller than the worst case analyzed above.

3.3 Storage of structured data in connectionist memories

One of the primary uses of connectionist representations is as objects of associations in associative memories. Because of its mathematical simplicity, it is possible to analyze the use of tensor product representations in such memories. Here I analyze pair association since it is simpler than content-addressed auto-association, which is perhaps a purer example of connectionist memory (e.g., Rumelhart, Hinton, and McClelland 1986).

Let us start with the simplest possible case.

(25) *Theorem.* Suppose $\psi_{F/R}$ is a tensor product realization of S induced by a decomposition with single-valued roles, with realizations of fillers and roles in which all filler vectors are mutually orthogonal, as are all role vectors. Let $\{\mathbf{s}^{(k)}\}$ be a subset of S, and let the vectors realizing these structures, $\{\mathbf{s}^{(k)}\}$, be associated in a connectionist network using the Hebb rule with the patterns $\{\mathbf{t}^{(k)}\}$. Then if the structures $\{\mathbf{s}^{(k)}\}$ share no common fillers (i.e., for each role, all structures have different fillers), the associator will function perfectly; otherwise, there will be cross-talk that is monotonic in the degree of shared fillers. In particular, the output associated with $\mathbf{s}^{(l)}$ is proportional to

$$\mathbf{t}^{(l)} + \sum_{k \neq l} \mu_{lk} \mathbf{t}^{(k)},$$

where

order for this vector to have unit length, the normalization constant C must be $N^{\frac{1}{2}}$. Now the inner product of this vector with any of the others is $C^{-1} = N^{-\frac{1}{2}}$.

$$\mu_{lk} = \frac{\sum_{i:\mathbf{f}_i^{(l)}=\mathbf{f}_i^{(k)}} \left\|\mathbf{f}_i^{(l)}\right\|^2 \|\mathbf{r}_i\|^2}{\sum_i \left\|\mathbf{f}_i^{(l)}\right\|^2 \|\mathbf{r}_i\|^2}.$$

It follows immediately that if the filler and role vectors are normalized to unit length, and the number of roles filled in $\mathbf{s}^{(l)}$ is n, then $\mu_{lk} = n_{lk}/n$, where n_{lk} is the number of roles in which $\mathbf{s}^{(l)}$ and $\mathbf{s}^{(k)}$ have the same filler. (Compare the discussion in Box 5:2 following (4).)

Proof. The Hebbian weights are

$$\mathbf{W} = \sum_k \mathbf{t}^{(k)}\mathbf{s}^{(k)\mathrm{T}}.$$

Thus, the output generated from the input realizing $\mathbf{s}^{(l)}$ is

$$\begin{aligned}
\mathbf{W}\mathbf{s}^{(l)} &= \sum_k \mathbf{t}^{(k)}\mathbf{s}^{(k)\mathrm{T}}\mathbf{s}^{(l)} \\
&= \sum_k \mathbf{t}^{(k)} \left[\sum_i \mathbf{f}_i^{(k)} \otimes \mathbf{r}_i\right] \cdot \left[\sum_j \mathbf{f}_j^{(l)} \otimes \mathbf{r}_j\right] \\
&= \sum_k \mathbf{t}^{(k)} \sum_i \sum_j \left(\mathbf{f}_i^{(k)} \cdot \mathbf{f}_j^{(l)}\right)\left(\mathbf{r}_i \cdot \mathbf{r}_j\right) \\
&= \sum_k \mathbf{t}^{(k)} \sum_i \sum_j \left(\delta_{\mathbf{f}_i^{(k)},\mathbf{f}_j^{(l)}} \left\|\mathbf{f}_i^{(k)}\right\|^2\right)\left(\delta_{\mathbf{r}_i,\mathbf{r}_j} \|\mathbf{r}_i\|^2\right) \\
&= \sum_k \mathbf{t}^{(k)} \sum_i \delta_{\mathbf{f}_i^{(k)},\mathbf{f}_i^{(l)}} \left\|\mathbf{f}_i^{(k)}\right\|^2 \|\mathbf{r}_i\|^2 \\
&= \left[\sum_i \left\|\mathbf{f}_i^{(l)}\right\|^2 \|\mathbf{r}_i\|^2\right]\mathbf{t}^{(l)} + \sum_{k \neq l}\left[\sum_i \left\|\mathbf{f}_i^{(l)}\right\|^2 \|\mathbf{r}_i\|^2 \delta_{\mathbf{f}_i^{(k)},\mathbf{f}_i^{(l)}}\right]\mathbf{t}^{(k)}.
\end{aligned}$$

The first term here is the correct associate $\mathbf{t}^{(l)}$ weighted by a positive coefficient. The second term is a sum of all other (incorrect) associates $\{\mathbf{t}^{(l)}\}_{k \neq l}$, each weighted by a non-negative coefficient. These coefficients will all vanish if there are no common fillers. Taking the ratio of the coefficient of $\mathbf{t}^{(k)}$ to that of $\mathbf{t}^{(l)}$ gives the claimed result.

The Hebb rule is capable of accurately learning associations to patterns that are orthogonal. If the patterns are not necessarily orthogonal but are still linearly independent, the associations can be accurately stored in a connectionist memory using the more complex Widrow and Hoff (1960) or delta learning procedure (Rumelhart, Hinton, and McClelland 1986). So the question is, what collection of symbolic structures have linearly independent realizations under the tensor product representation? To answer this question, it is useful to define the following concept:

(26) *Definition.* Let F/R be a role decomposition of S and let $k \mapsto \mathbf{s}^{(k)}$ be a sequence of elements in S. An **annihilator** of $k \mapsto \mathbf{s}^{(k)}$ with respect to F/R is a sequence of real numbers $k \mapsto \alpha^{(k)}$, not all 0, such that, for all fillers $\mathbf{f} \in F$, and all roles $r \in R$,

$$\sum_{k:\mathbf{f}/r\in\beta(s^{(k)})} \alpha^{(k)} = 0.$$

That is, for any binding $\mathbf{f}/r$, the structures $\mathbf{s}^{(k)}$ in the sequence that possess this binding have values $\alpha^{(k)}$, which sum to 0.

For example, consider the sequence of strings {**AX**, **BX**, **AY**, **BY**}. With respect to the positional role decomposition, this has an annihilator (+1 , −1 , −1 , +1), since for each filler/role binding in {$\mathbf{A}/r_1$, $\mathbf{B}/r_1$, $\mathbf{X}/r_2$, $\mathbf{Y}/r_2$}, the corresponding annihilator elements are {+1 , −1}, which sum to 0.

(27) *Theorem.* Suppose that ψ is a tensor product realization of the structures S, and that $k \mapsto \mathbf{s}^{(k)}$ is a sequence of distinct elements in S. Suppose that the filler vectors **f** realizing the fillers bound in the elements $\{\mathbf{s}^{(k)}\}$ are all linearly independent, and that the same is true of the role vectors **r** realizing the roles bound in the elements $\{\mathbf{s}^{(k)}\}$. If $k \mapsto \mathbf{s}^{(k)}$ has no annihilator with respect to F/R, then associations to the tensor product realizations $\{\psi(\mathbf{s}^{(k)})\}$ can all be simultaneously and accurately stored in a connectionist memory by using the Widrow-Hoff learning rule.

Proof. Let

$$\psi(\mathbf{s}^{(k)}) = \textstyle\sum_i \mathbf{f}_i^{(k)} \otimes \mathbf{r}_i .$$

Here we use the same set of roles $\{\mathbf{r}_i\}$ for all structures $\{\mathbf{s}^{(k)}\}$; this can always be done provided we allow the filler vector $\mathbf{f}_i^{(k)}$ to equal the zero vector $\mathbf{0}$ whenever the role r_i is unbound in structure $\mathbf{s}^{(k)}$.

By the remarks immediately preceding the definition of annihilator (26), it is sufficient to show that the patterns $\{\psi(\mathbf{s}^{(k)})\}$ are all linearly independent. Suppose on the contrary that there are coefficients $\{\alpha^{(k)}\}$, not all 0, such that

$$0 = \sum_k \alpha^{(k)} \psi(s^{(k)})$$

$$= \sum_k \alpha^{(k)} \left[\sum_i \mathbf{f}_i^{(k)} \otimes \mathbf{r}_i\right] = \sum_i \left[\sum_k \alpha^{(k)} \mathbf{f}_i^{(k)}\right] \otimes \mathbf{r}_i .$$

Then, because the role vectors $\{\mathbf{r}_i\}$ are linearly independent, this implies that for all i,

$$\textstyle\sum_k \alpha^{(k)} \mathbf{f}_i^{(k)} = \mathbf{0}.$$

Now we rewrite this as a sum over all distinct filler vectors:

$$\sum_\gamma \mathbf{f}_\gamma \sum_{k:\mathbf{f}_i^{(k)}=\mathbf{f}_\gamma} \alpha^{(k)} = \mathbf{0}.$$

Since the filler vectors $\{\mathbf{f}_\gamma\}$ are linearly independent, this implies, for all i and for all γ,

$$\sum_{k:\mathbf{f}_i^{(k)}=\mathbf{f}_\gamma} \alpha^{(k)} = 0.$$

This means exactly that $\{\alpha^{(k)}\}$ is an annihilator of the sequence of structures $k \mapsto \mathbf{s}^{(k)}$. Since by hypothesis such an annihilator does not exist, it must be that the representations $\{\psi(\mathbf{s}^{(k)})\}$ are linearly independent.

It was noted above that the strings {**AX**, **BX**, **AY**, **BY**} possess an annihilator with respect to the positional role decomposition. This means that the tensor product realizations of these strings are not linearly independent, even under the preceding theorem's assumptions of linearly independent filler and role vectors. They cannot therefore be accurately associated with arbitrary patterns even using the Widrow-Hoff learning rule. On the other hand, it is easy to see that the strings {**AX**, **BX**, **AY**} do *not* possess an annihilator; the preceding theorem shows that their tensor product realizations can therefore be accurately associated with arbitrary patterns.

3.4 Learning optimal role representations

The tensor product representation is constructed from connectionist representations of fillers and roles. As indicated in Section 2.3.2.3, distributed representation of fillers has been used in many connectionist models for some time; usually, these representations are built from an analysis of the fillers in terms of features relevant for the task being performed. But what about distributed representations of roles? This becomes a major question in tensor product representation. For many applications, it is easy to imagine task-appropriate features for roles that could serve well as the basis for distributed role representations. For example, Figure 2 shows a distributed representation of positional roles with the useful property that nearby positions are represented by similar patterns. Algorithms such as back-propagation (Rumelhart, Hinton, and Williams 1986) can also be adapted to learn role representations for a given task, using a network for performing tensor product binding and back-propagating through its multiplicative connections.

It is also possible to analyze the question of distributed representations for roles from a domain-independent perspective. In a general sense, a set of role vectors might be considered optimal if their fillers can be unbound in a way that minimizes the total unbinding error. Smolensky 1987b introduces such an error measure, gives algebraic and geometric characterizations of optimal sets of role vectors, and shows how a simple recurrent linear network can perform gradient descent in the error measure to find the optimal vectors. This learning algorithm is a 'recirculation algorithm' in which activity cycles in a loop, and the change in a weight $W_{\alpha\beta}$ from β to α is proportional to the activity at β times the *rate of change* of activity at α over time. See Smolensky 1987b for full detail.

4 Extension to Recursive Structures: Trees

While the tensor product technique is general enough to apply to virtually any kind of recursive symbolic structure, here we will examine only the case of binary trees, the basic data structure of formal syntax and of the classic symbolic programming language, Lisp.[12]

[12] With respect to formal languages, binary trees suffice for context-free languages (using Chomsky normal form). With respect to natural languages, tree binarity has long been one of the basic principles of generative syntax (e.g., Kayne 1984; Chomsky 1995). For Lisp binary trees, see Box 23:1.

Bound to tree nodes are atomic symbols from an alphabet A. A connectionist realization mapping ψ_A assigns to each atomic symbol $\mathbf{A} \in A$ a vector $\mathbf{A}$ in an atom-realizing vector space V_A. The set of vectors realizing atoms is $\mathcal{A} \equiv \{\mathbf{A} \in V_A \mid \exists \mathbf{A} \in A$ such that $\mathbf{A} = \psi_A(\mathbf{A})\}$. It will be assumed throughout this section that $\mathcal{A}$ is a linearly independent set (the independence assumption of Chapter 5 (9)). Another realization mapping ψ_R assigns to each role r a vector $\mathbf{r}$ in a role-vector space V_R. The set of vectors realizing all the tree roles is $\mathbf{R}$, also assumed to be a linearly independent set.

In this section, we will discuss two closely related filler/role decompositions for trees; 'filler' and 'role' are thus potentially ambiguous. In the first decomposition, the fillers are atomic symbols, and the roles are tree node positions: simple fillers, complex roles. In the second decomposition, the fillers are trees, and the roles are just left or right child of root: now the roles are simple but the fillers are complex. The most basic realization of roles concerns the two roles *left-* and *right-child*. For their realizations to be linearly independent, the role vector space must be at least two-dimensional. But two dimensions do suffice, and we will assume throughout this section that this space is in fact two-dimensional. This makes no difference for the algebra, but for producing schematic drawings for the realization vectors, it is helpful to adopt some concrete value for the dimensionality of the most basic role vectors. The two dimensions will be labeled 0 and 1.

In Section 4.1, we will construct a partially distributed, **stratified** connectionist realization for trees, in which each depth of a tree is realized over a distinct group of units; the vectors realizing all symbols at a given depth are superposed, however, so that within a depth this realization is completely distributed. An extension to a fully distributed, unstratified realization, in which all depths are superposed on one another, is introduced briefly in Section 4.4. Section 4.1 defines a general class $\mathcal{F}$ of recursive functions defined over trees and develops a general scheme for realizing them in feed-forward connectionist networks. Section 4.2 concerns Harmony-maximizing recurrent networks, developing a general method for realizing the rules of any context-free formal language—that is, for designing a weight matrix that defines the Harmony function realizing the harmonic grammar for that language. (Chapter 10 concerns the design of the harmonic grammar itself.)

4.1 Realizing recursive functions in feed-forward networks

4.1.1 Primitive operations on pseudotrees

To begin, we view a binary tree $\mathbf{s}$ as a structure defined by a large (unbounded) number of positions with varying locations relative to the root of the tree. These define a set of positional roles r_x that we can label by binary (or bit) strings such as x = 0101: reading left to right, this string labels the left child (0) of the right child (1) of the left child (0) of the right child (1) of the root of the tree $\mathbf{s}$. The tree operation that extracts the subtree at this location will be denoted $\mathbf{ex}_x$ = $\mathbf{ex}_{0101}$. Clearly, $\mathbf{ex}_{0101}(\mathbf{s})$ is equivalent to the nested sequence of operations $\mathbf{ex}_0(\mathbf{ex}_1(\mathbf{ex}_0(\mathbf{ex}_1(\mathbf{s}))))$.[13]

The bit string labeling the tree's root position is the empty string, which we will write ε. The function that extracts the filler of r_ε — the symbol at the root position — will be denoted $\mathbf{ex}_\varepsilon$. An atom **A** will be equated with the tree containing only the binding $\mathtt{A}/r_\varepsilon$: **A** at the root. $|x|$ denotes the number of bits in the string x, or the tree depth of the position r_x; $|\varepsilon| = 0$.

Decomposing the tree using these structural roles (positions) r_x, each constituent of a tree is one of a set of atoms A — for example, the filler **A** — bound to some role r_x specifying its location. A tree **s** with a set of atoms $\{\mathtt{A}_i\}$ at respective locations $\{x_i\}$ has the tensor product realization $\mathbf{s} = \Sigma_i\, \mathbf{A}_i \otimes \mathbf{r}_{x_i}$. Recalling that $\beta(\mathbf{s})$ denotes the set of all bindings in **s**, this can be written

(28) $$\mathbf{s} = \sum_{\mathtt{A}_i / r_{x_i} \in \beta(s)} \mathbf{A}_i \otimes \mathbf{r}_{x_i}.$$

It will actually prove extremely convenient to consider subsets of the bindings in a tree **s**, as well as the complete set $\beta(\mathbf{s})$ of all bindings. We will thus sometimes work with what will be called 'pseudotrees'; the basic concepts are defined in (29).

(29) *Definition.* Pseudotrees: Symbolic, vectorial, and hybrid

a. A **symbolic pseudotree t** over an alphabet A, or simply an **s-tree**, is a set of bindings $\{\mathtt{A}_i / r_{x_i}\}$ such that each role $r_{x_i} \in R$ is bound to at most one filler $\mathtt{A}_i \in A$. **t** can be represented as $\mathbf{t}^{\varnothing}$, a (standard) tree over the alphabet $A^{\varnothing} \equiv A \cup \{\varnothing\}$, that is, a tree in which some locations are bound to the pseudosymbol $\varnothing$.

b. Given connectionist realization mappings ψ_A: $A \rightarrow \mathbf{A} \subset V_A$ of the atoms A and ψ_R: $R \rightarrow \mathbf{R} \subset V_R$ of the positional roles R, a **vectorial pseudotree** or **v-tree** is a realization of an s-tree, that is, a vector

$$\mathbf{t} = \sum\nolimits_i \mathbf{A}_i \otimes \mathbf{r}_{x_i},$$

where there is at most one term for each role $r_{x_i} \in R$, and where each $\mathbf{A}_i \in \mathbf{A}$. The sum defining **t** will also be written $\Sigma_x\, \mathbf{A}_x \otimes \mathbf{r}_x$. Let $\varnothing$ be realized by the zero vector $\mathbf{0}_A$ of V_A; then **t** is also the realization of $\mathbf{t}^{\varnothing}$.

c. A **hybrid pseudotree** or **h-tree** t is a set of **hybrid bindings** $\{\mathbf{f}_x / r_x\}$ where each role r_x is bound to at most one filler $\mathbf{f}_x$, and each filler $\mathbf{f}_x \in V_A$ is a linear combination of the **atomic vectors** $\mathbf{A} \equiv \{\psi_A(\mathtt{A}) \mid \mathtt{A} \in A\}$ and the **dual vectors** $\mathbf{A}^+ \equiv \{\mathbf{A}^+ \mid \mathbf{A} \in \mathbf{A}\}$. When a role r_x is unbound in t, then $\mathbf{f}_x \equiv \mathbf{0}_A$, the zero vector of V_A. $\mathbf{A}^+$ is the dual basis corresponding to $\mathbf{A}$ (since we are assuming $\mathbf{A}$ to be a linearly independent set, a dual basis exists; Box 5:1 (8)).

[13] The conventional Lisp terminology is as follows. The basic tree operations are `car(s)` = left subtree of the binary tree **s**; `cdr(s)` = right subtree; `cons(u,v)` = the binary tree **s** constructed by joining **u** and **v**, so that **u** = `car(s)` and **v** = `cdr(s)`. Nested sequences of `car`/`cdr` operations are abbreviated as follows, with '`a`' and '`d`' abbreviating '`car`' and '`cdr`': `cadadr(s)` ≡ `car(cdr(car(cdr(s))))`, that is, the left child (`car`) of the right child (`cdr`) of the left child of the right child of the root of the tree **s**; this is our $\mathbf{ex}_{0101}$. In the traditional Lisp syntax, $f(x)$ is written $(f\ x)$; for example, `car(s)` is written `(car s)`.

d. Given two s-trees $\mathtt{t} = \{\mathbf{A}_x/r_x\}$ and $\mathtt{t}' = \{\mathbf{A}'_x/r_x\}$, their **unification** $\mathtt{t} \sqcup \mathtt{t}'$ is the s-tree determined by the union of their bindings,

$$\mathtt{t} \sqcup \mathtt{t}' \equiv \{\mathbf{A}_x/r_x\} \cup \{\mathbf{A}'_x/r_x\},$$

provided that this set of bindings is an s-tree; otherwise, $\mathtt{t} \sqcup \mathtt{t}'$ is undefined. ($\mathtt{t} \sqcup \mathtt{t}'$ is undefined iff there is some role for which $\mathtt{t}$ and $\mathtt{t}'$ have different fillers.)

e. Given two v-trees $\mathbf{t} = \Sigma_x \mathbf{A}_x \otimes \mathbf{r}_x$ and $\mathbf{t}' = \Sigma_x \mathbf{A}'_x \otimes \mathbf{r}_x$ realizing two s-trees $\mathtt{t}$ and $\mathtt{t}'$, their **unification** $\mathbf{t} \sqcup \mathbf{t}'$ is the realization of $\mathtt{t} \sqcup \mathtt{t}'$:

$$\mathbf{t} \sqcup \mathbf{t}' \equiv \Sigma_x \{\mathbf{A}''_x \otimes \mathbf{r}_x \mid \mathbf{A}''_x = \mathbf{f}_x \text{ or } \mathbf{A}''_x = \mathbf{f}'_x\}$$
$$= \mathbf{t} + \mathbf{t}' - \Sigma_x \{\mathbf{A}''_x \otimes \mathbf{r}_x \mid \mathbf{A}''_x = \mathbf{f}_x \text{ and } \mathbf{A}''_x = \mathbf{f}'_x\}.$$

$\mathbf{t} \sqcup \mathbf{t}'$ is undefined iff $\mathtt{t} \sqcup \mathtt{t}'$ is undefined.

f. Given two h-trees $\mathrm{t} = \{\mathbf{f}_x/r_x\}$ and $\mathrm{t}' = \{\mathbf{f}'_x/r_x\}$, define their sum to be

$$\mathrm{t} + \mathrm{t}' \equiv \{(\mathbf{f}_x + \mathbf{f}'_x)/r_x\}$$

(where $\mathbf{f}_x$ or $\mathbf{f}'_x$ is taken to be $\mathbf{0}_A$ if r_x is unbound in t or t', respectively). Other vector operations on V_A are carried over to h-trees similarly; in particular, the **dual** operation is defined by

$$\mathrm{t}^+ \equiv \{\Sigma_i (c_x{}^i \mathbf{A}_i{}^+ + d_x{}^i \mathbf{A}_i)/r_x\} \text{ iff } \mathrm{t} = \{\Sigma_i (c_x{}^i \mathbf{A}_i + d_x{}^i \mathbf{A}_i{}^+)/r_x\}.$$

g. Suppose $\mathtt{t} = \{\mathbf{A}_x/r_x\}$ is an s-tree. Define

$$\mathtt{cons}_0(\mathtt{t}) \equiv \{\mathbf{A}_x/r_{x0}\}; \quad \mathtt{cons}_1(\mathtt{t}) \equiv \{\mathbf{A}_x/r_{x1}\}$$

($\mathtt{cons}_0(\mathtt{t})$ is the s-tree obtained by sliding $\mathtt{t}$ as a whole 'down to the left' so that its root is moved to left-child-of-the-root position; for example, [**A** **B**] becomes [[**A** **B**] Ø].) Then

$$\mathtt{cons}(\mathtt{s}, \mathtt{t}) \equiv \mathtt{cons}_0(\mathtt{s}) \sqcup \mathtt{cons}_1(\mathtt{t}).$$

The roles bound in $\mathtt{cons}_0(\mathtt{t})$—seen below to be $\{r_{x0}\}$—and those bound in $\mathtt{cons}_1(\mathtt{t})$—$\{r_{x1}\}$—do not overlap, so this unification always exists. The realizations of $\mathtt{cons}$, $\mathtt{cons}_0$, and $\mathtt{cons}_1$—namely, **cons**, **cons**$_0$, and **cons**$_1$, respectively—are related by

$$\mathbf{cons}(\mathbf{s}, \mathbf{t}) = \mathbf{cons}_0(\mathbf{s}) + \mathbf{cons}_1(\mathbf{t}).$$

h. Suppose $\mathtt{t} = \{\mathbf{A}_x/r_x\}$ is an s-tree. Define the **0-shift** and **1-shift** functions by

$$\mathtt{sh}_0(\mathtt{t}) \equiv \{\mathbf{A}_x/r_{0x}\}; \quad \mathtt{sh}_1(\mathtt{t}) \equiv \{\mathbf{A}_x/r_{1x}\}$$

($\mathtt{sh}_0(\mathtt{t})$ is obtained by separately moving each atom in $\mathtt{t}$ to the node that was its left child. If $\mathtt{t}$ is a bona fide tree—not just a pseudotree—$\mathtt{sh}_0(\mathtt{t})$ will not be a tree; for example, [**A** **B**] becomes [[**A** Ø] [**B** Ø]].)

The simplest nonnull pseudotree is one consisting of a single binding, for example, $\mathbf{A}/r_{010}$: $\mathtt{t} = \{\mathbf{A}/r_{010}\}$. This can be represented as the tree

$$\mathtt{t}^{\varnothing} = [_{\varnothing}\, [_{\varnothing}\, \varnothing\, [_{\varnothing}\, \mathbf{A}\, \varnothing]]\, \varnothing].$$

Both $\mathtt{t}$ and $\mathtt{t}^{\varnothing}$ have the same realization, $\mathbf{A} \otimes \mathbf{r}_{010}$. The distinction between $\mathtt{t}$ and $\mathtt{t}^{\varnothing}$ will not generally be explicitly marked. Note that Ø is a 'pseudosymbol' in the sense that its realization is $\mathbf{0}_A$; in a faithful realization, this is not permitted of a genuine symbol (4). (Note that $\mathbf{0}_A$ is not linearly independent of any set of vectors.)

A more explicitly recursive view of a binary tree sees it as having only *two* constituents: the subtrees (or atoms) that are the left and right children of the root. In this **recursive role decomposition,** fillers may be either atoms or trees; the set of possible fillers F is the same as the original set of structures S (5).

For binary trees, a **recursive** realization ψ is one obeying, for all $\mathtt{s}, \mathtt{p}, \mathtt{q} \in S$,

(30) $\mathtt{s} = \mathtt{cons}(\mathtt{p}, \mathtt{q}) \Rightarrow \mathbf{s} = \mathbf{p} \otimes \mathbf{r}_0 + \mathbf{q} \otimes \mathbf{r}_1$.

Here, $\mathtt{s} = \mathtt{cons}(\mathtt{p}, \mathtt{q})$ is the tree with left subtree $\mathtt{p}$ and right subtree $\mathtt{q}$, while $\mathbf{s}$, $\mathbf{p}$, and $\mathbf{q}$ are the vectors realizing $\mathtt{s}$, $\mathtt{p}$, and $\mathtt{q}$ under ψ. The only two roles in this recursive decomposition are r_0, r_1: the left and right children of the root. These roles are realized by two vectors $\mathbf{r}_0$ and $\mathbf{r}_1$. The vectors themselves form a set called R°; they lie in a vector space V_{R°, which we are taking to be two-dimensional.

As stated in (29g), the **cons** operation can be decomposed into two elementary operations on pseudotrees; these can be characterized as in (31):

(31) $\mathtt{cons}_0(\mathtt{s}) \equiv \mathtt{cons}(\mathtt{s}, \varnothing)$; $\mathtt{cons}_1(\mathtt{s}) \equiv \mathtt{cons}(\varnothing, \mathtt{s})$.

A recursive realization obeying (30) can actually be constructed from the positional realization we began with, by assuming that the (unboundedly many) positional role vectors $\{\mathbf{r}_x\}$ are constructed recursively from the (two) recursive role vectors $\mathbf{r}_0$ and $\mathbf{r}_1$ according to (32):[14]

(32) $\mathbf{r}_{x0} = \mathbf{r}_x \otimes \mathbf{r}_0$; $\mathbf{r}_{x1} = \mathbf{r}_x \otimes \mathbf{r}_1$.

For example, $\mathbf{r}_{0101} = \mathbf{r}_0 \otimes \mathbf{r}_1 \otimes \mathbf{r}_0 \otimes \mathbf{r}_1$. The vectors realizing positions at depth d in the tree are tensors of rank d (taking the root to be depth 0).

To demonstrate that the role vectors recursively defined by (32) generate a realization that is recursive in the sense of (30), suppose that $\mathtt{s} = \mathtt{cons}(\mathtt{p}, \mathtt{q})$. Then if an atomic symbol $\mathtt{A}_i$ fills some role r_{x_i} in $\mathtt{p}$, that same symbol $\mathtt{A}_i$ fills the role r_{x_i0} in $\mathtt{s}$:

(33)

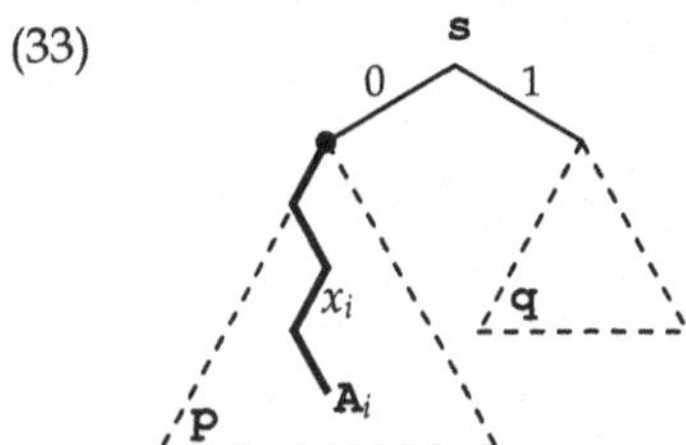

Similarly, if a symbol $\mathtt{A}_i$ fills some role r_{x_i} in $\mathtt{q}$, that same symbol $\mathtt{A}_i$ fills the role r_{x_i1} in $\mathtt{s}$. In other words,

(34) $\mathtt{A}_i / r_{x_i} \in \beta(\mathtt{p}) \;\Rightarrow\; \mathtt{A}_i / r_{x_i0} \in \beta(\mathtt{s})$; $\mathtt{A}_i / r_{x_i} \in \beta(\mathtt{q}) \;\Rightarrow\; \mathtt{A}_i / r_{x_i1} \in \beta(\mathtt{s})$.

[14] Adopting this definition (32) of $\mathbf{r}_x$ amounts to taking the recursive structure that is implicit in the subscripts x labeling the positional role vectors and mapping it into the structure of the vectors themselves, in such a way that this structure can be manipulated by connectionist processing mechanisms.

And conversely, if any symbol $\mathbf{A}_i$ fills some nonroot role r_{y_i} in **s**, then y_i falls either within **s**'s left subtree **p** or within its right subtree **q**. In the former case, $y_i = x_i0$ and $\mathbf{A}_i$ fills the role r_{x_i} in **p**; in the latter case, $y_i = x_i1$ and $\mathbf{A}_i$ fills the role r_{x_i} in **q**. Now we can compute, using (28) and (32),

(35) $$\mathbf{p}\otimes\mathbf{r}_0+\mathbf{q}\otimes\mathbf{r}_1=\left[\sum_{\mathbf{A}_i/r_{x_i}\in\beta(\mathbf{p})}\mathbf{A}_i\otimes\mathbf{r}_{x_i}\right]\otimes\mathbf{r}_0+\left[\sum_{\mathbf{A}_i/r_{x_i}\in\beta(\mathbf{q})}\mathbf{A}_i\otimes\mathbf{r}_{x_i}\right]\otimes\mathbf{r}_1$$
$$=\sum_{\mathbf{A}_i/r_{x_i}\in\beta(\mathbf{p})}\mathbf{A}_i\otimes[\mathbf{r}_{x_i}\otimes\mathbf{r}_0]+\sum_{\mathbf{A}_i/r_{x_i}\in\beta(\mathbf{q})}\mathbf{A}_i\otimes[\mathbf{r}_{x_i}\otimes\mathbf{r}_1]$$
$$=\sum_{\mathbf{A}_i/r_{x_i}\in\beta(\mathbf{p})}\mathbf{A}_i\otimes\mathbf{r}_{x_i0}+\sum_{\mathbf{A}_i/r_{x_i}\in\beta(\mathbf{q})}\mathbf{A}_i\otimes\mathbf{r}_{x_i1}$$
$$=\sum_{\mathbf{A}_i/r_{y_i}\in\beta(\mathbf{s})}\mathbf{A}_i\otimes\mathbf{r}_{y_i}$$
$$=\mathbf{s}.$$

The last steps follow from (34) and (28). This proves (30).

To pursue the example discussed in Section 5:1.3, consider the tree $\mathbf{s} \equiv$ [A [B C]]:

(36) $\mathbf{s}$ = cons(A, cons(B, C)) = cons(p, q),

where $\mathbf{p}$ = A (i.e., $\mathbf{p} = \{\mathrm{A}/r_\varepsilon\}$) and

(37) $\mathbf{q}$ = cons(B, C) = $\wedge$ (B C) = $\{\mathrm{B}/r_0, \mathrm{C}/r_1\}$.

Then by (32) $\mathbf{s} = \{\mathrm{A}/r_0, \mathrm{B}/r_{01}, \mathrm{C}/r_{11}\}$ is realized by the vector

(38) $$\mathbf{s} = \mathbf{A}\otimes\mathbf{r}_0+\mathbf{B}\otimes\mathbf{r}_{01}+\mathbf{C}\otimes\mathbf{r}_{11}$$
$$=\mathbf{A}\otimes\mathbf{r}_0+\mathbf{B}\otimes\mathbf{r}_0\otimes\mathbf{r}_1+\mathbf{C}\otimes\mathbf{r}_1\otimes\mathbf{r}_1$$
$$=\mathbf{A}\otimes\mathbf{r}_0+(\mathbf{B}\otimes\mathbf{r}_0+\mathbf{C}\otimes\mathbf{r}_1)\otimes\mathbf{r}_1$$
$$=\mathbf{p}\otimes\mathbf{r}_0+\mathbf{q}\otimes\mathbf{r}_1,$$

in accordance with (30).

Since we are now adding tensors of different rank, the vector space V of these recursive realizations is somewhat more complicated than the cases considered above: V is the **direct sum** of the spaces of tensors of different rank (Box 5:1 (19)). An element of V can be viewed as a vector whose elements are tensors of different ranks, or as one long vector, obtained by concatenating all the individual numbers constituting those tensors. In the first notation, the complete vector **s** is written

(39) $\mathbf{s} = (\mathbf{s}_{(0)}; \mathbf{s}_{(1)}; \mathbf{s}_{(2)}; \ldots);$

in the second notation,

(40) $$\mathbf{s}=\left\{\left[\mathrm{s}_{(0)}\right]_{\varphi},\left[\mathrm{s}_{(1)}\right]_{\varphi\rho_1},\left[\mathrm{s}_{(2)}\right]_{\varphi\rho_2\rho_1},\ldots\right\}.$$

Each $\mathbf{s}_{(d)}$ is a tensor of rank d+1 realizing depth d in the tree; for example, $\mathbf{s}_{(2)}$ is a rank-3 tensor built up by adding together tensor products of the form $\mathbf{A} \otimes \mathbf{r}_{x_1} \otimes \mathbf{r}_{x_2}$ for atoms $\mathbf{A}$ at depth-2 positions $x = x_2 x_1$ (where each of x_1 and x_2 is 0 or 1). The index φ ranges over the dimensions of the space V_A of vectors realizing atoms. Each index ρ_i ranges over the dimensions of the role space V_R; we are assuming that there are two such dimensions, labeled 0 and 1.

For example, consider the tree **s** in (38); here,

(41) $\mathbf{s}_{(2)} = \mathbf{B} \otimes \mathbf{r}_0 \otimes \mathbf{r}_1 + \mathbf{C} \otimes \mathbf{r}_1 \otimes \mathbf{r}_1.$

The numerical components making up $\mathbf{s}_{(2)}$ always have the form $[\mathbf{s}_{(2)}]_{\varphi\rho_2\rho_1}$; in (38), these numbers are

(42) $[\mathbf{s}_{(2)}]_{\varphi\rho_2\rho_1} = [\mathbf{B}]_\varphi[\mathbf{r}_0]_{\rho_2}[\mathbf{r}_1]_{\rho_1} + [\mathbf{C}]_\varphi[\mathbf{r}_1]_{\rho_2}[\mathbf{r}_1]_{\rho_1}$

(where $[\mathbf{r}_0]_{\rho_2}$ is of course the ρ_2th component in the vector $\mathbf{r}_0$). In (38), there is only one atom $\mathbf{A}$ at depth 1, so $\mathbf{s}_{(1)}$ is simply

(43) $\mathbf{s}_{(1)} = \mathbf{A} \otimes \mathbf{r}_0,$

which consists of the components

(44) $[\mathbf{s}_{(1)}]_{\varphi\rho_1} = [\mathbf{A}]_\varphi[\mathbf{r}_0]_{\rho_1}.$

In (38), there are no atoms at any depths other than 1 and 2, so all the other tensors $\mathbf{s}_{(d)}$ for $d \neq 1, 2$ are 0.

In general, the tensor $\mathbf{s}_{(d)}$ for depth d has one subscript φ for the filler vectors (e.g., **B** and **C**), and d subscripts $\rho_d \rho_{d-1} \cdots \rho_2 \rho_1$ for the depth-d role vectors

(45) $\mathbf{r}_x = \mathbf{r}_{x_d x_{d-1} \cdots x_2 x_1} = \mathbf{r}_{x_d} \otimes \mathbf{r}_{x_{d-1}} \otimes \cdots \otimes \mathbf{r}_{x_2} \otimes \mathbf{r}_{x_1}.$

Thus, $\mathbf{s}_{(d)}$ is rank-1 with respect to fillers, rank-d with respect to roles, and rank-(d+1) overall. The space of all such tensors $\mathbf{s}_{(d)}$ for tree depth d is called $S_{(d)}$.

The operation we have used to construct the complete representational vector space V from its subspaces is called the **direct sum**, written $\oplus$; V is S:

(46) *Definition.* $S \equiv S_{(0)} \oplus S_{(1)} \oplus S_{(2)} \oplus S_{(3)} \oplus \cdots.$

Because this construction realizes on separate units the symbols at different depths or strata of a tree, this realization is **stratified**. Section 4.4 introduces extensions of the techniques developed here that enable construction of a nonstratified, fully distributed representation, in which a given unit may participate in the realization of a symbol at any depth.

The tensorial representations in $S_{(d)}$ are all linear combinations of tensors of the form

(47) $\mathbf{A} \otimes \mathbf{r}_x = \mathbf{A} \otimes \mathbf{r}_{x_d x_{d-1} \cdots x_2 x_1} = \mathbf{A} \otimes \mathbf{r}_{x_d} \otimes \mathbf{r}_{x_{d-1}} \otimes \cdots \otimes \mathbf{r}_{x_2} \otimes \mathbf{r}_{x_1}.$

These vectors constitute the space $V_A \otimes V_{R^\circ} \otimes V_{R^\circ} \otimes \cdots \otimes V_{R^\circ}$, with d factors of V_{R°, the primitive role vector space V_{R° in which $\{\mathbf{r}_0, \mathbf{r}_1\}$ reside. These tensors have index structure

(48) $[\mathbf{s}_{(d)}]_{\varphi\rho_d\rho_{d-1}\cdots\rho_1}.$

There is a single index φ, placed leftmost by convention, which ranges over the dimensions of the atomic realization vector space V_A; then there is a sequence of d indices ρ_k ranging over the dimensions of V_{R°. Hence,

(49)
$$\begin{aligned} S &\equiv S_{(0)} \oplus S_{(1)} \oplus S_{(2)} \oplus S_{(3)} \oplus \cdots \\ &= [V_A] \oplus [V_A \otimes V_{R^\circ}] \oplus [V_A \otimes V_{R^\circ} \otimes V_{R^\circ}] \oplus [V_A \otimes V_{R^\circ} \otimes V_{R^\circ} \otimes V_{R^\circ}] \oplus \cdots \\ &= V_A \otimes [1 \oplus V_{R^\circ} \oplus V_{R^\circ} \otimes V_{R^\circ} \oplus V_{R^\circ} \otimes V_{R^\circ} \otimes V_{R^\circ} \oplus \cdots] \\ &\equiv V_A \otimes [\mathcal{R}_{(0)} \oplus \mathcal{R}_{(1)} \oplus \mathcal{R}_{(2)} \oplus \mathcal{R}_{(3)} \oplus \cdots] \\ &\equiv V_A \otimes \mathcal{R}. \end{aligned}$$

$\mathcal{R}_{(d)}$ is the vector space containing the *roles* for tree depth d; $S_{(d)} = V_A \otimes \mathcal{R}_{(d)}$ is the space containing the bindings of atomic symbols to roles at depth d. $\mathcal{R}$ contains the role vectors for all depths, S the binding vectors for symbols at all depths.

For ease of reference, (50) summarizes the concepts and notation, including those pertaining to matrices that will be defined in the next subsection. The right edge illustrates the concepts with our example tree [**A** [**B C**]]. As always, ψ labels realization mappings.

(50) Connectionist realizations of binary trees, S_{trees}

a. Primitives	
Atoms	
A: the set of atomic symbols	{**A**, …}
V_A, the atomic realization vector space, of dimension d_A	(large)
Realization mapping ψ_A: $A \to V_A$	$\mathbf{A} \mapsto \mathbf{A}, \ldots$
$\mathcal{M}_A$: Matrices over V_A	$[\mathbf{G}]_\varphi{}^{\varphi'}$
Primitive roles	
$R^\circ \equiv \{r_0, r_1\}$, the set of primitive roles	$\{r_0, r_1\}$
V_{R°, the primitive role vector space, of dimension d_{R°	≥ 2
Realization mapping ψ_{R°: $R^\circ \to V_{R^\circ}$	$r_0 \mapsto \mathbf{r}_0$; $r_1 \mapsto \mathbf{r}_1$
b. Positional role decomposition (F simple, R complex): tree **s**	[**A** [**B C**]]
$F = A$	**A**, **B**, **C**
$R = R^\infty \equiv \{r_x \mid x \text{ a bit-string tree-node address}\}$	r_0, r_{01}, r_{11}
$\psi_F = \psi_A$: $A \to V_A$	**A**, **B**, **C**
$\psi_R : R^\infty \to \mathcal{R} \equiv \mathcal{R}_{(0)} \oplus \mathcal{R}_{(1)} \oplus \mathcal{R}_{(2)} \oplus \cdots \equiv 1 \oplus V_{R^\circ} \oplus V_{R^\circ} \otimes V_{R^\circ} \oplus \cdots$	$\mathbf{r}_0, \mathbf{r}_{01}, \mathbf{r}_{11}$
constructed recursively from ψ_{R°	$\mathbf{r}_{01} \equiv \mathbf{r}_0 \otimes \mathbf{r}_1, \ldots$
$\psi_{F/R} \equiv \psi_F \otimes \psi_R$: $S_{\text{trees}} \to V_A \otimes \mathcal{R} = S$	$\mathbf{A} \otimes \mathbf{r}_0 + \mathbf{B} \otimes \mathbf{r}_{01} + \mathbf{C} \otimes \mathbf{r}_{11}$
Matrices to $\mathcal{R}_{(d)}$ from $\mathcal{R}_{(d')}$: $\mathcal{M}_d^{d'}$	$[\mathbf{M}]_{\rho_d\rho_{d-1}\cdots\rho_2\rho_1}{}^{\rho'_{d'}\rho'_{d'-1}\cdots\rho'_2\rho'_1}$
c. Recursive role decomposition (F complex, R simple): tree **s**	[**A** [**B C**]]
$F = S_{\text{trees}}$	**A**, [**B C**]

$R = R^{\circ}$ $\quad r_0, r_1$

$\psi_R = \psi_{R^{\circ}}: R^{\circ} \to V_{R^{\circ}}$ $\quad \mathbf{r}_0, \mathbf{r}_1$

$\psi_F: S_{\text{trees}} \to S \equiv S_{(0)} \oplus S_{(1)} \oplus S_{(2)} \oplus \cdots \equiv V_A \oplus V_A \otimes V_{R^{\circ}} \oplus \cdots$ $\quad \mathbf{A}, \mathbf{B} \otimes \mathbf{r}_0 + \mathbf{C} \otimes \mathbf{r}_1$

constructed recursively from ψ_A and $\psi_{R^{\circ}}$

$\psi_{F/R} \equiv \psi_F \otimes \psi_R: S_{\text{trees}} \to S \otimes V_{R^{\circ}} = S$ $\quad \mathbf{A} \otimes \mathbf{r}_0 + [\mathbf{B} \otimes \mathbf{r}_0 + \mathbf{C} \otimes \mathbf{r}_1] \otimes \mathbf{r}_1$

Matrices to $S_{(d)}$ from $S_{(d')}$: $\mathcal{W}_d^{\,d'}$ $\quad [\mathbf{W}]_{\varphi\rho_d\rho_{d-1}\cdots\rho_2\rho_1}^{\varphi'\rho'_{d'}\rho'_{d'-1}\cdots\rho'_2\rho'_1}$

The realizations of the two role decompositions (50b) and (50c) are built from the same primitive material: (50a). The two decompositions are different routes that end up constructing the same realization $\psi_{F/R}$.

4.1.2 Primitive matrices: Construction function cons

The vector operation **cons** for building the realization of a binary tree from that of its two subtrees is defined by (30), rewritten here as (51):

(51) $\mathbf{s} = \mathbf{cons}(\mathbf{p}, \mathbf{q}) \Rightarrow \mathbf{s} = \mathbf{p} \otimes \mathbf{r}_0 + \mathbf{q} \otimes \mathbf{r}_1 \equiv \mathbf{cons}(\mathbf{p}, \mathbf{q})$.

As an operation on S, this can be written

(52)
$$\mathbf{cons}: (\{[\mathbf{p}_{(0)}]_{\varphi}; [\mathbf{p}_{(1)}]_{\varphi\rho_1}; [\mathbf{p}_{(2)}]_{\varphi\rho_2\rho_1}; \ldots\}, \{[\mathbf{q}_{(0)}]_{\varphi}; [\mathbf{q}_{(1)}]_{\varphi\rho_1}; [\mathbf{q}_{(2)}]_{\varphi\rho_2\rho_1}; \ldots\}) \mapsto$$
$$\{\mathbf{0}_A; [\mathbf{p}_{(0)}]_{\varphi}[\mathbf{r}_0]_{\rho_1}; [\mathbf{p}_{(1)}]_{\varphi\rho_1}[\mathbf{r}_0]_{\rho_1}; \ldots\} + \{\mathbf{0}_A; [\mathbf{q}_{(0)}]_{\varphi}[\mathbf{r}_1]_{\rho_1}; [\mathbf{q}_{(1)}]_{\varphi\rho_1}[\mathbf{r}_1]_{\rho_1}; \ldots\},$$

or, more compactly,

(53)
$$\mathbf{cons}: \left((\mathbf{p}_{(0)}; \mathbf{p}_{(1)}; \mathbf{p}_{(2)}; \ldots), (\mathbf{q}_{(0)}; \mathbf{q}_{(1)}; \mathbf{q}_{(2)}; \ldots)\right) \mapsto$$
$$(\mathbf{0}_A; \mathbf{p}_{(0)} \otimes \mathbf{r}_0; \mathbf{p}_{(1)} \otimes \mathbf{r}_0; \ldots) + (\mathbf{0}_A; \mathbf{q}_{(0)} \otimes \mathbf{r}_1; \mathbf{q}_{(1)} \otimes \mathbf{r}_1; \ldots).$$

(Here, $\mathbf{0}_A$ denotes the zero vector in the filler space V_A for realizing the atoms A.)

The goal now is to identify matrices such that, using matrix multiplication '$\cdot$' in S, this mapping can simply be written, parallel to (51), as (54):

(54) $\mathbf{cons}(\mathbf{p}, \mathbf{q}) = \mathbf{W}_{\text{cons0}} \cdot \mathbf{p} + \mathbf{W}_{\text{cons1}} \cdot \mathbf{q}$.

To derive the matrix $\mathbf{W}_{\text{cons0}}$, note that for any binding $\mathbf{b} \equiv \mathbf{f}_x \otimes \mathbf{r}_x$ in $\mathbf{p}$, the effect of multiplying $\mathbf{b}$ by $\mathbf{W}_{\text{cons0}}$ must be to produce

(55) $\mathbf{W}_{\text{cons0}} \cdot \mathbf{b} \equiv \mathbf{b}' \equiv \mathbf{f}_x \otimes \mathbf{r}_{x0} = \mathbf{f}_x \otimes (\mathbf{r}_x \otimes \mathbf{r}_0) = (\mathbf{f}_x \otimes \mathbf{r}_x) \otimes \mathbf{r}_0 = \mathbf{b} \otimes \mathbf{r}_0$.

Suppose $\mathbf{b}$ is a depth-d binding; $|x| = d$ and $\mathbf{b} \in S_{(d)}$. Then $\mathbf{W}_{\text{cons0}} \cdot \mathbf{b} = \mathbf{b}' = \mathbf{b} \otimes \mathbf{r}_0$ is a depth-$d+1$ binding in $S_{(d+1)}$, with components

(56)
$$\begin{aligned}[\mathbf{b}']_{\varphi\rho_{d+1}\rho_d\cdots\rho_2\rho_1} &= \left[[\mathbf{W}_{\text{cons0}} \cdot \mathbf{b}]_{(d+1)}\right]_{\varphi\rho_{d+1}\rho_d\cdots\rho_2\rho_1} \\ &= [\mathbf{b} \otimes \mathbf{r}_0]_{\varphi\rho_{d+1}\rho_d\cdots\rho_2\rho_1} \\ &= [\mathbf{b}]_{\varphi\rho_{d+1}\rho_d\cdots\rho_2}[\mathbf{r}_0]_{\rho_1}.\end{aligned}$$

Thus, $\mathbf{W}_{\text{cons0}}$ must take $\mathbf{b} \in S_{(d)}$ into $\mathbf{b}' \in S_{(d+1)}$ in such a way as to retain all values of components except to multiply each by the ρ_1th component of $\mathbf{r}_0$, adding one additional index ρ_1. Thus, the nonzero elements of the matrix $\mathbf{W}_{\text{cons0}}$ must be

(57) $$[\mathbf{W}_{\text{cons}0}{}^{(d)}_{(d+1)}]_{\varphi\rho_{d+1}\rho_d\cdots\rho_2\rho_1}^{\varphi\rho_{d+1}\cdots\rho_2} = [\mathbf{r}_0]_{\rho_1}.$$

Clearly, $\mathbf{W}_{\text{cons1}}$ must obey the same equation, with $\mathbf{r}_1$ replacing $\mathbf{r}_0$.

In (57), and in the remainder of this chapter, it is convenient to adopt a notation for matrices in which the left matrix tag is set as a subscript, and the right matrix tag is set as a superscript: rather than the customary M_{jk} we will write M_j^k. It is further useful to treat strings of matrix indices such as $\rho_d \cdots \rho_2\rho_1$ as an **index vector** $\boldsymbol{\rho}$, a bit string like x but one that does not designate a tree position. As with x, $|\boldsymbol{\rho}|$ will denote the number of indices in $\boldsymbol{\rho}$. Finally, it is convenient to adopt a notational abbreviation (the **Einstein summation convention**): in a product of two factors containing identical indices, one set "upstairs" and the other "downstairs," there is an implicit summation over these common indices.

With these notational conventions, matrix multiplication can simply be written

(58) $$[\mathbf{A} \cdot \mathbf{B}]_{\boldsymbol{\alpha}}{}^{\boldsymbol{\beta}} \equiv [\mathbf{A}]_{\boldsymbol{\alpha}}{}^{\boldsymbol{\gamma}}[\mathbf{B}]_{\boldsymbol{\gamma}}{}^{\boldsymbol{\beta}}.$$

There is an implicit sum over the shared indices in the vector $\boldsymbol{\gamma}$; thus, (58) states that

(59) $$[\mathbf{A} \cdot \mathbf{B}]_{\alpha_a\cdots\alpha_2\alpha_1}^{\beta_b\cdots\beta_2\beta_1} = \sum\nolimits_{\gamma_c} \cdots \sum\nolimits_{\gamma_2} \sum\nolimits_{\gamma_1} [\mathbf{A}]_{\alpha_a\cdots\alpha_2\alpha_1}^{\gamma_c\cdots\gamma_2\gamma_1} [\mathbf{B}]_{\gamma_c\cdots\gamma_2\gamma_1}^{\beta_b\cdots\beta_2\beta_1}.$$

$\mathbf{B}$ is a matrix mapping tensors of rank b to tensors of rank c, while $\mathbf{A}$ is a matrix mapping tensors of rank c to tensors of rank a; thus, their product $\mathbf{A} \cdot \mathbf{B}$ is a matrix mapping tensors of rank b to tensors of rank a.

The definition of matrix-vector multiplication analogous to (58) is

(60) $$[\mathbf{A} \cdot \mathbf{b}]_{\boldsymbol{\alpha}} \equiv [\mathbf{A}]_{\boldsymbol{\alpha}}{}^{\boldsymbol{\gamma}}[\mathbf{b}]_{\boldsymbol{\gamma}};$$

that is,

(61) $$[\mathbf{A} \cdot \mathbf{b}]_{\alpha_a\cdots\alpha_2\alpha_1} = \sum\nolimits_{\gamma_c} \cdots \sum\nolimits_{\gamma_2} \sum\nolimits_{\gamma_1} [\mathbf{A}]_{\alpha_a\cdots\alpha_2\alpha_1}^{\gamma_c\cdots\gamma_2\gamma_1} [\mathbf{b}]_{\gamma_c\cdots\gamma_2\gamma_1}.$$

(57) defines $\mathbf{W}_{\text{cons0}}{}^{(d)}_{(d+1)}$, a submatrix of $\mathbf{W}_{\text{cons0}}$ that takes symbols at depth d in $\mathbf{p}$ and puts them at depth $d+1$ in the new tree $\mathbf{s} = \mathbf{cons}(\mathbf{p}, \mathbf{q})$. Since it maps vectors in $S_{(d)}$ to vectors in $S_{(d+1)}$, $\mathbf{W}_{\text{cons0}}{}^{(d)}_{(d+1)}$ is in the matrix space $\mathcal{W}_d^{d+1}$ (50c); it is only a small part of the full matrix $\mathbf{W}_{\text{cons0}}$. (62) shows the **block structure** of the matrix $\mathbf{W}_{\text{cons0}}$.

(62) $$\mathbf{W}_{\text{cons}0} = \begin{bmatrix} \mathbf{0} & \mathbf{0} & \mathbf{0} & \mathbf{0} \\ [\mathbf{W}_{\text{cons}0}]_{(1)}^{(0)} & \mathbf{0} & \mathbf{0} & \mathbf{0} \\ \mathbf{0} & [\mathbf{W}_{\text{cons}0}]_{(2)}^{(1)} & \mathbf{0} & \mathbf{0} \\ \mathbf{0} & \mathbf{0} & [\mathbf{W}_{\text{cons}0}]_{(3)}^{(2)} & \mathbf{0} \\ \vdots & \vdots & \mathbf{0} & \ddots \end{bmatrix}$$

The general block structure in (62) is not specific to $\mathbf{W}_{\text{cons0}}$; only the contents of the blocks (including **0**) are. For a general matrix **W** on *S*, the block $\mathbf{W}_{(d)}^{(d')}$ in row *d* and column *d'* is the submatrix mapping component vectors for depth *d'* of the tree into component vectors for depth *d*, as shown in (63).

$$(63)\quad \mathbf{W} = \begin{bmatrix} \mathbf{W}_{(0)}^{(0)} & \mathbf{W}_{(0)}^{(1)} & \mathbf{W}_{(0)}^{(2)} & \cdots \\ \mathbf{W}_{(1)}^{(0)} & \mathbf{W}_{(1)}^{(1)} & \mathbf{W}_{(1)}^{(2)} & \cdots \\ \mathbf{W}_{(2)}^{(0)} & \mathbf{W}_{(2)}^{(1)} & \mathbf{W}_{(2)}^{(2)} & \cdots \\ \vdots & \vdots & \vdots & \ddots \end{bmatrix}$$

Denoting the input $\mathbf{p} = (\mathbf{p}_{(0)}, \mathbf{p}_{(1)}, \ldots)$ and the output $\mathbf{W} \cdot \mathbf{p} = \mathbf{s} = (\mathbf{s}_{(0)}, \mathbf{s}_{(1)}, \ldots)$, we have

$$(64)\quad \mathbf{s}_{(d)} = \mathbf{W}_{(d)}^{(d')} \cdot \mathbf{p}_{(d')}.$$

Matrix multiplication mixes the block structure according to (65):

$$(65)\quad [\mathbf{A} \cdot \mathbf{B}]_{(d)}^{(d')} = \textstyle\sum_k \mathbf{A}_{(d)}^{(k)} \cdot \mathbf{B}_{(k)}^{(d')}.$$

In the case of $\mathbf{W} = \mathbf{W}_{\text{cons0}}$, all blocks $\mathbf{W}_{(d)}^{(d')}$ are zero matrices (**0**) except when $d = d' + 1$, because the **cons** operator just embeds trees one level down from the root, thereby increasing by one the depth of all symbols in the tree. Thus, all the nonzero blocks of $\mathbf{W}_{\text{cons0}}$ are just below the main block diagonal, which is shown in (62) and (63) between diagonal lines. The elements of the nonzero block matrices are specified in (57). For the example above of a vector **b** realizing a depth-*d* binding (i.e., $\mathbf{b} \in S_{(d)}$), utilizing (57) we get (66), where $\boldsymbol{\rho} \equiv \rho_{d+1}\rho_d \cdots \rho_2$ and $\boldsymbol{\rho}' \equiv \rho'_{d+1}\rho'_d \cdots \rho'_2$:

$$(66)\quad \begin{aligned} [\mathbf{b}']_{\varphi\boldsymbol{\rho}\rho_1} &\equiv [\mathbf{W}_{\text{cons}0}{}_{(d+1)}^{(d)} \cdot \mathbf{b}]_{\varphi\boldsymbol{\rho}\rho_1} && \mathbf{W}_{\text{cons}0}{}_{(d'')}^{(d)} = \mathbf{0} \text{ unless } d'' = d+1 \\ &\equiv [\mathbf{W}_{\text{cons}0}{}_{(d+1)}^{(d)}]_{\varphi\boldsymbol{\rho}\rho_1}^{\varphi'\boldsymbol{\rho}'} \mathbf{b}_{\varphi'\boldsymbol{\rho}'} && \text{by (58)} \\ &= [\mathbf{W}_{\text{cons}0}{}_{(d+1)}^{(d)}]_{\varphi\boldsymbol{\rho}\rho_1}^{\varphi\boldsymbol{\rho}} \mathbf{b}_{\varphi\boldsymbol{\rho}} && [\mathbf{W}_{\text{cons}0}{}_{(d+1)}^{(d)}]_{\varphi\boldsymbol{\rho}\rho_1}^{\varphi'\boldsymbol{\rho}'} = 0 \text{ if } \varphi' \neq \varphi \text{ or } \boldsymbol{\rho}' \neq \boldsymbol{\rho} \\ &= [\mathbf{r}_0]_{\rho_1} \mathbf{b}_{\varphi\boldsymbol{\rho}} && \text{by (57)} \\ &= \mathbf{b}_{\varphi\boldsymbol{\rho}}[\mathbf{r}_0]_{\rho_1} = [\mathbf{b} \otimes \mathbf{r}_0]_{\varphi\boldsymbol{\rho}\rho_1}. && \text{by (8)} \end{aligned}$$

This calculation verifies that, with the above definitions, the matrix-vector product $\mathbf{W}_{\text{cons}0}{}_{(d+1)}^{(d)} \cdot \mathbf{b}$ does indeed equal the tensor product $\mathbf{b} \otimes \mathbf{r}_0$: (55).

The elements of $\mathbf{W}_{\text{cons}0}{}_{(d)}^{(d')}$ can be displayed, in the case of $d' = 1$, as follows. According to (57), when $d' = 1$, the nonzero elements are

$$(67)\quad \left[\mathbf{W}_{\text{cons}0}{}_{(2)}^{(1)}\right]_{\varphi\rho_2\rho_1}^{\varphi\rho_2} = [\mathbf{r}_0]_{\rho_1}.$$

We are assuming a two-dimensional role vector space, $\mathbf{r}_0 = ([\mathbf{r}_0]_0, [\mathbf{r}_0]_1)$; and, as always, the Kronecker δ is defined by

$$\delta_i^j = \begin{cases} 1 & \text{if } i = j \\ 0 & \text{if } i \neq j \end{cases}.$$

Then (67) can be rewritten as follows:

(68) $$\left[\mathbf{W}_{\text{cons}0\binom{(1)}{(d)}}\right]^{\varphi'\rho_2'}_{\varphi\rho_2\rho_1} = \delta_d^2\, \delta_{\rho_2}^{\rho_2'}\, \delta_\varphi^{\varphi'}\, [\mathbf{r}_0]_{\rho_1}$$

$$= \begin{cases} [\mathbf{r}_0]_0 & \text{if } \rho_1 = 0 \text{ and } d = 2, \rho_2 = \rho_2', \varphi = \varphi' \\ [\mathbf{r}_0]_1 & \text{if } \rho_1 = 1 \text{ and } d = 2, \rho_2 = \rho_2', \varphi = \varphi' . \\ 0 & \text{otherwise} \end{cases}$$

That is,

(69) $$\left\{\left[\mathbf{W}_{\text{cons}0\binom{(1)}{(2)}}\right]^{\varphi\rho_2'}_{\varphi\rho_2\rho_1}\right\} = \begin{array}{c} \rho_2\rho_1 \\ 00 \\ 01 \\ 10 \\ 11 \end{array} \begin{array}{c} \rho_2' : 0 \quad\quad 1 \\ \left[\begin{array}{c|c} [\mathbf{r}_0]_0 & 0 \\ [\mathbf{r}_0]_1 & 0 \\ \hline 0 & [\mathbf{r}_0]_0 \\ 0 & [\mathbf{r}_0]_1 \end{array}\right] \end{array} = \left[\begin{array}{c|c} 1 & 0 \\ \hline 0 & 1 \end{array}\right] \otimes \begin{bmatrix} [\mathbf{r}_0]_0 \\ [\mathbf{r}_0]_1 \end{bmatrix} = \mathbf{1}_2 \otimes \mathbf{r}_0 .$$

(69) shows that $[\mathbf{W}_{\text{cons}0}]_{(2)}{}^{(1)}$ itself has an internal block structure, in which the diagonal vectors are $\mathbf{r}_0$ (in column vector form) and the off-diagonal vectors are $\mathbf{0}$. As we will see shortly, this means in fact that $[\mathbf{W}_{\text{cons}0}]_{(2)}{}^{(1)}$ is the tensor product of $\mathbf{r}_0$ with the 2×2 identity matrix $\mathbf{1}_2$: this is previewed in (69). (Recall that the space containing $\mathbf{r}_0$ and $\mathbf{r}_1$ is assumed to be two-dimensional, and that in an identity matrix, all elements are 0, except those along the main diagonal, where the elements are all 1.)

The special case of (68) ($d' = 1$) can be extended to the general case (57):

(70) $$[\mathbf{W}_{\text{cons}0\binom{(d)}{(d+1)}}]^{\varphi'\rho_{d+1}'\cdots\rho_2'}_{\varphi\rho_{d+1}\rho_d\cdots\rho_2\rho_1} = \delta_{\rho_{d+1}}^{\rho_{d+1}'}\delta_{\rho_d}^{\rho_d'}\cdots\delta_{\rho_2}^{\rho_2'}\delta_\varphi^{\varphi'}\,[\mathbf{r}_0]_{\rho_1} .$$

The elements $\{\delta_\varphi{}^{\varphi'}\}$ form the identity matrix $\mathbf{1}_A$ in the filler-vector space V_A of vectors realizing atoms, while the elements $\{\delta_\rho{}^{\rho'}\}$ constitute the identity matrix $\mathbf{1}_R$ in the space V_R of role vectors. Adopting henceforth the convention that unmarked '**1**' denotes $\mathbf{1}_R$, we can thus rewrite (70) as

(71) $$[\mathbf{W}_{\text{cons}0\binom{(d)}{(d+1)}}]^{\varphi'\rho_{d+1}'\cdots\rho_2'}_{\varphi\rho_{d+1}\rho_d\cdots\rho_2\rho_1} = [\mathbf{1}]_{\rho_{d+1}}^{\rho_{d+1}'}[\mathbf{1}]_{\rho_d}^{\rho_d'}\cdots[\mathbf{1}]_{\rho_2}^{\rho_2'}[\mathbf{1}_A]_\varphi^{\varphi'}\,[\mathbf{r}_0]_{\rho_1} .$$

Using an operation that we will formally define in the next subsection (78), the tensor product of matrices, we can write $\mathbf{W}_{\text{cons}0\binom{(d)}{(d+1)}}$ more succinctly, by expressing (71) as

(72) $$\mathbf{W}_{\text{cons}0\binom{(d)}{(d+1)}} = \mathbf{1} \otimes \cdots \otimes \mathbf{1} \otimes \mathbf{1}_A \otimes \mathbf{r}_0,$$

where there are d factors of $\mathbf{1}$; we will also write this as

(73) $\mathbf{W}_{\text{cons0}\,(d+1)}^{\;(d)} = \mathbf{1}^{\otimes d} \otimes \mathbf{1}_A \otimes \mathbf{r}_0$.

The full matrix $\mathbf{W}_{\text{cons0}}$ has one such block for each depth d:

(74) $\mathbf{W}_{\text{cons0}} = \mathbf{1}_A \otimes \mathbf{r}_0 + \mathbf{1} \otimes \mathbf{1}_A \otimes \mathbf{r}_0 + \mathbf{1}^{\otimes 2} \otimes \mathbf{1}_A \otimes \mathbf{r}_0 + \mathbf{1}^{\otimes 3} \otimes \mathbf{1}_A \otimes \mathbf{r}_0 + \cdots$.

This suggests the following definition:

(75) *Definition.* The **feed-forward recursion matrix** is

$$\mathbf{I} \equiv 1 + \mathbf{1} + \mathbf{1}^{\otimes 2} + \mathbf{1}^{\otimes 3} + \ldots$$
$$= \sum_{k=0}^{\infty} \mathbf{1}^{\otimes k}.$$

$\mathbf{I}$ is the identity matrix on the total role vector space, including all tree depths:

$$\mathcal{R} \equiv \mathcal{R}_{(0)} \oplus \mathcal{R}_{(1)} \oplus \mathcal{R}_{(2)} \oplus \mathcal{R}_{(3)} \oplus \cdots.$$

(And $\mathbf{I} \otimes \mathbf{1}_A$ is the matrix of the identity function for the entire representational space $S \equiv S_{(0)} \oplus S_{(1)} \oplus S_{(2)} \oplus S_{(3)} \oplus \cdots$.) The components of $\mathbf{I}$ are shown in (76).

(76) $\left[\mathbf{I}_{(d)}^{(d')}\right]_{\rho}^{\rho'} = \left[\mathbf{I}_{(d)}^{(d')}\right]_{\rho_d \cdots \rho_2 \rho_1}^{\rho'_{d'} \cdots \rho'_2 \rho'_1} = \delta_d^{d'} \delta_{\rho_d}^{\rho'_d} \cdots \delta_{\rho_2}^{\rho'_2} \delta_{\rho_1}^{\rho'_1}$

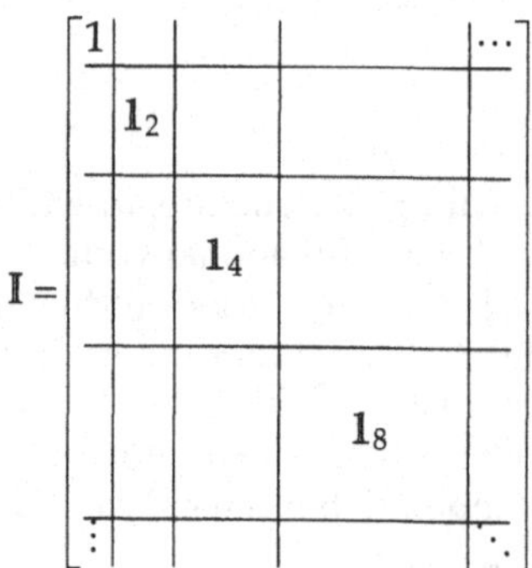

Here, $\mathbf{1}_k$ is the $k \times k$ identity matrix.

Using (75), we get a simple expression for $\mathbf{W}_{\text{cons0}}$ (74):

(77) $\mathbf{W}_{\text{cons0}} = \mathbf{I} \otimes \mathbf{1}_A \otimes \mathbf{r}_0$.

We can interpret this equation as stating that $\mathbf{W}_{\text{cons0}}$ is the recursive version of the operation of multiplying by $\mathbf{r}_0$; this weight matrix pushes or embeds a tensor realizing a tree into the role of left child of the root of a new tree. The matrix $\mathbf{W}_{\text{cons1}}$ satisfies the analogous equation, with 0 replaced by 1 (i.e., with $\mathbf{r}_0$ replaced by $\mathbf{r}_1$). Combining $\mathbf{W}_{\text{cons0}}$ and $\mathbf{W}_{\text{cons1}}$ gives the **cons** operation (54).

4.1.3 Matrix tensor products

Equations such as (72) and (79) involve the tensor product of matrices; this operation is defined so that (72) is equivalent to (71). A definition of this type of tensor product operation is given in (78).

(78) *Definition.* Tensor product of matrices

$$[\mathbf{B}\otimes(\mathbf{G}\otimes\mathbf{A})]_{\varphi\beta\alpha}^{\varphi'\beta'\alpha'} \equiv [\mathbf{G}]_{\varphi}^{\varphi'}[\mathbf{B}]_{\beta}^{\beta'}[\mathbf{A}]_{\alpha}^{\alpha'}$$

If $\mathbf{A}\in\mathcal{M}_a^{a'}$, $\mathbf{B}\in\mathcal{M}_b^{b'}$, $\mathbf{G}\in\mathcal{M}_A$, then $\mathbf{B}\otimes\mathbf{G}\otimes\mathbf{A}\in\ \mathcal{M}_A\otimes\mathcal{M}_{b+a}^{b'+a'}\equiv\mathcal{W}_{b+a}^{b'+a'}$.

The matrix tensor product is defined here in such a way as to produce a final matrix in one of the spaces $\mathcal{W}_d^{d'}$ of matrices operating on our representational vector space S; these matrices all have components of the form

$$[\mathbf{T}]_{\varphi\rho_d\rho_{d-1}\cdots\rho_2\rho_1}^{\varphi'\rho'_{d'}\rho'_{d'-1}\cdots\rho'_2\rho'_1}$$

where φ, φ' are indices ranging over the (many) dimensions of V_A, the vectors realizing atoms, while all the other indices ρ_j, ρ'_k range over the (two) dimensions of the primitive role space V_{R° hosting the realizations of $\{\mathbf{r}_0, \mathbf{r}_1\}$. In the tensor product of several matrices such as $\mathbf{B}\otimes\mathbf{G}\otimes\mathbf{A}$ in (78), only one matrix can operate over V_A—in (78), $\mathbf{G}$—while all others must operate over V_R. Regardless of where $\mathbf{G}$ is located in the product, the result is always a tensor in $\mathcal{W}_d^{d'}$, where our convention is to place the single V_A index downstairs (φ) and the single V_A index upstairs (φ') to the left of all the V_R indices (ρ_j, ρ'_k). Thus, for example, ($\mathbf{G} = \mathbf{1}_A$) (77):

(79) $\mathbf{W}_{\text{cons0}} = \mathbf{I}\otimes\mathbf{1}_A\otimes\mathbf{r}_0 = \mathbf{1}_A\otimes\mathbf{I}\otimes\mathbf{r}_0$.

A fundamental identity used frequently is expressed in (80).

(80) *Proposition.* Matrix multiplication of tensor products

Suppose V is a vector space with tag vectors $\boldsymbol{\rho}$, $\boldsymbol{\sigma}$ and $\mathbf{M}$ and $\mathbf{W}$ are matrices on V; suppose the same is true for V', $\boldsymbol{\rho}'$, $\boldsymbol{\sigma}'$, $\mathbf{M}'$, and $\mathbf{W}'$. Then

$$[\mathbf{M}\otimes\mathbf{M}']\cdot[\mathbf{W}\otimes\mathbf{W}'] = (\mathbf{M}\cdot\mathbf{W})\otimes(\mathbf{M}'\cdot\mathbf{W}').$$

Proof. From the definitions of '·' and '⊗':

$$\begin{aligned}
[(\mathbf{M}\otimes\mathbf{M}')\cdot(\mathbf{W}\otimes\mathbf{W}')]_{\rho\rho'}{}^{\sigma\sigma'} &\equiv [\mathbf{M}\otimes\mathbf{M}']_{\rho\rho'}{}^{\gamma\gamma'}[\mathbf{W}\otimes\mathbf{W}']_{\gamma\gamma'}{}^{\sigma\sigma'} && \text{by (58)}\\
&\equiv ([\mathbf{M}]_{\rho}{}^{\gamma}[\mathbf{M}']_{\rho'}{}^{\gamma'})([\mathbf{W}]_{\gamma}{}^{\sigma}[\mathbf{W}']_{\gamma'}{}^{\sigma'}) && \text{by (78)}\\
&\equiv ([\mathbf{M}]_{\rho}{}^{\gamma}[\mathbf{W}]_{\gamma}{}^{\sigma})([\mathbf{M}']_{\rho'}{}^{\gamma'}[\mathbf{W}']_{\gamma'}{}^{\sigma'}) &&\\
&\equiv ([\mathbf{M}\cdot\mathbf{W}]_{\rho}{}^{\sigma})([\mathbf{M}'\cdot\mathbf{W}']_{\rho'}{}^{\sigma'}) && \text{by (58)}\\
&\equiv [(\mathbf{M}\cdot\mathbf{W})\otimes(\mathbf{M}'\cdot\mathbf{W}')]_{\rho\rho'}{}^{\sigma\sigma'}. && \text{by (78)}
\end{aligned}$$

(81) *Corollary.* Matrix-vector multiplication over tensor products

Suppose V is a vector space with tag vector $\boldsymbol{\rho}$, $\mathbf{v}\in V$, and $\mathbf{M}$ is a matrix on V; suppose the same is true for V', $\boldsymbol{\rho}'$, $\mathbf{v}'$, and $\mathbf{M}'$. Then

$$[\mathbf{M}\otimes\mathbf{M}']\cdot(\mathbf{v}\otimes\mathbf{v}') = (\mathbf{M}\cdot\mathbf{v})\otimes(\mathbf{M}'\cdot\mathbf{v}').$$

> *Proof.* In the proof of (80), replace $\mathbf{W}$ by $\mathbf{b}$ and remove the indices σ, σ'; then the proof goes through identically, with (60) replacing (58). (Or, consider $\mathbf{b}$ as an $n \times 1$ matrix.)

Because of equations like (79), the following identity will be useful in much of what follows:

(82) *Proposition.* Suppose $\mathbf{M} \in \mathcal{M}_m^{\ m'}$. Then

$$[\mathbf{I} \otimes \mathbf{M}]_{(d)}^{(d')} = \begin{cases} [\mathbf{1}^{\otimes k} \otimes \mathbf{M}]_{(d)}^{(d')} & \text{if } \exists k \text{ s.t. } m+k=d \text{ and } m'+k=d' \\ \mathbf{0} & \text{otherwise} \end{cases}.$$

> *Proof.* By the definition of the recursion matrix $\mathbf{I}$ (75),
>
> $$\mathbf{I} \otimes \mathbf{M} = \left[\sum_{k=0}^{\infty} \mathbf{1}^{\otimes k}\right] \otimes \mathbf{M} = \sum_{k=0}^{\infty} [\mathbf{1}^{\otimes k} \otimes \mathbf{M}].$$
>
> The sought-after $[\mathbf{I} \otimes \mathbf{M}]_{(d)}^{(d')} \in \mathcal{M}_d^{\ d'}$. Since $\mathbf{M} \in \mathcal{M}_m^{\ m'}$, $\mathbf{1}^{\otimes k} \otimes \mathbf{M} \in \mathcal{M}_{m+k}^{\ m'+k'}$. For these to be the same space of matrices, it must be that $m+k=d$ and $m'+k=d'$; only this value of k, if it exists, contributes to $[\mathbf{I} \otimes \mathbf{M}]_{(d)}^{(d')}$; its contribution is $[\mathbf{1}^{\otimes k} \otimes \mathbf{M}]_{(d)}^{(d')}$. (Such a k exists iff the difference $m'-m$ is the same as $d'-d$; since $\mathbf{1}^{\otimes k}$ is a square matrix, taking its tensor product with $\mathbf{M}$ can increase the number of indices upstairs and downstairs, but only by the same amount; the difference between the number of up- and downstairs indices cannot change.)

4.1.4 Primitive matrices: Extraction functions $\mathbf{ex}_0$, $\mathbf{ex}_1$

Extracting a tree's left or right subtree is equivalent to **unbinding** r_0 or r_1. Assuming the role vectors to be linearly independent, then, as we saw in Section 3.1, these unbinding operations can be performed accurately, via linear operations $\mathbf{ex}_0$ and $\mathbf{ex}_1$: a kind of inner product of $\mathbf{s}$ with an **unbinding vector** $\mathbf{u}_0$ or $\mathbf{u}_1$. $\mathbf{ex}_0$ can be realized as multiplication in S by the matrix $\mathbf{W}_{\mathrm{ex0}}$, which has the following nonzero elements:

(83) $$[\mathbf{W}_{\mathrm{ex0}}{}_{(d)}^{(d+1)}]_{\varphi\rho_{d+1}\rho_d\cdots\rho_2}^{\varphi\rho_{d+1}\cdots\rho_2\rho_1} = [\mathbf{u}_0^{\mathrm{T}}]^{\rho_1} = [\mathbf{u}_0]_{\rho_1}.$$

$\mathbf{ex}_1$ is realized by the corresponding matrix $\mathbf{W}_{\mathrm{ex1}}$, with $\mathbf{u}_0$ replaced by $\mathbf{u}_1$. This matrix block maps tree depth $d+1$ in $\mathbf{s}$ to depth d in $\mathbf{ex}_0(\mathbf{s})$. Using the full identity matrix $\mathbf{I} \otimes \mathbf{1}_A$ on S, the full matrix $\mathbf{W}_{\mathrm{ex0}}$ for all depths can be written simply as

(84) $$\mathbf{W}_{\mathrm{ex0}} = \mathbf{I} \otimes \mathbf{1}_A \otimes \mathbf{u}_0^{\mathrm{T}}.$$

It is helpful to display the primitive matrices $\mathbf{W}_{\mathrm{ex}i}$ and $\mathbf{W}_{\mathrm{cons}i}$ in the format of (63). First consider $\mathbf{W}_{\mathrm{cons}i}$. It takes the form in (85); it can be simplified as shown, using the tensor product in (86).

Figure 4 Box 2

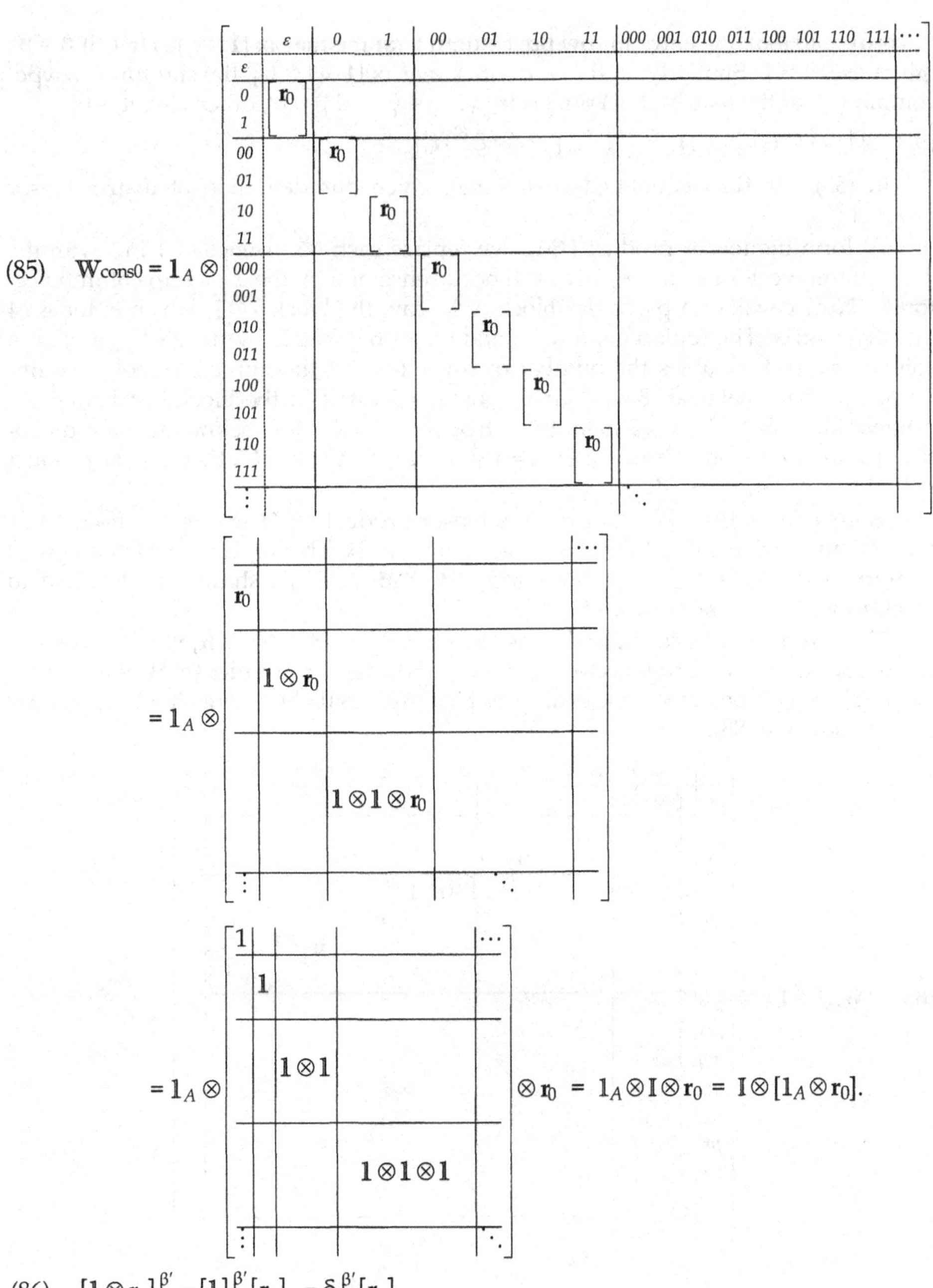

(86) $[\mathbf{1} \otimes \mathbf{r}_0]_{\beta\alpha}^{\beta'} = [\mathbf{1}]_{\beta}^{\beta'} [\mathbf{r}_0]_{\alpha} = \delta_{\beta}^{\beta'} [\mathbf{r}_0]_{\alpha}.$

According to (86), the entry in row βα, column β′ of the matrix $[\mathbf{1} \otimes \mathbf{r}_0]$ is $[\mathbf{r}_0]_\alpha$ if β = β′; otherwise, it is 0. Similarly, in the next block matrix $[\mathbf{1} \otimes \mathbf{1} \otimes \mathbf{r}_0]$, the entry in row γβα, column γ′β′ of the matrix $[\mathbf{1} \otimes \mathbf{1} \otimes \mathbf{r}_0]$ is $[\mathbf{r}_0]_\alpha$ if γ = γ′ and β = β′; otherwise, it is 0:

(87) $[\mathbf{1} \otimes \mathbf{1} \otimes \mathbf{r}_0]_{\gamma\beta\alpha}^{\gamma'\beta'} = [\mathbf{1}]_\gamma^{\gamma'} [\mathbf{1}]_\beta^{\beta'} [\mathbf{r}_0]_\alpha = \delta_\gamma^{\gamma'} \delta_\beta^{\beta'} [\mathbf{r}_0]_\alpha .$

In (85), the final equality is notational, given our definition of matrix tensor product (78).

To form the tensor product $\mathbf{I} \otimes \mathbf{r}_0$, we replace each occurrence of 1 in $\mathbf{I}$ with the 2×1 column vector $\mathbf{r}_0$, and replace each occurrence of 0 by the 2×1 zero column vector $\begin{bmatrix} 0 \\ 0 \end{bmatrix}$. Now consider a particular block of $\mathbf{I}$—say, the block $\mathbf{1} \otimes \mathbf{1}$, which is the 4×4 identity matrix. The replacement of 1s and 0s in this matrix by the 2×1 $\mathbf{r}_0$ and zero column matrices doubles the number of rows, leaving the number of columns unchanged. This creates an 8×4 matrix, which is located in the block just below the original location of the $\mathbf{1} \otimes \mathbf{1}$ identity matrix: this block is just below the main diagonal of $\mathbf{I}$. In other words, because $\mathbf{1} \otimes \mathbf{1} = \mathbf{I}_{(2)}^{(2)} \in \mathcal{M}_2^{\,2}$, and $\mathbf{r}_0 \in \mathcal{M}_1^{\,0}$, their tensor product is $\mathbf{1} \otimes \mathbf{1} \otimes \mathbf{r}_0 \in \mathcal{M}_{2+1}^{\,2+0} = \mathcal{M}_3^{\,2}$.

In general, if $\mathbf{M} \in \mathcal{M}_d^{\,d'}$, to form the tensor product $\mathbf{I} \otimes \mathbf{M}$ we replace each 1 in $\mathbf{I}$ with $\mathbf{M}$, and each 0 in $\mathbf{I}$ with the same size zero matrix. This replaces the kth diagonal identity block $\mathbf{1}^{\otimes k} \in \mathcal{M}_k^{\,k}$ with the matrix $\mathbf{1}^{\otimes k} \otimes \mathbf{M} \in \mathcal{M}_{k+d}^{\,k+d'}$, shifting its location to block-row $k + d$, block-column $k + d'$.

Thus, for example, consider the case $\mathbf{M} = \mathbf{u}_1{}^{\mathrm{T}} = \mathbf{u}_1{}^{\mathrm{T}}$ (84). Now $\mathbf{u}_1$ is a 2×1 column matrix, so $\mathbf{u}_1{}^{\mathrm{T}}$ is a 1×2 row vector: $\mathbf{M} \in \mathcal{M}_0^{\,1}$. In the tensor product $\mathbf{I} \otimes \mathbf{M}$, the identity blocks shift right one block: the change in block-row is 0, the change in block-column is 1, as shown in (88).

(88) $\mathbf{W}_{\mathrm{ex1}} = \mathbf{1}_A \otimes$

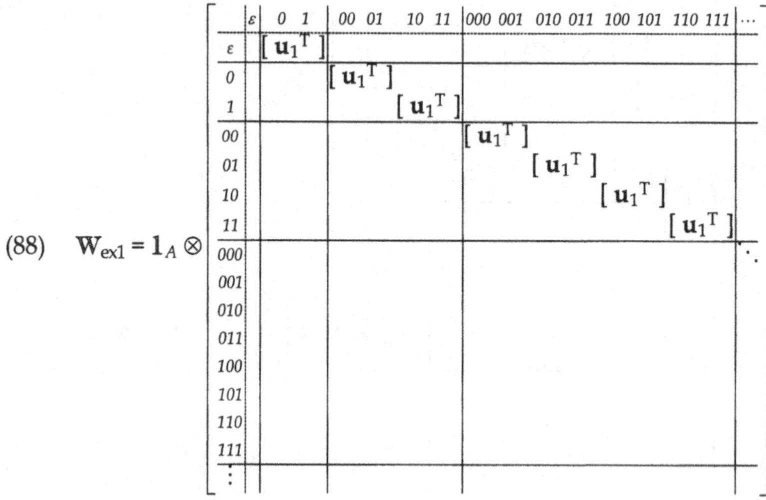

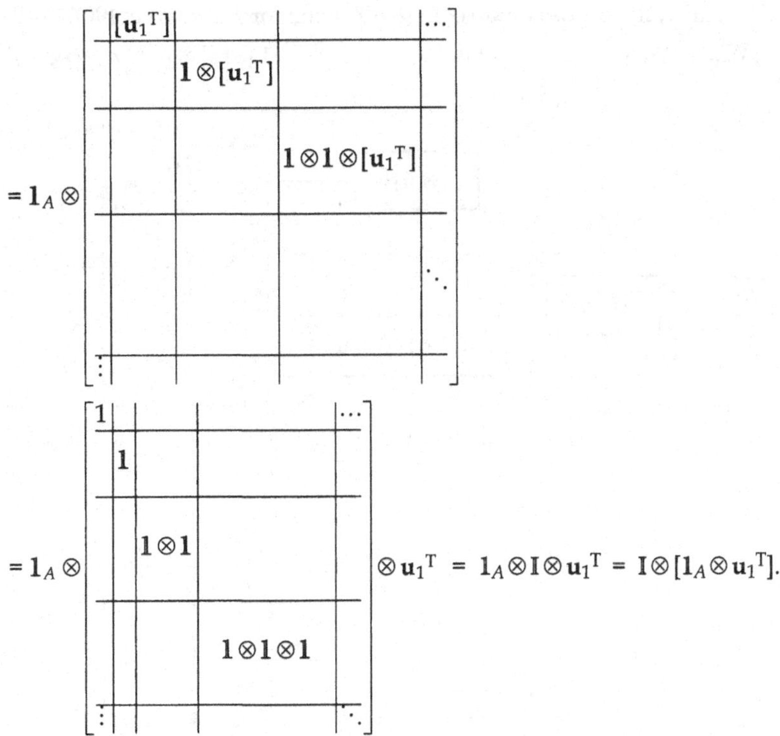

4.1.5 Products of primitive matrices

A crucial property of the primitive matrices shown above is that their form, $\mathbf{I}\otimes\mathbf{M}$, is preserved under matrix multiplication. An example is shown algebraically in (89).

(89) $\mathbf{W}_{\mathrm{cons0}}\cdot\mathbf{W}_{\mathrm{ex1}} = [\mathbf{1}_A\otimes\mathbf{I}\otimes\mathbf{r}_0]\cdot[\mathbf{1}_A\otimes\mathbf{I}\otimes\mathbf{u}_1^{\mathrm{T}}] = \mathbf{1}_A\otimes\mathbf{I}\otimes[\mathbf{r}_0\cdot\mathbf{u}_1^{\mathrm{T}}].$

Proof. Note, $\mathbf{r}_0 \in \mathcal{M}_1^0$ while $\mathbf{u}_1^{\mathrm{T}} \in \mathcal{M}_0^1$, so $\mathbf{r}_0\cdot\mathbf{u}_1^{\mathrm{T}} \in \mathcal{M}_1^1$.

$$
\begin{aligned}
[\mathbf{W}_{\mathrm{cons0}}\cdot\mathbf{W}_{\mathrm{ex1}}]_{(d)}^{(d')} &= \Sigma_k\,[\mathbf{W}_{\mathrm{cons0}}]_{(d)}^{(k)}\cdot[\mathbf{W}_{\mathrm{ex1}}]_{(k)}^{(d')} && \text{by (65)}\\
&= \Sigma_k\,[\mathbf{1}_A\otimes\mathbf{I}\otimes\mathbf{r}_0]_{(d)}^{(k)}\,\delta_{d-1}^{\;k}\cdot[\mathbf{1}_A\otimes\mathbf{I}\otimes\mathbf{u}_1^{\mathrm{T}}]_{(k)}^{(d')}\,\delta_k^{\;d'-1} && \text{by (79)}\\
&= (\mathbf{1}_A\cdot\mathbf{1}_A)\otimes[\mathbf{1}^{\otimes(d-1)}\otimes\mathbf{r}_0]\cdot[\mathbf{1}^{\otimes(d-1)}\otimes\mathbf{u}_1^{\mathrm{T}}]\,\delta_d^{\;d'} && \text{by (82)}\\
&= \mathbf{1}_A\otimes(\mathbf{1}\cdot\mathbf{1})^{\otimes(d-1)}\otimes(\mathbf{r}_0\cdot\mathbf{u}_1^{\mathrm{T}})\,\delta_d^{\;d'} && \text{by (80)}\\
&= \mathbf{1}_A\otimes\mathbf{1}^{\otimes(d-1)}\otimes(\mathbf{r}_0\cdot\mathbf{u}_1^{\mathrm{T}})\,\delta_d^{\;d'}. && \mathbf{1}\cdot\mathbf{1}=\mathbf{1}
\end{aligned}
$$

So

$$\mathbf{W}_{\mathrm{cons0}}\cdot\mathbf{W}_{\mathrm{ex1}} = \mathbf{1}_A\otimes\Sigma_k\,\mathbf{1}^{\otimes k}\otimes(\mathbf{r}_0\cdot\mathbf{u}_1^{\mathrm{T}}) = \mathbf{1}_A\otimes\mathbf{I}\otimes(\mathbf{r}_0\cdot\mathbf{u}_1^{\mathrm{T}}).$$

Pictorially, the product matrix in (89) has the form shown in (90).

(90) $\mathbf{W}_{\text{cons0}} \cdot \mathbf{W}_{\text{ex1}} = (\mathbf{1}_A \otimes \mathbf{I} \otimes \mathbf{r}_0) \cdot (\mathbf{1}_A \otimes \mathbf{I} \otimes \mathbf{u}_1^{\mathrm{T}}) = [\mathbf{1}_A \cdot \mathbf{1}_A] \otimes [(\mathbf{I} \otimes \mathbf{r}_0) \cdot (\mathbf{I} \otimes \mathbf{u}_1^{\mathrm{T}})]$

$= \mathbf{1}_A \otimes$

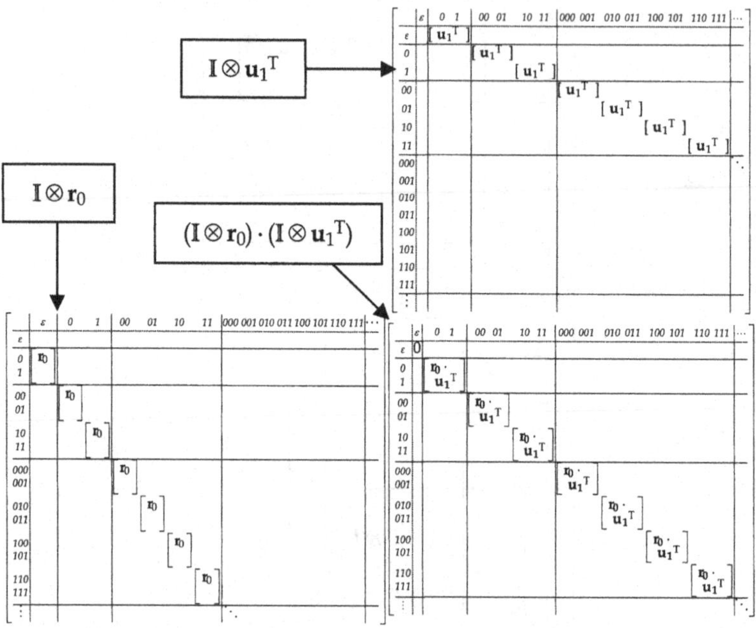

This matrix, $(\mathbf{I} \otimes \mathbf{r}_0) \cdot (\mathbf{I} \otimes \mathbf{u}_1^{\mathrm{T}})$, like the primitive matrices, can be generated directly from $\mathbf{I}$: we replace each 1 in the identity matrix in each diagonal block by the 2×2 matrix $\mathbf{r}_0 \cdot \mathbf{u}_1^{\mathrm{T}}$, sliding it down the diagonal one block (increasing the row by 1, and the column by 1, since $\mathbf{r}_0 \cdot \mathbf{u}_1^{\mathrm{T}} \in \mathcal{M}_1^{\,1}$). This is just the matrix $\mathbf{I} \otimes [\mathbf{r}_0 \cdot \mathbf{u}_1^{\mathrm{T}}]$ of (89).

4.1.6 The Feed-Forward Recursion Theorem

The remainder of Section 4.1 and all of Section 4.2 are sufficiently technical that it is best to present the material in a terse formal style consisting mostly of definitions, theorems, and proofs, with little commentary. The main results are the theorems presented with names in boldface.

In Section 4.1.5, we saw that $[\mathbf{I} \otimes \mathbf{r}_0] \cdot [\mathbf{I} \otimes \mathbf{u}_1^{\mathrm{T}}] = \mathbf{I} \otimes (\mathbf{r}_0 \cdot \mathbf{u}_1^{\mathrm{T}})$. This is general. The proof, however, requires considerable index bookkeeping: it occupies this subsection.

(91) Feed-Forward Recursion Theorem

Suppose $\mathbf{W} = \mathbf{I} \otimes \underline{\mathbf{W}}$ and $\mathbf{X} = \mathbf{I} \otimes \underline{\mathbf{X}}$, with $\underline{\mathbf{W}} \in \mathcal{M}_w^{\,w'}$, $\underline{\mathbf{X}} \in \mathcal{M}_x^{\,x'}$, and $w' - x \equiv \Delta > 0$. Then

$\mathbf{W} \cdot \mathbf{X} = \mathbf{I} \otimes \underline{\mathbf{Y}},$

where

$$\underline{\mathbf{Y}} \equiv \underline{\mathbf{W}} \cdot [1^{\otimes\Delta} \otimes \underline{\mathbf{X}}].$$

Proof.

$$\begin{aligned}[\mathbf{W}\cdot\mathbf{X}]_{(d)}^{(d')} &= \Sigma_k\, [\mathbf{I}\otimes\underline{\mathbf{W}}]_{(d)}^{(k)} \cdot [\mathbf{I}\otimes\underline{\mathbf{X}}]_{(k)}^{(d')} \\ &= \Sigma_k\, [\Sigma_u 1^{\otimes u}\otimes\underline{\mathbf{W}}]_{(d)}^{(k)} \cdot [\Sigma_v 1^{\otimes v}\otimes\underline{\mathbf{X}}]_{(k)}^{(d')}.\end{aligned}$$

A nonzero term in this sum is only possible if there are values of u, k, and v that enable the following to hold simultaneously:

$$1^{\otimes u}\otimes\underline{\mathbf{W}} \in \mathcal{M}_d^{\,k} \Leftrightarrow d = u + w \text{ and } k = u + w' \text{ (since } \underline{\mathbf{W}} \in \mathcal{M}_w^{\,w'});$$
$$1^{\otimes v}\otimes\underline{\mathbf{X}} \in \mathcal{M}_k^{\,d'} \Leftrightarrow k = v + x \text{ and } d' = v + x' \text{ (since } \underline{\mathbf{X}} \in \mathcal{M}_x^{\,x'}).$$

In this case, $[1^{\otimes u}\otimes\underline{\mathbf{W}}]_{(d)}^{(k)} \cdot [1^{\otimes v}\otimes\underline{\mathbf{X}}]_{(k)}^{(d')}$ is simply the product of a matrix in $\mathcal{M}_d^{\,k}$ and a matrix in $\mathcal{M}_k^{\,d'}$, that is, $[1^{\otimes u}\otimes\underline{\mathbf{W}}]\cdot[1^{\otimes v}\otimes\underline{\mathbf{X}}]$. These conditions on u, k, and v entail

$$\begin{aligned}
&d = u + w \Rightarrow \underline{u = d - w} && \\
&\qquad\quad \text{and } k = u + w' && \Rightarrow k = (d - w) + w', \\
&d' = v + x' \Rightarrow \underline{v = d' - x'} && \\
&\qquad\quad \text{and } k = v + x && \Rightarrow k = (d' - x') + x, \\
&k = d' - x' + x \text{ and } k = (d - w) + w' && \Rightarrow d - w + w' = d' - x' + x \\
& && \Rightarrow d' = x' - x + d - w + w' \\
& && \Rightarrow \underline{v} = \underline{d' - x'} = d - w + w' - x \\
& && \qquad = \underline{d - w + \Delta},
\end{aligned}$$

where, as defined in the theorem, $\Delta \equiv w' - x$. Thus,

$$\begin{aligned}[\mathbf{W}\cdot\mathbf{X}]_{(d)}^{(d')} &= \Sigma_k\, [\Sigma_u 1^{\otimes u}\otimes\underline{\mathbf{W}}]_{(d)}^{(k)} \cdot [\Sigma_v 1^{\otimes v}\otimes\underline{\mathbf{X}}]_{(k)}^{(d')} \\
&= \delta_{d-w+\Delta}^{\,d'-x'}\, [1^{\otimes(d-w)}\otimes\underline{\mathbf{W}}]\cdot[1^{\otimes(d-w+\Delta)}\otimes\underline{\mathbf{X}}] \\
&= \delta_{d-w+\Delta}^{\,d'-x'}\, [1^{\otimes(d-w)}\otimes\underline{\mathbf{W}}]\cdot[1^{\otimes(d-w)}\otimes 1^{\otimes\Delta}\otimes\underline{\mathbf{X}}] \\
&= \delta_{d-w+\Delta}^{\,d'-x'}\, (1^{\otimes(d-w)}\cdot 1^{\otimes(d-w)})\otimes(\underline{\mathbf{W}}\cdot[1^{\otimes\Delta}\otimes\underline{\mathbf{X}}]).\end{aligned}$$

The last line follows from the identity (80):

$$[\mathbf{A}\otimes\mathbf{B}]\cdot[\mathbf{A}'\otimes\mathbf{B}'] = (\mathbf{A}\cdot\mathbf{A}')\otimes(\mathbf{B}\cdot\mathbf{B}'),$$

with $\mathbf{A} \equiv 1^{\otimes(d-w)} \equiv \mathbf{A}'$. This same identity implies (letting $n \equiv d - w$)

$$\begin{aligned}\mathbf{A}\cdot\mathbf{A}' \equiv 1^{\otimes n}\cdot 1^{\otimes n} &\equiv [1\otimes 1\otimes\cdots\otimes 1]\cdot[1\otimes 1\otimes\cdots\otimes 1] \\
&= (1\cdot 1)\otimes(1\cdot 1)\otimes\cdots\otimes(1\cdot 1) \\
&= (1)\otimes(1)\otimes\cdots\otimes(1) \equiv 1^{\otimes n}.\end{aligned}$$

Finally, then, with $\underline{\mathbf{Y}} \equiv \mathbf{W}\cdot[1^{\otimes\Delta}\otimes\underline{\mathbf{X}}] \in \mathcal{M}_w^{\,x'+\Delta}$ as in the theorem,

$$\begin{aligned}[\mathbf{W}\cdot\mathbf{X}]_{(d)}^{(d')} &= \delta_{d-w+\Delta}^{\,d'-x'} \otimes (1^{\otimes(d-w)}\cdot 1^{\otimes(d-w)})\otimes(\underline{\mathbf{W}}\cdot[1^{\otimes\Delta}\otimes\underline{\mathbf{X}}]) \\
&= 1^{\otimes(d-w)}\otimes\underline{\mathbf{Y}},\end{aligned}$$

which is consistent since when $\delta_{d-w+\Delta}^{\,d'-x'} = 1$, $d{-}w{+}\Delta = d'{-}x'$, and then $1^{\otimes(d-w)}\otimes\underline{\mathbf{Y}} \in \mathcal{M}_{(d-w)+w}^{\,(d-w)+x'+\Delta} = \mathcal{M}_d^{\,d'}$. But, since $\underline{\mathbf{Y}} \in \mathcal{M}_w^{\,x'+\Delta}$, this is exactly the row-d, column-d' block of $\mathbf{I}\otimes\underline{\mathbf{Y}}$:

$$[\mathbf{W}\cdot\mathbf{X}]_{(d)}^{(d')} = 1^{\otimes(d-w)}\otimes\underline{\mathbf{Y}} = [\Sigma_k 1^{\otimes k}\otimes\underline{\mathbf{Y}}]_{(d)}^{(d')} = [\mathbf{I}\otimes\underline{\mathbf{Y}}]_{(d)}^{(d')}.$$

Since this is true for all d and d', we have $\mathbf{W}\cdot\mathbf{X} = \mathbf{I}\otimes\underline{\mathbf{Y}}$.

This theorem treats the case where $\underline{\mathbf{W}} \in \mathcal{M}_w^{\,w'}$, $\underline{\mathbf{X}} \in \mathcal{M}_x^{\,x'}$, and $w' - x \equiv \Delta > 0$, that is, where $\underline{\mathbf{X}}$ has Δ fewer rows than $\underline{\mathbf{W}}$ has columns; in this case, $\underline{\mathbf{X}}$ needs to be "expanded" before it can be multiplied by $\underline{\mathbf{W}}$. Taking the tensor product of $1^{\otimes\Delta}$ with $\underline{\mathbf{X}}$ adds Δ rows (and columns) to $\underline{\mathbf{X}}$.

The reverse case is also possible: $\underline{\mathbf{W}} \in \mathcal{M}_w^{\,w'}$, $\underline{\mathbf{X}} \in \mathcal{M}_x^{\,x'}$, and $x - w' \equiv \Delta' > 0$; that is, $\underline{\mathbf{X}}$ has Δ' *more* rows than $\underline{\mathbf{W}}$ has columns. In this case, it is now $\underline{\mathbf{W}}$ that must be expanded by taking its tensor product with $\mathbf{1}^{\otimes\Delta'}$ so that multiplication by $\underline{\mathbf{X}}$ is possible. The proof of the preceding theorem works exactly the same for this case, with the newly appropriate "expansion" factor Δ'.

(92) *Corollary.* Suppose $\mathbf{W} = \mathbf{I}\otimes\underline{\mathbf{W}}$ and $\mathbf{X} = \mathbf{I}\otimes\underline{\mathbf{X}}$, with $\underline{\mathbf{W}} \in \mathcal{M}_w^{\ w'}$, $\underline{\mathbf{X}} \in \mathcal{M}_x^{\ x'}$, and $x - w' \equiv \Delta' > 0$. Then

$$\mathbf{W}\cdot\mathbf{X} = \mathbf{I}\otimes\underline{\mathbf{Y}},$$

where $\underline{\mathbf{Y}} \equiv [\mathbf{1}^{\otimes\Delta'}\otimes\underline{\mathbf{W}}]\cdot\underline{\mathbf{X}}$.

The preceding theorem and corollary make the following definition quite useful:

(93) *Definition.* Given $\underline{\mathbf{W}} \in \mathcal{M}_w^{\ w'}$ and $\underline{\mathbf{X}} \in \mathcal{M}_x^{\ x'}$, their **circle product** $\underline{\mathbf{W}}\circ\underline{\mathbf{X}}$ is defined as follows:

a. If $w' - x \equiv \Delta > 0$, $\underline{\mathbf{W}}\circ\underline{\mathbf{X}} \equiv \underline{\mathbf{W}}\cdot[\mathbf{1}^{\otimes\Delta}\otimes\underline{\mathbf{X}}] \in \mathcal{M}_w^{\ x'+\Delta}$.

b. If $x - w' \equiv \Delta' > 0$, $\underline{\mathbf{W}}\circ\underline{\mathbf{X}} \equiv [\mathbf{1}^{\otimes\Delta'}\otimes\underline{\mathbf{W}}]\cdot\underline{\mathbf{X}} \in \mathcal{M}_{w+\Delta'}^{\ x'}$.

Given $\mathbf{G}\otimes\underline{\mathbf{W}} \in \mathcal{M}_A\otimes\mathcal{M}_w^{\ w'} \equiv \mathcal{W}_w^{\ w'}$ and $\mathbf{G}'\otimes\underline{\mathbf{X}} \in \mathcal{W}_x^{\ x'}$, their circle product is

c. $(\mathbf{G}\otimes\underline{\mathbf{W}})\circ(\mathbf{G}'\otimes\underline{\mathbf{X}}) \equiv (\mathbf{G}\cdot\mathbf{G}')\otimes\underline{\mathbf{W}}\circ\underline{\mathbf{X}}$.

Now (91) and (92) can be simply stated:

(94) **Feed-Forward Recursion Theorem**

If $\underline{\mathbf{W}} \in \mathcal{M}_w^{\ w'}$ and $\underline{\mathbf{W}'} \in \mathcal{M}_x^{\ x'}$, or if $\underline{\mathbf{W}} \in \mathcal{W}_w^{\ w'}$ and $\underline{\mathbf{W}'} \in \mathcal{W}_x^{\ x'}$ (for any values of x, x', w, w'), then

$$(\mathbf{I}\otimes\underline{\mathbf{W}})\cdot(\mathbf{I}\otimes\underline{\mathbf{W}'}) = \mathbf{I}\otimes(\underline{\mathbf{W}}\circ\underline{\mathbf{W}'}).$$

4.1.7 Finite specification of PC functions

This subsection defines a class of recursive symbolic functions mapping binary trees to binary trees. It characterizes a sense in which this infinite behavior derives from a finite specification. The analysis addresses a set of functions where the fate of each binding in the input tree is independent of the other bindings in the input.

(95) *Definition.* A function f on s-trees is **first order** iff $f(\varnothing) = \varnothing$ and

$$f(\sqcup_i\{\mathbf{A}_i/r_i\}) = \sqcup_i\{f(\mathbf{A}_i/r_i)\}.$$

(96) *Proposition.* The primitive functions $\mathbf{ex}_i$, $\mathbf{cons}_i$ are first order.

Proof. By definition, for either $i = 0$ (and $\bar{\imath} = 1$) or $i = 1$ (and $\bar{\imath} = 0$),

$$\mathbf{ex}_i(\sqcup_x\{\mathbf{A}_{xi}/r_{xi}\}\sqcup\sqcup_y\{\mathbf{A}_{y\bar{\imath}}/r_{y\bar{\imath}}\}) \equiv \sqcup_x\{\mathbf{A}_{xi}/r_x\} \equiv \sqcup_x\{\mathbf{ex}_i(\mathbf{A}_{xi}/r_{xi})\};$$

$$\mathbf{cons}_i(\sqcup_x\{\mathbf{A}_x/r_x\}) \equiv \sqcup_x\{\mathbf{A}_x/r_{xi}\} \equiv \sqcup_x\{\mathbf{cons}_i(\mathbf{A}_x/r_x)\}.$$

(97) *Definition.* $\mathcal{F}$ is the class of partial functions from A, the set of atoms, to A.

'Partial' means that for a function $g \in \mathcal{F}$, there may be some symbol **A** $\in A$ such that $g(\mathbf{A})$ is undefined; this will be interpreted to mean that g deletes **A**.

(98) *Definition.* $\mathcal{B}$ is the set of functions h: $S \rightarrow S$ satisfying the following conditions.

a. h is first order.

b. For all $\mathbf{s} \in S$, $h(\mathbf{s}) = \mathbf{cons}(h(\mathbf{ex}_0(\mathbf{s})), h(\mathbf{ex}_1(\mathbf{s}))) \sqcup h(\mathbf{ex}_\varepsilon(\mathbf{s}))/r_\varepsilon$.

c. There is a $g \in \mathcal{F}$ such that $\forall \mathbf{A} \in A$, $h(\mathbf{A}/r_\varepsilon) = g(\mathbf{A})/r_\varepsilon$. Write $h = h_g$.

As (99) asserts, h_g simply replaces every atom **A** in **s** by $g(\mathbf{A})$.

(99) *Proposition.* Let **s** be the pseudotree with bindings $\{\mathbf{A}_x/r_x\}$. Then $h_g(\mathbf{s})$ is the pseudotree $\{g(\mathbf{A}_x)/r_x\}$.

Proof. This follows immediately from the first-order property of h_g (98a) and Lemma (100).

(100) *Lemma.* $h_g(\mathbf{A}/r_x) = g(\mathbf{A})/r_x$

Proof. By induction. If $|x| = 0$, then $x = \varepsilon$, and the proposition holds by definition (98c). Make the inductive hypothesis that the proposition holds for all x with $|x| \le d$. Now given a y with $|y| = d+1$, either $y = x0$ or $y = x1$, where $|x| = d$. Suppose $y = x0$; then $\mathbf{A}/r_y = \mathbf{cons}(\mathbf{A}/r_x, \varnothing)$. Thus,

$$\begin{aligned} h_g(\mathbf{A}/r_y) &= h_g(\mathbf{cons}(\mathbf{A}/r_x, \varnothing)) \\ &= \mathbf{cons}(h(\mathbf{A}/r_x), h(\varnothing)) && \text{by (98b)} \\ &= \mathbf{cons}(g(\mathbf{A})/r_x, \varnothing) && \text{by the inductive hypothesis and } h(\varnothing) = \varnothing \text{ (95)} \\ &= g(\mathbf{A})/r_{x0} = g(\mathbf{A})/r_y. \end{aligned}$$

Similarly, if $y = x1$, $\mathbf{A}/r_y = \mathbf{cons}(\varnothing, \mathbf{A}/r_x)$ and the same conclusion follows by the analogous argument.

(101) *Definition.* $\mathscr{F}$ is the function class defined by the following recursive definition:

a. Base case: $h \in \mathcal{B} \Rightarrow h \in \mathscr{F}$.

b. Recursion

i. If $h \in \mathcal{B}$ and $f \in \mathscr{F}$, then $h \circ f \equiv h(f) \in \mathscr{F}$.

ii. If $f, f' \in \mathscr{F}$, then $\mathbf{ex}_0(f)$, $\mathbf{ex}_1(f)$, and $\mathbf{cons}(f, f') \in \mathscr{F}$.

c. No other functions are in $\mathscr{F}$.

((101b.i) uses '$\circ$' in the standard sense of function composition: $h \circ f(x) \equiv h(f(x))$.) $\mathscr{F}$ is the closure under finite composition of the primitive functions $\mathbf{ex}_i$, **cons**. A function in $\mathscr{F}$ will be called **PC** ('primitives' closure').

(102) **Finite Specification Theorem for PC Functions**

For any $f \in \mathscr{F}$, there is a depth d such that if x is the bit-string address of a tree position at depth at least d, (i.e., $|x| \ge d$), then

$$f(\mathbf{sh}_i(\mathbf{A}/r_x)) = \mathbf{sh}_i(f(\mathbf{A}/r_x)), \qquad \text{for all } i \in \{0, 1\}, \mathbf{A} \in A$$

where the shift functions $\mathbf{sh}_i$ are defined by (29h). That is, if $f(\mathbf{A}/r_x) = \{\mathbf{B}_y/r_y\}$, then $f(\mathbf{A}/r_{ix}) = \{\mathbf{B}_y/r_{iy}\}$ for all $i \in \{0, 1\}$, $\mathbf{A}, \mathbf{B} \in A$ (very roughly: "the image of the child is the child of the image").

Proof. By induction. Every function $f \in \mathcal{F}$ is derived by a finite combination of the recursive operations in (101b) acting upon the base functions in (101a). Thus, the proposition is proved if (i) it is true for each base function and (ii) it is preserved by the recursive operations. In the proof, we derive the values for d for the base cases ($d = 0$) and derive the change in value of d under the recursive operations (**cons** takes the maximum of the d values of its arguments, and $\mathbf{ex}_i$ increases d by 1).

We begin with the base case. If $f \in \mathcal{B}$, then there is a $g \in \mathcal{F}$ such that $f = h_g$. Then by (100), for any x and $\mathbf{A} \in A$,

$$f(\mathbf{A}/r_x) = g(\mathbf{A})/r_x \text{ and } f(\mathbf{A}/r_{ix}) = g(\mathbf{A})/r_{ix}.$$

This establishes the result for $f \in \mathcal{B}$, with $d = 0$.

For the first recursive clause (101b.i), consider $f' = h_g \circ f$. Suppose inductively that f satisfies the proposition for some value d, and consider an x with $|x| \geq d$; let $f(\mathbf{A}/r_x) = \{\mathbf{B}_y/r_y\}$. Then, again by (100),

$$f'(\mathbf{A}/r_{ix}) \equiv h_g(f(\mathbf{A}/r_{ix})) = h_g(\{\mathbf{B}_y/r_{iy}\}) = \{g(\mathbf{B}_y)/r_{iy}\}$$

and

$$f'(\mathbf{A}/r_x) \equiv h_g(f(\mathbf{A}/r_x)) = h_g(\{\mathbf{B}_y/r_y\}) = \{g(\mathbf{B}_y)/r_y\}.$$

Thus, f' satisfies the proposition with the same value d as f.

Now consider the other recursive clause (101b.ii), as it pertains to **cons**. Suppose inductively that f and f' obey the proposition with values d and d'. Let d'' be the maximum of d and d'. Define $f'' \equiv \mathbf{cons}(f, f')$. Consider an x with $|x| \geq d''$; we then have $|x| \geq d$ and $|x| \geq d'$, so both f and f' satisfy the proposition for x. Let $f(\mathbf{A}/r_x) = \{\mathbf{B}_y/r_y\}$. Now by (29g), $\mathbf{cons}(f, f') = \mathbf{cons}_0(f) \sqcup \mathbf{cons}_1(f')$; to verify the proposition for f'', it will suffice to verify it for $\mathbf{cons}_0(f)$, since the analogous argument will verify the proposition for $\mathbf{cons}_1(f')$, and $\sqcup$ merely takes the union of bindings. Now since f obeys the proposition, and by the definition of $\mathbf{cons}_0$ (29g),

$$\mathbf{cons}_0(f(\mathbf{A}/r_{ix})) = \mathbf{cons}_0(\{\mathbf{B}_y/r_{iy}\}) = \{\mathbf{B}_y/r_{iy0}\}$$

while

$$\mathbf{cons}_0(f(\mathbf{A}/r_x)) = \mathbf{cons}_0(\{\mathbf{B}_y/r_y\}) = \{\mathbf{B}_y/r_{y0}\},$$

so the proposition holds.

Finally, consider (101b.ii) as it applies to $\mathbf{ex}_k$. Suppose inductively that f obeys the proposition for value d; consider x such that $|x| \geq d$, and let

$$f(\mathbf{A}/r_x) = \{\mathbf{B}_y/r_y\} \equiv \mathbf{B}_\varepsilon/r_\varepsilon \sqcup \{\mathbf{B}_{z0}/r_{z0}\} \sqcup \{\mathbf{B}_{w1}/r_{w1}\},$$

where the various bit strings y have been separated into those with final bit 0 ($y = z0$), those with final bit 1 ($y = w1$), and the null string ($y = \varepsilon$; if there is no symbol at the root, we can take $\mathbf{B}_\varepsilon = \varnothing$). By the inductive hypothesis, f satisfies the theorem, so

$$f(\mathbf{A}/r_{ix}) = \{\mathbf{B}_y/r_{iy}\} \equiv \mathbf{B}_\varepsilon/r_i \sqcup \{\mathbf{B}_{z0}/r_{iz0}\} \sqcup \{\mathbf{B}_{w1}/r_{iw1}\}.$$

Since $\mathbf{ex}_k$ is first order (96),

$$\mathbf{ex}_k[f(\mathbf{A}/r_{ix})] = \mathbf{ex}_k[\{\mathbf{B}_y/r_{iy}\}] = \mathbf{ex}_k[\mathbf{B}_\varepsilon/r_i] \sqcup \mathbf{ex}_k[\{\mathbf{B}_{z0}/r_{iz0}\}] \sqcup \mathbf{ex}_k[\{\mathbf{B}_{w1}/r_{iw1}\}]$$
$$= \begin{cases} \mathbf{B}_z/r_{iz} & \text{if } k = 0 \\ \mathbf{B}_w/r_{iw} & \text{if } k = 1 \\ \varnothing & \text{if } k = \varepsilon \end{cases}.$$

And

$$\mathbf{ex}_k[f(\mathbf{A}/r_x)] = \mathbf{ex}_k[\{\mathbf{B}_y/r_y\}] = \mathbf{ex}_k[\mathbf{B}_\varepsilon/r_\varepsilon] \sqcup \mathbf{ex}_k[\{\mathbf{B}_{z0}/r_{z0}\}] \sqcup \mathbf{ex}_k[\{\mathbf{B}_{w1}/r_{iw1}\}]$$

Figure 4 Box 2

$$= \begin{cases} \mathbf{B}_z / r_z & \text{if } k = 0 \\ \mathbf{B}_w / r_w & \text{if } k = 1 \\ \mathbf{B}_\varepsilon / r_\varepsilon & \text{if } k = \varepsilon \end{cases}.$$

The relationship required by the theorem holds for $\mathbf{ex}_k(f)$, for $k = 0$ or 1, but not for $k = \varepsilon$, unless $\mathbf{B}_\varepsilon = \emptyset$. Thus, $f(\mathbf{A}/r_x) = \{\mathbf{B}_y/r_y\}$ must not have a symbol at the root. This can be ensured if $|x| \geq d+1$. Then we can write $x = jq$ for $j = 0$ or 1, and q a bit string with $|q| \geq d$. Then since f satisfies the proposition for all such bit strings q, we must have

$$f(\mathbf{A}/r_x) = f(\mathbf{A}/r_{jq}) = \{\mathbf{C}_y/r_{jq}\}, \text{ where } \{\mathbf{C}_y/r_q\} = f(\mathbf{A}/r_q).$$

But $\{\mathbf{C}_y/r_{jq}\}$ can include no binding $\mathbf{C}_\varepsilon/r_\varepsilon$ because for all q, $jq \neq \varepsilon$. Thus, if the proposition holds of f for d, it holds of $\mathbf{ex}_k(f)$ for $d+1$.

This theorem shows how a function f in $\mathcal{F}$ is finitely specified; beyond a certain finite depth d, the image under f of any symbol is strictly determined by the image of its parent. Thus, specifying f for the finite set of trees of depth at most d completely determines the output of f for any input tree, no matter its depth.

The example in (103) illustrates these ideas.

(103) Example

Define the function f: $\mathbf{s} \mapsto [\mathbf{s}\ \mathbf{s}]$. For example,

$$f([\mathbf{A}\ [\mathbf{B}\ \mathbf{A}]]) = [[\mathbf{A}\ [\mathbf{B}\ \mathbf{A}]]\ [\mathbf{A}\ [\mathbf{B}\ \mathbf{A}]]].$$

Then f can be constructed as $f(\mathbf{s}) = \mathbf{cons}(\mathrm{Id}_S(\mathbf{s}), \mathrm{Id}_S(\mathbf{s}))$; that is,

$$f = \mathbf{cons}(f', f''),\ f' \equiv \mathrm{Id}_S \equiv f'',$$

where Id_S is the identity function on S. Id_S is h_g, where g is the identity function on A; hence, $f' = f'' \in \mathcal{F}$. Then it follows that $f = \mathbf{cons}\ (\mathrm{Id}_S, \mathrm{Id}_S) \in \mathcal{F}$: f is PC. Now in terms of individual bindings,

$$f(\mathbf{A}/r_x) = \mathbf{cons}(\{\mathbf{A}/r_x\}, \{\mathbf{A}/r_x\}) = \{\mathbf{A}/r_{x0}, \mathbf{A}/r_{x1}\},$$

so therefore

$$\mathbf{sh}_i(f(\mathbf{A}/r_x)) = \mathbf{sh}_i(\{\mathbf{A}/r_{x0}, \mathbf{A}/r_{x1}\}) = \{\mathbf{A}/r_{ix0}, \mathbf{A}/r_{ix1}\}.$$

In accord with the Finite Specification Theorem (102), this equals

$$f(\mathbf{sh}_i(\mathbf{A}/r_x)) = f(\mathbf{A}/r_{ix}) \equiv \mathbf{cons}(\{\mathbf{A}/r_{ix}\}, \{\mathbf{A}/r_{ix}\}) = \{\mathbf{A}/r_{ix0}, \mathbf{A}/r_{ix1}\}.$$

4.1.8 Connectionist realization of PC functions

(104) *Proposition.* Let f be the function such that $f(\mathbf{s}) = \mathbf{B}/r_y$ if $\mathbf{A}/r_x \in \beta(\mathbf{s})$, and $f(\mathbf{s}) = \emptyset$ otherwise, where $\mathbf{A}/r_x$ and $\mathbf{B}/r_y$ are any two bindings of atomic symbols. Then f is realized by the matrix

$$\mathbf{M} \equiv [\mathbf{B} \otimes \mathbf{r}_y]\ [\mathbf{A}^+ \otimes \mathbf{u}_x]^T.$$

Recall that $\mathbf{A}^+$ is the dual basis vector corresponding to $\mathbf{A}$, a basis vector in A, the set of all realizations of atomic symbols (29c). This means $\mathbf{A}^+ \cdot \mathbf{C} = \delta_{\mathbf{A},\mathbf{C}}$: if $\mathbf{A}$ and $\mathbf{C}$ realize the same symbol, the dot product is 1; otherwise, it is 0 (Box 5:1 (8)). Likewise, $\mathbf{u}_x$ is the dual vector corresponding to $\mathbf{r}_x$ ($\mathbf{u}_x \equiv \mathbf{r}_x^+$). Thus, $\mathbf{u}_x \cdot \mathbf{r}_y = \delta_{x,y}$: 1 if $\mathbf{u}_x$ corresponds to the same role as $\mathbf{r}_y$ (i.e., $x = y$), and 0 otherwise.

> *Proof.*
> $$\begin{aligned}\mathbf{M}\cdot\mathbf{s} = \mathbf{M}\cdot\Sigma_z \mathbf{a}_z\otimes\mathbf{r}_z &= [\mathbf{B}\otimes\mathbf{r}_y]\,\Sigma_z[\mathbf{A}^{+}\otimes\mathbf{u}_x]^{\mathrm{T}}\mathbf{a}_z\otimes\mathbf{r}_z\\ &= [\mathbf{B}\otimes\mathbf{r}_y]\,\Sigma_z[\mathbf{A}^{+}\otimes\mathbf{u}_x]\cdot[\mathbf{a}_z\otimes\mathbf{r}_z]\\ &= [\mathbf{B}\otimes\mathbf{r}_y]\,\Sigma_z[\mathbf{A}^{+}\cdot\mathbf{a}_z][\mathbf{u}_x\cdot\mathbf{r}_z] \qquad \text{by (80)}\\ &= [\mathbf{B}\otimes\mathbf{r}_y]\,\Sigma_z[\mathbf{A}^{+}\cdot\mathbf{a}_z]\,\delta_{xz}\\ &= [\mathbf{B}\otimes\mathbf{r}_y]\,[\mathbf{A}^{+}\cdot\mathbf{a}_x].\end{aligned}$$
> $[\mathbf{A}^{+}\cdot\mathbf{a}_x]$ is 1 if $\mathbf{a}_x = \mathbf{A}$, and 0 otherwise; thus, $\mathbf{M}\cdot\mathbf{s} = \mathbf{B}\otimes\mathbf{r}_y$ if $\mathtt{A}/r_x$ is one of **s**'s bindings, and 0 otherwise.

(105) *Proposition.* If $\mathbf{M} \equiv \mathbf{D}\,\mathbf{A}^{+\mathrm{T}}\otimes\mathbf{I}$, then $\mathbf{M}\cdot\mathbf{C}/\mathbf{r}_y = \mathbf{D}/\mathbf{r}_y$ if $\mathbf{C} = \mathbf{A}$, and 0 if $\mathbf{C}\in A$ is the realization of any symbol other than **A**. (**M** is an "**A** to **D** converter.")

> *Proof.* Recall that **I** is the identity matrix on the entire role space $\mathcal{R}$. $\mathbf{A}^{+\mathrm{T}}$ is just $(\mathbf{A}^{+})^{\mathrm{T}}$.
> $$\begin{aligned}\mathbf{M}\cdot\mathbf{C}/\mathbf{r}_y &= (\mathbf{D}\,\mathbf{A}^{+\mathrm{T}}\otimes\mathbf{I})\cdot(\mathbf{C}\otimes\mathbf{r}_y) = (\mathbf{D}\,\mathbf{A}^{+\mathrm{T}}\cdot\mathbf{C})\otimes(\mathbf{I}\cdot\mathbf{r}_y)\\ &= (\mathbf{D}[\mathbf{A}^{+}\cdot\mathbf{C}])\otimes\mathbf{r}_y = [\mathbf{A}^{+}\cdot\mathbf{C}](\mathbf{D}\otimes\mathbf{r}_y),\end{aligned}$$
> using (81) and $\mathbf{A}^{+\mathrm{T}}\cdot\mathbf{C} = \mathbf{A}^{+}\cdot\mathbf{C}$, where the left side uses matrix-vector multiplication and the right side uses the inner product of vectors (Box 5:1 (16)). If $\mathbf{C} = \mathbf{A}$, then $\mathbf{A}^{+}\cdot\mathbf{C} = 1$, and the result is $\mathbf{D}\otimes\mathbf{r}_y$; if **C** realizes a symbol other than **A**, then $\mathbf{A}^{+}\cdot\mathbf{C} = 0$.

(106) *Definition.* The function $f \mapsto \underline{\mathbf{W}}_f$ maps an $f \in \mathcal{F}$ to its **realization kernel** $\underline{\mathbf{W}}_f$, a matrix over a recursive tensor product representational space *S*. $f \mapsto \underline{\mathbf{W}}_f$ is defined recursively as follows:

a. Base case

If $f = h_g \in \mathcal{B}$, where $g\colon A \to A$ is a function in $\mathcal{F}$, then

$\underline{\mathbf{W}}_f \equiv \underline{\mathbf{W}}_g \in \mathcal{M}_A$, $\underline{\mathbf{W}}_g \equiv \Sigma_{\mathbf{A}\in A}\, \psi(g(\mathbf{A}))\, \psi(\mathbf{A})^{+\mathrm{T}} \equiv \Sigma_{\mathbf{A}\in A}\, \mathbf{g}(\mathbf{A})\, \mathbf{A}^{+\mathrm{T}}$.

b. Recursion

If $f = h(f')$, $h \in \mathcal{B}$, then $\underline{\mathbf{W}}_f \equiv \underline{\mathbf{W}}_h \circ \underline{\mathbf{W}}_{f'}$.

If $f = \mathbf{ex}_i(f')$, then $\underline{\mathbf{W}}_f \equiv \underline{\mathbf{W}}_{\mathrm{ex}i} \circ \underline{\mathbf{W}}_{f'}$,

where $\underline{\mathbf{W}}_{\mathrm{ex}_i} \equiv \underline{\mathbf{W}}_{\mathrm{ex}i} \equiv \mathbf{1}_A \otimes \mathbf{u}_i^{\mathrm{T}} \in \mathcal{W}_0^{\,1}$ for $i = 0, 1$.

If $f = \mathtt{cons}(f', f'')$ then $\underline{\mathbf{W}}_f \equiv \underline{\mathbf{W}}_{\mathrm{cons}0} \circ \underline{\mathbf{W}}_{f'} + \underline{\mathbf{W}}_{\mathrm{cons}1} \circ \underline{\mathbf{W}}_{f''}$,

where $\underline{\mathbf{W}}_{\mathrm{cons}i} \equiv \mathbf{1}_A \otimes \mathbf{r}_i \in \mathcal{W}_1^{\,0}$, $i = 0, 1$.

(107) *Proposition.* For any $f \in \mathcal{F}$, the realization kernel $\underline{\mathbf{W}}_f$ is a finite matrix.

> *Proof.* By induction. Every $f \in \mathcal{F}$ is built from the base functions $\mathcal{B}$ by a finite set of recursive operations (101); for the base functions $f \in \mathcal{B}$, $\underline{\mathbf{W}}_f$ is finite (106a), and under the recursive operations (106b), a finite matrix is transformed into another finite matrix.

(108) **Realization Theorem for PC Functions**

For any $f \in \mathcal{F}$, f is realized by the weight matrix

$\mathbf{W}_f = \mathbf{I}\otimes\underline{\mathbf{W}}_f$,

where I is the (unbounded) feed-forward recursion matrix (75) and $\underline{\mathbf{W}}_f$ is the (finite) realization kernel of f (106).

Proof. By induction. Throughout the proof, let $\mathbf{s}$ be an s-tree with bindings $\beta(\mathbf{s}) = \{\mathbf{s}_x/r_x\}$, realized by the v-tree $\mathbf{s} \equiv \psi(\mathbf{s}) = \Sigma_x \mathbf{s}_x \otimes \mathbf{r}_x$; let $f(\mathbf{s}) \equiv \mathbf{t} \equiv \{\mathbf{t}_x/r_x\}$ and let $\mathbf{t} \equiv \psi(\mathbf{t}) = \Sigma_x \mathbf{t}_x \otimes \mathbf{r}_x$. We proceed through the base case and recursive operations of $\mathcal{F}$.

Base case: if $f = h_g \in \mathcal{B}$, then $\mathbf{t}_x = g(\mathbf{s}_x)$, and so, using (105),

$$\begin{aligned}\mathbf{W}_f \cdot \mathbf{s} &\equiv (\mathbf{I} \otimes \underline{\mathbf{W}}_f) \cdot \mathbf{s} \equiv (\mathbf{I} \otimes \underline{\mathbf{W}}_g) \cdot \Sigma_x \mathbf{s}_x \otimes \mathbf{r}_x \equiv (\underline{\mathbf{W}}_g \otimes \mathbf{I}) \cdot \Sigma_x \mathbf{s}_x \otimes \mathbf{r}_x \qquad \text{by (78)}\\ &= \Sigma_x (\underline{\mathbf{W}}_g \cdot \mathbf{s}_x) \otimes (\mathbf{I} \cdot \mathbf{r}_x)\\ &= \Sigma_x \Sigma_{\mathbf{A} \in A} ([\mathbf{g}(\mathbf{A})\, \mathbf{A}^{+T}] \cdot \mathbf{s}_x) \otimes \mathbf{r}_x\\ &= \Sigma_x \mathbf{g}(\mathbf{s}_x) \otimes \mathbf{r}_x\\ &= \Sigma_x \mathbf{t}_x \otimes \mathbf{r}_x = \mathbf{t}.\end{aligned}$$

For the first recursive operation, suppose $f = h(f')$ and $h = h_g \in \mathcal{B}$, and make the inductive hypothesis that the theorem holds for f'. That is, $\mathbf{W}_{f'}$ realizes f'; if $\mathbf{u} \equiv f'(\mathbf{s})$, then

$$\mathbf{u} = \mathbf{W}_{f'} \cdot \mathbf{s}.$$

We have from the base case that $\mathbf{W}_h$ realizes h, so if $\mathbf{t} = h(\mathbf{u})$, then

$$\mathbf{t} = \mathbf{W}_h \cdot \mathbf{u} = \mathbf{W}_h \cdot (\mathbf{W}_{f'} \cdot \mathbf{s}) = (\mathbf{W}_h \cdot \mathbf{W}_{f'}) \cdot \mathbf{s}.$$

Since $\mathbf{t} = h(\mathbf{u}) = h(f'(\mathbf{s})) = f(\mathbf{s})$, f is realized by $\mathbf{W}_h \cdot \mathbf{W}_{f'}$. It remains to prove that

$$[\mathbf{I} \otimes \underline{\mathbf{W}}_h] \cdot [\mathbf{I} \otimes \underline{\mathbf{W}}_{f'}] = \mathbf{W}_h \cdot \mathbf{W}_{f'} = \mathbf{W}_f \equiv \mathbf{I} \otimes \underline{\mathbf{W}}_f \equiv \mathbf{I} \otimes [\underline{\mathbf{W}}_h \circ \underline{\mathbf{W}}_{f'}],$$

but this is just the Feed-Forward Recursion Theorem (94).

For the next recursive case, suppose $f = \mathbf{ex}_i(f')$ and assume inductively that $\mathbf{W}_{f'}$ realizes f'. By (84), $\mathbf{ex}_0$ is realized by $\mathbf{I} \otimes \underline{\mathbf{W}}_{ex0}$, where $\underline{\mathbf{W}}_{ex0} \equiv \mathbf{1}_A \otimes \mathbf{u}_0^{\mathrm{T}}$. Thus, by exactly the same reasoning as was just used for the case $f = h(f')$, if we now define $\underline{\mathbf{W}}_f \equiv \underline{\mathbf{W}}_{ex0} \circ \underline{\mathbf{W}}_{f'}$, it follows that $\mathbf{I} \otimes \underline{\mathbf{W}}_f$ realizes $f \equiv \mathbf{ex}_0(f')$. The analogous result holds for $f \equiv \mathbf{ex}_1(f')$.

For the final recursive case, suppose $f = \mathbf{cons}(f', f'')$ and assume inductively that $\mathbf{W}_{f'}$ and $\mathbf{W}_{f''}$ respectively realize f' and f''. Here, we use the result (79) that $\mathbf{I} \otimes [\mathbf{1}_A \otimes \mathbf{r}_0] \equiv \mathbf{I} \otimes \underline{\mathbf{W}}_{cons0}$ is $\mathbf{cons}_0$, the realization of $\mathbf{cons}_0$; the analogous result for $\mathbf{cons}_1$; and the expansions (29g):

$$\begin{aligned}\mathbf{cons}(\mathbf{u}, \mathbf{v}) &= \mathbf{cons}_0(\mathbf{u}) \sqcup \mathbf{cons}_1(\mathbf{v})\,;\\ \mathbf{cons}(\mathbf{u}, \mathbf{v}) &= \mathbf{cons}_0(\mathbf{u}) + \mathbf{cons}_1(\mathbf{v})\\ &= [\mathbf{I} \otimes \underline{\mathbf{W}}_{cons0}] \cdot \mathbf{u} + [\mathbf{I} \otimes \underline{\mathbf{W}}_{cons1}] \cdot \mathbf{v}.\end{aligned}$$

By the same argument we have used in the previous recursive cases, the theorem holds for $\underline{\mathbf{W}}_f \equiv \underline{\mathbf{W}}_{cons0} \circ \underline{\mathbf{W}}_{f'} + \underline{\mathbf{W}}_{cons1} \circ \underline{\mathbf{W}}_{f''}$ because of the following identity:

$$\begin{aligned}\mathbf{I} \otimes \underline{\mathbf{W}}_f &\equiv \mathbf{I} \otimes [\underline{\mathbf{W}}_{cons0} \circ \underline{\mathbf{W}}_{f'} + \underline{\mathbf{W}}_{cons1} \circ \underline{\mathbf{W}}_{f''}]\\ &= \mathbf{I} \otimes [\underline{\mathbf{W}}_{cons0} \circ \underline{\mathbf{W}}_{f'}] + \mathbf{I} \otimes [\underline{\mathbf{W}}_{cons1} \circ \underline{\mathbf{W}}_{f''}]\\ &= [\mathbf{I} \otimes \underline{\mathbf{W}}_{cons0}] \cdot [\mathbf{I} \otimes \underline{\mathbf{W}}_{f'}] + [\mathbf{I} \otimes \underline{\mathbf{W}}_{cons1}] \cdot [\mathbf{I} \otimes \underline{\mathbf{W}}_{f''}].\end{aligned}$$

If $\mathbf{u} \equiv f'(\mathbf{s})$, $\mathbf{v} \equiv f''(\mathbf{s})$, and $\mathbf{t} \equiv f(\mathbf{s}) \equiv \mathbf{cons}(f'(\mathbf{s}), f''(\mathbf{s})) \equiv \mathbf{cons}(\mathbf{u}, \mathbf{v})$, then

$$\begin{aligned}\mathbf{t} &= \mathbf{cons}(\mathbf{u}, \mathbf{v}) = \mathbf{cons}_0(\mathbf{u}) + \mathbf{cons}_1(\mathbf{v})\\ &= [\mathbf{I} \otimes \underline{\mathbf{W}}_{cons0}] \cdot ([\mathbf{I} \otimes \underline{\mathbf{W}}_{f'}] \cdot \mathbf{s}) + [\mathbf{I} \otimes \underline{\mathbf{W}}_{cons1}] \cdot ([\mathbf{I} \otimes \underline{\mathbf{W}}_{f''}] \cdot \mathbf{s})\\ &= ([\mathbf{I} \otimes \underline{\mathbf{W}}_{cons0}] \cdot [\mathbf{I} \otimes \underline{\mathbf{W}}_{f'}] + [\mathbf{I} \otimes \underline{\mathbf{W}}_{cons1}] \cdot [\mathbf{I} \otimes \underline{\mathbf{W}}_{f''}]) \cdot \mathbf{s}\\ &= [\mathbf{I} \otimes \underline{\mathbf{W}}_f] \cdot \mathbf{s}.\end{aligned}$$

Since every $f \in \mathcal{F}$ derives from a finite set of recursive operations upon base functions, the above results establish that any such f is realized by $\mathbf{I} \otimes \underline{\mathbf{W}}_f$.

4.1.9 Examples

4.1.9.1 Exchange

The function f_{exchange} exchanges the left and right subtrees of its argument, deleting any symbol that may reside at the root. For example, f_{exchange}([[**A B**] **C**]) = [**C** [**A B**]]. In terms of primitive functions, f_{exchange} can be written

(109) $f_{\text{exchange}}(\mathbf{s}) \equiv \mathbf{cons}(\mathbf{ex}_1(\mathbf{s}), \mathbf{ex}_0(\mathbf{s}))$.

According to the Realization Theorem (108), this function is realized by the matrix

(110) $\mathbf{W}_{\text{exchange}} = \mathbf{I} \otimes \underline{\mathbf{W}}_{\text{exchange}}$,

where, following (106), $\underline{\mathbf{W}}_{\text{exchange}}$ is

(111) $\underline{\mathbf{W}}_{\text{exchange}} \equiv \underline{\mathbf{W}}_{\text{cons0}} \circ \underline{\mathbf{W}}_{f'} + \underline{\mathbf{W}}_{\text{cons1}} \circ \underline{\mathbf{W}}_{f''}$.

Here, $f' = \mathbf{ex}_1$ and $f'' = \mathbf{ex}_0$, so $\underline{\mathbf{W}}_{f'} = \underline{\mathbf{W}}_{\text{ex1}}$ and $\underline{\mathbf{W}}_{f''} = \underline{\mathbf{W}}_{\text{ex0}}$. Then

(112) $\underline{\mathbf{W}}_{\text{exchange}} \equiv \underline{\mathbf{W}}_{\text{cons0}} \circ \underline{\mathbf{W}}_{\text{ex1}} + \underline{\mathbf{W}}_{\text{cons1}} \circ \underline{\mathbf{W}}_{\text{ex0}}$.

By (106b), $\underline{\mathbf{W}}_{\text{cons}i} \equiv \mathbf{1}_A \otimes \mathbf{r}_i \in \mathcal{M}_1^{\ 0}$ and $\underline{\mathbf{W}}_{\text{ex}_i} \equiv \underline{\mathbf{W}}_{\text{ex}i} \equiv \mathbf{1}_A \otimes \mathbf{u}_i^{\text{T}} \in \mathcal{M}_0^{\ 1}$ for $i = 0, 1$. Since these matrices can be multiplied directly, the circle product $\underline{\mathbf{W}}_{\text{cons}i} \circ \underline{\mathbf{W}}_{\text{ex}j}$ is simply the matrix product $\underline{\mathbf{W}}_{\text{cons}i} \cdot \underline{\mathbf{W}}_{\text{ex}j}$ (in the circle product definition (93), $\Delta = 0$). Thus,

(113) $\underline{\mathbf{W}}_{\text{exchange}} \equiv \underline{\mathbf{W}}_{\text{cons0}} \cdot \underline{\mathbf{W}}_{\text{ex1}} + \underline{\mathbf{W}}_{\text{cons1}} \cdot \underline{\mathbf{W}}_{\text{ex0}}$.

This matrix can be depicted using the scheme of (90):

(114) $\mathbf{W}_{\text{exchange}}$ =

	ε	0 1	00 01	10 11	000 001	010 011	100 101	110 111	…
ε	0								
0 1		$\mathbf{r}_0 \cdot \mathbf{u}_1^{\text{T}} + \mathbf{r}_1 \cdot \mathbf{u}_0^{\text{T}}$							
00 01			$\mathbf{r}_0 \cdot \mathbf{u}_1^{\text{T}} + \mathbf{r}_1 \cdot \mathbf{u}_0^{\text{T}}$						
10 11				$\mathbf{r}_0 \cdot \mathbf{u}_1^{\text{T}} + \mathbf{r}_1 \cdot \mathbf{u}_0^{\text{T}}$					
000 001					$\mathbf{r}_0 \cdot \mathbf{u}_1^{\text{T}} + \mathbf{r}_1 \cdot \mathbf{u}_0^{\text{T}}$				
010 011						$\mathbf{r}_0 \cdot \mathbf{u}_1^{\text{T}} + \mathbf{r}_1 \cdot \mathbf{u}_0^{\text{T}}$			
100 101							$\mathbf{r}_0 \cdot \mathbf{u}_1^{\text{T}} + \mathbf{r}_1 \cdot \mathbf{u}_0^{\text{T}}$		
110 111								$\mathbf{r}_0 \cdot \mathbf{u}_1^{\text{T}} + \mathbf{r}_1 \cdot \mathbf{u}_0^{\text{T}}$	
⋮									⋱

Figure 4 Box 2

4.1.9.2 Reverse

The function f_{reverse} reverses the left and right subtrees of its argument and does the same for all the embedded subtrees. For example, $f_{\text{reverse}}([[\mathbf{A}\ \mathbf{B}]\ \mathbf{C}]) = [\mathbf{C}\ [\mathbf{B}\ \mathbf{A}]]$. This function has a simple recursive definition:

(115) f_{reverse}: Recursive definition

$$f_{\text{reverse}}(\mathbf{s}) \equiv \begin{cases} \mathbf{s} & \text{if } \mathbf{s} \in A \\ \mathbf{cons}(f_{\text{reverse}}(\mathbf{ex}_1(\mathbf{s})), f_{\text{reverse}}(\mathbf{ex}_0(\mathbf{s}))) & \text{otherwise} \end{cases}.$$

(Recall that A is the set of atomic symbols.) This function is first order. In fact,

(116) $f_{\text{reverse}}(\sqcup_x \mathbf{A}_x/r_x) = \sqcup_x \mathbf{A}_x/r_{\bar{x}}$,

where $\bar{x}$ is the bit-wise complement of x, with 0s and 1s interchanged. For example,

(117) $f_{\text{reverse}}([[\mathbf{A}\ \mathbf{B}]\ \mathbf{C}]) = f_{\text{reverse}}(\{\mathbf{A}/r_{00},\ \mathbf{B}/r_{10},\ \mathbf{C}/r_1\})$
$= \{\mathbf{A}/r_{11},\ \mathbf{B}/r_{01},\ \mathbf{C}/r_0\}) = [\mathbf{C}\ [\mathbf{B}\ \mathbf{A}]]$.

Is f_{reverse} a PC function? If it were PC, the Finite Specification Theorem (102) would apply, telling us that beyond some depth d,

$$f(\mathbf{sh}_i(a/r_x)) = \mathbf{sh}_i(f(a/r_x)),$$

where $f \equiv f_{\text{reverse}}$ and $i = 0, 1$. But this cannot hold for any d:

$$f(\mathbf{sh}_i(\mathbf{A}/r_x)) = f(\mathbf{A}/r_{ix}) = \mathbf{A}/r_{\bar{i}\bar{x}},$$

while

$$\mathbf{sh}_i(f(\mathbf{A}/r_x)) = \mathbf{sh}_i(\mathbf{A}/r_{\bar{x}}) = \mathbf{A}/r_{i\bar{x}}.$$

These are never equal; for example, if $i = 0$ and $x = 010$, then the bit-string tag for the first binding is 1101 and that for the second is 0101.

The function f_{reverse} is interesting because it enables us to prove (118).

(118) *Proposition.* There exist functions that are first order but not realizable as $\mathbf{I} \otimes \underline{\mathbf{M}}$.

> *Proof.* We have seen that the function f_{reverse} is first order, yet it is not PC, so we have no guarantee from the Realization Theorem for PC Functions that it can be realized by a matrix $\mathbf{I} \otimes \underline{\mathbf{M}}$. And indeed it cannot be so realized. If $\mathbf{W}$ is a matrix realizing f_{reverse}, then it must obey the following recursion relation, the matrix equivalent of the recursive definition (115):
>
> (1) $\mathbf{W} = \mathbf{W}_{\text{cons0}} \cdot \mathbf{W} \cdot \mathbf{W}_{\text{ex1}} + \mathbf{W}_{\text{cons1}} \cdot \mathbf{W} \cdot \mathbf{W}_{\text{ex0}}$.
>
> If $\mathbf{W} = \mathbf{I} \otimes \underline{\mathbf{M}}$, then by the recursion theorem (91), it would follow that
>
> (2) $\mathbf{I} \otimes \underline{\mathbf{M}} = \mathbf{I} \otimes (\underline{\mathbf{W}}_{\text{cons0}} \circ \underline{\mathbf{M}} \circ \underline{\mathbf{W}}_{\text{ex1}} + \underline{\mathbf{W}}_{\text{cons1}} \circ \underline{\mathbf{M}} \circ \underline{\mathbf{W}}_{\text{ex0}})$.
>
> Unless $\underline{\mathbf{M}}$ is zero, there must exist within $\underline{\mathbf{M}}$ at least one nonzero block matrix $\underline{\mathbf{M}}_d{}^{d'} \in \mathcal{M}_d{}^{d'}$. Representing explicitly the dimensionality of all matrices, (2) becomes
>
> (3) $[\mathbf{I} \otimes \underline{\mathbf{M}}]_{d+1}{}^{d'+1} = [\underline{\mathbf{W}}_{\text{cons0}}]_1{}^0 \circ [\underline{\mathbf{M}}]_d{}^{d'} \circ [\underline{\mathbf{W}}_{\text{ex1}}]_0{}^1 + [\underline{\mathbf{W}}_{\text{cons1}}]_1{}^0 \circ [\underline{\mathbf{M}}]_d{}^{d'} \circ [\underline{\mathbf{W}}_{\text{ex0}}]_0{}^1$
> $= (\mathbf{1}^{\otimes d} \otimes [\underline{\mathbf{W}}_{\text{cons0}}]_1{}^0) \cdot [\underline{\mathbf{M}}]_d{}^{d'} \cdot (\mathbf{1}^{\otimes d'} \otimes [\underline{\mathbf{W}}_{\text{ex1}}]_0{}^1)$
> $+ (\mathbf{1}^{\otimes d} \otimes [\underline{\mathbf{W}}_{\text{cons1}}]_1{}^0) \cdot [\underline{\mathbf{M}}]_d{}^{d'} \cdot (\mathbf{1}^{\otimes d'} \otimes [\underline{\mathbf{W}}_{\text{ex0}}]_0{}^1)$.
>
> This matrix is in $\mathcal{M}_{d+1}{}^{d'+1}$. By the left side of (2), it must be a block of $\mathbf{I} \otimes \underline{\mathbf{M}}$. Thus, it could be $\mathbf{1} \otimes [\underline{\mathbf{M}}]_d{}^{d'}$, or $\mathbf{1}^{\otimes 2} \otimes [\underline{\mathbf{M}}]_{d-1}{}^{d'-1}$, or $\mathbf{1}^{\otimes (k+1)} \otimes [\underline{\mathbf{M}}]_{d-k}{}^{d'-k}$ for a larger value of k. For

now, we assume the first: $[\mathbf{I}\otimes\underline{\mathbf{M}}]_{d+1}{}^{d'+1} = \mathbf{1}\otimes[\underline{\mathbf{M}}]_d{}^{d'}$. Then the components of $\underline{\mathbf{M}}$ obey

$$\begin{aligned}\delta_{\gamma_1}^{\xi'_1} M_{\gamma_2\gamma_3\cdots\gamma_d\rho}^{\xi'_2\xi'_3\cdots\xi'_{d'}\zeta} &= \delta_{\gamma_1}^{\gamma'_1}\delta_{\gamma_2}^{\gamma'_2}\cdots\delta_{\gamma_d}^{\gamma'_d}\,\mathbf{r}_{0\rho} M_{\gamma'_1\gamma'_2\cdots\gamma'_d}^{\xi_1\xi_2\cdots\xi_{d'}}\delta_{\xi_1}^{\xi'_1}\delta_{\xi_2}^{\xi'_2}\cdots\delta_{\xi_{d'}}^{\xi'_{d'}}\,\mathbf{u}_1{}^\zeta \\ &\quad + \delta_{\gamma_1}^{\gamma'_1}\delta_{\gamma_2}^{\gamma'_2}\cdots\delta_{\gamma_d}^{\gamma'_d}\,\mathbf{r}_{1\rho} M_{\gamma'_1\gamma'_2\cdots\gamma'_d}^{\xi_1\xi_2\cdots\xi_{d'}}\delta_{\xi_1}^{\xi'_1}\delta_{\xi_2}^{\xi'_2}\cdots\delta_{\xi_{d'}}^{\xi'_{d'}}\,\mathbf{u}_0{}^\zeta \\ &= \mathbf{r}_{0\rho} M_{\gamma_1\gamma_2\cdots\gamma_d}^{\xi'_1\xi'_2\cdots\xi'_{d'}}\mathbf{u}_1{}^\zeta + \mathbf{r}_{1\rho} M_{\gamma_1\gamma_2\cdots\gamma_d}^{\xi'_1\xi'_2\cdots\xi'_{d'}}\mathbf{u}_0{}^\zeta \\ &= M_{\gamma_1\gamma_2\cdots\gamma_d}^{\xi'_1\xi'_2\cdots\xi'_{d'}}\left(\mathbf{r}_{0\rho}\mathbf{u}_1{}^\zeta + \mathbf{r}_{1\rho}\mathbf{u}_0{}^\zeta\right).\end{aligned}$$

Now let $f_\rho{}^\zeta \equiv (\mathbf{r}_{0\rho}\mathbf{u}_1{}^\zeta + \mathbf{r}_{1\rho}\mathbf{u}_0{}^\zeta)$. In the general distributed case, these are all nonzero; we can certainly specifically choose the role vectors to make this so. Now

$$\delta_{\gamma_1}^{\xi'_1} M_{\gamma_2\gamma_3\cdots\gamma_d\rho}^{\xi'_2\xi'_3\cdots\xi'_{d'}\zeta} = M_{\gamma_1\gamma_2\cdots\gamma_d}^{\xi'_1\xi'_2\cdots\xi'_{d'}} f_\rho{}^\zeta.$$

If $\gamma_1 \neq \xi'_1$, the left side is zero, and since $f_\rho{}^\zeta$ is not zero, $M_{\gamma_1\gamma_2\cdots\gamma_d}^{\xi'_1\xi'_2\cdots\xi'_{d'}}$ must be zero whenever its leftmost indices are unequal. So consider the components where $\xi'_1 = \gamma_1 = \eta_1$:

$$M_{\gamma_2\gamma_3\cdots\gamma_d\rho}^{\xi'_2\xi'_3\cdots\xi'_{d'}\zeta} = M_{\eta_1\gamma_2\cdots\gamma_d}^{\eta_1\xi'_2\cdots\xi'_{d'}} f_\rho{}^\zeta.$$

The left side is independent of η_1, so $M_{\eta_1\gamma_2\cdots\gamma_d}^{\eta_1\xi'_2\cdots\xi'_{d'}}$ must be the same for $\eta_1 = 0$ and $\eta_1 = 1$. On the left side, $M_{\gamma_2\gamma_3\cdots\gamma_d\rho}^{\xi'_2\xi'_3\cdots\xi'_{d'}\zeta}$ is zero if the first pair of indices are not equal (i.e., if $\gamma_2 \neq \xi'_2$); again, since $f_\rho{}^\zeta$ is not zero, $M_{\eta\gamma_2\cdots\gamma_d}^{\eta\xi'_2\cdots\xi'_{d'}}$ must be zero unless its *second* pair of indices (from the left) are equal. Furthermore, since $M_{\gamma_2\gamma_3\cdots\gamma_d\rho}^{\xi'_2\xi'_3\cdots\xi'_{d'}\zeta}$ has the same value whether its first pair of indices are both 0 or both 1, it must be that $M_{\eta\gamma_2\cdots\gamma_d}^{\eta\xi'_2\cdots\xi'_{d'}}$ has the same value whether the second pair of indices are both 0 or both 1. So suppose $\gamma_2 = \xi'_2 = \eta_2$. Then

$$M_{\eta_2\gamma_3\cdots\gamma_d\rho}^{\eta_2\xi'_3\cdots\xi'_{d'}\zeta} = M_{\eta_1\eta_2\gamma_3\cdots\gamma_d}^{\eta_1\eta_2\xi'_3\cdots\xi'_{d'}} f_\rho{}^\zeta.$$

And again, since on the left, the component vanishes if the second pair of indices are unequal, then if $\gamma_3 \neq \xi'_3$, $M_{\eta_1\eta_2\gamma_3\cdots\gamma_d}^{\eta_1\eta_2\xi'_3\cdots\xi'_{d'}}$ is zero, so the *third* pair of indices of $\mathbf{M}$ must be equal if a component is to be nonzero. Once again, when the third pair of indices are equal, the value of the component is the same whether the indices are both 0 or both 1. Clearly, this can continue until we get to the conclusion that the component vanishes unless all pairs of indices are equal, and the component is the same for any common value of the index pairs.

Suppose for now that $d' > d$. Then we have

$$M_{\eta_2\eta_3\cdots\eta_d\rho}^{\eta_2\eta_3\cdots\eta_d\xi'_{d+1}\cdots\xi'_{d'}\zeta} = M_{\eta_1\eta_2\eta_3\cdots\eta_d}^{\eta_1\eta_2\eta_3\cdots\eta_d\xi'_{d+1}\cdots\xi'_{d'}} f_\rho{}^\zeta,$$

and this vanishes unless the dth pair of indices on the left side are equal: $\xi'_{d+1} = \rho$,

$$M_{\eta_2\eta_3\cdots\eta_d\rho}^{\eta_2\eta_3\cdots\eta_d\rho\xi'_{d+2}\cdots\xi'_{d'}\zeta} = M_{\eta_1\eta_2\eta_3\cdots\eta_d}^{\eta_1\eta_2\eta_3\cdots\eta_d\rho\xi'_{d+2}\cdots\xi'_{d'}} f_\rho{}^\zeta,$$

and this value must be the same for $\rho = 0$ and $\rho = 1$. Now let $\boldsymbol{\alpha} \equiv \eta_2\eta_3\cdots\eta_d$, let $\boldsymbol{\mu} \equiv \xi'_{d+2}\cdots\xi'_{d'}$, and let $\eta \equiv \eta_1$. Then we get (with no summation over ρ)

(4) $M_{\alpha\rho}^{\alpha\rho\mu\zeta} = M_{\eta\alpha}^{\eta\alpha\rho\mu} f_\rho{}^\zeta.$

We will examine this for two special cases. In the first, $\boldsymbol{\alpha} = 00\cdots0$, $\rho = 0$, and $\eta = 0$; later, we will replace all 0s with 1s. The two results must actually be equal, since the value of $M_{\alpha\rho}^{\alpha\rho\mu\zeta}$ is the same for any set of values for the indices $\boldsymbol{\alpha}$ and ρ.

In the 0 case, note that $\boldsymbol{\alpha}0 = 0\boldsymbol{\alpha} = 00\cdots0$. Then (4) becomes

(5) $M_{\alpha0}^{\alpha0\mu\zeta} = M_{0\alpha}^{0\alpha0\mu} f_0{}^\zeta.$

Into this, substitute $\boldsymbol{\mu} = \mu_1\zeta_1$; ζ_1 is the last bit of $\boldsymbol{\mu}$, either 0 or 1.

(6) $M_{\alpha0}^{\alpha0\mu_1\zeta_1\zeta} = M_{0\alpha}^{0\alpha0\mu_1\zeta_1} f_0{}^\zeta.$

The M component on the right side of (6) matches the M component on the left side of (5), with ζ, $\boldsymbol{\mu}$ of (5) equal to ζ_1, $0\boldsymbol{\mu}_1$ of (6) (recall that $\boldsymbol{\alpha}0 = 0\boldsymbol{\alpha}$). Substituting (5) into the right side of (6) gives

$$M_{\boldsymbol{\alpha}0}^{\boldsymbol{\alpha}0\boldsymbol{\mu}_1\zeta_1\zeta} = M_{0\boldsymbol{\alpha}}^{0\boldsymbol{\alpha}00\boldsymbol{\mu}_1} \mathrm{f}_0^{\zeta_1} \mathrm{f}_0^{\zeta}.$$

This equation matches the one we started with, (5), except that on the right side there is an additional factor $\mathrm{f}_0^{\zeta_1}$; ζ_1 has left the upper index of M and an additional 0 has appeared there. The index vector $\boldsymbol{\mu}$ has been shortened by one to $\boldsymbol{\mu}_1$. Iterating this logic then ultimately replaces all indices in $\boldsymbol{\mu}$ with 0, producing multiple f factors:

$$M_{\boldsymbol{\alpha}0}^{\boldsymbol{\alpha}0\zeta_{n-1}\cdots\zeta_1\zeta} = M_{0\boldsymbol{\alpha}}^{0\boldsymbol{\alpha}00\cdots0} \mathrm{f}_0^{\zeta_{n-1}} \cdots \mathrm{f}_0^{\zeta_1} \mathrm{f}_0^{\zeta},$$

where $n = d' - d$ is the number of 0s following $\boldsymbol{\alpha}$ in the upstairs matrix tag. Now recalling that $\boldsymbol{\alpha} = 00\cdots0$, if we define the constant $m_0 \equiv M_{00\cdots0}^{00\cdots00}$ (with d 0s downstairs and d' upstairs), then we get

$$(7)\quad M_{00\cdots0}^{00\cdots0\zeta_{n-1}\cdots\zeta_1\zeta} = m_0 \mathrm{f}_0^{\zeta_{n-1}} \cdots \mathrm{f}_0^{\zeta_1} \mathrm{f}_0^{\zeta}.$$

With all 0s replaced by 1s, exactly the same logic gives

$$(8)\quad M_{11\cdots1}^{11\cdots1\zeta_{n-1}\cdots\zeta_1\zeta} = m_1 \mathrm{f}_1^{\zeta_{n-1}} \cdots \mathrm{f}_1^{\zeta_1} \mathrm{f}_1^{\zeta},$$

where the constant $m_1 \equiv M_{11\cdots1}^{11\cdots11}$. Now as noted above, the two values (7) and (8) must in fact be the same:

$$(9)\quad m_0 \mathrm{f}_0^{\zeta_{n-1}} \cdots \mathrm{f}_0^{\zeta_1} \mathrm{f}_0^{\zeta} = m_1 \mathrm{f}_1^{\zeta_{n-1}} \cdots \mathrm{f}_1^{\zeta_1} \mathrm{f}_1^{\zeta}.$$

And at last we have reached a contradiction, because in general there is no pair of constants m_0, m_1 that meet this condition, for all values $\zeta_{n-1}\cdots\zeta_1\zeta$, except $m_0 = m_1 = 0$. From (7) and (8) we conclude that all components of **M** must be zero. This is indeed a solution of the original recursion relation (1)—but not a solution that realizes f_{reverse}.

After deriving (3), we made a provisional assumption that has proven to lead to a contradiction; we must now consider the alternatives. (3) tells us that if there is a nonzero block in $\underline{\mathbf{M}}$ somewhere, $\underline{\mathbf{M}}_d^{d'} \in \mathcal{M}_d^{d'}$, then there must be a nonzero block from $\mathcal{M}_{d+1}^{d'+1}$ in $\mathbf{I}\otimes\underline{\mathbf{M}}$: call this **B**. This requires that for some $k \geq 0$, $\mathbf{1}^{\otimes(k+1)} \otimes [\underline{\mathbf{M}}]_{d-k}^{d'-k} = \mathbf{B}$. The assumption made above was that $k = 0$: that it is from $\underline{\mathbf{M}}_d^{d'}$ itself that **B** arises. Alternatively, it could be that **B** arises from a different block in $\underline{\mathbf{M}}$, necessarily, one that is smaller in both dimensions: $[\underline{\mathbf{M}}]_{d-k}^{d'-k}$ with $k > 0$. In that case, (3) is no longer an equation relating elements of the same block, and the argument above, leading to a contradiction, cannot be made. However, if **B** does derive from another block $[\underline{\mathbf{M}}]_{d-k}^{d'-k}$ with $k > 0$, then we can start all over again with this smaller block in place of the original block $\underline{\mathbf{M}}_d^{d'}$. Since the argument above does not depend on the values of d and d', it applies again: (3) holds again, but now with a smaller matrix. The conclusion again arises that there must be a nonzero block **B′** in $\mathbf{I}\otimes\underline{\mathbf{M}}$; and as before the question arises what block of $\underline{\mathbf{M}}$ this derives from. Perhaps it is the same block, in which case the argument above leads to a contradiction. Or perhaps it's a smaller block, in which case we take *that* block and start all over yet again. But each time the block is getting smaller in both dimensions, and this can't go on forever. If there is indeed a nonzero solution, at some point there must be a nonzero block that itself gives rise to the bigger block in $\mathbf{I}\otimes\underline{\mathbf{M}}$ that (3) requires. Yet we have seen above that this too is not possible. So no nonzero solution exists.

Thus, the theorems (108) and (118) together establish that (i) a large set of recursive functions ($\mathcal{F}$) can be realized with a recursive matrix of the form $\mathbf{I}\otimes\underline{\mathbf{W}}$, but (ii) not all recursive functions can be realized this way—and not even all first-order functions can be so realized.

4.2 Feedback networks: Grammars

In Section 4.1, we derived a simple form for weight matrices realizing a class of recursive functions in feed-forward networks. In this section, we derive a simple form for weight matrices that realize grammars in recurrent networks—in the sense that the network's Harmony-maximizing states are realizations of grammatical structures.

(119) *Definition.* **Dualizer** matrix **D**

Define the vectors

$$\mathbf{d}_0 \equiv [\mathbf{u}_0]_0\,\mathbf{u}_0 + [\mathbf{u}_1]_0\,\mathbf{u}_1; \quad \mathbf{d}_1 \equiv [\mathbf{u}_0]_1\,\mathbf{u}_0 + [\mathbf{u}_1]_1\,\mathbf{u}_1.$$

Define the matrix **D** so that $\mathbf{D}^T = [\mathbf{d}_0\ \mathbf{d}_1]$, that is, row 0 of **D** is $\mathbf{d}_0$ and row 1 of **D** is $\mathbf{d}_1$.[15]

(120) *Proposition.* **D** is symmetric: $\mathbf{D}^T = \mathbf{D}$.

Proof.

$$\mathbf{D}^T \equiv \left[\begin{bmatrix} \\ \mathbf{d}_0 \\ \\ \end{bmatrix} \begin{bmatrix} \\ \mathbf{d}_1 \\ \\ \end{bmatrix} \right] = \begin{bmatrix} [\mathbf{d}_0]_0 & [\mathbf{d}_1]_0 \\ [\mathbf{d}_0]_1 & [\mathbf{d}_1]_1 \end{bmatrix}$$

and

$$\mathbf{D} \equiv \begin{bmatrix} [\quad \mathbf{d}_0^T \quad] \\ [\quad \mathbf{d}_1^T \quad] \end{bmatrix} = \begin{bmatrix} [\mathbf{d}_0]_0 & [\mathbf{d}_0]_1 \\ [\mathbf{d}_1]_0 & [\mathbf{d}_1]_1 \end{bmatrix};$$

hence, $\mathbf{D}^T = \mathbf{D}$ iff $[\mathbf{d}_0]_1 = [\mathbf{d}_1]_0$. But

$$[\mathbf{d}_0]_1 \equiv [[\mathbf{u}_0]_0\mathbf{u}_0 + [\mathbf{u}_1]_0\mathbf{u}_1]_1 = [\mathbf{u}_0]_0\,[\mathbf{u}_0]_1 + [\mathbf{u}_1]_0\,[\mathbf{u}_1]_1$$

and

$$[\mathbf{d}_1]_0 \equiv [[\mathbf{u}_0]_1\mathbf{u}_0 + [\mathbf{u}_1]_1\mathbf{u}_1]_0 = [\mathbf{u}_0]_1\,[\mathbf{u}_0]_0 + [\mathbf{u}_1]_1\,[\mathbf{u}_1]_0.$$

Clearly, these are indeed equal.

(121) *Proposition.* Let x be a bit string with $|x| = k > 0$. Then

$$\mathbf{D}^{\otimes k} \cdot \mathbf{r}_x = \mathbf{u}_x$$

(**D** is an "**r** to $\mathbf{r}^+ \equiv \mathbf{u}$ converter.")

Proof. First we show that $\mathbf{D} \cdot \mathbf{r}_0 = \mathbf{u}_0$ and $\mathbf{D} \cdot \mathbf{r}_1 = \mathbf{u}_1$, the case $k = 1$. Since row i of **D** is $\mathbf{d}_i$, the ith component of $\mathbf{D} \cdot \mathbf{r}_0$ is

$$\begin{aligned} [\mathbf{D} \cdot \mathbf{r}_0]_i = \mathbf{d}_i \cdot \mathbf{r}_0 &= ([\mathbf{u}_0]_i\,\mathbf{u}_0 + [\mathbf{u}_1]_i\,\mathbf{u}_1) \cdot \mathbf{r}_0 \\ &= [\mathbf{u}_0]_i\,(\mathbf{u}_0 \cdot \mathbf{r}_0) + [\mathbf{u}_1]_i\,(\mathbf{u}_1 \cdot \mathbf{r}_0) \end{aligned}$$

[15] Within the vector space V_{R° containing $\{\mathbf{r}_0, \mathbf{r}_1\}$, we are interested only in the subspace spanned by these two vectors. If the dimension of V_{R° is greater than two, choose additional vectors $\mathbf{r}_2, \mathbf{r}_3, \ldots$ to fill out a basis for V_{R° and let $\{\mathbf{u}_i\}$ be the dual basis. For defining **D**, we let the additional rows be defined by $\mathbf{d}_k \equiv [\mathbf{u}_0]_k\mathbf{u}_0 + [\mathbf{u}_1]_k\mathbf{u}_1$; then proposition (121) holds.

$= [\mathbf{u}_0]_i(1) + [\mathbf{u}_1]_i(0) = [\mathbf{u}_0]_i.$

Hence, $\mathbf{D}\cdot\mathbf{r}_0 = \mathbf{u}_0$. Identical argumentation shows $\mathbf{D}\cdot\mathbf{r}_1 = \mathbf{u}_1$.

Now the proposition follows by induction. Assume it holds for some value of k; we show that it then holds for $k+1$. Suppose $x = iy$, where $i = 0$ or 1 and $|x| = k+1$, $|y| = k$. Then

$$\begin{aligned}\mathbf{D}^{\otimes(k+1)}\cdot\mathbf{r}_x &= (\mathbf{D}\otimes\mathbf{D}^{\otimes k})\cdot\mathbf{r}_{iy} \equiv (\mathbf{D}\otimes\mathbf{D}^{\otimes k})\cdot(\mathbf{r}_i\otimes\mathbf{r}_y)\\ &= (\mathbf{D}\cdot\mathbf{r}_i)\otimes(\mathbf{D}^{\otimes k}\otimes\mathbf{r}_y)\\ &= \mathbf{u}_i\otimes\mathbf{u}_y \equiv \mathbf{u}_{iy} \equiv \mathbf{u}_x.\end{aligned}$$

(122) *Proposition.* Let $\mathbf{M} \equiv \mathbf{X}^+\mathbf{A}^{+\mathrm{T}}\otimes[\mathbf{u}_j{}^{\mathrm{T}}\otimes\mathbf{D}^{\otimes k}] \in \mathcal{W}_k^{k+1}$; let x be a bit string with $|x| = k$; and let $i = 0$ or 1. Then $\mathbf{M}\cdot\mathbf{C}\otimes\mathbf{r}_{ix} = \mathbf{X}^+\otimes\mathbf{u}_x$ if $\mathbf{C} = \mathbf{A}$ and $i = j$, and $\mathbf{M}\cdot\mathbf{C}\otimes\mathbf{r}_{ix} = \mathbf{0}$ if $i \neq j$ or if $\mathbf{A} \neq \mathbf{C} \in \mathcal{A}$ realizes a symbol other than **A**.

Proof.

$$\begin{aligned}(\mathbf{X}^+\mathbf{A}^{+\mathrm{T}}\otimes[\mathbf{u}_j{}^{\mathrm{T}}\otimes\mathbf{D}^{\otimes k}])\cdot\mathbf{C}\otimes\mathbf{r}_{ix} &= \mathbf{X}^+(\mathbf{A}^{+\mathrm{T}}\mathbf{C})\otimes([\mathbf{u}_j{}^{\mathrm{T}}\otimes\mathbf{D}^{\otimes k}]\cdot[\mathbf{r}_i\otimes\mathbf{r}_x])\\ &= \mathbf{X}^+(\mathbf{A}^+\cdot\mathbf{C})\otimes([\mathbf{u}_j{}^{\mathrm{T}}\cdot\mathbf{r}_i]\otimes[\mathbf{D}^{\otimes k}\cdot\mathbf{r}_x])\\ &= \mathbf{X}^+(\mathbf{A}^+\cdot\mathbf{C})\otimes([\delta_{ij}]\otimes[\mathbf{u}_x]).\end{aligned}$$

The proposition follows from the fact that $\mathbf{A}^+\cdot\mathbf{C} = 1$ if $\mathbf{C} = \mathbf{A}$, and $\mathbf{A}^+\cdot\mathbf{C} = 0$ if **C** is some symbol other than **A**.

(123) *Definition.* Define the **recurrent recursion matrix**:

$$\mathbf{R} \equiv \mathbf{1} + \mathbf{D} + \mathbf{D}\otimes\mathbf{D} + \mathbf{D}\otimes\mathbf{D}\otimes\mathbf{D} + \cdots = \Sigma_k\,\mathbf{D}^{\otimes k}.$$

(124) *Proposition.* Let

$$\mathbf{M} \equiv \mathbf{X}^+\mathbf{A}^{+\mathrm{T}}\otimes[\mathbf{u}_j{}^{\mathrm{T}}\otimes\mathbf{R}],\ j = 0 \text{ or } 1.$$

Then if $\mathbf{s} = \psi(\mathbf{s})$ is the realization of **s**,

$$\mathbf{M}\cdot\mathbf{s} = \Sigma\,\{\mathbf{X}^+\otimes\mathbf{u}_x \mid \mathbf{A}/r_{jx} \in \mathbf{s}\}.$$

Proof. The function $\mathbf{s} \mapsto \mathbf{M}\cdot\mathbf{s}$ is first order, so it suffices to compute its output for any single binding $\mathbf{s} = \mathbf{C}/\mathbf{r}_y \in S_{(n)}$, where $n \equiv |y|$. If the proposition is correct, the value of $\mathbf{M}\cdot\mathbf{C}/\mathbf{r}_y$ should be zero unless $\mathbf{C} = \mathbf{A}$ and $y = jx$, in which case the value should be $\mathbf{X}^+\otimes\mathbf{u}_x$. Now

$$\begin{aligned}\mathbf{M} \equiv \mathbf{X}^+\mathbf{A}^{+\mathrm{T}}\otimes[\mathbf{u}_j{}^{\mathrm{T}}\otimes\mathbf{R}] &\equiv \mathbf{X}^+\mathbf{A}^{+\mathrm{T}}\otimes[\mathbf{u}_j{}^{\mathrm{T}}\otimes\Sigma_k\,\mathbf{D}^{\otimes k}]\\ &= \Sigma_k\mathbf{X}^+\mathbf{A}^{+\mathrm{T}}\otimes[\mathbf{u}_j{}^{\mathrm{T}}\otimes\mathbf{D}^{\otimes k}].\end{aligned}$$

The kth matrix in this sum is in $\mathcal{M}_k^{k+1}$; it is the matrix with $k = n-1$, in $\mathcal{M}_{n-1}{}^n$, that contributes a nonzero value to $\mathbf{M}\cdot\mathbf{C}/\mathbf{r}_y$, since $\mathbf{C}/\mathbf{r}_y \in S_{(n)}$. By (122),

$$\mathbf{X}^+\mathbf{A}^{+\mathrm{T}}\otimes[\mathbf{u}_j{}^{\mathrm{T}}\otimes\mathbf{D}^{\otimes k}]\cdot\mathbf{C}/\mathbf{r}_y = \mathbf{0}$$

unless $\mathbf{C} = \mathbf{A}$ and $y = jx$; in that case,

$$\mathbf{X}^+\mathbf{A}^{+\mathrm{T}}\otimes[\mathbf{u}_j{}^{\mathrm{T}}\otimes\mathbf{D}^{\otimes k}]\cdot\mathbf{C}/\mathbf{r}_y = \mathbf{X}^+\otimes\mathbf{u}_x.$$

For this **M**, the symbolic function realized by $\mathbf{s} \mapsto \mathbf{M}\cdot\mathbf{s} \equiv \mathbf{t}$ takes each **A** in **s** that is a left child and replaces it with an $\mathbf{X}^+$ bound to the unbinding vector for its parent's location. Thus, the resulting **t** will have dot product 1 with a binding of **X** to the parent position, and dot product 0 with any other symbol binding $\mathbf{C}\otimes\mathbf{r}_x$. Thus, the sum of terms defining $\mathbf{t}\cdot\mathbf{s}$ will include a 1 for each **A** that is a left child of **X**; the number of such **X/A** pairs is called $v_{X\to A-}(\mathbf{s})$ in the following proposition.

(125) *Proposition.* Define

$$\mathbf{M_{X/A}} \equiv \mathbf{X^{+}A^{+T}} \otimes [\mathbf{u_0}^T \otimes \mathbf{R}] = (\mathbf{X^{+}A^{+T}} \otimes \mathbf{u_0}^T) \otimes \mathbf{R} \equiv \underline{\mathbf{M}}_{\mathbf{X/A}} \otimes \mathbf{R};$$
$$\mathbf{M_{X\backslash B}} \equiv \mathbf{X^{+}B^{+T}} \otimes [\mathbf{u_1}^T \otimes \mathbf{R}] = (\mathbf{X^{+}B^{+T}} \otimes \mathbf{u_1}^T) \otimes \mathbf{R} \equiv \underline{\mathbf{M}}_{\mathbf{X\backslash B}} \otimes \mathbf{R}.$$

Let

$$\mathbf{W_{X\to A-}} \equiv \tfrac{1}{2}(\mathbf{M_{X/A}} + [\mathbf{M_{X/A}}]^T);$$
$$\mathbf{W_{X\to -B}} \equiv \tfrac{1}{2}(\mathbf{M_{X\backslash B}} + [\mathbf{M_{X\backslash B}}]^T).$$

Then

$$\mathbf{s}^T\cdot\mathbf{W_{X\to A-}}\cdot\mathbf{s} = |\{x \mid \mathbf{X}/r_x \in \mathbf{s} \text{ and } \mathbf{A}/r_{0x} \in \mathbf{s}\}| \equiv v_{X\to A-}(\mathbf{s}),$$
$$\mathbf{s}^T\cdot\mathbf{W_{X\to -B}}\cdot\mathbf{s} = |\{x \mid \mathbf{X}/r_x \in \mathbf{s} \text{ and } \mathbf{B}/r_{1x} \in \mathbf{s}\}| \equiv v_{X\to -y}(\mathbf{s}),$$

and

$$\mathbf{W_{X\to A-}} = \tfrac{1}{2}(\underline{\mathbf{M}}_{\mathbf{X/A}} + [\underline{\mathbf{M}}_{\mathbf{X/A}}]^T) \otimes \mathbf{R} \equiv \underline{\mathbf{W}}_{\mathbf{X\to A-}} \otimes \mathbf{R},$$
$$\mathbf{W_{X\to -B}} = \tfrac{1}{2}(\underline{\mathbf{M}}_{\mathbf{X\backslash B}} + [\underline{\mathbf{M}}_{\mathbf{X\backslash B}}]^T) \otimes \mathbf{R} \equiv \underline{\mathbf{W}}_{\mathbf{X\to -B}} \otimes \mathbf{R}.$$

Proof. By (124),

$$\begin{aligned}
\mathbf{s}^T\cdot\mathbf{M_{X/A}}\cdot\mathbf{s} &= \mathbf{s}^T\cdot\Sigma\{\mathbf{X}^+\otimes\mathbf{u}_x \mid \mathbf{A}/r_{0x}\in\mathbf{s}\}\\
&= \Sigma_y \mathbf{s}_y\otimes\mathbf{r}_y\cdot\Sigma\{\mathbf{X}^+\otimes\mathbf{u}_x \mid \mathbf{A}/r_{0x}\in\mathbf{s}\}\\
&= \Sigma\{\Sigma_y \mathbf{s}_y\otimes\mathbf{r}_y\cdot\mathbf{X}^+\otimes\mathbf{u}_x \mid \mathbf{A}/r_{0x}\in\mathbf{s}\}\\
&= \Sigma\{\Sigma_y (\mathbf{s}_y\cdot\mathbf{X}^+)(\mathbf{r}_y\cdot\mathbf{u}_x) \mid \mathbf{A}/r_{0x}\in\mathbf{s}\}\\
&= \Sigma\{\Sigma_y (\mathbf{s}_y\cdot\mathbf{X}^+)(\delta_{yx}) \mid \mathbf{A}/r_{0x}\in\mathbf{s}\}\\
&= \Sigma\{\mathbf{s}_x\cdot\mathbf{X}^+ \mid \mathbf{A}/r_{0x}\in\mathbf{s}\}\\
&= \Sigma\{1 \mid \mathbf{A}/r_{0x}\in\mathbf{s} \text{ and } \mathbf{s}_x=\mathbf{X}\} = v_{X\to A-}(\mathbf{s}).
\end{aligned}$$

Now in general, $\mathbf{v}^T\cdot\mathbf{A}\cdot\mathbf{v} = \mathbf{v}^T\cdot\mathbf{A}^T\cdot\mathbf{v}$: since $\mathbf{v}^T\cdot\mathbf{A}\cdot\mathbf{v}$ is simply a number (a 1×1 matrix), it equals its "transpose," so

$$\mathbf{v}^T\cdot\mathbf{A}\cdot\mathbf{v} = (\mathbf{v}^T\cdot\mathbf{A}\cdot\mathbf{v})^T = \mathbf{v}^T\cdot\mathbf{A}^T\cdot(\mathbf{v}^T)^T = \mathbf{v}^T\cdot\mathbf{A}^T\cdot\mathbf{v}.$$

Thus, $\mathbf{s}^T\cdot\mathbf{M_{X/A}}^T\cdot\mathbf{s} = \mathbf{s}^T\cdot\mathbf{M_{X/A}}\cdot\mathbf{s} = v_{X\to A-}(\mathbf{s})$. Hence,

$$\begin{aligned}
\mathbf{s}^T\cdot\mathbf{W_{X\to A-}}\cdot\mathbf{s} &\equiv \mathbf{s}^T\cdot\tfrac{1}{2}(\mathbf{M_{X/A}} + [\mathbf{M_{X/A}}]^T)\cdot\mathbf{s}\\
&= \tfrac{1}{2}\,\mathbf{s}^T\cdot\mathbf{M_{X/A}}\cdot\mathbf{s} + \tfrac{1}{2}\,\mathbf{s}^T\cdot\mathbf{M_{X/A}}^T\cdot\mathbf{s}\\
&= \tfrac{1}{2}\,v_{X\to A-}(\mathbf{s}) + \tfrac{1}{2}\,v_{X\to A-}(\mathbf{s}) = v_{X\to A-}(\mathbf{s}).
\end{aligned}$$

That $\mathbf{s}^T\cdot\mathbf{W_{X\to -B}}\cdot\mathbf{s} = v_{X\to -B}(\mathbf{s})$ follows by the analogous argument.

For the remaining claims of the proposition, note that the symmetry of $\mathbf{D}$ (120) implies

$$\begin{aligned}
[\mathbf{M_{X/A}}]^T \equiv [\underline{\mathbf{M}}_{\mathbf{X/A}}\otimes\mathbf{R}]^T &= [\underline{\mathbf{M}}_{\mathbf{X/A}}]^T\otimes[\Sigma_k \mathbf{D}^{\otimes k}]^T\\
&= [\underline{\mathbf{M}}_{\mathbf{X/A}}]^T\otimes\Sigma_k [\mathbf{D}^T]^{\otimes k}\\
&= [\underline{\mathbf{M}}_{\mathbf{X/A}}]^T\otimes\Sigma_k [\mathbf{D}]^{\otimes k} \equiv [\underline{\mathbf{M}}_{\mathbf{X/A}}]^T\otimes\mathbf{R},
\end{aligned}$$

so

$$\begin{aligned}
\mathbf{W_{X\to A-}} &\equiv \tfrac{1}{2}(\mathbf{M_{X/A}} + [\mathbf{M_{X/A}}]^T)\\
&= \tfrac{1}{2}(\underline{\mathbf{M}}_{\mathbf{X/A}}\otimes\mathbf{R} + [\underline{\mathbf{M}}_{\mathbf{X/A}}]^T\otimes\mathbf{R})\\
&= \tfrac{1}{2}(\underline{\mathbf{M}}_{\mathbf{X/A}} + [\underline{\mathbf{M}}_{\mathbf{X/A}}]^T)\otimes\mathbf{R}.
\end{aligned}$$

The analogous result for $\mathbf{W_{X\to -B}}$ follows from the same logic.

(126) *Corollary.* Let $\mathbf{W_{X\to AB}} \equiv \mathbf{W_{X\to A-}} + \mathbf{W_{X\to -B}}$. Then

$$\mathbf{s}^{\mathrm{T}} \cdot w\mathbf{W}_{\mathbf{X}\to\mathbf{AB}} \cdot \mathbf{s} = w\mathrm{v}_{\mathbf{X}\to\mathbf{A}-}(\mathbf{s}) + w\mathrm{v}_{\mathbf{X}\to-\mathbf{B}}(\mathbf{s}).$$

Hence, if the weight matrix of a network is $\mathbf{W} \equiv w\mathbf{W}_{\mathbf{X}\to\mathbf{AB}}$, the Harmony of $\mathbf{s}$, $H(\mathbf{s}) \equiv \mathbf{s}^{\mathrm{T}} \cdot \mathbf{W} \cdot \mathbf{s}$, is the Harmony assessed to $\mathbf{s}$ by the Harmonic Grammar soft constraints

$R_{\mathbf{X}\to\mathbf{A}-}$: The left child of $\mathbf{X}$ is $\mathbf{A}$ (*strength: w*);

$R_{\mathbf{X}\to-\mathbf{B}}$: The right child of $\mathbf{X}$ is $\mathbf{B}$ (*strength: w*).

The Harmonic Grammar rules of (126)—and those of (127)—were introduced in Section 6:2; they are developed more fully in Chapter 10.

(127) *Proposition.* Let $\mathbf{W}_{\mathbf{X}} \equiv \mathbf{X}^{+}\mathbf{X}^{+\mathrm{T}} \otimes \mathbf{R} \equiv \underline{\mathbf{W}}_{\mathbf{X}} \otimes \mathbf{R}$. Then if the weight matrix of a network is $\mathbf{W} \equiv -w\mathbf{W}_{\mathbf{X}}$, the Harmony of $\mathbf{s}$, $H(\mathbf{s}) \equiv \mathbf{s}^{\mathrm{T}} \cdot \mathbf{W} \cdot \mathbf{s}$, is the Harmony assessed to $\mathbf{s}$ by the Harmonic Grammar soft rule

$R_{\mathbf{X}}$: No $\mathbf{X}$ (*strength: w*).

Proof. Suppose $|x| = n$; then

$$\begin{aligned}\mathbf{W}_{\mathbf{X}} \cdot \mathbf{C}/\mathbf{r}_x = \mathbf{X}^{+}\mathbf{X}^{+\mathrm{T}} \otimes \mathbf{R} \cdot \mathbf{C}/\mathbf{r}_x &= [\mathbf{X}^{+}\mathbf{X}^{+\mathrm{T}} \otimes \Sigma_k \mathbf{D}^{\otimes k}] \cdot \mathbf{C}/\mathbf{r}_x \\ &= \mathbf{X}^{+}[\mathbf{X}^{+} \cdot \mathbf{C}] \otimes [\mathbf{D}^{\otimes n}] \cdot \mathbf{r}_x \\ &= \mathbf{X}^{+}[\mathbf{X}^{+} \cdot \mathbf{C}] \otimes \mathbf{u}_x\end{aligned}$$

by (121). This equals $\mathbf{0}$ if $\mathbf{C} \neq \mathbf{X}$, and $\mathbf{X}^{+} \otimes \mathbf{u}_x$ if $\mathbf{C} = \mathbf{X}$. Thus,

$$\mathbf{W}_{\mathbf{X}} \cdot \mathbf{s} = \Sigma\,\{\mathbf{X}^{+} \otimes \mathbf{u}_x \mid \mathbf{s}_x = \mathbf{X}\}.$$

Then

$$\begin{aligned}\mathbf{s}^{\mathrm{T}} \cdot \mathbf{W}_{\mathbf{X}} \cdot \mathbf{s} &= \mathbf{s}^{\mathrm{T}} \cdot \Sigma\,\{\mathbf{X}^{+} \otimes \mathbf{u}_x \mid \mathbf{s}_x = \mathbf{X}\} \\ &= [\Sigma_y \mathbf{s}_y \otimes \mathbf{r}_y]^{\mathrm{T}} \cdot \Sigma\,\{\mathbf{X}^{+} \otimes \mathbf{u}_x \mid \mathbf{s}_x = \mathbf{X}\} \\ &= \Sigma\,\{\Sigma_y[\mathbf{s}_y \otimes \mathbf{r}_y] \cdot [\mathbf{X}^{+} \otimes \mathbf{u}_x] \mid \mathbf{s}_x = \mathbf{X}\} \\ &= \Sigma\,\{\Sigma_y[\mathbf{s}_y \cdot \mathbf{X}^{+}] \otimes [\mathbf{r}_y \cdot \mathbf{u}_x] \mid \mathbf{s}_x = \mathbf{X}\} \\ &= \Sigma\,\{\Sigma_y[\mathbf{s}_y \cdot \mathbf{X}^{+}] \otimes [\delta_{yx}] \mid \mathbf{s}_x = \mathbf{X}\} \\ &= \Sigma\,\{[\mathbf{s}_x \cdot \mathbf{X}^{+}] \mid \mathbf{s}_x = \mathbf{X}\} \\ &= \Sigma\,\{1 \mid \mathbf{s}_x = \mathbf{X}\} \equiv \mathrm{v}_{\mathbf{X}}(\mathbf{s}),\end{aligned}$$

that is, the number of times $\mathbf{X}$ appears in $\mathbf{s}$. Then

$$\mathbf{s}^{\mathrm{T}} \cdot \mathbf{W} \cdot \mathbf{s} \equiv \mathbf{s}^{\mathrm{T}} \cdot (-w\mathbf{W}_{\mathbf{X}}) \cdot \mathbf{s} = -w\mathrm{v}_{\mathbf{X}}(\mathbf{s}),$$

which is indeed the Harmony of $\mathbf{s}$ as assessed by $R_{\mathbf{X}}$.

This gives us as an immediate corollary the following theorem:

(128) **Context-Free Harmonic Grammar Realization Theorem**

Let $\mathcal{G}$ be a harmonic grammar for a context-free language $\mathcal{L}$, consisting of soft rules $\{R_r\}$ of types $R_{\mathbf{X}\to\mathbf{A}-}$, $R_{\mathbf{X}\to-\mathbf{B}}$, and $R_{\mathbf{X}}$, with their respective weights $\{w_r\}$. For each soft rule R_r, define the corresponding matrix $\underline{\mathbf{W}}_r$ as in (125)–(126); let

$$\underline{\mathbf{W}}_{\mathcal{G}} \equiv \Sigma_r\, w_r \underline{\mathbf{W}}_r\,.$$

Then in the network with weight matrix $\mathbf{W}_{\mathcal{G}} \equiv \underline{\mathbf{W}}_{\mathcal{G}} \otimes \mathbf{R}$, the Harmony of $\mathbf{s} = \psi(\mathbf{s})$ is the same as the Harmony of $\mathbf{s}$ as defined by $\mathcal{G}$.

This was the method used to realize the simple grammar in Box 2:2.

(129) *Corollary.* Let C be the Harmonic Grammar constraint $*[\mathbf{X}/r_\varepsilon\ \&\ \mathbf{A}/r_x]$ with

strength $-w$. That is, C contributes $-w$ to the Harmony for each pair **X**, **A** for which the tree position of **A** relative to **X** is that labeled by the bit string x (i.e., for each pair $\mathbf{X}/r_y$, $\mathbf{A}/r_{xy}$). Then C is realized by the weight matrix

$$-w\mathbf{W}_C = -w\underline{\mathbf{W}}_C \otimes \mathbf{R} \equiv -\tfrac{1}{2}w[\mathbf{X}^+\mathbf{A}^{+\mathrm{T}} \otimes \mathbf{u}_x^{\mathrm{T}} + \mathbf{A}^+\mathbf{X}^{+\mathrm{T}} \otimes \mathbf{u}_x] \otimes \mathbf{R}.$$

Proof. This generalizes the results (125) for $\underline{\mathbf{W}}_{\mathrm{X}\to\mathrm{A}-} \equiv \tfrac{1}{2}([\mathbf{X}^+\mathbf{A}^{+\mathrm{T}} \otimes \mathbf{u}_0^{\mathrm{T}}] + [\mathbf{X}^+\mathbf{A}^{+\mathrm{T}} \otimes \mathbf{u}_0^{\mathrm{T}}]^{\mathrm{T}})$ $(x = 0)$, $\underline{\mathbf{W}}_{\mathrm{X}\to-\mathrm{B}} \equiv \tfrac{1}{2}([\mathbf{X}^+\mathbf{B}^{+\mathrm{T}} \otimes \mathbf{u}_1^{\mathrm{T}}] + [\mathbf{X}^+\mathbf{B}^{+\mathrm{T}} \otimes \mathbf{u}_1^{\mathrm{T}}]^{\mathrm{T}})$ $(x = 1)$, and (127) $\underline{\mathbf{W}}_{\mathrm{X}} \equiv \mathbf{X}^+\mathbf{X}^{+\mathrm{T}}$ $(x = \varepsilon)$; the proofs of those results generalize directly to the case of arbitrary x.

(130) *Definition.* The weight matrix **W** of a symmetric recurrent network is **recursive** if it obeys the recursion equation

$$\mathbf{W} = \underline{\mathbf{W}} + \mathbf{W} \otimes \mathbf{D},$$

where $\underline{\mathbf{W}}$ is a finite **root matrix** with this defining property: for all **C**, **t**,

$$\mathbf{C}/\mathbf{r}_x^{\mathrm{T}} \cdot \underline{\mathbf{W}} \cdot \mathbf{t} = 0 \;\text{ unless } x = \varepsilon.$$

(131) **Embedding Invariance Theorem**

Let a symmetric recurrent network have a recursive weight matrix **W**. Then the Harmony is **embedding invariant**; that is, for all nonroot positions $x \neq \varepsilon$, the Harmony of any **s** at the root is the same as the Harmony of **s** displaced to x:

$$H(\mathbf{s}) = H(\mathbf{s} \otimes \mathbf{r}_x).$$

Proof. First consider $x = i = 0$ or 1 $(|x| = 1)$.

$$\begin{aligned} H(\mathbf{s} \otimes \mathbf{r}_i) &\equiv (\mathbf{s} \otimes \mathbf{r}_i)^{\mathrm{T}} \cdot \mathbf{W} \cdot (\mathbf{s} \otimes \mathbf{r}_i) \\ &= (\mathbf{s} \otimes \mathbf{r}_i)^{\mathrm{T}} \cdot [\underline{\mathbf{W}} + \mathbf{W} \otimes \mathbf{D}] \cdot (\mathbf{s} \otimes \mathbf{r}_i) \\ &= (\mathbf{s} \otimes \mathbf{r}_i)^{\mathrm{T}} \cdot \underline{\mathbf{W}} \cdot (\mathbf{s} \otimes \mathbf{r}_i) + (\mathbf{s} \otimes \mathbf{r}_i)^{\mathrm{T}} \cdot [\mathbf{W} \otimes \mathbf{D}] \cdot (\mathbf{s} \otimes \mathbf{r}_i). \end{aligned}$$

Since $\underline{\mathbf{W}}$ is a root matrix, and $x = i \neq \varepsilon$, the first term vanishes, as $\mathbf{s} \otimes \mathbf{r}_i$ can have no root bindings $\mathbf{C}/\mathbf{r}_\varepsilon$. Then, using $\mathbf{D} \cdot \mathbf{r}_i = \mathbf{u}_i$ (121),

$$\begin{aligned} H(\mathbf{s} \otimes \mathbf{r}_i) &= (\mathbf{s} \otimes \mathbf{r}_i)^{\mathrm{T}} \cdot [\mathbf{W} \otimes \mathbf{D}] \cdot (\mathbf{s} \otimes \mathbf{r}_i) \\ &= [\mathbf{s}^{\mathrm{T}} \cdot \mathbf{W} \cdot \mathbf{s}]\, [\mathbf{r}_i^{\mathrm{T}} \cdot \mathbf{D} \cdot \mathbf{r}_i] \\ &= H(\mathbf{s})\, [\mathbf{r}_i \cdot \mathbf{u}_i] = H(\mathbf{s}). \end{aligned}$$

Now recurse: for $|x| = 2$, $x = ij$, where i and j are 0 or 1, we have

$$H(\mathbf{s} \otimes \mathbf{r}_x) = H(\mathbf{s} \otimes \mathbf{r}_{ij}) = H(\mathbf{s} \otimes [\mathbf{r}_i \otimes \mathbf{r}_j]) = H([\mathbf{s} \otimes \mathbf{r}_i] \otimes \mathbf{r}_j) = H(\mathbf{s} \otimes \mathbf{r}_j) = H(\mathbf{s}).$$

Clearly, this can be continued to positions x at any depth $d = |x|$.

(132) **Recursive Weight Matrix Theorem**

A recursive weight matrix **W** of a symmetric recurrent network has the form

$$\mathbf{W} = \underline{\mathbf{W}} \otimes \mathbf{R},$$

where $\underline{\mathbf{W}}$ is a root matrix and **R** is the recursion matrix (123), which solves the recursion equation

$$\mathbf{R} = \mathbf{1} + \mathbf{R} \otimes \mathbf{D}.$$

Figure 4 Box 2

Proof. The recursion equation (130) defining a recursive weight matrix W is

$$\mathbf{W} = \underline{\mathbf{W}} + \mathbf{W} \otimes \mathbf{D}.$$

Substituting the equation into itself recursively yields

$$\begin{aligned}
\mathbf{W} &= \underline{\mathbf{W}} + \mathbf{W} \otimes \mathbf{D} \\
&= \underline{\mathbf{W}} + [\underline{\mathbf{W}} + \mathbf{W} \otimes \mathbf{D}] \otimes \mathbf{D} \\
&= \underline{\mathbf{W}} + \underline{\mathbf{W}} \otimes \mathbf{D} + \mathbf{W} \otimes \mathbf{D} \otimes \mathbf{D} \\
&= \underline{\mathbf{W}} + \underline{\mathbf{W}} \otimes \mathbf{D} + [\underline{\mathbf{W}} + \mathbf{W} \otimes \mathbf{D}] \otimes \mathbf{D} \otimes \mathbf{D} \\
&= \underline{\mathbf{W}} + \underline{\mathbf{W}} \otimes \mathbf{D} + \underline{\mathbf{W}} \otimes \mathbf{D} \otimes \mathbf{D} + \mathbf{W} \otimes \mathbf{D} \otimes \mathbf{D} \otimes \mathbf{D} \\
&= \cdots \\
&= \underline{\mathbf{W}} + \underline{\mathbf{W}} \otimes \mathbf{D} + \underline{\mathbf{W}} \otimes \mathbf{D} \otimes \mathbf{D} + \cdots \\
&= \underline{\mathbf{W}} \otimes (\mathbf{1} + \mathbf{D} + \mathbf{D} \otimes \mathbf{D} + \cdots) \\
&\equiv \underline{\mathbf{W}} \otimes \mathbf{R}.
\end{aligned}$$

Similar computation verifies that R itself solves $\mathbf{R} = \mathbf{1} + \mathbf{R} \otimes \mathbf{D}$ (applying $\underline{\mathbf{W}} \otimes$ to both sides of this equation and letting $\mathbf{W} \equiv \underline{\mathbf{W}} \otimes \mathbf{R}$ yields the recursion relation (130) for W).

In (125) and (127), we have seen examples of recursive weight matrices of just this form, $\mathbf{W} \equiv \underline{\mathbf{W}} \otimes \mathbf{R}$.

Equation (132) is rather easy to interpret: it says that to create a recursive weight matrix **W**, take the relatively small number of basic weights in $\underline{\mathbf{W}}$ that determine the well-formedness of structures in root position, and copy each of them to all the homologous locations throughout the network that correspond to all possible embedding positions. Thus, this equation gives rise to embedding invariance in a way analogous to how translation invariance is often achieved in connectionist networks for vision: a relatively small number of weights determine the processing of the patch of image at the origin, and each of these is copied to all the homologous locations in the network that correspond to translating the patch away from the origin (e.g., Fukushima 1980; also Minsky and Papert 1969). Equation (132) characterizes a low-level invariance structure imposed on the network, in which individual connection weights in homologous network locations are required to be equal. It has the high-level consequence that the well-formedness of pairs of symbolic constituents—the crucial Harmony values $H(\mathbf{c}_1, \mathbf{c}_2)$ for Harmonic Grammar—depends only on their relative, not their absolute, positions in the tree. And this in turn is just what is needed for *H* to specify a recursive measure of well-formedness, such as that required to characterize context-free languages (Chapter 10).

For harmonic recurrent networks, the recursivity requirement on the weight matrix is that it take the form $\mathbf{W}_{\mathrm{H}} \equiv \underline{\mathbf{W}} \otimes \mathbf{R}$; for feed-forward networks realizing the recursive functions in $\mathscr{F}$, the required form is $\mathbf{W}_{\mathrm{FF}} \equiv \mathbf{I} \otimes \underline{\mathbf{W}}$ (108). There are two differences to be understood. First, the harmonic net matrix uses the matrix **R**, the unbounded extension of the dualizer matrix **D**; the feed-forward net uses **I**, the extension of the identity matrix **1**. This is because in the feed-forward case, the output of the matrix is to be a particular tree, with a particular set of bindings specified by $\underline{\mathbf{W}}$; $\mathbf{W}_{\mathrm{FF}}$ must map bindings $\mathbf{f} \otimes \mathbf{r}_x$ to other bindings $\mathbf{f}' \otimes \mathbf{r}_{x'}$. In contrast, the output **o** of $\mathbf{W}_{\mathrm{H}}$ must have a given *inner product* with certain bindings—it must yield a given *Harmony* value. Thus, it must map bindings $\mathbf{f}\otimes\mathbf{r}_x$ to other bindings $\mathbf{f}'\otimes\mathbf{u}_{x'}$. Because these involve $\mathbf{u}_{x}'$, the basic matrix needed is $\mathbf{D}$, which converts role vectors $\mathbf{r}_x$ to dual (unbinding) vectors $\mathbf{u}_x$. But $\mathbf{W}_{\mathrm{FF}}$ maps $\mathbf{r}_x$-bindings to $\mathbf{r}_{x'}$-bindings, so the identity matrix $\mathbf{1}$ is the relevant basic matrix.

The other difference is that in the harmonic case, $\mathbf{W}_{\mathrm{H}}\equiv\underline{\mathbf{W}}\otimes\mathbf{R}$, $\underline{\mathbf{W}}$ appears on the left, while in the feed-forward case, $\mathbf{W}_{\mathrm{FF}}\equiv\mathbf{I}\otimes\underline{\mathbf{W}}$, it appears on the right. This arises from a difference in the recursivity requirements: whether, essentially, what gets moved down is the tree as a whole (operating on the root) or just the lowest nodes of the tree (operating on each node independently). In the harmonic case, the requirement is that moving a tree, in its entirety, down to a deeper embedding depth must have the correct effect (no change in H): the Embedding Invariance Theorem (131). In the feed-forward case, the requirement (124) is that the correct effect result from moving down the lowest part of a tree (below some depth dependent on the function being realized; the image in the output must also move down in the corresponding way). In the harmonic case, the requirement involves taking the role vector $\mathbf{r}_x$ of each binding in the input tree and demoting it to, say, $\mathbf{r}_{x0}$; appending 0 to the *right* edge of the location index x involves multiplying $\mathbf{r}_x$ on the *right* (by $\mathbf{R}$); the input is multiplied by the appropriate recursion matrix ($\mathbf{R}$) before it is processed by the grammar-specific matrix $\underline{\mathbf{W}}$. In the feed-forward case, the requirement involves taking the role vector $\mathbf{r}_x$ of an individual binding in the input and demoting it to, say, $\mathbf{r}_{0x}$; appending 0 on to the *left* edge of x involves multiplying $\mathbf{r}_x$ on the *left* by the appropriate recursion matrix, $\mathbf{I}$.

4.3 TPPL: Tensor Product Programming Language

The stratified connectionist realization of trees developed above enables massively parallel processing. Whereas in the traditional sequential implementation of Lisp, symbol processing consists of a long sequence of $\mathbf{ex}_0$, $\mathbf{ex}_1$, and **cons** operations, here we can compose the corresponding sequence of $\mathbf{W}_{\mathrm{ex0}}$, $\mathbf{W}_{\mathrm{ex1}}$, $\mathbf{W}_{\mathrm{cons0}}$, and $\mathbf{W}_{\mathrm{cons1}}$ operations into a single matrix operation.

By adding some minimal nonlinearity, it is possible to compose more complex operations incorporating the equivalent of conditional branching. The idea has just begun to be explored. One example has been worked out, a network shown in Figure 5 called **Active/PassiveNet** (or APNet) (Legendre, Miyata, and Smolensky 1991). We already saw part of this network, PassiveNet, in Section 5:2.2.

APNet computes a function f^{AP} which can be expressed symbolically as in (133).

(133) Function computed by Active/PassiveNet

```
fAP(s) = IF    [ex0(ex1(ex1(s)))=Aux]
         THEN  cons(ex1(ex0(cdr(s))),
                    cons(ex1(ex1(ex1(s))), ex0(s)))
         ELSE  cons(ex0(ex1(s)),
                    cons(ex0(s), ex1(ex1(s))))
```

Figure 5. Active / PassiveNet

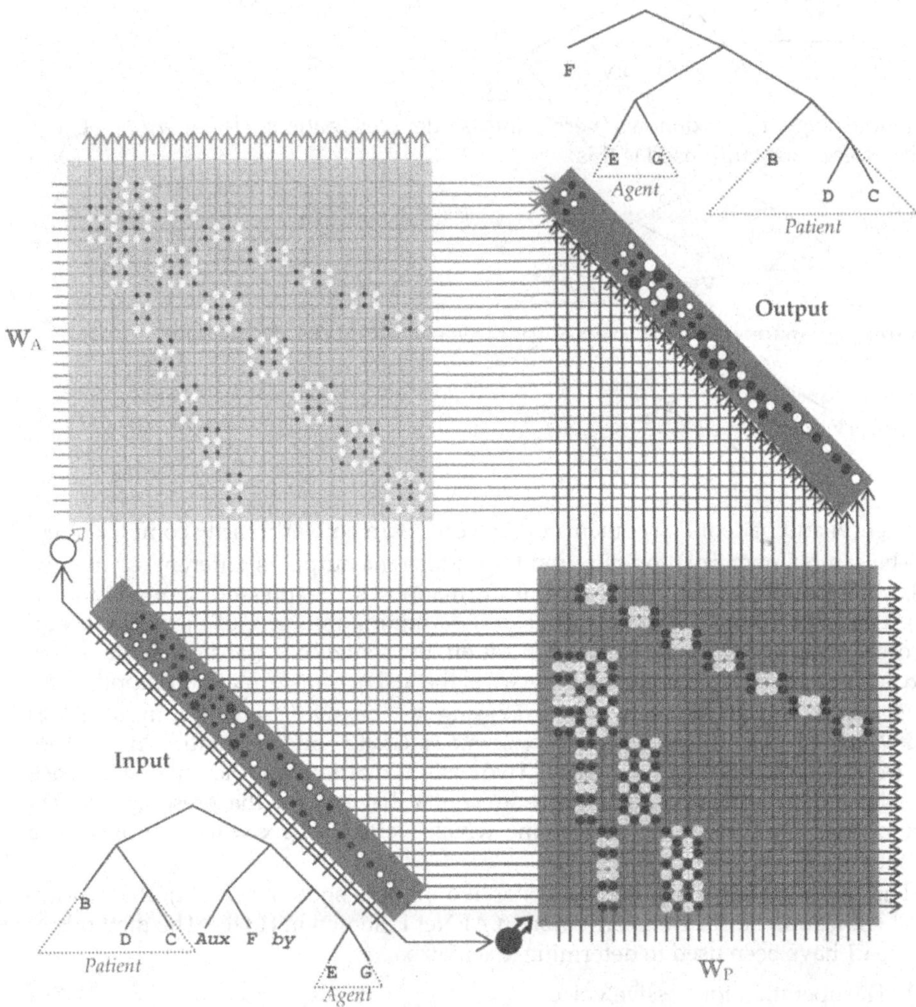

APNet takes as input a distributed pattern of activity realizing the tree structure of an English sentence, conducts a simple inspection of the structure to determine whether the form is that of a stylized "active" or "passive" sentence, and, accordingly, produces as output a distributed pattern realizing a tree structure encoding a predicate-calculus form of the "semantic interpretation" of the input sentence. The crude tree structures used for the input include the "passive" form already seen in Chapter 5:

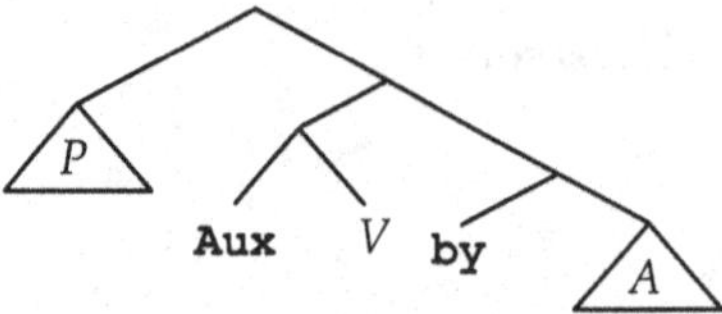

'A' denotes 'agent', 'V' denotes 'verb', and 'P' denotes 'patient': *P is V-ed by A*. The "active voice" structure used is this:

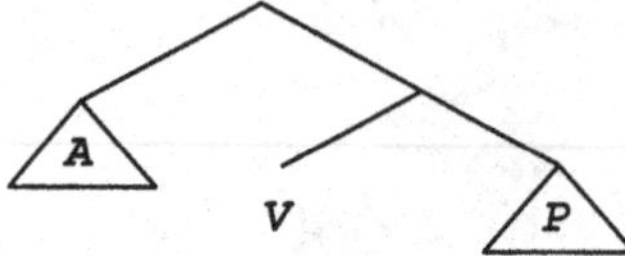

Both trees are mapped by $\mathbf{f}$ into an output tree encoding *V*(*A*, *P*), namely,

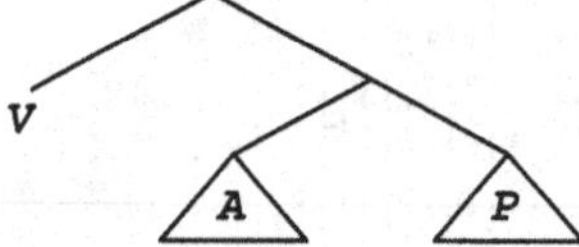

The agent *A* and patient *P* arguments of the verb *V* are both arbitrarily complex trees.

The symbol manipulation required to produce the output is different for the two kinds of input sentences. The two transformations are expressed symbolically in (133). The test for **Aux** is a crude means of determining the voice of the input: if **Aux** is present at its appropriate structural position, the sentence is transformed in a way appropriate for a passive sentence; otherwise, the active transformation is applied.

Figure 5 shows the network processing a "passive" sentence input [[**A B**] [[**Aux V**] [**by C**]]]—as in *Few leaders are admired by George*—and generating the output [**V** [**C** [**A B**]]]—*admire(George, few leaders)*. Two weight matrices are shown, one for each voice-dependent transformation. There are units that test for the presence and absence of **Aux**, and these units determine which weight matrix will be applied to a given input.

The transformation required for a passive input is shown in (134a); the connectionist realization of this transformation in APNet is shown in (134b). The methods of Section 4.1 have been used to determine this matrix.

(134) The operation for passive voice

a. $\mathbf{f}_P(\mathbf{s}) = \mathbf{cons}(\mathbf{ex}_1(\mathbf{ex}_0(\mathbf{ex}_1(\mathbf{s}))),$
$\qquad \mathbf{cons}(\mathbf{ex}_1(\mathbf{ex}_1(\mathbf{ex}_1(\mathbf{s}))), \mathbf{ex}_0(\mathbf{s})))$.

b. $\mathbf{W}_P = \mathbf{W}_{cons0}[\mathbf{W}_{ex1}\mathbf{W}_{ex0}\mathbf{W}_{ex1}] +$
$\qquad \mathbf{W}_{cons1}[\mathbf{W}_{cons0}(\mathbf{W}_{ex1}\mathbf{W}_{ex1}\mathbf{W}_{ex1}) + \mathbf{W}_{cons1}(\mathbf{W}_{ex0})]$.

The unit that becomes active for a passive input checks whether $\mathbf{ex}_0(\mathbf{ex}_1(\mathbf{ex}_1(\mathbf{s}))) =$ **Aux**. This condition unit can be a linear threshold element whose activity is 1 when

Figure 5 *Box 2*

its net input $\iota \geq 0$, and 0 otherwise; its net input $\iota \equiv -\|\mathbf{W}_{ex0}\mathbf{W}_{ex1}\mathbf{W}_{ex1} \cdot \mathbf{s} - \mathbf{Aux}\|^2$ is always negative, except that $\iota = 0$ when the desired condition $\mathbf{ex_0}(\mathbf{ex_1}(\mathbf{ex_1}(\boldsymbol{s}))) = \mathbf{Aux}$ is satisfied. The connections from input to output are all multiplied or **gated** by this unit: when it is active, the connections for the passive matrix, $\mathbf{W}_P$, apply; otherwise, the connections for the active matrix apply.

The methods developed above suggest the possibility of an explicit symbolic formalism—call it **TPPL** for 'Tensor Product Programming Language'—enabling high-level formal characterization of the computations performed by feed-forward connectionist networks processing tensor product representations.[16] TPPL would contain analogues of simple programming language control structures (like IF—THEN—ELSE) and basic symbolic computation operators (like $\mathbf{ex_0}$, $\mathbf{ex_1}$, **cons**) that are formally defined using elements of the tensor calculus. TPPL would enable both a formal higher-level symbolic description of the connectionist networks and a calculus for proving their correctness.

To illustrate the idea, APNet might be described in TPPL by the program in (135):

(135) APNet in TPPL

$$\begin{aligned}
AP(\boldsymbol{s}) &\equiv \texttt{if } PassiveP(\boldsymbol{s}) \texttt{ then } PassiveF(\boldsymbol{s}) \texttt{ else } ActiveF(\boldsymbol{s}) \\
PassiveP(\boldsymbol{s}) &\equiv [PassiveMarkerF(\boldsymbol{s}) = \mathbf{Aux}] \\
PassiveMarkerF(\boldsymbol{s}) &\equiv \mathbf{ex_0}(\mathbf{ex_0}(\mathbf{ex_1}(\boldsymbol{s}))) \\
PassiveF(\boldsymbol{s}) &\equiv \mathbf{cons}(\mathbf{ex_1}(\mathbf{ex_0}(\mathbf{ex_1}(\boldsymbol{s}))), \\
&\qquad \mathbf{cons}(\mathbf{ex_1}(\mathbf{ex_1}(\mathbf{ex_1}(\boldsymbol{s}))), \ \mathbf{ex_0}(\boldsymbol{s}))) \\
ActiveF(\boldsymbol{s}) &\equiv \mathbf{cons}(\mathbf{ex_0}(\mathbf{ex_1}(\boldsymbol{s})), \\
&\qquad \mathbf{cons}(\mathbf{ex_0}(\boldsymbol{s}), \ \mathbf{ex_1}(\mathbf{ex_1}(\boldsymbol{s}))))
\end{aligned}$$

The primitive operations **cons** and $\mathbf{ex_{0/1}}$ are defined as above in (83) and (57). As illustrated for *PassiveF* in (134), the matrix realizations of these operations are straightforwardly combined to produce a single matrix that performs the entire function *PassiveF*, which can then be implemented in one layer of connection weights. The same applies to the other functions, *ActiveF* and *PassiveMarkerF*.

Predicates like *PassiveP* of the general form[17] $[s = r]$ might be defined by the function $\theta(\|s - r\|)$, where $\theta(x)$ is 1 if $x = 0$ and 0 otherwise (or some smoothed version, such as the Gaussian $\theta(x) = \exp(-cx^2)$). This can then be conveniently implemented in the connectionist network by a linear threshold unit, or, perhaps more naturally, by a radial basis function unit.

Finally, the construct 'if P then F_1 else F_2' could be defined as the function

$$P \cdot \mathbf{F}_1 + (1 - P) \cdot \mathbf{F}_2 = P \cdot (\mathbf{F}_1 - \mathbf{F}_2) + \mathbf{F}_2.$$

This is in turn implemented either (i) by having the output of the unit u implementing P gate (through multiplicative connections) the connections implementing $\mathbf{F}_1$,

[16] Multiple-level specification of a computational system is discussed extensively in Chapter 23.
[17] Note that this allows conditions such as $\mathbf{ex_0}(\mathbf{ex_1}(\mathbf{ex_1}(\mathbf{s}))) = \mathbf{ex_0}(\mathbf{ex_1}(\mathbf{r}))$ in which neither element of the comparison is a constant.

while $1 - u$ gates the connections implementing $\mathbf{F}_2$; or (ii) by having u gate connections implementing $\mathbf{F}_1 - \mathbf{F}_2$ while connections implementing $\mathbf{F}_2$ are ungated.

In such a setting, TPPL provides a third language for formally describing networks like APNet for processing recursive tensor product representations. The lowest-level 'language' is that provided by the equations governing individual units and connections of a connectionist network that employs fairly traditional machinery such as radial basis function units and multiplicative connections to perform fully distributed, massively parallel computation. A higher-level 'language' uses tensor calculus and θ functions to concisely but precisely describe the numerical vector processing the net carries out. Finally, TPPL provides a still more abstract, yet formally precise, language for high-level description of the system as performing symbolic structure processing. These TPPL programs describe the symbolic function being computed using expressions like

$$\mathbf{cons}(\mathbf{ex}_1(\mathbf{ex}_0(\mathbf{ex}_1(\mathbf{s}))),\ \mathbf{cons}(\mathbf{ex}_1(\mathbf{ex}_1(\mathbf{ex}_1(\mathbf{s}))),\mathbf{ex}_0(\mathbf{s}))),$$

but the actual computation does *not* involve sequential application of $\mathbf{ex}_0$, $\mathbf{ex}_1$, and **cons**. It is possible to precisely define each description language in terms of the next most abstract language (TPPL in terms of tensorial equations; tensorial equations in terms of equations governing individual units and connections)—precisely enough to allow proofs of correctness which ensure that the network computes the symbolic function defined by the TPPL program.

4.4 Fully distributed recursive representations

The recursive realization of binary trees described in Section 4.1 has been called a *stratified* realization: different levels of the tree are realized separately (over different connectionist units)—they are essentially *concatenated* by the direct sum in the construction of the vector space V, rather than truly superimposed, as in fully distributed representations. Among other things, this means that a finite-sized network will have a sharp cutoff in the depth of trees it can realize, rather than displaying graceful saturation—where the accuracy with which information in a tree is realized gracefully degrades beyond a certain depth (see Section 3.2). We will now see how to overcome this limitation, without sacrificing the recursive character of the realization. The representation space is actually somewhat simpler than in the stratified representation, and the equations are basically the same, but the operators involved are somewhat more complex. The new technique, as before, can be studied by a combination of mathematical analysis and computer simulation.

The crux of the idea is to add to the fundamental role vectors $\{\mathbf{r}_0, \mathbf{r}_1\}$ of the stratified representation a third vector $\mathbf{v}$ that serves basically as a placeholder, like the digit 0 in numerals. Instead of representing an atom **B** at position r_{01} by $\mathbf{B} \otimes \mathbf{r}_0 \otimes \mathbf{r}_1$, we use $\mathbf{B} \otimes \mathbf{v} \otimes \mathbf{v} \otimes \cdots \otimes \mathbf{v} \otimes \mathbf{r}_0 \otimes \mathbf{r}_1$, using as many **v**s as necessary to pad the total tensor product out to produce a tensor of some selected rank $D+1$. Now, atoms at all depths are realized by tensors of the same rank; the new vector space of representations of binary trees is just a space V' of tensors of rank $D+1$, and the realizations of all atoms can fully superimpose: this representation is *fully distributed*.

Trees up to depth D can now be realized with complete accuracy (assuming the three vectors $\{\mathbf{r}_0, \mathbf{r}_1, \mathbf{v}\}$ are linearly independent). The stratified realization of Section 4.1 can be straightforwardly embedded as a special case of this new fully distributed representation by mapping $\mathbf{r}_0 \to (\mathbf{r}_0, 0)$, $\mathbf{r}_1 \to (\mathbf{r}_1, 0)$ and by setting $\mathbf{v} \equiv (\mathbf{0}, 1)$, where $\mathbf{0}$ is the zero vector with the same dimensionality as $\mathbf{r}_0$ and $\mathbf{r}_1$. That is, the special case in which $\{\mathbf{r}_0, \mathbf{r}_1, \mathbf{v}\}$ is decomposed as the direct sum of the two-dimensional space spanned by the old vectors $\{\mathbf{r}_0, \mathbf{r}_1\}$ and the one-dimensional space spanned by $\mathbf{v}$ reduces the new fully distributed representation to the direct-sum-across-depths stratified representation. But in the *general* case, $\{\mathbf{r}_0, \mathbf{r}_1, \mathbf{v}\}$ are three linearly independent vectors, each with nonzero components along all coordinate axes; in this case, every unit in the connectionist network will take part in the realization of every atom, regardless of its depth in the tree. As before, for extracting tree elements, we need the unbinding vectors $\{\mathbf{u}_0, \mathbf{u}_1, \mathbf{u}\}$ that form the basis dual to $\{\mathbf{r}_0, \mathbf{r}_1, \mathbf{v}\}$.

The recursive characterization of this new representation requires the following new operations:

(136)
$$\mathbf{w} \odot \mathbf{T} \equiv \sum_{\rho_D} w_{\rho_D} T_{\varphi\rho_D \cdots \rho_2\rho_1} \qquad \mathbf{T} \odot \mathbf{w} \equiv \sum_{\rho_1} T_{\varphi\rho_D \cdots \rho_2\rho_1} w_{\rho_1}$$

$$\mathbf{T} \circledcirc \mathbf{w} \equiv \mathbf{v} \otimes (\mathbf{T} \odot \mathbf{w}) \qquad \mathbf{T} \circledast \mathbf{w} \equiv (\mathbf{u} \odot \mathbf{T}) \otimes \mathbf{w}$$

$\mathbf{w} \odot \mathbf{T}$ is an inner product of $\mathbf{w}$ with the leftmost (deepest-level) role index of $\mathbf{T}$, and $\mathbf{T} \odot \mathbf{w}$ an inner product with the rightmost (highest-level); the resulting tensor has rank one less than that of $\mathbf{T}$. $\mathbf{T} \circledcirc \mathbf{w}$ is a rank-preserving inner product, a version of $\mathbf{T} \odot \mathbf{w}$ in which a right inner product with $\mathbf{w}$ is taken, and an extra $\mathbf{v}$ is added to pad the new tensor back up to full rank.[18] $\mathbf{T} \circledast \mathbf{w}$ is a rank-preserving outer product, a version of $\mathbf{T} \otimes \mathbf{w}$ in which the tensor product with $\mathbf{w}$ is taken only after "unpadding" $\mathbf{T}$ via an inner product with $\mathbf{u}$, the vector dual to $\mathbf{v}$. (This operation should not be confused with the circular convolution operator of Section 7:6.2.1, also denoted '$\circledast$'.)

Now the new equations generalizing those of Section 4.1 are

(137)
$$\begin{aligned}
\mathbf{s} = \mathbf{cons}(\mathbf{p}, \mathbf{q}) &\Rightarrow \mathbf{s} = \mathbf{p} \circledast \mathbf{r}_0 + \mathbf{q} \circledast \mathbf{r}_1;\\
\mathbf{p} = \mathbf{ex}_0(\mathbf{s}) &\Rightarrow \mathbf{p} = \mathbf{s} \circledcirc \mathbf{u}_0;\\
\mathbf{q} = \mathbf{ex}_1(\mathbf{s}) &\Rightarrow \mathbf{q} = \mathbf{s} \circledcirc \mathbf{u}_1.
\end{aligned}$$

The equations, like (30), characterizing the recursive properties of the stratified representation still hold except that the rank-altering inner- and outer-product operations $\odot$ and $\otimes$ are now replaced by their rank-preserving counterparts $\circledcirc$ and $\circledast$. As before, all operations can be readily realized as matrix operations on the representational vector space, now V'. Active/PassiveNet has been reimplemented with this new technique, using a representation in which all connectionist units participate in the

[18] In these equations, it is understood that the leftmost element in every tensor product is a vector like $\mathbf{B}$ representing an atomic symbol like B. So, for example, if $D = 4$ and $\mathbf{T} = \mathbf{B} \otimes \mathbf{v} \otimes \mathbf{v} \otimes \mathbf{r}_0 \otimes \mathbf{r}_1$, then $\mathbf{T} \circledcirc \mathbf{u}_1 \equiv \mathbf{B} \otimes \mathbf{v} \otimes \mathbf{v} \otimes \mathbf{v} \otimes \mathbf{r}_0 (\mathbf{r}_1 \cdot \mathbf{u}_1)$.

realization of all tree depths (Miyata, Smolensky, and Legendre 1993). As before, the network behaves perfectly, as indeed it provably must.

Now that a fully distributed recursive representation has been produced, it remains to develop specific ways to exploit the full advantages of distributed representation. As one example, consider the issue of graceful saturation with depth. One general technique is to take a high- (perhaps infinite-) dimensional, fully accurate representational space and project onto a lower-dimensional subspace. Here, we want to pick such a subspace so that less accuracy is associated with greater depth. A promising idea for how to achieve this comes from revisiting the means described above for specializing the fully distributed representation to the stratified representation. Strict depth stratification arises from choosing $\mathbf{v} = (0, 1)$ because $\mathbf{v}$ is orthogonal to the subspace spanned by $\{\mathbf{r}_0, \mathbf{r}_1\}$. If instead we choose $\mathbf{v}$ to have small but nonzero projection onto this subspace, each depth will have small but nonzero realization on subspaces that are primarily dedicated to the realization of lesser depths. We can therefore set up a fully distributed representation with some large depth limit *D* (possibly infinite) and then project onto a lower-dimensional subspace, achieving a soft depth limit beyond which the representation saturates gracefully.

Figure 5 Box 2

References

Chomsky, N. 1995. *The Minimalist Program*. MIT Press.

Dolan, C. P., and M. G. Dyer. 1987. Symbolic schemata, role binding, and the evolution of structure in connectionist memories. *IEEE International Conference on Neural Networks* 1, 287–98.

Dolan, C. P., and M. G. Dyer. 1988. Parallel retrieval of conceptual knowledge. In *Proceedings of the 1988 Connectionist Models Summer School.*

Dolan, C. P., and P. Smolensky. 1988. Implementing a connectionist production system using tensor products. In *Proceedings of the 1988 Connectionist Models Summer School.*

Dolan, C. P., and P. Smolensky. 1989. Tensor product production system: A modular architecture and representation. *Connection Science* 1, 53–68.

Fukushima, K. 1980. Neocognitron: A self-organizing neural network model for a mechanism of pattern recognition unaffected by shift in position. *Biological Cybernetics* 36, 193–202.

Hinton, G. E., J. L. McClelland, and D. E. Rumelhart. 1986. Distributed representation. In *Parallel distributed processing: Explorations in the microstructure of cognition*. Vol. 1, *Foundations*, D. E. Rumelhart, J. L. McClelland, and the PDP Research Group. MIT Press.

Jordan, M. I. 1986. An introduction to linear algebra in parallel distributed processing. In *Parallel distributed processing: Explorations in the microstructure of cognition*. Vol. 1, *Foundations*, D. E. Rumelhart, J. L. McClelland, and the PDP Research Group. MIT Press.

Kayne, R. S. 1984. *Connectedness and binary branching*. Foris .

Lachter, J., and T. G. Bever. 1988. The relation between linguistic structure and associative theories of language learning – a constructive critique of some connectionist learning models. *Cognition* 28, 195–247.

Legendre, G., Y. Miyata, and P. Smolensky. 1991. Distributed recursive structure processing. In *Advances in neural information processing systems* 3, eds. R. P. Lippman, J. E. Moody, and D. S. Touretzky. Morgan Kaufmann.

Loomis, L. H., and S. Sternberg. 1968. *Advanced calculus*. Addison-Wesley.

McClelland, J. L., and A. H. Kawamoto. 1986. Mechanisms of sentence processing: Assigning roles to constituents. In *Parallel distributed processing: Explorations in the microstructure of cognition*. Vol. 2, *Psychological and biological models*, J. L. McClelland, D. E. Rumelhart, and the PDP Research Group. MIT Press.

Minsky, M., and S. Papert. 1969. *Perceptrons*. MIT Press.

Miyata, Y., P. Smolensky, and G. Legendre. 1993. Distributed representation and parallel processing of recursive structures. In *Proceedings of the Cognitive Science Society 15*.

Nelson, E. 1967. *Tensor analysis*. Princeton University Press.

Pinker, S., and A. Prince. 1988. On language and connectionism: Analysis of a parallel distributed processing model of language acquisition. *Cognition* 28, 73–193.

Prince, A., and S. Pinker. 1988. Wickelphone ambiguity. *Cognition* 30, 188–90.

Rumelhart, D. E., G. E. Hinton, and J. L. McClelland. 1986. A general framework for parallel distributed processing. In *Parallel distributed processing: Explorations in the microstructure of cognition*. Vol. 1, *Foundations*, D. E. Rumelhart, J. L. McClelland, and the PDP Research Group. MIT Press.

Rumelhart, D. E., G. E. Hinton, and R. J. Williams. 1986. Learning internal representations by error propagation. In *Parallel distributed processing: Explorations in the microstructure of cognition*. Vol. 1, *Foundations*, D. E. Rumelhart, J. L. McClelland, and the PDP Research Group. MIT Press.

Rumelhart, D. E., and J. L. McClelland. 1986. On learning the past tenses of English verbs. In *Parallel distributed processing: Explorations in the microstructure of cognition*. Vol. 2, *Psychological and biological models*, J. L. McClelland, D. E. Rumelhart, and the PDP Research Group. MIT Press.

Smolensky, P. 1986a. Information processing in dynamical systems: Foundations of Harmony Theory. In *Parallel distributed processing: Explorations in the microstructure of cognition.* Vol. 1, *Foundations,* D. E. Rumelhart, J. L. McClelland, and the PDP Research Group. MIT Press.

Smolensky, P. 1986b. Neural and conceptual interpretations of parallel distributed processing models. In *Parallel distributed processing: Explorations in the microstructure of cognition.* Vol. 2, *Psychological and biological models,* J. L. McClelland, D. E. Rumelhart, and the PDP Research Group. MIT Press.

Smolensky, P. 1987a. Connectionist AI, symbolic AI, and the brain. *AI Review* 1, 95–109.

Smolensky, P. 1987b. On variable binding and the representation of symbolic structures in connectionist systems. Technical report CU-CS-355-87, Computer Science Department, University of Colorado at Boulder.

Smolensky, P. 1988. On the proper treatment of connectionism. *Behavioral and Brain Sciences* 11, 1–74.

Smolensky, P. 1990. Tensor product variable binding and the representation of symbolic structures in connectionist networks. *Artificial Intelligence* 46, 159–216.

Smolensky, P. 1995. Constituent structure and explanation in an integrated connectionist/symbolic cognitive architecture. In *Connectionism.* Vol. 2, *Debates on psychological explanation,* eds. C. Macdonald and G. Macdonald. Blackwell.

Smolensky, P., G. Legendre, and Y. Miyata. 1992. Principles for an integrated connectionist/symbolic theory of higher cognition. Technical report CU-CS-600-92, Computer Science Department, and 92–8, Institute of Cognitive Science, University of Colorado at Boulder.

Warner, F. W. 1971. *Foundations of differentiable manifolds and Lie groups.* Scott, Foresman.

Widrow, G., and M. E. Hoff. 1960. Adaptive switching circuits. In *Institute of Radio Engineers, Western Electronic Show and Convention, Convention Record, part 4.*

Willshaw, D. 1981. Holography, associative memory, and inductive generalization. In *Parallel models of associative memory,* eds. G. E. Hinton and J. A. Anderson. Erlbaum.

9

Optimization in Neural Networks: Harmony Maximization

Paul Smolensky

A fundamental principle of the Integrated Connectionist/Symbolic Cognitive Architecture (ICS) is Harmony maximization. This principle, P3: HMax, identifies optimization as a key characteristic of higher cognition generally, and of the language faculty especially. The mathematical content of this principle is presented here. The results discussed cover a wide range of connectionist network architectures: deterministic and stochastic networks, Boolean and continuous-valued activations, feed-forward and symmetric recurrent connectivity. Stochastic networks and the relation between Harmony and probability are briefly introduced (Boltzmann machines, Harmony Theory). This analysis concerns ⑧ of Figure 5, and ③–⑤ in Figure 8, in Chapter 2's ICS map.

Contents

Neural networks are dynamical systems which compute functions that best capture the statistical regularities in training data. Thus, for the purposes of mathematical analysis, it is useful to regard neural networks from three broad perspectives: the computational, the dynamical, and the statistical (Smolensky 1996a, 2; see also Golden 1996).

From a computational perspective, the activation equations of a neural network define a parallel numerical algorithm for computing a function; the weights are parameter values specifying the function. From a dynamical perspective, neural networks are dynamical systems, whose states are activation vectors that move through state space on trajectories defined by the dynamical equations for spreading activation; the weights specify the coupling strength between state variables. From a statistical perspective, activation values are truth values or probabilities assigned to propositions about the world external to the network, and activation spread implements statistical inference from input propositions (givens) to output propositions (unknowns); the weights encode the parameter values of a joint probability distribution over input and output propositions.

In this chapter, we will examine a class of neural networks—**harmonic** networks—for which each of these perspectives makes an important contribution. From a computational perspective, harmonic networks compute optimal values: they perform optimization; the function being optimized—Harmony—is defined by the connection weights, which are the strengths of soft constraints between variables. From a dynamical systems perspective, the dynamics of harmonic networks continuously increases the value of a function—Harmony—and therefore ultimately converges to an equilibrium state. From a statistical perspective, activation spread in stochastic networks assigns propositions those truth values that describe the state of the problem domain that optimizes (maximizes) log probability—Harmony—given the input propositions.

The characteristics of harmonic networks mentioned above concern spreading activation: this is the topic of the chapter. Learning will enter the discussion only marginally, although for learning too the computational, dynamical, and statistical perspectives all have crucial contributions to make. And in learning too, optimization plays a central role. For instance, from the computational perspective, many learning algorithms are explicitly derived as means of optimizing (minimizing) the network's performance error over a set of training examples. From the statistical perspective, the weights learned by stochastic harmonic networks encode the parameters of a probability distribution of a particular form, whose values specify, of those distributions that are consistent with training data, the one that makes the fewest additional assumptions (i.e., contains minimal information or maximum entropy). For presentations of many facets of learning-as-optimization in neural networks, see Golden 1996; Smolensky 1996c; Hinton and Sejnowski 1999, among many other sources.

This chapter is divided into two main sections. After two preliminary sections, the first primary section, Section 3, analyzes **deterministic** harmonic networks, that is, networks lacking randomness in which the activation value of each unit at any moment is completely determined by the activation values of its neighbors. Section 4 takes up **stochastic** networks, where the activation value of a unit α is a random variable: the activation values of α's neighbors influence the *probability* that α's activation will assume various values, but do not completely determine α's activation—an irreducible element of randomness remains. A statistical perspective will be central to the analysis of stochastic harmonic networks, and computational and dynamical perspectives will be important throughout the chapter.

In this chapter, we will analyze processing in harmonic neural networks exhibiting several architectural variations. Despite the variation, processing in these networks will maximize the value of a Harmony function of a consistent form.

(1) General form of the Harmony function

a. For harmonic networks, the **total Harmony** H is the sum of two terms:
$H(\mathbf{a}) = H_0(\mathbf{a}) + H_1(\mathbf{a})$.

b. The **core Harmony** H_0 is defined as
$H_0(\mathbf{a}) = \mathbf{a}^{\mathrm{T}}\,\mathbf{W}\,\mathbf{a} = \Sigma_{\alpha\beta}\, \mathrm{a}_\alpha\, \mathrm{W}_{\alpha\beta}\, \mathrm{a}_\beta$.

c. The **unit Harmony** H_1 is defined via an **individual unit Harmony function** h^f specific to the activation function f of unit α:
$H_1(\mathbf{a}) = \Sigma_\alpha h^f(\mathrm{a}_\alpha)$.

The core Harmony function H_0 has been discussed at some length in Section 6:1.2, and the intuitions it formalizes will not be repeated here. To summarize that discussion: core Harmony is the sum over all connections in the network of the Harmony cost at each connection, which equals the weight of that connection times the product of the activation values of the two units it connects. H_0 is the part of the Harmony function that measures the *compatibility* between the activation values of pairs of connected units: it evaluates the extent to which the **soft constraints** encoded in the connections are satisfied by the current activation pattern **a**. It is only core Harmony that is sensitive to the weights—the knowledge—in a particular network.

The unit Harmony function H_1, on the other hand, does not depend on the weights in the network. It evaluates each unit individually and sums the individual Harmony costs of all units. The individual Harmony cost of a unit α is determined by its activation level a_α, via a function h^f that is specific to the activation function f operating at unit α. Since core Harmony has already been introduced intuitively in Section 6:1.2, much of the intuitive exposition presented here will concern unit Harmony, which is presented in Section 3.2.2.1.

1 GROUNDWORK

In this section, we set up the basic apparatus for analyzing deterministic Harmonic networks. Much of this will carry over to the stochastic case as well, but until Section 4 we will restrict attention to deterministic networks.

In all networks studied in this chapter, the following properties are assumed:

(2) Basic architectural assumptions

a. The number of units is finite.

b. Input to the network is provided by clamping an activation pattern **i** on a set of input units; these units retain fixed activation values the entire time the network processes that input. Every possible state vector **a** of the network is thus a **completion** of the input vector **i**: the portion of the pattern **a** defined by the input units' activations equals **i**.[1]

c. Every noninput unit is updated repeatedly: there is never a time beyond which some unit is no longer updated. If the network reaches an equilibrium state, then all subsequent updates simply maintain the equilibrium activation values—that is, have no effect.

1.1 Discrete-update and continuous-update networks

There are two ways that activation change is modeled in neural network theory: the discrete-update and the continuous-update modes. In **discrete-update** networks, time consists of a series of discrete instants—'ticks of the clock'—separated by a uniform interval Δt: $t = 0, \Delta t, 2\Delta t, 3\Delta t$, and so on. When a unit's state is updated at one instant t, its activation value instantaneously jumps to an activation level determined by the input it receives from neighboring units, which depends on their activation levels at the previous tick $t - \Delta t$. The new activation level after such an update is in general not close to the previous value. If such a network is interpreted as a model of a physical system (biological or electronic), then Δt must correspond to a sufficiently *long* interval of time: whatever the underlying physical process that actually effects the change of state modeled by activation updating, that process must have completed its response to input at time $t - \Delta t$ by time t.

By contrast, in **continuous-update** networks, activation values change smoothly in time. In such networks, time can be formalized as a continuum, the values of t ranging over an interval of the real numbers. This is often convenient for formal analysis. But for computer simulations—and sometimes for expository simplicity—the continuum is replaced by a series of 'clock ticks' $t = 0, \Delta t, 2\Delta t, \ldots$ where now, crucially, Δt is as *small* as necessary to guarantee that only very small changes in activation values will occur from one clock tick to the next. Networks of this sort will be called 'continuous-update' networks, even though the time continuum has been

[1] Some network models have 'input lines' that carry activation e_α to unit α. Such a network is equivalent to a network with input units instead of input lines; for each input line to a unit α, create a new input unit i_α, connected only to α, with a weight of 1, and assign i_α the activation value e_α.

modeled discretely. As we will see, the major analytic divide concerns not the discreteness of the variable t, but the nature of activation change: jumpy or smooth. These two models of activation spread require different modes of analysis, but the two variants of continuous-update networks—with real-valued t or a discrete approximation to it—can usually be analyzed together, with real-valued t being the case of infinitesimal Δt (sometimes written dt, a stand-in for the limit as $\Delta t \to 0$).

Activation update equations will typically be written in the following form:

(3) $\Delta a_\alpha = \Delta t \, F(a_\alpha, \iota_\alpha)$.

When unit α is updated, this equation specifies that it should change its activation value a_α by an amount Δa_α that equals the intertick interval Δt times some function F of its current value a_α and the input it is currently receiving from other units, ι_α. For a continuous-update system, Δt is some small constant, small enough to ensure that Δa_a is small. For a continuous-time system, (3) should be understood as stating

(4) $da_\alpha = dt \, F(a_\alpha, \iota_\alpha)$.

That is, the continuous-time interpretation of the update equation (3) is the differential equation

(5) $$\frac{da_\alpha}{dt} = F(a_\alpha, \iota_\alpha).$$

1.2 Feed-forward and symmetric connectivity architectures

In this chapter, the harmonic networks analyzed fall into two broad classes of network architecture defined by their pattern of connectivity: feed-forward nets and symmetric nets.

(6) Network architectures defined by restricted connectivity

a. A network is **symmetric** if all connections are two-way; that is, the weight on the connection *to* α *from* β, $W_{\alpha\beta}$, is equal to the weight of the reciprocal connection, *to* β *from* α, $W_{\beta\alpha}$:

$W_{\alpha\beta} = W_{\beta\alpha}$ for all units α, β.

b. A network is **feed-forward** if there are no closed loops of activation flow.[2]

Connectivity in symmetric networks is in a sense just the opposite of connectivity in feed-forward nets. A symmetric network contains a closed loop between every pair of (nonzero-)connected units: if activation flows to γ from α along a connection of (nonzero) strength $W_{\gamma\alpha}$, then activation flows back to α from γ along a connection of exactly equal (nonzero) strength $W_{\alpha\gamma} = W_{\gamma\alpha}$. In a feed-forward network, by contrast, if activation flows along a nonzero connection to γ from α, $W_{\gamma\alpha} \neq 0$, then activation cannot flow back to α from γ, so we must have $W_{\alpha\gamma} = 0$. (As a special case, when $\alpha = \gamma$, it follows that $W_{\gamma\gamma} = 0$: no self-connections are possible in a feed-forward network.)

[2] That is, there is no sequence of units $\alpha, \beta, \gamma, \ldots, \xi, \omega$ such that the following weights are all nonzero: $W_{\beta a}, W_{\gamma\beta}, \ldots, W_{\omega\xi}, W_{a\omega}$.

A feed-forward network can always be divided into **layers** of units. These layers will be numbered, from 0 for the input layer to some value L for the output layer. The layers are defined in such a way that activation flows from units in layer l to units in layers numbered higher than l, but not to layers numbered l or lower. It is helpful to visualize the input layer at the bottom of the network, with successively higher layers moving to the top of the network, where the output layer resides. Thus, activation flows vertically upward.

In the case of discrete-update networks, the feed-forward nets we study operate as follows. All unit activations are initially zero. At time $t = 0$, an activation pattern is imposed on the input units. Activation flows from the input units along one connection, arriving, at time $t = \Delta t$, at a set of units including those that form 'layer 1' of the network.[3] Upon receiving their input, the units in layer 1 adopt their activation values, jumping from activity 0 directly to their final activation values. Activation then flows from the now-active units in layer 1 to another set of units, including those making up layer 2, which then jump to their final activation values at time $t = 2\Delta t$. This continues until the output units, layer L, jump to their final values at $t = L\Delta t$. The activation values of the units in these networks may be discrete (e.g., 0 or 1) or continuous (e.g., in the interval of real numbers from 0 to 1).

In continuous-update feed-forward networks, the situation is the same, except that units continuously adjust their activation values by small changes, thus requiring an extended period of time to reach their final values.

In a symmetric network, there are no layers; activation circulates around the net for an unlimited period of time. In a discrete-update network, units jump from one value to another to another in response to the jumping inputs they receive as other units update their own activation values. A final equilibrium will result if the network reaches a state in which the activation of every unit is the one appropriate to the input it is receiving. In a continuous-update network, the same holds; the only difference is that units' activations move smoothly over time rather than jumping about.

By studying these two classes of (deterministic) network architecture—feed-forward and symmetric—and two different modes of activation spread—discrete- and continuous-update—we will sample several quite different places in the space of network architectures. Understanding Harmony maximization in these types of networks provides a good foundation; while Harmony maximization can be studied in other architectures as well, that work goes beyond the scope of this chapter.

The table in (7) depicts the portion of the space of deterministic neural network architectures that we explore in this chapter. The last column gives the number of the appropriate section.

Harmonic analysis of neural computation was developed by many people. Citations to original sources are provided when the relevant results are discussed.

[3] Layer 1 is the set of units receiving input *only* from layer 0, the input units; then, iteratively, layer n is the set of units receiving input only from units in layers less than n.

(7) Architectures analyzed in this chapter

	Activation values	Update mode	Connectivity	f	Example	Section
Quasi-linear nets	Discrete (Boolean)	Discrete	Symmetric	Linear threshold function	Hopfield net	3.1.1
			Feed-forward		Perceptron	3.1.2
	Continuous	Discrete	Feed-forward	Linear, no hiddens	Linear associator	3.2.2.2
				Logistic	Backprop net	3.2.2.4
		Continuous	Symmetric	sign( )	Brain-state-in-a-box	3.2.3.4
				Increasing	Additive nets	3.2.3.5
			Feed-forward	Linear	Cascade model	3.2.3.6

1.3 Harmony maximization in static and dynamic networks

In discrete-update feed-forward networks, units' final activations are determined in 'one shot': each unit is updated only once. Such networks will be called **static**. By contrast, in discrete-update symmetric networks, and in all continuous-update networks, units update their values repeatedly before achieving a final equilibrium state (if they ever do); these will be called **dynamic** nets.

Harmony maximization is conceptually rather different in static and dynamic networks. The dynamic case is most intuitive: the network's activation state is evolving over time, moving through its state space, 'seeking out', as it were, a point of rest, an equilibrium. In this context, Harmony maximization means that the Harmony value of the network state steadily increases during this 'search'. Prototypically (although not always), the final equilibrium state is a **local maximum** of Harmony; in that state, the Harmony would decrease if any single unit were to change its activation value (by a small amount, in the case of continuous activation values).

As activation propagates in a Harmony-maximizing dynamic network, Harmony will increase on some updates, but on others it will remain unchanged; what is assured is that Harmony will never decrease. This behavior will be described as follows:

(8) A function $F(x)$ is **monotonically weakly increasing** if F never decreases as x increases:

$$x > y \Rightarrow F(x) \geq F(y).$$

If the stronger inequality holds, namely,

$$x > y \Rightarrow F(x) > F(y),$$

then F is said to be **monotonically strictly increasing**.

In a static network, there is no 'search' for a final state: each unit, when updated, goes immediately to it. Yet the final activation pattern of the network maximizes Harmony—in a nondynamical sense. The final activation pattern of a static network is a local Harmony maximum if, as in the dynamical case, no single unit's activation value *could* be changed (by a small amount, in the continuous case) without lowering the network's Harmony. In the dynamical case, if in the final state **a** there *were* a change to a unit that would increase Harmony, then that unit *would* change its activation when updated, and the state **a** wouldn't have been a final state after all. The same cannot be said of a static network: the network has no dynamics that would move the state to higher Harmony if that were possible. It is the *analyst* rather than the *network* that examines the neighborhood of the final state **a** to discover that indeed no higher Harmony *could* have been achieved locally. In a commonly used metaphor, Harmony can be thought of as a landscape. In the dynamical case, the network explores this landscape, continually seeking higher ground: Harmony causally drives activation change (although this is achieved indirectly through the local activation equation of the network, which does not involve actually computing the global Harmony). But the Harmony landscape can also be thought of as a roadmap for the analyst rather than for the network, a roadmap that picks out the very special locations where the network can end up: the local maxima. And this conception is as valid for a static as for a dynamic network. In the dynamic case, the network slides up to the summit of Harmony Hill, pulled by a rope-tow; in the static case, the network is dropped by helicopter directly onto the peak.

1.4 Quasi-linear units

In this chapter, we will consider a large class of networks that embraces the architectures of many of the connectionist models that have been proposed in cognitive science. These networks all consist of **quasi-linear** units (Smolensky 1986b): their input is a linear combination of the activations of their neighbors.

(9) Quasi-linear and semilinear units

A connectionist unit α is a **quasi-linear unit with activation function** f iff its **equilibrium activation level** a_α^{eq} is related to the activation values of its neighbors by

$$a_\alpha^{eq} = f(\iota_\alpha) \quad \text{(i.e., } a_\alpha^{eq}(t) = f(\iota_\alpha(t))\text{)},$$

where ι_α is the **input** to α:

$$\iota_\alpha = \Sigma_\beta W_{\alpha\beta} a_\beta \quad \text{(i.e., } \iota_\alpha(t) = \Sigma_\beta W_{\alpha\beta} a_\beta(t - \Delta t)\text{)}.$$

If f is differentiable, the unit is called **semilinear** (Rumelhart, Hinton, and Williams 1986).

The time variable t is indicated explicitly in the rightmost equations in (9): the equilibrium activation level a_α^{eq} of a unit α at time t is determined by its input ι_α at that moment, and the input at time t is in turn determined by the activations of all the units at the previous time, $t - \Delta t$, where as always Δt is the time interval between updates of the units' states.

The phrase 'equilibrium activation level' in (9) allows the definition to apply to both discrete-update and continuous-update units. In the former case, the activation level of the quasi-linear unit jumps directly to the value $f(\iota_\alpha)$, immediately achieving its 'equilibrium activation value'. In the continuous case, in a single update, only a small activation change occurs. When a continuous unit α's actual activation value equals its equilibrium value, $a_\alpha = f(\iota_\alpha)$, then α does not change its activation. If a continuous-valued quasi-linear unit always moves toward its equilibrium value, we will call it *monotonic*.

(10) A continuously updated quasi-linear unit α is **monotonic** iff its activation equation obeys the following condition:[4]

$$\text{sign}[\Delta a_\alpha] = \text{sign}[f(\iota_\alpha) - a_\alpha].$$

That is, when the equilibrium activation value $a_\alpha^{eq}(t) = f(\iota_\alpha(t))$ exceeds the current activation $a_\alpha(t)$, that activation increases; when the equilibrium activation value $f(\iota_\alpha)$ is less than a_α, a_α decreases.

A simple but important type of static unit is the **linear unit**; in this case, the unit's activation value is a linear function of its input. Linear units are a special case of semilinear units (and therefore a special case of quasi-linear units); they have an activation function that is linear: $f^{lin}(\iota) = k\iota$. There is no loss of generality in taking the constant k to be unity (the effect of $k = 2$ is identical to the effect of $k = 1$ with weights twice as large).

(11) Linear activation function

$$f^{lin}(\iota) = \iota.$$

1.5 Thresholds and the bias unit B

It will simplify the mathematics to dispense with 'thresholds' of units via a standard trick of the trade. Intuitively, a threshold is a value that the input to a unit must exceed if the unit is to become active. This is modeled simply by taking the input to a unit α, $\iota_\alpha = \Sigma_\beta W_{\alpha\beta} a_\beta$, and subtracting the threshold θ_α. This difference $\iota_\alpha - \theta_\alpha$ is what determines the activation level, via the activation function f_α of the unit; the equilibrium activation level of α is thus

(12) $a_\alpha^{eq} = f_\alpha(\iota_\alpha - \theta_\alpha) = f_\alpha(\Sigma_\beta W_{\alpha\beta} a_\beta - \theta_\alpha)$.

Now the trick is to create a new **bias unit** B that always has unit activation level $a_B(t) \equiv 1$, for all t. Then we connect the bias unit B to unit α with a connection of strength $W_{\alpha B} \equiv -\theta_\alpha$. Now the input flowing into α from B is

(13) $W_{\alpha B} a_B = (-\theta_\alpha)(1) = -\theta_\alpha$.

So the bias unit is providing a constant input to α that the input from other units

[4] The value of sign(x) is +1 when $x > 0$, −1 when $x < 0$, and 0 when $x = 0$.

must exceed if the total (or net) input to α is to be positive; the bias unit does the work of the original threshold, which we now dispense with. Assuming now that α has a threshold of 0, its equilibrium activation with the bias unit B is

(14) $a_\alpha^{eq} = f_\alpha(\iota_\alpha) = f_\alpha(\Sigma_\beta W_{\alpha\beta} a_\beta) = f_\alpha(\Sigma_{\beta \neq B} W_{\alpha\beta} a_\beta + W_{\alpha B} a_B) = f_\alpha(\Sigma_{\beta \neq B} W_{\alpha\beta} a_\beta - \theta_\alpha)$.

Thus, a network containing units with thresholds can always be replaced by an equivalent network of units with no thresholds (i.e., thresholds of 0), as long as we allow the possibility of a unit B with constant activation value 1. In this chapter, then, we assume no thresholds on the units: the equilibrium activation value of unit α will be defined as in (9), with the understanding that one of the units β in this sum is a bias unit B.

2 Expansion of the Core Harmony Function

How do activation level changes affect Harmony? To determine the relation between activation changes of a particular unit γ and the corresponding changes in Harmony, we need to know the contribution of unit γ to the total Harmony of a network state. For the core Harmony, we compute this by expanding the double sum over all units α and β in (1b), separating out the terms in which α = γ and those in which β = γ.

(15) Contribution of unit γ to the core Harmony of network $\mathcal{N}$

$$H_0(\mathbf{a}) = \sum_{\alpha,\beta} a_\alpha W_{\alpha\beta} a_\beta$$

$$= a_\gamma W_{\gamma\gamma} a_\gamma + a_\gamma \left[\sum_{\beta \neq \gamma} W_{\gamma\beta} a_\beta \right] + \left[\sum_{\alpha \neq \gamma} a_\alpha W_{\alpha\gamma} \right] a_\gamma + \sum_{\alpha \neq \gamma, \beta \neq \gamma} a_\alpha W_{\alpha\beta} a_\beta$$

$$= H_\gamma^{self} + a_\gamma \left[\bar{\iota}_\gamma \right] + \left[\bar{\iota}_\gamma^{T} \right] a_\gamma + H_0^{\mathcal{N}-\gamma},$$

where

$H_\gamma^{self} \equiv a_\gamma W_{\gamma\gamma} a_\gamma$ – self-Harmony of γ,

$\bar{\iota}_\gamma \equiv \sum_{\beta \neq \gamma} W_{\gamma\beta} a_\beta$ – proper input to γ,

$\bar{\iota}_\gamma^{T} \equiv \sum_{\alpha \neq \gamma} a_\alpha W_{\alpha\gamma}$ – proper transpose input to γ,

$H_0^{\mathcal{N}-\gamma} \equiv \sum_{\alpha \neq \gamma, \beta \neq \gamma} a_\alpha W_{\alpha\beta} a_\beta$ – core Harmony of $\mathcal{N}$ without γ.

The total core Harmony consists of three terms that depend on the activation value of γ and a final term that does not: this last is the core Harmony of the rest of the network, that is, of the whole network $\mathcal{N}$ less the unit γ: $\mathcal{N}-\gamma$.

The three terms dependent on γ can be understood as follows. The first is the **self-Harmony**, which depends *only* on γ: it equals a_γ^2 times $W_{\gamma\gamma}$, the weight of the connection from γ to itself.

The second term is the key term: a_γ times ι_γ, the **proper input** to γ, that is, the input from all the units other than itself. This term, $a_\gamma \iota_\gamma$, will be called **the core Harmony at** γ.

The third term dependent upon γ is similar to the second: a_γ times a quantity that will be called ι_γ^T. The quantity ι_γ^T is the sum $\Sigma_{\alpha \neq \gamma} a_\alpha W_{\alpha\gamma}$, which can be thought of in two ways. First, it is the sum over units α of the product of a_α times $W_{\alpha\gamma}$—the strength of a connection *to* α *from* γ times the activation of the *receiving* unit, a_α. Thus, ι_γ^T is the input that γ *would* receive if all connections in the network were reversed (leaving weight values unchanged)—that is, it is the input γ would receive in the **transpose network** in which the weight matrix is $\mathbf{W}^T$, the transpose of the actual weight matrix $\mathbf{W}$ (in $\mathbf{W}^T$, each element $W_{\alpha\gamma}$ of $\mathbf{W}$ has been replaced by the element $W_{\gamma\alpha}$). Thus, ι_γ^T will be called the **transpose input** of γ.

There is a second way of conceiving of the third Harmony term,

$$\iota_\gamma^T a_\gamma \equiv [\Sigma_{\alpha \neq \gamma} a_\alpha W_{\alpha\gamma}] a_\gamma.$$

This term can be seen as *the contribution of* γ *to the Harmony of its neighbors*. To see this, consider one of γ's neighbors, α. The core Harmony at α is $a_\alpha \iota_\alpha$. Unit γ contributes to this Harmony via its contribution to ι_α, the input to α; to this it contributes $W_{\alpha\gamma} a_\gamma \equiv \iota_{\alpha \leftarrow \gamma}$, and thus it contributes $a_\alpha \iota_{\alpha \leftarrow \gamma}$ to the Harmony at α. This Harmony contribution is $a_\alpha \iota_{\alpha \leftarrow \gamma} = a_\alpha W_{\alpha\gamma} a_\gamma$. The sum of this quantity, over all units α other than γ, is exactly the third Harmony term, $\Sigma_{\alpha \neq \gamma} [a_\alpha W_{\alpha\gamma} a_\gamma] = \iota_\gamma^T a_\gamma$.

Thus, we can gloss the Harmony expansion (15) as follows:

(16) Contribution of unit γ to the core Harmony of network $\mathcal{N}$: Gloss

$H = H_0^{\text{self}} +$	[self-Harmony of γ] +
$a_\gamma \iota_\gamma +$	[Harmony at γ] +
$\iota_\gamma^T a_\gamma +$	[Harmony contributed by γ to its neighbors] +
$H_0^{\mathcal{N}-\gamma}$	[Harmony of the network excluding γ].

This expression provides a first glimpse of the crucial difficulty of maximizing Harmony via local activation propagation. The activation value of unit γ must be based exclusively on locally available information. Available at γ is the information needed to maximize self-Harmony and the Harmony at γ: the first two terms of H_0 pose no difficulty. For $H_0^{\text{self}} = W_{\gamma\gamma} a_\gamma^2$, and the Harmony at γ is $a_\gamma \iota_\gamma$, and all these quantities are locally available at γ: the weight from γ to itself ($W_{\gamma\gamma}$), its activation (a_γ), and the proper input it receives (ι_γ). The fourth term, $H_0^{\mathcal{N}-\gamma}$, is none of γ's concern: it will be up to other units to maximize this. The problem is the third term, $\iota_\gamma^T a_\gamma$, which has been boxed in (16): the Harmony that γ contributes to its neighbors requires information available only at the neighbors, and not at γ. This term is the sum over neighbors α of $a_\alpha W_{\alpha\gamma} a_\gamma$, which requires knowledge of the neighbor's activation value a_α. This problem does not arise for the Harmony at γ itself (the second term) because for that term, $\Sigma_{\alpha \neq \gamma} a_\gamma W_{\gamma\alpha} a_\alpha = a_\gamma \iota_\gamma$, what matters is not the neighbors' activations per se, but the quantity $\Sigma_{\alpha\neq\gamma} W_{\gamma\alpha} a_\gamma \equiv \bar{\iota}_\gamma$ – the proper input to γ, which is available locally at γ. To compute the problematic third term $\bar{\iota}_\gamma^T a_\gamma$, it would suffice for γ to have local access to the *transpose* input, $\bar{\iota}_\gamma^T$ – but this is a *hypothetical* input, the input γ *would* receive in the transpose network, were all connections to be reversed. It cannot play a causal role itself in determining the activation of γ.

It is to solve this problem that restrictions on connectivity are imposed. The special connectivity restrictions defining the feed-forward and the symmetric architectures each allow the problematic term $\bar{\iota}_\gamma^T a_\gamma$ – the contribution of γ to the Harmony of its neighbors – to be computed locally at γ. In the feed-forward case, the proper transpose input $\bar{\iota}_\gamma^T$ is zero, and in the symmetric case, it equals the actual proper input $\bar{\iota}_\gamma^T$. These claims will be established in the next section.

The expansion (15) has been discussed at some length because it figures centrally in virtually all of the analyses we now develop.

3 Deterministic Neural Networks as Dynamical Systems

In this section, we will examine Harmony maximization in deterministic networks. Networks composed of units with discrete or continuous activation values are analyzed in Sections 3.1 and 3.2, respectively. Section 3.3 summarizes the results, while Section 3.4 briefly describes extensions of the results.

3.1 Boolean networks

In the simplest networks, activation values are simply 1 and 0, encoding a Boolean active/inactive contrast. Since activations cannot vary continuously, these networks necessarily employ discrete updating.

For networks of Boolean units, Harmony computation is simplified. Let's consider a particular unit γ, and compute the two Harmony values arising from its two possible activation values, assuming that all other units' activation values are not changing. For γ active (i.e., $a_\gamma = 1$), (15) gives

(17) $$H_0(\mathbf{a})\big|_{a_\gamma=1} = H_\gamma^{\text{self}} + a_\gamma\left[\bar{\iota}_\gamma\right] + \left[\bar{\iota}_\gamma^T\right]a_\gamma + H_0^{\mathcal{N}-\gamma}$$
$$= W_{\gamma\gamma} + \bar{\iota}_\gamma \qquad + \bar{\iota}_\gamma^T \qquad + H_0^{\mathcal{N}-\gamma}.$$

For γ inactive (i.e., $a_\gamma = 0$), $H_\gamma^{\text{self}} = 0$, so we have simply

(18) $$H_0(\mathbf{a})\big|_{a_\gamma=0} = H_0^{\mathcal{N}-\gamma}.$$

Subtracting (18) from (17) yields the Harmony difference between the two possible states of γ:

(19) $$\Delta_\gamma H_0(\mathbf{a}) \equiv H_0(\mathbf{a})\big|_{a_\gamma=1} - H_0(\mathbf{a})\big|_{a_\gamma=0} = W_{\gamma\gamma} + \bar{\iota}_\gamma + \bar{\iota}_\gamma^T.$$

If this difference is positive, Harmony is maximized when γ is active; if the difference is negative, Harmony is maximized when γ is inactive. If the difference is exactly zero, either activity level can be adopted: in such an exceptional case, it will be assumed that the unit is inactive, which is regarded as the default value.

(20) Condition on activation rule: Boolean networks

To maximize Harmony, γ should be active if

$$\Delta_\gamma H_0(\mathbf{a}) = H_0(\mathbf{a})\big|_{a_\gamma=1} - H_0(\mathbf{a})\big|_{a_\gamma=0}$$

is positive; otherwise, it should be inactive.

Now, the activation level of γ must be determined by its input ι_γ, as in any neural network; but equation (19) has two terms on the right-hand side in addition to the proper net input: the self-Harmony term $W_{\gamma\gamma}$ and the proper transpose input $\bar{\iota}_\gamma^T$.

Consider first the self-Harmony term $W_{\gamma\gamma}$. This term can be eliminated by adding $W_{\gamma\gamma}$ to the bias weight $W_{\gamma B}$, increasing the proper input to γ by $W_{\gamma\gamma}$ (because the bias unit B always has activation value 1). Thus, as far as Harmony computation is concerned, there is no need for self-connections in a Boolean network. So let us suppose henceforth that our Boolean network contains no self-connections. Then there is no difference between the proper input to γ, $\bar{\iota}_\gamma$, and the total input, ι_γ. So equation (19) simplifies to

(21) $\Delta_\gamma H_0(\mathbf{a}) = \iota_\gamma + \iota_\gamma^T$ – if no self-connections.

Thus, the activation rule in (20) becomes (22):

(22) Condition on activation rule: Boolean networks, no self-connections

To maximize Harmony, γ should be active if

$$\Delta_\gamma H_0(\mathbf{a}) = \iota_\gamma + \iota_\gamma^T$$

is positive; otherwise, it should be inactive.

As explained in the previous section, the second term, $\bar{\iota}_\gamma$, is problematic, because in general it is not locally computable at γ, so γ's activation rule cannot refer to it. Thus, we examine two special architectures where this problem can be finessed: these constitute harmonic networks.

3.1.1 Symmetric networks

The first harmonic architecture is the symmetric network (Section 1.2). In the symmetric case, the transpose network is the same as the original network, since $W_{\alpha\gamma} = W_{\gamma\alpha}$ for all pairs of units (i.e., $\mathbf{W}^T = \mathbf{W}$). Thus, ι_γ^T, the transpose input to γ, is the same as the actual input to γ, ι_γ, and (21) simplifies to

(23) $\Delta_\gamma H_0(\mathbf{a}) = 2\iota_\gamma$ – if symmetric and no self-connections.

With the transpose input ι_γ^T eliminated, the activation rule for γ (22) can make reference only to its input: if the input is positive, it should be active; otherwise, it should be inactive. (The factor of 2 obviously has no effect on this rule. In the case of continuous-valued units, however, this factor of 2 must be taken into account.)

(24) Harmony-maximizing activation rule: Symmetric Boolean network, no self-connections

To maximize core Harmony, a unit γ should be active if and only if its net input ι_γ is positive.

Intuitively, the crucial role played by the assumption of symmetric weights is this: symmetry ensures that the (hypothetical) transpose input ι^T_γ to a unit γ equals the actual input to the unit, ι_γ, so the activation decision made using the actual input can never be contrary to the decision that would be made by consulting the transpose input, were it available. Alternatively expressed, symmetry ensures that the Harmony at γ equals the contribution of γ to the Harmony of its neighbors, so the activation decision based on ι_γ not only maximizes the Harmony at γ, it also maximizes the contribution γ makes to the Harmony of its neighbors.

Throughout this computation of Harmony in Boolean nets, we have asked what activation value γ should have to maximize Harmony, assuming that all other units' activation values are held constant. As we will see shortly (Section 3.1.4), this assumption is crucial. So to maximize Harmony in a symmetric network, the unit activation function must be specified as in (24), and units must change their activation values *one at a time*. This ensures that while γ computes the value that it should adopt to maximize Harmony, no other units change their activity. After γ applies its activation rule, its new activation value determines the input it sends to all other units, including the unit that updates its activation value next.

Examination of the logic shows that what is actually crucial is that two *connected* units must not be updated simultaneously. For if units γ and α are not connected (i.e., if $W_{\gamma\alpha} = W_{\alpha\gamma} = 0$), neither contributes to the Harmony of the other. Then, if α changes its activation while γ computes its Harmony-maximizing change, α's change cannot invalidate the computation of the Harmony at γ. Thus, the following definition is convenient:

(25) A network updates **asynchronously** if no two connected units α and γ ($W_{\alpha\gamma} \neq 0$ or $W_{\gamma\alpha} \neq 0$) are updated simultaneously.

What we have shown above is that in an asynchronously updated Boolean network with no self-connections obeying (24), updating a unit puts it into the state that gives the higher Harmony. If the unit was already in that state, then no activation change results and so no Harmony change results. If the unit was not already in that state, then it moves from the state of lower Harmony to the state of higher Harmony, and the Harmony increases. In the exceptional case where the two states of the network have equal Harmony, the unit adopts (or retains) the default inactive state, and no Harmony change occurs. Thus, while an activation change from 1 to 0 may occur with no Harmony difference resulting, a change from 0 to 1 necessarily brings an increase in Harmony.

Must the spreading activation process reach a final, unchanging, equilibrium state? It must, basically because each change of activation value causes Harmony to increase, and that cannot continue forever. This basic idea needs to be spelled out with a bit of care, however.

In a finite Boolean network, there are only a finite number of possible states, and thus only a finite number of possible Harmony values. This has two consequences. First, there must be a maximum possible value, M. Second, there must be a smallest nonzero difference in Harmony values, δ. Every time a unit changes its activation from 0 to 1, it increases Harmony—at least by δ, the minimum possible difference in Harmony values. Now, if activation changes continue forever, there must be an infinite number of changes of activation from 0 to 1; but since each of these changes increases Harmony by at least δ, this would mean Harmony would eventually grow beyond M, contradicting M's definition as the maximum possible Harmony value. Thus, it cannot be that activation changes forever: there must be a point in time after which no further changes occur. The network has **settled** into an equilibrium.

The equilibrium state must be a *local maximum* of core Harmony.

(26) **Maxima**

a. **Local** Harmony maximum: an activation state **a** such that no small change in the activation of a single unit would increase Harmony. (In the case of Boolean activations, the requirement that the change be small is waived.)

b. **Global** Harmony maximum: an activation state **a** such that no other activation state has higher Harmony.

Suppose there were a unit γ such that changing γ's activation would increase core Harmony. Then on its next update, γ would change its activation to increase Harmony, and by the definition of an equilibrium state, such changes never in fact occur. (It might be, however, that simultaneously changing multiple connected units in the network *would* increase Harmony beyond that of the equilibrium state: since the network updates asynchronously, such a large-scale simultaneous change could never actually occur. Thus, while the equilibrium state is a *local* Harmony maximum, it may not be a *global* Harmony maximum.)

We have now established the simplest case of Harmony maximization.

(27) *Theorem.* HMax: Boolean symmetric nets

Suppose $\mathcal{N}$ is a network with the following properties:

a. *Updating* is asynchronous (25).

b. *Connectivity* is symmetric, with no self-connections.

c. *Activation function:* Activation values are Boolean (0 or 1). A unit is active if and only if its input is positive (24).

Then, as activation spreads, the core Harmony of $\mathcal{N}$ monotonically weakly increases until $\mathcal{N}$ reaches an equilibrium state that is a local maximum of core Harmony.

This theorem was published in an extremely influential paper, Hopfield 1982. Networks with the architecture of this theorem are often called **Hopfield networks**.

3.1.2 Feed-forward networks

The other type of harmonic network we will examine here is the feed-forward architecture (Section 1.2). By definition, for any unit γ in layer l, input ι_γ comes exclusively from units in lower layers; activation flows upward. Thus, its transpose input ι_γ^T comes only from units in higher layers: in the transpose network, with all connections reversed, activation flows downward. This means that a version of Harmony maximization applies in feed-forward networks: *sequential* Harmony maximization.

(28) Sequential Harmony maximization in a feed-forward network

An activation pattern in a feed-forward network **sequentially maximizes Harmony** if the activation pattern at layer l is the one that maximizes Harmony given the activation values of units in lower layers only – with the activation of all units in higher layers set to zero.

This sense of maximization is quite natural for a feed-forward network. At time $t = 0$, an activation pattern is imposed on the input units, layer 0, and all other units have activation 0. At time $t = \Delta t$, an activation pattern arises on the units in layer 1; this pattern maximizes Harmony given the activation pattern on the input layer, and the activation in layers above 1, which is zero. Then at time $t = 2\Delta t$, an activation pattern arises on the units in layer 2, which maximizes Harmony given the activation already established in layers 0 and 1, and given the zero activation in layers higher than 2. And so on, until finally, at $t = L\Delta t$, an activation pattern arises on the layer-L output units that maximizes Harmony given the activation in all other layers.

Sequential Harmony maximization occurs because in this sequential feed-forward propagation of activation, when a unit γ determines its activation, the transpose input ι_γ^T is zero: this is the input γ would receive, given the current activation pattern in the network, if all the connections were reversed. This vanishes because the transpose input would come entirely from layers *higher* than l, but the activation in these layers is zero at the moment when γ's activation is determined. Since $\iota_\gamma^T = 0$, the activation rule for (sequentially) maximizing Harmony (22) becomes simply this:

(29) Harmony-maximizing activation rule: Feed-forward Boolean net

To maximize Harmony, a unit should be active if and only if its net input ι_γ is positive.

A form of feed-forward Boolean net architecture called the **perceptron** was the topic of a landmark book, Minsky and Papert 1969. This book's demonstration of the limitations of computation by perceptrons is often "credited" with turning the attention of artificial intelligence researchers in the 1970s and early 1980s away from neural networks.

3.1.3 Linear threshold units

The activation rule for both symmetric (24) and feed-forward (29) Boolean networks is the same:

(30) Harmony-maximizing activation function: Linear threshold unit

$$a_\alpha = \begin{cases} 1 & \text{if } \iota_\alpha > 0 \\ 0 & \text{otherwise} \end{cases}.$$

This is perhaps the simplest interesting neural network activation rule, and it defines the simplest type of unit: the **linear threshold unit**. (The 'threshold' here is fixed at 0 because of the introduction in Section 1.1 of the bias unit B to eliminate any nonzero thresholds.) If we define the threshold function

(31) Linear threshold function

$$f^{\mathrm{LTU}}(\iota) = \begin{cases} 1 & \text{if } \iota > 0 \\ 0 & \text{otherwise} \end{cases},$$

then the linear threshold unit activation rule can be written in the standard form for a quasi-linear unit (9): $a_\gamma = f^{\mathrm{LTU}}(\iota_\gamma)$.

The preceding analysis has established the following theorem:

(32) *Theorem.* HMax: Boolean networks

Suppose $\mathcal{N}$ is a network with the following properties:

a. *Updating* in $\mathcal{N}$ is asynchronous (in the feed-forward case, all the units in layer l are updated before those in higher layers).

b. *Connectivity* in $\mathcal{N}$ is either symmetric or feed-forward, and there are no self-connections.

c. *Activation function:* $\mathcal{N}$ consists of Boolean-valued linear threshold units, with activation function defined by (30).

Then, given any input pattern **i**, activation spread in $\mathcal{N}$ monotonically weakly increases core Harmony H_0, ultimately achieving an equilibrium activation pattern that maximizes H_0, among all those activation patterns that are completions of **i**. The type of maximum achieved is as follows:

i. If $\mathcal{N}$ is symmetric, the final activation pattern **a** is a local maximum of H_0 (26a).

ii. If $\mathcal{N}$ is feed-forward, the final activation pattern sequentially maximizes H_0, as defined in (28).

3.1.4 Asynchrony

In the Harmony maximization theorem (32), networks are required to update asynchronously. One might wonder whether a stronger analysis could demonstrate Harmony maximization without this restriction. But the extremely simple example in (33) shows this to be impossible.

(33) Oscillation in a symmetric network with synchronous updating

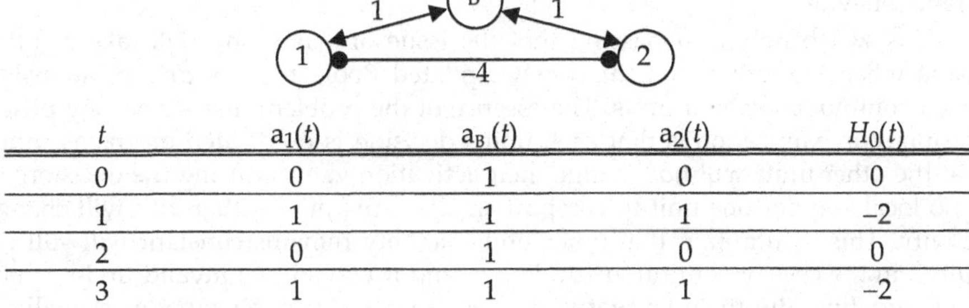

t	$a_1(t)$	$a_B(t)$	$a_2(t)$	$H_0(t)$
0	0	1	0	0
1	1	1	1	–2
2	0	1	0	0
3	1	1	1	–2

In the initial state ($t = 0$), the two units labeled 1 and 2 are inactive; the bias unit B is of course active, as always. The core Harmony is 0: every connection involves an inactive unit so all Harmony terms $a_\alpha W_{\alpha\beta} a_\beta$ vanish. But the input to unit 1, ι_1, is 1, which is positive, so according to the linear threshold unit activation function, after updating, unit 1 is active: $a_1(1) = 1$.

Now if updating were asynchronous, this would be the final state: Harmony would have increased to 1 ($= a_1 W_{1B} a_B$), and the input to unit 2 would be negative ($W_{2B} a_B + W_{21} a_1 = -3$), so it would remain inactive.

But with synchronous updating, unit 2 updates at the same time as unit 1, not after it. But 2's connections are identical to 1's, so its update will produce the same result: 2 will become active. Thus, after both 1 and 2 are synchronously updated, at $t = \Delta t$, all units are active. This represents a *decrease* in Harmony, from 0 to –2. The inhibitory connection between 1 and 2 encodes a constraint that these units should not both be active; this is violated in the state $\mathbf{a}(1)$, producing a Harmony cost of –4, the strength of this constraint. This negative cost exceeds the positive Harmony reward for satisfying the constraints between B and the other units: with positive weights, these connections encode constraints stating that both 1 and 2 should be active, because B is. But the summed benefit of these two satisfied constraints, both of strength 1, cannot overcome the –4 penalty from violation of the constraint between 1 and 2, so the resulting total Harmony is negative. (See Box 1:4 for interpretation of connections as constraints.)

The next synchronous update, at $t = 2\Delta t$, returns the network to its initial state: the inhibition units 1 and 2 receive from each other exceeds the excitation they receive from B. It is now clear that the network will oscillate forever between these two states, $\mathbf{a}(0) = (a_1(0), a_B(0), a_2(0)) = (0, 1, 0)$ and $\mathbf{a}(1) = (1, 1, 1)$. The Harmony value oscillates accordingly between $H_0(0) = 0$ and $H_0(1) = -2$. Harmony is not maximized, and the network does not converge to a final equilibrium state.

The oscillation of this network between two states entails that there is no way to modify the definition of Harmony so that the network will maximize Harmony under the new definition. Convergence to an equilibrium on the one hand and oscillation on the other are simply two quite different asymptotic behaviors for dynamical systems, and changing the mode of updating from asynchronous to synchronous changes the asymptotic behavior from Harmony maximization to a qualitatively different behavior.

It is worth noting in passing that the issue of synchrony will take a different shape when we move from discretely updated Boolean units to continuously updated continuous-valued units. The essence of the problem that synchrony poses for Harmony maximization is that each unit's decision is predicated on the assumption that the other units will not change their activation values during the decision; there is no local way for one unit to compute in advance how another unit will change its activity. This assumption that other units' activity remains constant will still be required in the case of continuous updating, and it will still be invalid under synchronous updating. But the quantitative degree of invalidity can be made as small as desired by ensuring that the continuous activations can only change by a small amount at each update. This will allow Harmony maximization to apply in the continuous case even under synchronous updating.

3.1.5 Asymmetry

It is useful to see how, when symmetry fails, Harmony maximization can fail also, even with asynchronous updating. A simple example is shown in (34), where W_{12} (–4) does not equal W_{21} (2).

(34) Oscillation with asymmetric connections

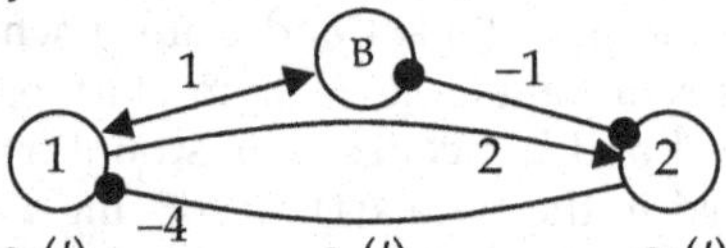

t	$a_1(t)$	$a_B(t)$	$a_2(t)$	$H_0(t)$
0	0	1	0	0
1	1	1	0	1
2	1	1	1	–2
3	0	1	1	–1
4	0	1	0	0

In the initial state, both unit 1 and unit 2 are inactive. The positive bias weight for 1 means that once it is updated, it will become active (the negative bias for 2 means that if updated from the initial state, it will simply remain inactive). Once unit 1 is active, it excites unit 2 more strongly than the bias unit inhibits it, so 2 will become active when it is updated. Now 2's inhibition of 1 is stronger than 1's positive bias, so 1 becomes inactive. Now that 1's excitation of 2 is gone, its negative bias is unchallenged, so 2 becomes inactive. After four updates, the network is back where it started. Clearly, the force for this oscillation comes from the asymmetry of connections between units 1 and 2: 1 *excites* 2, turning it on, then 2 *inhibits* 1, turning it off. As in the case of synchronous updating described above, this oscillation will continue forever, with Harmony cycling up and down.

3.2 Continuous-valued networks

While Boolean networks provide a simple context in which to understand Harmony maximization, for our purposes we need to go further. The entire approach to distributed representations presented in Chapter 5 depends upon the notion that two patterns of activation each representing an item are superimposed to form the representation of the set consisting of those two items together: this superposition operation is vector addition. The representational space of interest then is a vector space in which arbitrary additions are allowed. Thus, activation values cannot be Boolean; we've taken them to be real numbers. We therefore turn our attention to networks of units taking continuous values, more specifically, quasi-linear networks as defined in (9), where $a_\alpha = f_\alpha(\iota_\alpha)$. The activation function f will now be a real-valued function, rather than the Boolean-valued function f^{LTU} for linear threshold units.

3.2.1 The gradient of core Harmony

Thus, we return to the expansion (15) of the core Harmony function in terms of the contributions of a single unit γ, repeated here as (35):

(35) Contribution of γ to the core Harmony

$$\begin{aligned} H_0(\mathbf{a}) &= \sum_{\alpha,\beta} a_\alpha W_{\alpha\beta} a_\beta \\ &= a_\gamma W_{\gamma\gamma} a_\gamma + a_\gamma \left[\sum_{\beta\neq\gamma} W_{\gamma\beta} a_\beta \right] + \left[\sum_{\alpha\neq\gamma} a_\alpha W_{\alpha\gamma} \right] a_\gamma + \sum_{\alpha\neq\gamma,\beta\neq\gamma} a_\alpha W_{\alpha\beta} a_\beta \\ &= H_\gamma^{\mathrm{self}} + a_\gamma \left[\iota_\gamma \right] + \left[\iota_\gamma^{\mathrm{T}} \right] a_\gamma + H_0^{\mathcal{N}-\gamma}. \end{aligned}$$

For Boolean networks, we compared the value of H_0 for the two possible activation values of γ; now, with continuous activations, we evaluate the rate at which H_0 changes as a_γ changes its value continuously. This quantity—the partial derivative of H_0 with respect to a_γ, $\partial H_0 / \partial a_\gamma$—is computed in (37). It is sometimes convenient to collect all these partial derivatives into a vector, the **gradient** of H_0, written ∇H_0:

(36) $$\nabla H_0 \equiv \nabla H_0 \equiv \left(\frac{\partial H_0}{\partial a_1}, \frac{\partial H_0}{\partial a_2}, \frac{\partial H_0}{\partial a_3}, \ldots \right).$$

Computing the γth component of this vector from (35) gives

(37) Gradient of core Harmony

$$\begin{aligned}\frac{\partial}{\partial a_\gamma} H_0(\mathbf{a}) &= W_{\gamma\gamma}\frac{\partial}{\partial a_\gamma}{a_\gamma}^2 + \left(\frac{\partial}{\partial a_\gamma}a_\gamma\right)\left[\sum_{\beta\neq\gamma} W_{\gamma\beta}\, a_\beta\right] + \left[\sum_{\alpha\neq\gamma} a_\alpha\, W_{\alpha\gamma}\right]\left(\frac{\partial}{\partial a_\gamma}a_\gamma\right) \\ &\quad + \frac{\partial}{\partial a_\gamma}\sum_{\alpha\neq\gamma,\beta\neq\gamma} a_\alpha\, W_{\alpha\beta}\, a_\beta \\ &= W_{\gamma\gamma}\left(2a_\gamma\right) + (1)\left[\sum_{\beta\neq\gamma} W_{\gamma\beta}\, a_\beta\right] + \left[\sum_{\alpha\neq\gamma} a_\alpha\, W_{\alpha\gamma}\right](1) \\ &\quad + 0 \\ &= 2W_{\gamma\gamma}a_\gamma + \bar{\iota}_\gamma + \bar{\iota}_\gamma^{T}.\end{aligned}$$

This result is identical to its Boolean counterpart (19), except that the first term here is $2W_{\gamma\gamma}a_\gamma$, whereas its Boolean counterpart was simply $W_{\gamma\gamma}$. We can break $2W_{\gamma\gamma}a_\gamma$ into two equal terms ($W_{\gamma\gamma}a_\gamma + a_\gamma W_{\gamma\gamma}$), which, when added to the proper input terms ($\bar{\iota}_\gamma + \bar{\iota}_\gamma^{T}$), convert them to total inputs:

(38) Input and core Harmony change

$$\begin{aligned}\frac{\partial}{\partial a_\gamma} H_0(\mathbf{a}) &= \left(W_{\gamma\gamma}a_\gamma + \bar{\iota}_\gamma\right) + \left(a_\gamma W_{\gamma\gamma} + \bar{\iota}_\gamma^{T}\right) \\ &= \left[W_{\gamma\gamma}a_\gamma + \sum_{\beta\neq\gamma} W_{\gamma\beta}\, a_\beta\right] + \left[a_\gamma W_{\gamma\gamma} + \sum_{\alpha\neq\gamma} a_\alpha\, W_{\alpha\gamma}\right] \\ &= \sum_{\beta} W_{\gamma\beta}\, a_\beta + \sum_{\alpha} a_\alpha\, W_{\alpha\gamma} \\ &\equiv \iota_\gamma + \iota_\gamma^{T}.\end{aligned}$$

Since the self-connection term (involving $W_{\gamma\gamma}$) can here be reabsorbed into the input terms, Harmony maximization does not require a prohibition on self-connections, unlike the Boolean case. (And indeed negative self-connections are often used in continuous-valued networks to cause activation to decay to zero in the absence of input from other units.)

What (38) says is that as the activation of γ increases, the rate at which core Harmony changes is $\iota_\gamma^{T} + \iota_\gamma$: if this is positive, γ should become more active if Harmony is to be maximized; if $\iota_\gamma^{T} + \iota_\gamma$ is negative, γ should become less active.

All the remarks made about the implications of the transpose input ι_γ^{T} in the Boolean counterpart of (38) apply here. This purely hypothetical input cannot itself be directly involved in activation computation, so we specialize to the two cases discussed previously: feed-forward networks and symmetric networks. These connectivity restrictions have exactly the same consequences as in Boolean networks. In the feed-forward case, with respect to sequential Harmony maximization, the transpose input vanishes (i.e., $\iota_\gamma^{T} = 0$) because when updating γ, the units in higher layers have zero activation, and these are the units that would be sending γ input in the transpose network. And in the symmetric case, the transpose input equals the actual input (i.e., $\iota_\gamma^T = \iota_\gamma$), so the actual input can also do the work of the transpose input in determining the activation change that will increase Harmony. Thus:

(39) For both symmetric networks and feed-forward networks,

$$\frac{\partial}{\partial a_\gamma} H_0(\mathbf{a}) = c\,\iota_\gamma,$$

where c is a positive constant: $c = 2$ for symmetric networks, $c = 1$ for feed-forward networks. (In the feed-forward case, we assume here and henceforth that initial activations are zero and that all units in layer l are updated before those of higher layers.)

3.2.2 Discrete-update, static networks

As discussed in Section 1.1, continuous-valued units can be updated in two quite different ways. In the continuous-update mode, activation values are dynamic: they change by a small amount at each update, and it takes multiple updates for a unit to reach an equilibrium value, even if it is receiving constant input. In the discrete-update mode, units jump directly to the equilibrium activation value determined by their current input. The latter mode is often deployed in feed-forward architectures—for example, the prototypical 3-layer backprop net (Rumelhart, Hinton, and Williams 1986): activation passes from the input layer to the hidden layer, where units jump directly to the value given by their nonlinear activation function; activation then passes from the hidden layer to the output layer, where again the units jump directly to their final values. Such architectures are not dynamic, but static, in that units need be updated only once to achieve their final values. (Updating a unit a second time would have no effect in a feed-forward network.)

It is expositorily convenient to begin with this architecture: static, feed-forward, discrete-update networks. As discussed in Section 1.3, however, Harmony maximization in static networks needs to be understood somewhat differently than in dynamic networks: the network does not climb Harmony Hill, it leaps directly to Harmony Peak.

3.2.2.1 Unit Harmony

Among the limitations imposed upon activations in Boolean networks is a lower (0) and upper (1) limit on activities. In the analysis of Harmony maximization in continuous-valued networks, a problem arises from potentially unbounded activation values.

Suppose an activation pattern $\mathbf{a}$ has positive core Harmony $H_0(\mathbf{a})$. Then the same pattern with twice the magnitude, $\mathbf{a}' \equiv 2\mathbf{a}$, has even greater core Harmony:

(40) $H_0(\mathbf{a}') = \mathbf{a}'^T \mathbf{W} \mathbf{a}' = (2\mathbf{a})\,\mathbf{W}\,(2\mathbf{a}) = 4\,\mathbf{a}^T \mathbf{W}\,\mathbf{a} = 4\,H_0(\mathbf{a})$.

This shows that if the activation of units can grow without limit, there can be no maximum of core Harmony (except in the trivial case where the zero activation vector is a maximum).[5]

There are two general responses to this fact. The most obvious, and most popular, is to impose strict lower and upper limits on activation values. This approach will be developed in Section 3.2.2.3, but for now we simply note that imposing such limits prevents the activation space of the network from truly being a vector space, because the sum of two states, or the result of multiplying a state by a number, might not be a state because it would require activation values outside the limits. By contrast, the second response to the problem of unbounded activation values allows the state space to be a true vector space, with unrestricted activation values. This response is to modify the Harmony function so as to add to the core Harmony another term—**unit Harmony** H_1—that assigns a Harmony penalty to large activation values, rather than to declare them impossible by fiat. That is, the second approach is to impose a *soft* limit on activation in place of the *hard* limit adopted in the first approach. The total Harmony function H now becomes the sum of the core Harmony H_0 and the unit Harmony H_1.

3.2.2.2 Linear associators

For a first introduction to unit Harmony, we will examine the simplest and arguably purest case of a neural network: the linear associator (Section 5:2.1). Such a network has only an input layer and an output layer, is feed-forward, and consists of output units with the simple activation rule

(41) Linear activation equation

$$a_\gamma = \iota_\gamma = \sum_\beta W_{\gamma\beta} a_\beta .$$

In the weight matrix for a linear associator, $W_{\gamma\beta} = 0$ except when γ is an output unit and β is an input unit.

As pointed out above (11), this is the special case of a quasi-linear unit—$a_\gamma = f(\iota_\gamma)$—in which the activation function is the identity function:

(42) Linear activation function

$$f^{\text{lin}}(\iota) \equiv \iota.$$

If we partition the total activation vector $\mathbf{a}$ into its two subvectors, the input activation vector over the input units, $\mathbf{i}$, and the vector of output unit activations, $\mathbf{o}$ ($\mathbf{a} = \mathbf{i} + \mathbf{o}$), we can write the linear activation in matrix form:

(43) Linear associator

$$\mathbf{o} = \mathbf{W}\,\mathbf{i}.$$

[5] If $H(\mathbf{a}) > 0$, $\mathbf{a}$ cannot be a maximum, since $\mathbf{a}' \equiv 2\mathbf{a}$ has higher Harmony; so there can be no maximum as long as any pattern has positive Harmony. And if no pattern has positive Harmony, the Harmony maximum must be zero, achieved by the null activation vector $\mathbf{a}'' \equiv \mathbf{0}$.

The activation values of a linear unit can be arbitrarily large, which, as we have just seen, means there can be no interesting maximum of core Harmony: Harmony can be made larger and larger by increasing the magnitude of activations in any positive-Harmony pattern. The strategy under development in this section adds a second term to the core Harmony, a term H_1 that penalizes large vectors:

(44) Total Harmony

$$H = H_0 + H_1$$

(i.e., [total Harmony] = [core Harmony] + [unit Harmony]).

A simple way to define the length penalty H_1 is to assess a penalty proportional to the squared Euclidean length of the vector:

(45) Unit Harmony function, linear network

a. $$H_1^{\text{lin}}(\mathbf{a}) \equiv -\tfrac{1}{2}\|\mathbf{a}\|^2 \equiv -\tfrac{1}{2}\sum_{\gamma} \mathrm{a}_\gamma{}^2 = -\tfrac{1}{2}\left(\|\mathbf{i}\|^2 + \|\mathbf{o}\|^2\right);$$

b. $$H_1^{\text{lin}}(\mathbf{a}) = \sum_{\gamma} h^{\text{lin}}(\mathbf{a}_\gamma);$$

c. $$h^{\text{lin}}(a) \equiv -\tfrac{1}{2}a^2.$$

The length penalty H_1 is expressed in several equivalent forms in (45). In (45a), H_1 is defined as the square of the Euclidean length of the total activation vector **a**, times negative ½. The negative sign is what makes this term a *penalty*, and the factor of ½ will prove convenient below. The Euclidean length of **a** is the square root of the sum of the squares of the numbers a_γ; the *squared* Euclidean length conveniently eliminates the square root. The sum of squares defining the squared Euclidean length can be partitioned into two sums, over the input and output unit activations, respectively; this leads to an expression for H_1 as the sum of the squared lengths of the input and output vectors, times −½.

In (45b), H_1 is expressed in a form that will generalize to nonlinear networks: as the sum of terms, one for each unit. Thus, the crucial difference between the core Harmony H_0 and the unit Harmony H_1 is that H_1 consists of a sum of contributions from each unit independently, while H_0 consists of a sum of contribution from each *pair* of units (or equivalently, each connection). And the contribution of each individual unit γ to the unit Harmony—denoted $h_\gamma^{\text{lin}}(\mathrm{a}_\gamma)$ in (45b)—is a simply $\mathrm{a}_\gamma{}^2$, times −½ (45c). H_1 penalizes each unit individually, proportionally to the square of its activation level.

The intuition behind defining total Harmony to be the sum of H_0 and H_1 is rather simple. By itself, H_0 maximization corresponds to force in a preferred *direction* in activation space; and left to itself, the force would push the activation vector **a** in that direction indefinitely, to infinity. By itself, H_1 maximization corresponds to a force pushing **a** straight back toward zero, the origin. In fact, H_1 is defined so that this force is exactly that of an ideal spring pulling back to an equilibrium position at the origin. Maximization of the *sum* of these, $H_0 + H_1 \equiv H$, corresponds to setting up a conflict between these two forces, which determines an equilibrium point where they exactly balance. This is the activation vector that points in the direction favored by H_0, but with a length that is held in check by H_1; this length depends on the magnitude of the weights and the magnitude of the input vector, which together provide the force for H_0 maximization—the larger the weights or the input activations, the further from the origin is the equilibrium point where the spring's inward force pulling **a** to the origin exactly balances the outward force driven by H_0.

To locate this equilibrium point quantitatively, we must find the location of the maximum of H. At this point, the partial derivative of H with respect to each output activation value a_γ (= o_γ) must vanish (input activities are fixed). This is the point at which the derivative of H_0 (the outward force) is exactly equal and opposite to the derivative of H_1 (the inward force):

$$(46)\quad 0 = \frac{\partial H}{\partial a_\gamma} = \frac{\partial H_0}{\partial a_\gamma} + \frac{\partial H_1}{\partial a_\gamma} \quad \Rightarrow \quad \frac{\partial H_0}{\partial a_\gamma} = -\frac{\partial H_1}{\partial a_\gamma}.$$

For feed-forward nets like our linear associator, we have already computed the partial derivative of H_0 with respect to the activation of an output unit γ (39): it is simply ι_γ.

$$(47)\quad \frac{\partial H_0}{\partial o_\gamma} = \iota_\gamma = \sum_\beta W_{\gamma\beta} i_\beta .$$

This is the outward force. To express it as a vector, we employ the gradient, consisting of all the partial derivatives $\partial H_0 / \partial o_\gamma$: ∇H_0.

$$(48)\quad \nabla H_0 = \boldsymbol{\iota} = \mathbf{W}\,\mathbf{i} \qquad \text{— outward force.}$$

The inward force is easily computed (and the factor of ½ now does its work):

$$(49)\quad \frac{\partial}{\partial o_\gamma} H_1^{\text{lin}}(\mathbf{a}) = \frac{\partial}{\partial o_\gamma} \sum_\alpha h^{\text{lin}}(a_\alpha) = \frac{\partial}{\partial o_\gamma} h^{\text{lin}}(o_\gamma) = \frac{\partial}{\partial o_\gamma}(-\tfrac{1}{2} o_\gamma{}^2) = -o_\gamma .$$

In vector notation, it is evident that this force on **o** is indeed directed toward the origin:

$$(50)\quad \nabla H_1 = -\mathbf{o} \qquad \text{— inward force.}$$

Inserting (49) and (47) into (46) gives the condition for balance between the two forces:

$$(51)\quad \frac{\partial H_0}{\partial o_\gamma} = -\frac{\partial H_1}{\partial o_\gamma} \quad \Rightarrow \quad \iota_\gamma = o_\gamma .$$

In vector notation:

$$(52)\quad \nabla H_0 = -\nabla H_1 \quad \Rightarrow \quad \boldsymbol{\iota} = \mathbf{o}.$$

Thus, the point where **o** equals **ι** is a critical point of *H*: its first partial derivatives all vanish. To determine whether this critical point is a local maximum of *H*, we need to compute its second partial derivatives:

(53) $$\frac{\partial}{\partial o_\beta}\frac{\partial H}{\partial o_\gamma} = \frac{\partial}{\partial o_\beta}\frac{\partial H_0}{\partial o_\gamma} + \frac{\partial}{\partial o_\beta}\frac{\partial H_1}{\partial o_\gamma} = \frac{\partial}{\partial o_\beta}\iota_\gamma + \frac{\partial}{\partial o_\beta}(-o_\gamma).$$

The first term vanishes, as does the second unless $\beta = \gamma$, in which case it equals –1. The matrix of partial derivatives is thus –**1**, where **1** is the identity matrix. Because this matrix is negative definite, the *H* surface is everywhere concave downward;[6] our balance point **ι** = **o** is a local maximum of total Harmony. (In fact, in the case of the linear associator, the Harmony function is quadratic and has only one maximum, so the local maximum is also a global maximum.)

And of course **o** = **ι** is precisely the equation for the output of a linear associator (43). Thus, we have established the following result:

(54) *Theorem.* HMax: Linear associator

Among all activation states **a** that are completions of a given input **ι**, the output of a linear associator given input **ι** is the vector achieving the global maximum of total Harmony:

$$H \equiv H_0 + H_1^{\text{lin}} = \mathbf{a}^T \mathbf{W} \mathbf{a} - \tfrac{1}{2}\,\|\mathbf{a}\|^2.$$

Linear associators are of particular relevance to ICS, because parallel symbol-manipulating tensor networks like those discussed in Section 5:2 and Chapter 8 use linear associators to perform complex transformations of tensor product realizations of symbolic structures.

3.2.2.3 Harmony maximization in feed-forward quasi-linear networks

The analysis we have carried out for linear associators can be generalized to other nonlinear networks governed by the quasi-linear activation equation $a_\alpha^{eq} = f(\iota_\alpha)$ (9): specifically, to feed-forward networks in which the activation function *f* is invertible. This is normally the case in a continuous-valued network, where *f* is typically a monotonically increasing and therefore invertible function.

The inverse of *f*, f^{-1}, allows us to express the input in terms of the activation:

[6] For any function *H*, the first approximation to the *H*-surface is the plane with slope on the a_γ-axis equal to the first partial derivative $\partial H/\partial a_\gamma$. At a critical point, by definition, all these vanish, so the plane is horizontal: to first approximation, at a critical point, *H* is constant. To second approximation, the *H*-surface is a paraboloid. The intersection of the surface with a vertical plane through the critical point, with direction **Δa** in the horizontal **a**-plane, is a parabola $H = \kappa x^2$, where *x* is the distance from the critical point along **Δa** and κ is the curvature of the parabola. This curvature is $\kappa = \Delta\mathbf{a}^T \mathbf{J}\, \Delta\mathbf{a}$, where **J** is the Jacobian matrix consisting of all second derivatives $\partial^2 H/\partial a_\alpha \partial a_\gamma$. **J** is negative definite if $\mathbf{v}^T \mathbf{J} \mathbf{v} < 0$ for all nonzero vectors **v**; in this case, the curvature $\kappa < 0$ and the parabola is concave downward. Here, since **J** = –**1**, we have $\mathbf{v}^T \mathbf{J} \mathbf{v} = -\|\mathbf{v}\|^2 < 0$. Because **J** = –**1** *everywhere* for a linear associator, this parabola is not merely an approximation, it is the actual surface. A concave-downward paraboloid has one maximum. Indeed, it may be verified that $H = -\tfrac{1}{2}\|\mathbf{o} - \boldsymbol{\iota}\|^2 + \tfrac{1}{2}(\|\boldsymbol{\iota}\|^2 - \|\mathbf{i}\|^2)$, with fixed **i** and **ι**, has a unique global maximum at **o** = **ι**.

(55) Inverting the quasi-linear activation equation

$\iota_\gamma = f^{-1}(a_\gamma)$.

Here and henceforth, a_γ^{eq} is simply written a_γ, since the analysis here always concerns equilibrium activation values.

To demonstrate Harmony maximization, it is only necessary to generalize the expression for the unit Harmony H_1 so that it applies for all activation functions f, and not just f^{lin}. As before, the total Harmony will be a sum of the core Harmony and the unit Harmony: $H \equiv H_0 + H_1^f$, where H_1^f is the unit Harmony for units with activation function f.

A maximum of the total Harmony function H must be a critical point—a point where all its partial derivatives vanish. At such a point,

(56) $$0 = \frac{\partial H}{\partial a_\gamma} = \frac{\partial H_0}{\partial a_\gamma} + \frac{\partial H_1^f}{\partial a_\gamma} \quad \Rightarrow \quad \frac{\partial H_1^f}{\partial a_\gamma} = -\frac{\partial H_0}{\partial a_\gamma}.$$

Using the fact that $\partial H_0/\partial a_\gamma = c\,\iota_\gamma$ (39) for feed-forward networks, with $c = 1$, it follows that at a critical point of H,

(57) $$\frac{\partial H_1^f}{\partial a_\gamma} = -\frac{\partial H_0}{\partial a_\gamma} = -c\iota_\gamma.$$

We retain the constant c because the algebra here also applies to symmetric networks, with $c = 2$; these results will be used below in the analysis of continuous-update networks that are either feed-forward or symmetric.

As in the special case of the linear associator, so in the general case the unit Harmony H_1^f is a sum of contributions from each unit individually:

(58) $$H_1^f \equiv \sum_\beta h^f(a_\beta).$$

Inserting this into (57) yields

(59) $$-c\iota_\gamma = \frac{\partial H_1^f}{\partial a_\gamma} = \frac{\partial}{\partial a_\gamma}\sum_\beta h^f(a_\beta) = \frac{d}{da_\gamma} h^f(a_\gamma).$$

If this critical point is to satisfy the quasi-linear activation equation $a_\gamma = f(\iota_\gamma)$, then at this point we must have $\iota_\gamma = f^{-1}(a_\gamma)$ (55):

(60) $$\frac{dh^f}{da_\gamma} = -c\iota_\gamma = -cf^{-1}(a_\gamma).$$

This equation states that the derivative of h^f is $-cf^{-1}$; so to find h^f itself, we simply apply the inverse operation to differentiation—integration—to the quantity $-cf^{-1}$:

(61) $$h^f(a) = -c\int_{a0}^{a} f^{-1}(x)dx + C.$$

Here, a_0 is an arbitrary, fixed constant in the range of activation values output by f, and C is another constant. These simply determine a constant quantity that is added to the unit Harmony function: this quantity has no consequence for determining the activation vector that maximizes Harmony, as it affects the Harmony of all states equally. Thus, we drop C and let it be understood that a_0 can be chosen to be any convenient value.

(62) Unit activation function: Feed-forward ($c = 1$) or symmetric ($c = 2$)

$$h^f(a) = -c\int_{a_0}^{a} f^{-1}(x)dx.$$

As a useful check on this result, we can take the special case of a linear associator, where $c = 1$, and f is the identity function: $f^{\text{lin}}(\iota) \equiv \iota$ (11). The identity function is its own inverse—$f^{\text{lin}\,-1}(a) = a$—so the integral in (61) is

(63) $$h^{f^{\text{lin}}}(a) = -c\int_{a_0}^{a} f^{\text{lin}-1}(x)dx = -\int_{0}^{a} x\,dx = -\tfrac{1}{2}x^2$$

(where $a_0 = 0$ has been chosen for convenience). This agrees with our earlier analysis of the linear case (45c).

We have found a formal expression for the unit Harmony function h^f determined by an invertible function f. The total Harmony thus defined has a critical point at the activation pattern satisfying the activation equation of a quasi-linear network. To determine whether this is a maximum, we evaluate the second partial derivatives of H:

(64) $$\frac{\partial}{\partial \mathrm{a}_\alpha}\left(\frac{\partial}{\partial \mathrm{a}_\gamma}H\right) = \frac{\partial}{\partial \mathrm{a}_\alpha}\left(\frac{\partial H_0^f}{\partial \mathrm{a}_\gamma} + \frac{\partial H_1^f}{\partial \mathrm{a}_\gamma}\right) = \frac{\partial}{\partial \mathrm{a}_\alpha}\iota_\gamma + \frac{\partial}{\partial \mathrm{a}_\alpha}\left[\frac{\partial}{\partial \mathrm{a}_\gamma}\sum_\beta h^f(\mathrm{a}_\beta)\right]$$
$$= \frac{\partial}{\partial \mathrm{a}_\alpha}\sum_\beta \mathrm{W}_{\gamma\beta}\mathrm{a}_\beta + \frac{\partial}{\partial \mathrm{a}_\alpha}\left[\frac{d}{d\mathrm{a}_\gamma}h^f(\mathrm{a}_\gamma)\right]$$
$$= \mathrm{W}_{\gamma\alpha} + \frac{\partial}{\partial \mathrm{a}_\alpha}\left[-cf^{-1}(\mathrm{a}_\gamma)\right].$$

For sequential Harmony maximization, at any one time the units in one layer are updated: the pattern of activation in layer l maximizes Harmony among those overall network patterns in which the activity of levels lower than l is fixed to the pattern already computed for them, and the activity of units in layers higher than l is fixed at 0. So the relevant case is when the two units α and γ in equation (64) are both in layer l. In that case, $\mathrm{W}_{\alpha\gamma}$ vanishes, since the network is feed-forward and there are by definition no nonzero connections within a single layer. And the second term vanishes unless $\alpha = \gamma$. In that case,

(65) $$\frac{\partial}{\partial \mathrm{a}_\gamma}\left(\frac{\partial}{\partial \mathrm{a}_\gamma}H\right) = \frac{d}{d\mathrm{a}_\gamma}\left[-cf^{-1}(\mathrm{a}_\gamma)\right] = -c\Big/\frac{df}{d\iota_\gamma}.$$

If f is a strictly increasing function, its derivative $df/d\iota_\gamma$ is strictly positive, so the overall expression for $\partial^2 H/\partial a_\gamma \partial a_\gamma$ is negative. Thus, H is concave downward and the critical point is a local maximum.

(66) *Theorem.* HMax: Feed-forward quasi-linear networks

Suppose $\mathcal{N}$ is a network with the following properties:

a. *Updating* is discrete.

b. *Connectivity* is feed-forward.

c. *Activation equation*: The units are quasi-linear units, with activation function f.

Let the total Harmony be defined by

$$H = H_0 + H_1^f\,;\; H_1^f \equiv \sum_\beta h^f(a_\beta);\;\; h^f(a) \equiv -\int_{a_0}^{a} f^{-1}(x)dx.$$

Then the result of spreading activation in $\mathcal{N}$ sequentially maximizes the total Harmony, given the input.

3.2.2.4 Logistic sigmoid

As one example of the computation of the unit Harmony for a nonlinear unit, consider a nonlinear activation function commonly used in backprop nets, the logistic sigmoid:

(67) $$f^{\log}(\iota) \equiv \frac{1}{1-e^{-\iota}}.$$

Logistic units have activation values between 0 and 1.

First the inverse of f — $f^{\log\,-1}$ — must be computed:

$$a = f^{\log}(\iota) = 1/_{1+e^{-\iota}} \;\Rightarrow\; a^{-1} = 1 + e^{-\iota} \;\Rightarrow\; e^{-\iota} = a^{-1} - 1 = \frac{1-a}{a} \;\Rightarrow$$

$$\ln\left(\frac{1-a}{a}\right) = -\iota = -f^{\log\,-1}(a) \;\Rightarrow$$

(68) $$f^{\log\,-1}(a) = -\ln(1-a) + \ln(a).$$

The logistic unit Harmony function h is thus defined to be

(69) $$h^{f^{\log}}(a) = -\int_{a_0}^{a} f^{\log\,-1}(x)dx = -\int_{a_0}^{a} [-\ln(1-x) + \ln(x)]dx$$

$$= -\int_{1-a_0}^{1-a} \ln(y)dy - \int_{a_0}^{a} \ln(x)dx,$$

where a change of variables $y = 1-x$ has been used in the first term. Now the integral of the natural logarithm function, which we will denote F, is

(70) $$\int_b^c \ln(x)dx = [x\ln x - x]_b^c = F(c) - F(b);$$

$$F(x) \equiv x\ln x - x.$$

Substituting this into (69) yields

(71) $$h^{f^{\log}}(a) = -\int_{1-a_0}^{1-a} \ln(y)dy - \int_{a_0}^{a} \ln(x)dx$$
$$= -[F(1-a) - F(1-a_0)] - [F(a) - F(a_0)]$$
$$= -F(1-a) - F(a) + C,$$

where $C \equiv F(1 - a_0) + F(a_0)$. As discussed above, a constant such as C (which depends on the arbitrary choice of the constant a_0) can be discarded in the definition of a Harmony function. Then, evaluating F,

(72) $$h^{f^{\log}}(a) = -F(1-a) - F(a)$$
$$= -[(1-a)\ln(1-a) - (1-a)] - [a\ln a - a]$$
$$= -(1-a)\ln(1-a) - a\ln a + 1.$$

Finally, discarding the constant 1, we get an expression for the unit Harmony function for the logistic activation function:

(73) $$h^{f^{\log}}(a) = -(1-a)\ln(1-a) - a\ln a.$$

This function grows to infinity as the activation value a approaches either of its limits, 0 or 1. Thus, it provides a force pushing toward smaller activation values, a force that grows infinitely strong as the activation vector approaches the edge of the space of allowed states. This force exactly balances the force provided by core Harmony when the activation value of γ equals $1/(1+e^{-\iota_\gamma})$:

$$0 = \frac{\partial H}{\partial a_\gamma} = \frac{\partial H_0}{\partial a_\gamma} + \frac{\partial H_1^f}{\partial a_\gamma}$$
$$= \iota_\gamma + \frac{\partial}{\partial a_\gamma}\{-(1-a_\gamma)\ln(1-a_\gamma) - a_\gamma \ln a_\gamma\}$$
$$= \iota_\gamma + \{\ln(1-a_\gamma) - \ln a_\gamma\}$$
$$= \iota_\gamma + \ln\left(\frac{1}{a_\gamma} - 1\right)$$
$$\Leftrightarrow \quad \iota_\gamma = -\ln\left(\frac{1}{a_\gamma} - 1\right) \quad \Leftrightarrow \quad a_\gamma = \frac{1}{1+e^{-\iota_\gamma}}.$$

3.2.3 Continuous-update, dynamic networks

Turning to continuous-update quasi-linear networks, we will now see that much of the analysis of discrete-update networks is relevant. As discussed in Section 1.3, for continuous-update networks, Harmony maximization is a dynamical property: as activation spreads, Harmony never decreases.

3.2.3.1 Harmony dynamics

The basic characterization of dynamic Harmony maximization is that change in Harmony over time—that is, dH/dt, the rate of change of Harmony over time—is never negative. The quantity dH/dt depends upon the rates of change of H with respect to the activation values a_γ, $\partial H/\partial a_\gamma$, according to the basic equation of multivariate differential calculus:

(74) Chain rule for partial derivatives

$$\frac{dH}{dt} = \sum_\gamma \frac{\partial H}{\partial a_\gamma} \frac{da_\gamma}{dt}.$$

This time rate of change of H cannot be negative if none of the terms in this sum are negative. And that will be true if the activation change $\Delta a_\gamma = \Delta t\, da_\gamma/dt$ of each unit γ is in the same 'direction' (positive or negative) as the partial derivative $\partial H/\partial a_\gamma$:

(75) Harmony maximization condition on dynamics

$$\text{sign}(\Delta a_\gamma) = \text{sign}\left[\frac{\partial H}{\partial a_\gamma}\right].$$

That is, if $\partial H/\partial a_\gamma$ is positive, Δa_γ is positive; if $\partial H/\partial a_\gamma$ is negative, so is Δa_γ; if $\partial H/\partial a_\gamma$ is zero, neither type of change is implicated, and $\Delta a_\gamma = 0$. Then each term in the sum (74) is either (i) the product of two positive numbers, if $\partial H/\partial a_\gamma > 0$; (ii) the product of two negative numbers, if $\partial H/\partial a_\gamma < 0$; or (iii) 0 times 0, if $\partial H/\partial a_\gamma = 0$. In every case, the product is positive or zero.

The condition (75) is intuitively clear. If $\partial H/\partial a_\gamma$ is negative, then as a_γ increases, H decreases; so to increase H, a_γ must decrease. The reverse holds if $\partial H/\partial a_\gamma$ is positive.

One simple way to satisfy the condition (75) is to make Δa_γ proportional to $\partial H/\partial a_\gamma$ (with a positive constant of proportionality):

(76) Gradient ascent dynamics

$$\Delta a_\gamma = k\Delta t \frac{\partial H}{\partial a_\gamma} \qquad \text{(i.e., } \Delta\mathbf{a} = k\Delta t \nabla H \ (k > 0)).$$

This activation equation sets the change in the activation vector $\Delta\mathbf{a}$ proportional to the gradient ∇H. It causes the network to climb directly up Harmony Hill, in the direction of steepest ascent: the gradient.

In order to make the condition (75)—or the equation (76)—usable, we now need to compute the gradient of H.

3.2.3.2 Harmony gradient

The total Harmony H is defined exactly as in the static case (66):

(77) $H = H_0 + H_1^f$.

This implies

(78) $[\nabla H]_\gamma \equiv \frac{\partial H}{\partial a_\gamma} = \frac{\partial H_0}{\partial a_\gamma} + \frac{\partial H_1^f}{\partial a_\gamma}.$

Since the unit Harmony H_1^f is a sum of contributions from each unit individually,

(79) $H_1^f \equiv \sum_\beta h^f(a_\beta),$

we have

(80) $[\nabla H]_\gamma \equiv \frac{\partial H_0}{\partial a_\gamma} + \frac{\partial H_1^f}{\partial a_\gamma} = \frac{\partial H_0}{\partial a_\gamma} + \frac{\partial}{\partial a_\gamma}\sum_\beta h^f(a_\beta) = \frac{\partial H_0}{\partial a_\gamma} + \frac{\partial h^f(a_\gamma)}{\partial a_\gamma}.$

For the first term (the gradient of H_0), (39) states

(81) $\frac{\partial}{\partial a_\gamma} H_0(\mathbf{a}) = c\iota_\gamma$

in the special cases of feed-forward (c = 1) and symmetric (c = 2) networks. The second term of (80) (the gradient of H_1) is given in (60):

(82) $\frac{dh^f}{da_\gamma} = -cf^{-1}(a_\gamma).$

This was the differential equation that *defined* the unit Harmony function h^f for a unit with activation function f. The solution is (61),

(83) $h^f(a) = -c\int_{a_0}^{a} f^{-1}(x)dx,$

up to an arbitrary constant dependent on the choice of a_0.

Inserting (81) and (82) into (80) gives the gradient of total Harmony:

(84) $[\nabla H]_\gamma \equiv \frac{\partial H}{\partial a_\gamma} = \frac{\partial H_0}{\partial a_\gamma} + \frac{\partial h^f(a_\gamma)}{\partial a_\gamma} = c\iota_\gamma - cf^{-1}(a_\gamma).$

What this says is that Harmony will be increased by increasing the activation of a unit γ—a positive partial derivative: $\partial H/\partial a_\gamma \equiv [\nabla H]_\gamma > 0$—if the input to γ, ι_γ, exceeds $f^{-1}(a_\gamma)$, the level of input for which the current activation level a_γ would be the equilibrium value.

3.2.3.3 Harmony maximization in continuous-update networks

Inserting the expression for the Harmony gradient (84) into the condition for the Harmony-maximizing activation equation (75), we have

(85) $\text{sign}(\Delta a_\gamma) = \text{sign}\left(\frac{\partial H}{\partial a_\gamma}\right) = \text{sign}\left(\iota_\gamma - f^{-1}(a_\gamma)\right).$

Now the activation function f is virtually always monotonically increasing; let us assume this is true. This means that $a > b$ iff $f(a) > f(b)$. Thus, $\iota_\gamma > f^{-1}(a_\gamma)$ iff $f(\iota_\gamma) > f[f^{-1}(a_\gamma)] \equiv a_\gamma$. That is,

(86) $\text{sign}(\iota_\gamma - f^{-1}(a_\gamma)) = \text{sign}(f(\iota_\gamma) - a_\gamma)$ – f monotonically increasing.

So this means the Harmony-maximizing condition (85) can be written

(87) $\text{sign}(\Delta a_\gamma) = \text{sign}(f(\iota_\gamma) - a_\gamma)$.

This condition is exactly what defines a monotonic activation equation for a semilinear unit with activation function f (10). Thus, we have proved the following theorem:

(88) *Theorem.* HMax: Feed-forward and symmetric continuous-update nets
Suppose $\mathcal{N}$ is a network with the following properties:
a. *Updating* is continuous.
b. *Connectivity* is feed-forward or symmetric.
c. *Activation equation*: The units are monotonic quasi-linear units (10), with a monotonically increasing activation function f.
Let the total Harmony be defined by

$$H = H_0 + H_1^f;\ H_1^f \equiv \sum_\beta h^f(a_\beta);\ h^f(a) \equiv -c\int_{a0}^{a} f^{-1}(x)dx,$$

where $c \equiv 1$ if $\mathcal{N}$ is feed-forward and $c \equiv 2$ if $\mathcal{N}$ is symmetric.
Then the total Harmony monotonically weakly increases as activation propagates in $\mathcal{N}$.

There are many examples of network models proposed in the literature that fall under the purview of this theorem. The following three subsections illustrate two important examples.

3.2.3.4 Brain-state-in-a-box model

A historically important psychological model with continuous-valued units is the **brain-state-in-a-box (BSB) model** (Anderson et al. 1977). The state space for the BSB network is an n-dimensional 'box', within which the activations of all n units are restricted to the interval [–1, 1]. The equilibrium activation levels are defined by the sign function, f^{BSB}:

(89) $$f^{\text{BSB}}(\iota) \equiv \begin{cases} 1 & \text{if } \iota > 0 \\ -1 & \text{if } \iota < 0 \end{cases}.$$

The units are monotonic, so when positive input is received, activation increases; when negative input is received, activation decreases. (When $\iota = 0$, there is no activation change.) The activation change is given by

(90) Brain-state-in-a-box dynamics

$$a_\gamma + \Delta a_\gamma = \begin{cases} a_\gamma + k\Delta t\, \iota_\gamma & \text{if this result } r \text{ is in the interval } [-1,1] \\ 1 & \text{if } r > 1 \\ -1 & \text{if } r < -1 \end{cases}$$

That is, each unit changes its activation by a small amount proportional to its input, except when such a change would take the state outside the box; in that case, the activation value is limited to ±1.

The connections in a BSB network must be symmetric.

Golden (1986) showed that, away from the edges of the box, the BSB dynamics does gradient ascent in core Harmony. This can be seen from (39), which states that, for symmetric networks, the gradient of H_0 is proportional to $\boldsymbol{\iota}$; the dynamics (90) sets $\boldsymbol{\Delta a}$ proportional to $\boldsymbol{\iota}$ as well (interior to the box).

3.2.3.5 Additive nets

The most straightforward approach to Harmony maximization with nonlinear units is simply to employ symmetric connections and to achieve the Harmony maximization condition (87)

(91) $\text{sign}(\Delta a_\gamma) = \text{sign}\big(f(\iota_\gamma) - a_\gamma\big)$

by simply setting Δa_γ proportional to $f(\iota_\gamma) - a_\gamma$:

(92) $\Delta a_\gamma = k\Delta t\big[f(\iota_\gamma) - a_\gamma\big].$

This dynamical system is the **continuous Hopfield network** (Hopfield 1987). It is commonly written in another form that describes the network state in terms of the input variables $\{\iota_\gamma\}$ rather than the activation variables $\{a_\gamma\}$. To make this change of variables, we multiply equation (92) by $W_{\beta\gamma}$ and sum over γ:

(93) $$\sum_\gamma W_{\beta\gamma}\Delta a_\gamma = k\Delta t \sum_\gamma W_{\beta\gamma}\big[f(\iota_\gamma) - a_\gamma\big] = k\Delta t\left[\sum_\gamma W_{\beta\gamma} f(\iota_\gamma) - \sum_\gamma W_{\beta\gamma} a_\gamma\right].$$

Rewriting this in terms of the variables $\{\iota_\beta\}$ gives

(94) $$\Delta\iota_\beta = \Delta\left[\sum_\gamma W_{\beta\gamma} a_\gamma\right] = \sum_\gamma W_{\beta\gamma}\Delta a_\gamma = k\Delta t\left[\sum_\gamma W_{\beta\gamma} f(\iota_\gamma) - \iota_\beta\right].$$

This is the dynamics of an **additive net**. It is usually treated analytically, as a differential equation in continuous time; letting Δt become the infinitesimal quantity dt, we get

(95) Additive net dynamics

$$\frac{d\iota_\beta}{dt} = -k\iota_\beta + k\sum_\gamma W_{\beta\gamma} f(\iota_\gamma).$$

One of the earliest proofs that network dynamics optimize a function is due to the seminal paper Cohen and Grossberg 1983, which analyzed a class of systems of which these additive networks are a special case.

(96) Cohen-Grossberg Theorem

A network with the dynamics

$$\frac{d\iota_\beta}{dt} = A_\beta(\iota)\left[B_\beta(\iota) + \sum_\gamma W_{\beta\gamma} f_\gamma(\iota_\gamma)\right]$$

maximizes the function

$$H = 2\sum_\gamma \int_0^{\iota_\gamma} B_\gamma(\iota) f_\gamma{}'(\iota)d\iota + \sum_{\alpha\beta} a_\alpha W_{\alpha\beta} a_\beta,$$

where $a_\gamma \equiv f_\gamma(\iota_\gamma)$, provided **W** is symmetric, A_β is positive, and the derivatives of f_γ are positive.

The additive dynamics (95) is the case $B_\gamma(\iota) = -\iota_\gamma$; in this case, the more general expression for H given in (96) reduces to our earlier expression (88) (with $c = 2$) under a change of variables in the integral from $\iota = f^{-1}(a)$ to $a = f(\iota)$ (so $f'(\iota) = da/d\iota$):

(97) $$2\int_0^{\iota_\gamma} B(\iota) f'(\iota) d\iota = 2\int_0^{\iota_\gamma} (-\iota)\frac{da}{d\iota} d\iota = -2\int_{f(0)}^{a_\gamma} f^{-1}(a)da.$$

This result is one of a class of more general theorems concerning Harmony maximization in continuous-valued neural networks.[7] For an expository presentation of these results, and others concerning the analysis of neural networks as dynamical systems, see Hirsch 1996. In dynamical systems theory, the standard name for a function like Harmony that over time is monotonically weakly increasing (or decreasing) (8) is **Lyapunov function**.

3.2.3.6 Cascade model

An example of a feed-forward, continuous-valued harmonic network architecture is the **cascade model** (McClelland 1979), which played an important role in the transition from serial to parallel processing models of cognition. The dynamics is given by (92), where f is the identity function, leading to linear dynamics:

(98) $f^{\text{Cascade}}(\iota) \equiv \iota.$

McClelland 1979 provides an analytic solution for this dynamics.

[7] For further results concerning additive nets, see, for example, Wang and Zou 2002, Lu and Chen 2003, and the references therein.

3.3 Summary

Let us collect all the particular Harmony maximization results in Section 3: (27), (32), (54), (66), (88). The general result, which was stated less precisely in Section 6:1.2, applies to a diverse class of networks:

(99) *Definition.* Harmonic network architecture

A neural network $\mathcal{N}$ is **harmonic** if it possesses the following properties:

a. *Updating:* The units in $\mathcal{N}$ are updated either
  discretely and asynchronously (25), or
  continuously and synchronously (Section 1.1).

b. *Activation function:* The units in $\mathcal{N}$ are quasi-linear units with a monotonically increasing activation function f defining the equilibrium values of a unit α as in (9)to be

$$a_\alpha = f(\iota_\alpha) \qquad \text{(i.e., } a_\alpha(t) = f(\iota_\alpha(t))\text{)},$$

where ι_α is the input to the unit

$$\iota_\alpha = \Sigma_\beta W_{\alpha\beta}\, a_\beta \qquad \text{(i.e., } \iota_\alpha(t) = \Sigma_\beta W_{\alpha\beta}\, a_\beta(t-\Delta t)\text{)}.$$

If the units are discretely updated, they are assigned their equilibrium value directly. If the units are continuously updated, their dynamics are monotonic (10)—activation changes are directed toward the unit's current equilibrium value:

$$\text{sign}[\Delta a_\alpha] = \text{sign}[f(\iota_\alpha) - a_\alpha].$$

c. *Connectivity:* The connectivity of $\mathcal{N}$ is either
  i. feed-forward or
  ii. symmetric (Section 1.2). (In the discrete-update case, $\mathcal{N}$ must have no self-connections.)

Examples of harmonic network architectures include Hopfield networks (Section 3.1.1), perceptrons (3.1.2), linear associators (3.2.2.2), prototypical backprop nets (3.2.2.3), brain-state-in-a-box models (3.2.3.4), additive nets (3.2.3.5), and the cascade model (3.2.3.6).

The general statement of the HMax principle is then as follows:

(100) *Theorem.* HMax: General formulation

Let $\mathcal{N}$ be a harmonic network with activation function f. Define the total Harmony of an activation vector **a** to be the sum of the core Harmony $H_0(\mathbf{a})$ and the unit Harmony $H_1(\mathbf{a})$:

$$H(\mathbf{a}) \equiv H_0(\mathbf{a}) + H_1(\mathbf{a}) \equiv \Sigma_{\alpha\beta}\, a_\alpha W_{\alpha\beta}\, a_\beta + \Sigma_\alpha h^f(a_\alpha),$$

where the individual unit Harmony function is defined by (62),

$$h^f(a) = -c \int_{a_0}^{a} f^{-1}(x)dx,$$

with a_0 an arbitrary constant in the range of f.

Then $\mathcal{N}$ maximizes H, in a sense appropriate to its architecture:

a. If $\mathcal{N}$ is feed-forward, the final state is a sequential maximum: the activation pattern on each layer of $\mathcal{N}$ is a local maximum of H given the activation on all lower layers, and zero activation on all higher layers (28).

b. If $\mathcal{N}$ is dynamic (Section 1.3), H monotonically weakly increases as activation propagates.

3.4 Extensions: Beyond Harmony maximization

Convergence to an equilibrium while increasing a function is a restricted yet surprisingly powerful type of dynamics; Šíma and Orponen (2003) even establish that this dynamics possesses a type of computational universality. Yet such convergence is only one of several general types of behavior exhibited by dynamical systems (Skarda and Freeman 1987; Banerjee 2001; Hansel and Mato 2003). A central component of dynamical systems theory is the typology of long-term or asymptotic behaviors. These include not only convergence to an equilibrium (with or without optimization), but also periodic behavior (endlessly repeating a sequence of states) and chaotic wandering through subspaces of often highly intricate shapes. It is my hope that, in addition to Harmony maximization, other general principles characterizing typical global behavior of large classes of neural networks can be exploited in future work to further the development of the ICS cognitive architecture. For a tutorial presentation of dynamical systems theory, with applications to neural networks, see Hirsch 1996, which is summarized in Smolensky 1996b.

4 STOCHASTIC NEURAL NETWORKS AS PROBABILISTIC MENTAL MODELS

In Section 3, deterministic neural networks were analyzed as dynamical systems, and a large class of them—harmonic networks—were shown to respect the HMax principle, maximizing Harmony in different senses appropriate to their various architectures. The principle has greater applicability, however: it also extends to a number of important architectures of *stochastic* networks. First, we will discuss the utility of stochastic algorithms for computing Harmony maxima (Section 4.1). Then we will take a different direction, starting with the characterization of a general cognitive problem at a level higher than that of network algorithms. This problem is one of statistical inference; a general approach to its solution leads ultimately to a stochastic network implementation (Section 4.2).

4.1 Stochastic global Harmony maximization: Boltzmann networks

As we have seen, a deterministic harmonic network maximizes Harmony in a sense appropriate to its architecture. Feed-forward nets sequentially maximize Harmony; at each layer, a global Harmony maximum is achieved. Dynamic symmetric nets, however, monotonically weakly increase Harmony until reaching a stable point that may be a local Harmony maximum, but is not a global Harmony maximum in general.

In the seminal paper Kirkpatrick and Gelatt 1983, a technique for achieving global Harmony maximization by employing randomness was presented. The method is called **simulated annealing** because of its formal similarity to the process of gradually cooling a metal. In their landmark work, Hinton and Sejnowski (Hinton and Sejnowski 1983a, b, 1986; Ackley, Hinton, and Sejnowski 1985) applied simulated annealing to compute global Harmony maxima in symmetric neural networks, thereby creating the **Boltzmann machine**. Such machines are the topic of this section.

In a **stochastic** algorithm like simulated annealing, the steps of the algorithm determine not the exact values of variables, but the *probabilities* that variables will have various values. To analyze these algorithms, these probability distributions are computed over time. To simulate these algorithms on a traditional (deterministic) computer, the probability distributions are sampled: at each step in the simulation of an algorithm, the value of each variable is determined by computing its probability distribution and then 'randomly' selecting a specific value, the 'random' choice being characterized by the computed probability distribution. The 'random' selection is made with the help of a pseudo-random-number generator, a separate standard deterministic algorithm provided by the computer for generating a sequence of numbers with random-like behavior.

In the case of stochastic networks like the Boltzmann machine, the equations defining the network determine the probability that the activation level of each unit will adopt various possible values. The equations can also be thought of as defining the probability that the global state of the network—the entire activation *vector* **a**—will adopt various values, or equivalently, the probability that the state of the network will fall at various locations in the network's state space. The initial state of a Boltzmann network is 'highly random'; that is, the probability distribution will assign more or less equal probability to all the points in a large portion of the state space, this portion being dependent on the input. As the network processes the input, the distribution becomes more and more focused: more and more of the state space has essentially zero probability. Eventually, the distribution may be focused entirely on a single state, which is then the network's output. Alternatively, at the end of computation some randomness may still remain in the network state; then the output is a set of states, with their respective probabilities.

The probability that a Boltzmann machine will be in an activation state **a** is always governed by the **Boltzmann distribution**, named after the physicist Ludwig Boltzmann who proposed it as a description of the probabilities of microscopic physical states at some temperature T:

(101) $$pr(\mathbf{a}) = \frac{e^{H(\mathbf{a})/T}}{Z_T}.$$

Z_T is a number that normalizes the probability distribution so that the sum of the probabilities of all states is 1; it depends on T but not on **a**. (In the analogy with physics, H corresponds to the negative of energy, $-E$; Harmony maximization corresponds to energy minimization. Building on Hopfield's demonstration that symmetric asynchronous Boolean networks compute a local minimum of the function Hopfield called 'energy', Hinton and Sejnowski adopted this terminology and described Boltzmann machines as computing global energy minima. For consistency with the rest of the book, I will continue the terminology of Harmony maximization.)

In the Boltzmann probability distribution, the probability of a state is determined entirely by its Harmony: states with greater Harmony have greater probability. The relation is exponential, so that small Harmony differences can correspond to large probability differences. A convenient alternative formulation of the Boltzmann distribution is

$$(102)\quad \frac{pr(\mathbf{a}_1)}{pr(\mathbf{a}_2)} = \frac{e^{H(\mathbf{a}_1)/T}}{e^{H(\mathbf{a}_2)/T}} = e^{[H(\mathbf{a}_1)-H(\mathbf{a}_2)]/T} = e^{\Delta H/T}.$$

Thus, the *ratio* of the probabilities of two states is determined by the *difference* in their Harmonies, ΔH. This correspondence is regulated by the **temperature** parameter T: at extremely high temperature, all states have equal probability, because the Harmony differences between them are tiny compared to T, so $\Delta H/T$ is essentially zero and the ratio of probabilities of any two states is therefore $e^0 = 1$. At extremely low temperature, all states have essentially zero probability except the one (or ones) with highest Harmony; for if $\mathbf{a}_1$ is a maximum-Harmony state and $\mathbf{a}_2$ is a state with a lower Harmony value—lower by a Harmony difference ΔH —then state $\mathbf{a}_1$ is overwhelmingly more probable: the ratio of its probability to that of $\mathbf{a}_2$ is $e^{\Delta H/T}$, which is huge when T is much smaller than ΔH. The simulated annealing process involves gradually 'cooling' the network from high T to very low T; thus, the network moves from an initial condition in which all states are equally probable to one where only the state(s) of highest Harmony have nonzero probability. This is global Harmony maximization. That this result follows formally, if cooling is done sufficiently slowly, was shown in an extremely important paper by Geman and Geman 1984 (in their theorem, 'sufficiently slowly' is of course defined precisely).

Using the heat bath method of computational statistical physics, the formal basis of which was established in the seminal paper Metropolis et al. 1953 (see Smolensky 1986a, 277), it turns out that translating the Boltzmann distribution into a local rule for updating the activations of individual units is surprisingly easy—provided we consider the architecture that, in the deterministic case, Hopfield showed (locally) maximizes core Harmony: Boolean, asynchronous, symmetric nets with no self-connections. In this case, the core Harmony difference between the two possible states of a single unit γ, with all other activations fixed, is given in (23), repeated here:

$$(103)\quad \Delta_\gamma H_0(\mathbf{a}) = H_0(\mathbf{a})\big|_{a_\gamma=1} - H_0(\mathbf{a})\big|_{a_\gamma=0} = 2\iota_\gamma,$$

where ι_γ is the input to γ: as always, $\Sigma_\beta W_{\gamma\beta} a_\beta$ (9). Inserting this into (102) gives

$$(104)\quad \frac{pr(\mathbf{a}_1)}{pr(\mathbf{a}_0)} = e^{\Delta_\gamma H/T} = e^{2\iota_\gamma/T} = e^{\iota_\gamma/T'},$$

where $\mathbf{a}_1$ is the state of the network were γ made active ($a_\gamma = 1$) and $\mathbf{a}_0$ is the same state were γ inactive ($a_\gamma = 0$). Here, $T' \equiv T/2$ is a rescaling of the temperature parameter, which is of no consequence: the prime will now be dropped.

Equation (104) defines a **stochastic update rule** for γ: when γ is updated, a random decision is made in which the ratio of the probabilities of the two outcomes is $e^{\iota_\gamma/T}$. Since the probabilities of the two outcomes must sum to unity, (104) can readily be shown to entail

(105) $$pr(a_\gamma \text{ is active}) = \frac{1}{1+e^{-\iota_\gamma/T}} = f^{\log}(\iota_\gamma/T),$$

where $f^{\log}$ is the logistic sigmoid function defined in (67). Thus, if the input to γ is large and positive, the probability is very close to 1 that the unit will be active; if large and negative, inactive. And if the unit receives zero net input, it is equally likely to be active or inactive.

Putting all the preceding discussion together, we have the following result:

(106) *Theorem.* HMax: Boltzmann machines

Suppose $\mathcal{N}$ is a network with the following properties:

a. *Updating* is asynchronous.
b. *Connectivity* is symmetric, with no self-connections.
c. *Activation equation*: The units are Boolean, updating their values stochastically according the equation

$$pr(a_\gamma = 1) = f^{\log}(\iota_\gamma/T),$$

where $f^{\log}$ is the logistic sigmoid (67).

Then if T starts at a sufficiently high value and is lowered to zero sufficiently slowly, with probability 1 as $t \to \infty$ the state of $\mathcal{N}$ globally maximizes core Harmony (1b).

For a tutorial introduction to optimization computation by Boltzmann machines—and simulated annealing generally—see Aarts, Korst, and Zwietering 1996.

4.2 Modeling a stochastic environment: Harmonium networks

It is useful to adopt another perspective on stochastic networks, a perspective that motivated the approach to neural network analysis developed in Smolensky 1983, 1986a: Harmony Theory. Although Harmony Theory originally developed independently of the Boltzmann machine, very close formal connections will ultimately be established. The discussion here will be very brief and general.

Mapping input vectors to output vectors can be conceived as a case of the more general **completion problem.** The network is given a partial description of an input-output pair, the input portion; it is asked to complete this partial description by computing the missing bit, the output portion. More generally, networks can receive partial descriptions of what can often be construed as states of an external world; they are then asked to complete the description. Such completion might involve, for instance, determining the location of hidden edges of an object partially occluded by another object, or filling in events in a story that are not explicitly mentioned but important for comprehension. In general, it is not known in advance which parts of the description of the external world state will be given as input to the network. And in stochastic environments, completion can only be done probabilistically: the given partial description will in general determine not the exact values of the missing variables, but only their probabilities.

One approach to the problem is to have the network build, through experience with the environment, an internal (and highly incomplete) **model** of the environment, which it can use to internally simulate the environment. An accurate simulation is one in which the probability of an internal activation state **a** is the same as the probability of the external world state that it describes. Given such an internal model, a network can perform the completion task by simulation: with the input variables held fixed, the unknown variables stochastically adopt values that describe possible completions of the input. The frequency with which different completions occur provide the network's output: the network infers as most probable those completions that it most frequently adopts. Alternatively, such a network could output a single completion, the one that it infers to be most probable—what we will call the **maximum-likelihood completion**.

With this highly general starting point, Harmony Theory assumes that there is a measure *H* of the 'goodness' of internal states, with two properties: (i) the probability of a state **a** is entirely determined by its *H* value—the higher *H*(**a**), the more likely the state; and (ii) if a network consists of two disconnected subnets, the *H* value for a total state is the *sum* of the *H* values for states of the two subnets. From this it mathematically follows that the relation between *H*—Harmony, of course—and probability must be of the form

(107) $pr(\mathbf{a}) = k e^{H/T}$,

where *T* is an arbitrary positive constant and *k* the constant needed to normalize total probability to 1. (This result was generalized in Golden 1988.)

Next, Harmony Theory assumes that there is a set of 'observables' characterizing what information the network can 'observe' about the environment. Environmental states are internally represented as the activation values of a set of **representational feature** units; the vector of activation values for these units will be written **r**. An **observable** is a set of activation values for a subset of these units. For example, observing the aspects of the environment described by the states of three units {α, β, γ}, the network may encode the fact that (–1, 1, –1) occurs with high frequency, while (1, 1, 1) never occurs at all. It is convenient to characterize the first of these observables by a function $\chi_1(\mathbf{r})$ that gives the value of this observable in state **r**: $\chi_1(\mathbf{r}) = 1$ if, in state **r**, the units α, β, γ have values (–1, 1, –1) (in this case, we will say the observable 'occurs' in state **r**); otherwise, $\chi_1(\mathbf{r}) = 0$. The information encoded in the network is the frequency with which the observables occur in the environment. From such fragmentary knowledge, the network is to perform the completion task.

What probability should the network assign to the state **r** if what is known is only the probability of observables, each of which records the correlations among a small subset of the units? This is a typical kind of question addressed in the theory of statistical inference. One general answer is the **Principle of Minimum Information**: don't assume any information you don't have. That is, the network should infer the probability distribution that maximizes the *missing* information, among those distributions that are consistent with all information it has. Information theory provides a quantitative measure of missing information, or **entropy**. The information the network has is the probabilities of the observables in the environment. What distribution the network should infer is then formally determinate. When computed, the result turns out to be

(108) $pr(\mathbf{r}) = k\, e^{\sum_i \lambda_i \chi_i(\mathbf{r})}$

(Stuart Geman, personal communication, 1984). For each observable *i*, there is a coefficient λ_i that encodes (indirectly) the frequency with which the observable occurs in the environment; very roughly, a larger frequency of *i* means a larger value for λ_i. (This is a **log-linear** probability model, since $\ln(pr(\mathbf{r})) = \Sigma_i \lambda_i \chi_i(\mathbf{r}) + \ln(k)$.)

The probability distribution (108) gives the inferred probability for any completion of an input. A stochastic network could probabilistically adopt multiple completions with this probability, thereby simulating the environment as discussed above. Or, given an input, it could compute a maximum-likelihood completion.[8]

It turns out that maximum-likelihood completions can be computed simply in a network with a special **bipartite** structure. This architecture was dubbed **harmonium** after the important early parallel-processing model, pandemonium (Selfridge and Neisser 1960). A harmonium network has two layers, with symmetric connections between layers and no connections within layers (see Figure 1, which illustrates the observables χ_1, χ_2 above). The lower layer contains the representational feature units with activation vector **r**. The upper layer has one unit for each observable. Each of these units—called **knowledge atoms** in Smolensky 1986a—is connected so that the net input it receives from the lower layer (including bias) is positive exactly when the corresponding observable occurs in **r**. This entails that activating a knowledge atom will increase core Harmony—defined as always by (1b)—by becoming active if and only if the corresponding observable occurs. And when such a unit is on, Harmony is increased when units in **r** adopt the values of the observable, filling in missing representational features that are not provided in the input.

Intuitively, the states of maximum Harmony are thus those in which **r** consists of a combination of observables that have high frequency in the environment. Thus, these networks embody a kind of connectionist version of the **combinatorial strategy** described in Chapter 1 (3), a central component of symbolic cognitive theory. The activity pattern realizing a good (i.e., probable) image is thus a combination of the sub-

[8] See Goldwater and Johnson 2003 for processing and learning in a statistical version of Optimality Theory based on this maximum-entropy approach.

patterns that represent good objects; the pattern realizing a good (probable) syllable is thus a combination of the subpatterns that realize a good onset, a good nucleus, and a good coda (Chapter 13); the pattern realizing a good (probable) sentence is one that combines subpatterns representing good constituents.

Figure 1. Harmony Theory: A harmonium network

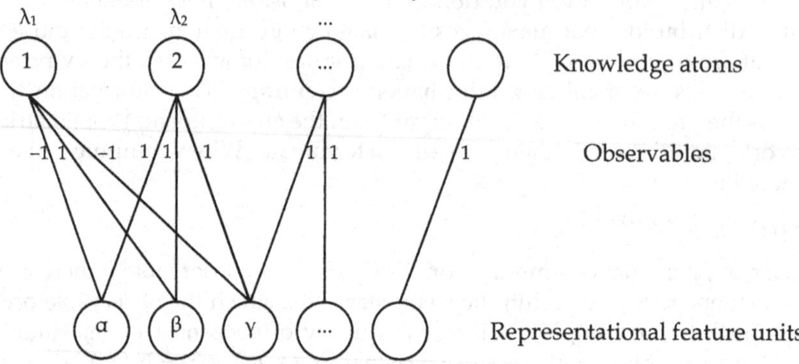

The bipartite structure of the network means that all units in one layer can update at once, and this will count as 'asynchronous' by the definition (25) as long as no unit in the other layer updates at the same time: for according to that definition, asynchronous updating requires that no two *connected* units update simultaneously, and the units in a single layer have no interconnections. Thus, the entire network, no matter how large, can be asynchronously updated in two time-steps.

The desired output is the maximum-likelihood completion of the input. But since probability is the exponential of Harmony, this is equivalent to computing the global Harmony maximum. Independently of the work of Hopfield, Kirkpatrick, and Hinton and Sejnowski, I proposed elsewhere (Smolensky 1983) to achieve this through heat-bath simulation with a T value that goes from an initial high to a final low value according to a 'cooling schedule'. The resulting stochastic activation equation is equivalent to that of the Boltzmann machine. The corresponding Harmony maximization theorem is given in (109).

(109) *Theorem.* HMax: Harmonium network (Harmony Theory)

Suppose $\mathcal{N}$ is a network with the following properties:

a. *Updating* is done one layer at a time, with all the units in one layer updating simultaneously.

b. *Connectivity* is symmetric and bipartite: there are two layers with symmetric connections between layers and no connections within a layer.

c. *Activation equation*: The units are Boolean, updating their values stochastically according the equation

Figure 1

$$pr(a_\gamma = 1) = f^{\log}(\iota_\gamma / T),$$

where $f^{\log}$ is the logistic sigmoid (67).

Then if T starts at a sufficiently high value and is lowered to zero sufficiently slowly, with probability 1 as $t \to \infty$ the state of $\mathcal{N}$ globally maximizes core Harmony (1b). For suitable choice of connection weights, the result is the maximum-likelihood completion with respect to the maximum-entropy distribution determined by a set of observables.

The connections between harmonium and Boltzmann networks are very strong. Harmonium can be seen as a more restricted Boltzmann architecture, with the requirement of bipartite connectivity imposed. Less obviously, but more instructively, Boltzmann machines can be seen as a special case of harmonium. In this special case, all the observables involve no more than two representational features: only first- and second-order statistics of the environment can be observed. These statistics are, respectively, the average values of the features individually and the correlation between any two features.

With this restriction, all units in the upper layer are connected to at most two units in the lower layer. The λ_i value of an upper-level unit connected to lower-level units α and β is directly proportional to the weight $W_{\alpha\beta}$ in the corresponding Boltzmann machine. These two networks can then be shown to compute the same output for any input.

Learning in the two systems is intimately related as well. Boltzmann machine learning was a revolutionary proposal, providing the first published method for training networks with hidden units (units that are never assigned values externally during training). The algorithm (which we will invoke in Chapter 21) has two phases, P^+ and P^-. In P^+, complete representations of environmental states (complete vectors **r**) are given to the network, drawn from the probability distribution characterizing the environment. The network processes each input for a period of time, cooling to $T = 1$ and then measuring how often every pair of connected units are active at the same time. After the network responds to a set of inputs, each weight is then increased in proportion to this measure of simultaneous activation: this is simple Hebbian learning. Then, in the second phase P^-, similar processing occurs, but no inputs are given. (This is often colorfully described as the "dream" or "sleep" phase.) Correlations are again measured. But at the end of P^-, each connection is *decreased* in proportion to the degree of simultaneous activation: *anti*-Hebbian learning. If the network's model of the environment is accurate (with respect to all second-order statistics), then a state will be "dreamed up" by the network in P^- just as often as it is presented by the environment in P^+, and the decrement to each weight in P^- will exactly cancel the increment in P^+: no net change will result, and the network will have found the desired weights. (To achieve such an equilibrium, the match between the model and the environment need not actually be perfect: only the first- and second-order statistics need match.)

This learning algorithm—like nearly all effective learning procedures—was explicitly designed as an optimization algorithm. The algorithm performs gradient descent in a measure of the **error** made by the network: an information-theoretic measure G of the difference between the probability distribution comprising the network's internal model and the actual probability distribution defining the external environment. For learning in harmonium networks, the two-phase procedure introduced by Hinton and Sejnowski for Boltzmann machine learning was adapted. The desired probabilistic model is the one that maximizes missing information F. It turns out that gradient descent in F moves the harmonium strength parameters λ_i along a trajectory that corresponds exactly to the way gradient descent in G moves the weight parameters in the Boltzmann network.

The harmonium learning procedure that results is straightforward. During P^+, environmental input is presented in the lower-layer activation vector **r**; in response, the upper-layer units corresponding to the observables present in the **r** become active. Each time an upper-layer unit becomes active, its strength is incremented slightly. During P^-, when no environmental input is present, the network generates its own values for **r**, and the corresponding upper-level units become active. Now, each time the unit is activated, its strength is *decremented*. Thus, the upper-level units act as memory traces for subpatterns observed in the environment, becoming stronger each time the subpattern is observed. The second phase holds the first in check, so that strengths do not grow beyond the point where the model best fits the environment. (See Freund and Haussler 1992 and Hinton 2002 for the computational advantages of the bipartite connectivity structure of harmonium networks for analysis of learning according to a new error measure.)

5 Conclusion

The chapter has attempted to convey the intuitive basis of Harmony maximization, and the wide range of network architectures that exhibit it. Of course, convergence to an equilibrium point, while monotonically weakly increasing some function, is certainly not the only behavior exhibited by networks, and the chapter attempted to shed light on which architectural features lead a network to be harmonic in this sense. The claim is that Harmony maximization is a robust enough property of a range of network architectures to recommend it as *one* higher-level characterization of neural computation on which principle-centered cognitive theories may be built (see Chapter 3). It is hoped that the analysis of other classes of activation dynamics can provide other principles like HMax that can be used to inform the theory of cognitive processing. It is further hoped that high-level principles governing *learning* dynamics can also be identified and used to build principle-centered, connectionist-grounded theories of human learning.

Figure 1

References

Aarts, E. H. L., J. H. M. Korst, and P. J. Zwietering. 1996. Deterministic and randomized local search. In *Mathematical perspectives on neural networks*, eds. P. Smolensky, M. C. Mozer, and D. E. Rumelhart. Erlbaum.

Ackley, D. H., G. E. Hinton, and T. J. Sejnowski. 1985. A learning algorithm for Boltzmann machines. *Cognitive Science* 9, 147–69.

Anderson, J. A., J. W. Silverstein, S. A. Ritz, and R. S. Jones. 1977. Distinctive features, categorical perception, and probability learning: Some applications of a neural model. *Psychological Review* 84, 413–51.

Banerjee, A. 2001. On the phase-space dynamics of systems of spiking neurons. II: Formal analysis. *Neural Computation* 13, 195–225.

Cohen, M. A., and S. Grossberg. 1983. Absolute stability of global pattern formation and parallel memory storage by competitive neural networks. *IEEE Transactions on Systems, Man, and Cybernetics* 13, 815–25.

Freund, Y., and D. Haussler. 1992. Unsupervised learning of distributions on binary vectors using two layer networks. In *Advances in neural information processing systems* 4, eds. J. E. Moody, S. J. Hanson, and R. P. Lippmann. Morgan Kaufmann.

Geman, S., and D. Geman. 1984. Stochastic relaxation, Gibbs distributions, and the Bayesian restoration of images. *IEEE Transactions on Pattern Analysis and Machine Intelligence* 6, 721–41.

Golden, R. M. 1986. The "brain-state-in-a-box" neural model is a gradient descent algorithm. *Mathematical Psychology* 30–31, 73–80.

Golden, R. M. 1988. A unified framework for connectionist systems. *Biological Cybernetics* 59, 109–20.

Golden, R. M. 1996. *Mathematical methods for neural network analysis and design*. MIT Press.

Goldwater, S., and M. Johnson. 2003. Learning OT constraint rankings using a maximum entropy model. In *Proceedings of the Stockholm Workshop on Variation within Optimality Theory*.

Hansel, D., and G. Mato. 2003. Asynchronous states and the emergence of synchrony in large networks of interacting excitatory and inhibitory neurons. *Neural Computation* 15, 1–56.

Hinton, G. E. 2002. Training products of experts by minimizing contrastive divergence. *Neural Computation* 14, 1771–800.

Hinton, G. E., and T. J. Sejnowski. 1983a. Analyzing cooperative computation. In *Proceedings of the Cognitive Science Society 5*.

Hinton, G. E., and T. J. Sejnowski. 1983b. Optimal perceptual inference. In *Proceedings of the IEEE Computer Society Conference on Computer Vision and Pattern Recognition*.

Hinton, G. E., and T. J. Sejnowski. 1986. Learning and relearning in Boltzmann machines. In *Parallel distributed processing: Explorations in the microstructure of cognition*. Vol. 1, *Foundations*, D. E. Rumelhart, J. L. McClelland, and the PDP Research Group. MIT Press.

Hinton, G. E., and T. J. Sejnowski, eds. 1999. *Unsupervised learning*. MIT Press.

Hirsch, M. W. 1996. Dynamical systems. In *Mathematical perspectives on neural networks*, eds. P. Smolensky, M. C. Mozer, and D. E. Rumelhart. Erlbaum.

Hopfield, J. J. 1982. Neural networks and physical systems with emergent collective computational abilities. *Proceedings of the National Academy of Sciences USA* 79, 2554–8.

Hopfield, J. J. 1984. Neurons with graded response have collective computational properties like those of two-state neurons. *Proceedings of the National Academy of Sciences USA* 81, 3088–92.

Kirkpatrick, S., and C. D. Gelatt, Jr. 1983. Optimization by simulated annealing. *Science* 220, 671–80.

Lu, W., and T. Chen. 2003. New conditions on global stability of Cohen-Grossberg neural networks. *Neural Computation* 15, 1173–89.

McClelland, J. L. 1979. On the time-relations of mental processes: An examination of systems of processes in cascade. *Psychological Review* 86, 287–330.

Metropolis, M., A. Rosenbluth, M. Rosenbluth, A. Teller, and E. Teller. 1953. Equations of state calculations by fast computing machines. *Journal of Chemical Physics* 21, 1087–92.

Minsky, M., and S. Papert. 1969. *Perceptrons*. MIT Press.

Rumelhart, D. E., G. E. Hinton, and R. J. Williams. 1986. Learning internal representations by error propagation. In *Parallel distributed processing: Explorations in the microstructure of cognition*. Vol. 1, *Foundations*, D. E. Rumelhart, J. L. McClelland, and the PDP Research Group. MIT Press.

Selfridge, O. G., and U. Neisser. 1960. Pattern recognition by machine. *Scientific American* 203, 60–8.

Šíma, J., and P. Orponen. 2003. Continuous-time symmetric Hopfield nets are computationally universal. *Neural Computation* 15, 693–733.

Skarda, C. A., and W. J. Freeman. 1987. How brains make chaos to make sense of the world. *Behavioral and Brain Sciences* 10, 161–95.

Smolensky, P. 1983. Schema selection and stochastic inference in modular environments. In *Proceedings of the National Conference on Artificial Intelligence 3*.

Smolensky, P. 1986a. Information processing in dynamical systems: Foundations of Harmony Theory. In *Parallel distributed processing: Explorations in the microstructure of cognition*. Vol. 1, *Foundations*, D. E. Rumelhart, J. L. McClelland, and the PDP Research Group. MIT Press.

Smolensky, P. 1986b. Neural and conceptual interpretations of parallel distributed processing models. In *Parallel distributed processing: Explorations in the microstructure of cognition*. Vol. 2, *Psychological and biological models*, J. L. McClelland, D. E. Rumelhart, and the PDP Research Group. MIT Press.

Smolensky, P. 1996a. Computational, dynamical, and statistical perspectives on the processing and learning problems in neural network theory. In *Mathematical perspectives on neural networks*, eds. P. Smolensky, M. C. Mozer, and D. E. Rumelhart. Erlbaum.

Smolensky, P. 1996b. Dynamical perspectives on neural networks. In *Mathematical perspectives on neural networks*, eds. P. Smolensky, M. C. Mozer, and D. E. Rumelhart. Erlbaum.

Smolensky, P. 1996c. Statistical perspectives on neural networks. In *Mathematical perspectives on neural networks*, eds. P. Smolensky, M. C. Mozer, and D. E. Rumelhart. Erlbaum.

Wang, L., and X. Zou. 2002. Exponential stability of Cohen-Grossberg neural networks. *Neural Networks*, 415–22.

10

Harmonic Grammars and Harmonic Parsers for Formal Languages

John Hale and Paul Smolensky

Harmonic Grammar (HG) is a connectionist-based grammar formalism central to the Integrated Connectionist/Symbolic Cognitive Architecture (ICS). The expressive power of HG is evaluated here by comparison with symbolic rewrite-rule grammars. HG is shown to possess a kind of Turing machine equivalence: its descriptive power is shown to be equivalent, in an appropriate sense, to that of the most complex symbolic grammars in the Chomsky hierarchy—despite its restriction to elementary second-order constraints with simple additive interaction. A parser for context-free languages, realized in a local connectionist network, is constructed, exploiting HG representations of these languages. This work provides part of the bridge between symbolic grammars and connectionist networks: see ⑤ of Figure 5, and (27c), in the ICS map of Chapter 2.

Sections 1 and 2 are revised and expanded versions of Smolensky 1993 and Hale and Smolensky 2001, respectively.

Contents

1 CONTEXT-FREE HARMONIC GRAMMARS

The principles defining the Integrated Connectionist/Symbolic Cognitive Architecture (ICS) characterize the mental representations subserving language processing as activation patterns possessing tensor product structure, and characterize grammatical knowledge as connection weight matrices possessing corresponding tensor product structure (Chapters 2, 5, 7, 8). These principles yield **Harmonic Grammar (HG)** as a higher-level description of this knowledge (Chapters 2 and 6).

Are these connectionist systems actually adequate for subserving the power of symbolic computation? One way to approach this question is to ask what class of languages HG has the expressive power to specify. With 'language' construed as **formal language** (Box 6:1), this is a classic means within computer science of evaluating the power of a computational formalism.

Can any, say, context-free language $\mathcal{L}$ be specified by a harmonic grammar? The specifications defining harmonic grammars are highly restricted: they are **soft rules** of the form in (1) (Section 6:2)

(1) R_{ij}: If s simultaneously contains the constituents $\mathbf{c}_i$ and $\mathbf{c}_j$, then add the numerical quantity $H(\mathbf{c}_i, \mathbf{c}_j)$ to H.

or, equivalently, **soft constraints** of the form in (2)

(2) C_{ij}: s must/must *not* simultaneously contain the constituents $\mathbf{c}_i$ and $\mathbf{c}_j$ (strength: w_{ij}).

(with 'must' if $H(\mathbf{c}_i, \mathbf{c}_j) > 0$, 'must not' if $H(\mathbf{c}_i, \mathbf{c}_j) < 0$, and $w_{ij} \equiv |H(\mathbf{c}_i, \mathbf{c}_j)|$). Can a set of such simple soft constraints be specified so that a string $\mathbf{s} \in \mathcal{L}$ if and only if the maximum-Harmony tree with $\mathbf{s}$ as terminals has, say, nonnegative Harmony: $H(\mathbf{s}) \geq 0$?[1]

A crucial limitation of these soft constraints is that each may refer only to a *pair* of constituents: in this sense, they are only **second order**. (It simplifies the exposition to describe as 'pairs' cases in which both constituents are the same, $\mathbf{c}_i = \mathbf{c}_j$; these actually correspond to first-order soft rules, which also exist in HG.) As pointed out in Section 6:2.2, the limitation to second order arises because soft constraints are realized in connection weights of networks in which connections link only two units. But do second-order interactions suffice for specifying context-free languages?

For a context-free language (**CFL**), a tree is well formed if and only if all of its **local trees** are—where a local tree is just some node and all its children. Thus, the HG rules need only refer to pairs of nodes that fall in a single local tree, that is, par-

[1] This gives an HG definition in terms of the *absolute* value of the Harmony of a parse that is optimal in *comprehension-directed optimization*, where the terminal string is fixed and the parse tree of its derivation needs to be determined. This may seem inconsistent with the Optimality Theory definition of grammaticality in terms of *production-directed* optimization with respect to *relative* Harmony: surface structures (here, parsed terminal strings) compete as means of expressing a fixed interpretation (here, the start symbol; see Chapter 12). Actually, the two definitions are mutually compatible; see Section 20:1.4.

ent-child pairs and/or sibling pairs. The H value of the entire tree is just the sum of all the numbers for each such pair of nodes given by the soft rules defining the harmonic grammar.

It is clear that for a general **context-free grammar (CFG)**, pairwise evaluation doesn't suffice. For example, consider the CFG fragment $\mathcal{G}_1 \equiv \{\mathbf{A} \to \mathbf{B}\ \mathbf{C},\ \mathbf{A} \to \mathbf{D}\ \mathbf{E},\ \mathbf{F} \to \mathbf{B}\ \mathbf{E}\}$ and the ill-formed local tree $[_{\mathbf{A}}\ \mathbf{B}\ \mathbf{E}]$ (here, **A** is the parent, **B** and **E** the two children). Pairwise well-formedness checks fail to detect the ill-formedness, since the first rule says **B** can be a left child of **A**, the second that **E** can be a right child of **A**, and the third that **B** can be a left sibling of **E**. The ill-formedness can be detected only by examining *all three* nodes simultaneously, and seeing that this triple as a whole is not licensed by any single rule.

One possible approach would be to extend HG to rules higher than second order, involving more than two constituents; this corresponds to H functions of degree higher than 2. Such H functions go beyond standard connectionist networks with pairwise connectivity, requiring networks defined over hypergraphs rather than ordinary graphs. There is a natural alternative, however, that requires no change at all in HG, but instead adopts a special kind of grammar for the CFL. The basic trick is a modification of an idea taken from Generalized Phrase Structure Grammar (Gazdar et al. 1985), a theory that adapts CFGs to the study of natural languages.

It is useful to introduce a new normal form for CFGs, **harmonic normal form (HNF)**. In HNF, all rules are one of three types: **A[i]** → **B C**, **A** → **a**, **A** → **A[i]**. Moreover, the **Unique Branching Condition** holds: there can be only one branching rule with a given left-hand side.[2] Here, lowercase letters denote terminal symbols, and there are two sorts of nonterminals: general symbols like **A** and **subcategorized** symbols like **A[1]**, **A[2]**, …, **A[i]**, …, **A[n]**. To see that every CFL $\mathcal{L}$ indeed has an HNF grammar, it suffices to first take a CFG for $\mathcal{L}$ in **Chomsky normal form (CNF)**[3] and, for each (necessarily binary) branching rule **A** → **B C**, (i) replace the symbol **A** on the left-hand side with **A[i]**, using a different value of **i** for each branching rule with a given left-hand side, and (ii) add the rule **A** → **A[i]**. (A unary-branching node will be taken to have only a left child.)

Subcategorizing the general category **A**, which may have several legal branching expansions, into the specialized subcategories **A[i]**, each of which has only one legal branching expansion, makes it possible to determine the well-formedness of an entire tree simply by examining each parent-child pair separately: an entire tree is well formed if and only if every parent-child pair is. To see the import of the Unique Branching Condition, reconsider the grammar fragment $\mathcal{G}_1$ defined above. This violates the condition because **A** has two branching rules; **A** needs to be subcategorized into **A[1]** and **A[2]**. Thus, the corresponding HNF grammar fragment is $\mathcal{G}_{\text{HNF}} \equiv$

[2] This condition, which does not restrict the set of CFGs that can be treated, is also known as invertibility (e.g., Harrison 1978).

[3] A grammar is in CNF if every rule is either of the form A → B C or of the form A → a (where, as always, uppercase denotes nonterminal symbols, and lowercase, terminals). Every CFL has a grammar in CNF (Hopcroft and Ullman 1979, 92).

{**A** → **A[1]**, **A[1]** → **B C**, **A** → **A[2]**, **A[2]** → **D E**, **F** → **F[1]**, **F[1]** → **B E**}. Now reconsider the ill-formed tree [$_{\mathbf{A}}$ **B E**]: its ill-formedness is apparent from checking only two tree nodes at a time. According to $\mathcal{G}_{\mathrm{HNF}}$, **B** and **E** are both missing a legal parent and **A** is missing two legal children. Introducing a now-necessary subcategorized version of **A** does not suffice: in [$_{\mathbf{A}}$ [$_{\mathbf{A[1]}}$ [**B E**]]], the pair **A[1]**, **E** is not legal according to $\mathcal{G}_{\mathrm{HNF}}$, and in [$_{\mathbf{A}}$ [$_{\mathbf{A[2]}}$ [**B E**]]], the pair **A[2]**, **B** is illicit. But the correct parse of the string **B E**—namely, [$_{\mathbf{F}}$ [$_{\mathbf{F[1]}}$ [**B E**]]]—has no ill-formed pairs.

HNF enables us to evaluate the Harmony of a tree simply by adding a collection of numbers (specified by the soft rules of a harmonic grammar), one for each node and one for each link of the tree. Now, any CFL $\mathcal{L}$ can be specified by a harmonic grammar. First, find an HNF grammar $\mathcal{G}_{\mathrm{HNF}}$ for $\mathcal{L}$; from it, generate a set of soft rules defining a harmonic grammar $\mathcal{G}_{\mathrm{H}}$ via the correspondences in (3) (see Figure 1).

(3) From harmonic normal form to a harmonic grammar

$\mathcal{G}_{\mathrm{HNF}}$	$\mathcal{G}_{\mathrm{H}}$
a	$R_{\mathbf{a}}$: If **a** is at any node, add –1 to H.
A	$R_{\mathbf{A}}$: If **A** is at any node, add –2 to H.
A[*i*]	$R_{\mathbf{A[i]}}$: If **A[*i*]** is at any node, add –3 to H.
start symbol **S**	R_{root}: If **S** is at the root, add +1 to H.
A → Γ (Γ = **a** or **A[*i*]**)	If Γ is a left child of **A**, add +2 to H.
A[*i*] → **B C**	If **B** is a left child of **A[*i*]**, add +2 to H. If **C** is a right child of **A[*i*]**, add +2 to H.

The soft rules $R_{\mathbf{a}}$, $R_{\mathbf{A}}$, $R_{\mathbf{A[i]}}$, and R_{root} are first order and evaluate tree nodes; the remaining second-order soft rules are **legal domination** rules evaluating tree links.

(4) *Theorem.* This harmonic grammar assigns $H = 0$ to any legal parse tree (with **S** at the root), and $H < 0$ to any other tree. Thus, $\boldsymbol{s} \in \mathcal{L}$ if and only if the maximum-Harmony completion of $\boldsymbol{s}$ to a tree has $H \geq 0$.

Proof. We evaluate the Harmony of any tree by conceptually breaking up its nodes and links into pieces each of which contributes either +1 or –1 to H. (See the recasting of Figure 1 as Figure 2; each '+' or '–' represents ±1.) In legal trees, the positive and negative contributions will completely cancel; illegal trees will have uncanceled –1s, leading to a total $H < 0$.

The decomposition of nodes and links proceeds as follows. We replace each (undirected) link in the tree with a pair of directed links, one pointing up to the parent, the other down to the child. If the link joins a legal parent-child pair, the corresponding legal domination rule will contribute +2 to H; we break this +2 into two contributions of +1, one for each of the directed links. We similarly break up the nonterminal nodes into subnodes. A nonterminal node labeled **A[*i*]** has two children in legal trees, and we break such a node into three subnodes, one corresponding to each downward link to a child and one corresponding to the upward link to the parent of

A[i]. According to soft rule $R_{\mathbf{A[i]}}$, the contribution of this node **A[i]** to H is –3; this is distributed as three contributions of –1, one for each subnode. Similarly, a nonterminal node labeled **A** has only one child in a legal tree, so we break it into two subnodes, one for the downward link to the only child, one for the upward link to the parent of **A**. The contribution of –2 dictated by soft rule $R_{\mathbf{A}}$ is similarly decomposed into two contributions of –1, one for each subnode. There is no need to break up terminal nodes, which in legal trees have only one outgoing link, upward to the parent; the contribution from $R_{\mathbf{a}}$ is already just –1.

We can evaluate the Harmony of any tree by examining each node, now decomposed into a set of subnodes, and determining the contribution to H made by the node and its *outgoing* directed links. This way, we will not double-count link contributions; half the contribution of each original undirected link is counted at each of the nodes it connects.

Consider first a nonterminal node n labeled by **A[i]**. If n has a legal parent, it will have an upward link to the parent that contributes +1, which cancels the –1 contributed by n's corresponding subnode. If n has a legal left child, the downward link to it will contribute +1, canceling the –1 contributed by n's corresponding subnode. Similarly for the right child. Thus, the total contribution of this node will be 0 if it has a legal parent and two legal children. For each *missing* legal child or parent, the node contributes an uncanceled –1, so the contribution of this node n in the general case is

(1) H_n = –(the number of missing legal children and parents of node n).

The same result (1) holds of the nonbranching nonterminals labeled **A**; the only difference is that now the only child that could be missing is a legal left child. If **A** happens to be a legal start symbol in root position, then the –1 of the subnode corresponding to the upward link to a parent is canceled not by a legal parent, as usual, but by the +1 of the soft rule R_{root}. The result (1) still holds even in this case, if we simply agree to count the root position itself as a legal 'parent' for start symbols. And finally, (1) holds of a terminal node n labeled **a**; such a node can have no missing child, but might have a missing legal parent.

Thus, the total Harmony of a tree is $H = \Sigma_n H_n$, with H_n given by (1). That is, H is *minus* the total number of missing legal children and parents for all nodes in the tree. Thus, $H = 0$ if each node has a legal parent and all its required legal children; otherwise, $H \leq 0$. Because the grammar is in HNF, a parse tree is legal if and only if every node has a legal parent and its required number of legal children, where 'legal' parent-child dominations are defined only pairwise, in terms of the parent and one child, blind to any other children that might be present or absent. Thus, we have established the desired result, that the maximum-Harmony parse of a string **s** has $H \geq 0$ if and only if **s** $\in \mathcal{L}$.

We can also now see how to understand the soft rules of $\mathcal{G}_{\text{H}}$, which will allow us to generalize beyond CFLs. The soft rules say that each node makes a negative contribution equal to its valence, while each link makes a positive contribution equal to its valence, 2, where the 'valence' of a node (or link) is just the number of links (or nodes) it is attached to in a legal tree. The negative contributions of the nodes are made any time the node is present; these are canceled by positive contributions from the links only when the link constitutes a legal domination, sanctioned by the grammar.

To apply this strategy to unrestricted grammars, we will set the magnitude of the (negative) contributions of a node equal to its valence, as determined by the grammar.

Figure 1. Harmonic grammar for context-free rewrite rules

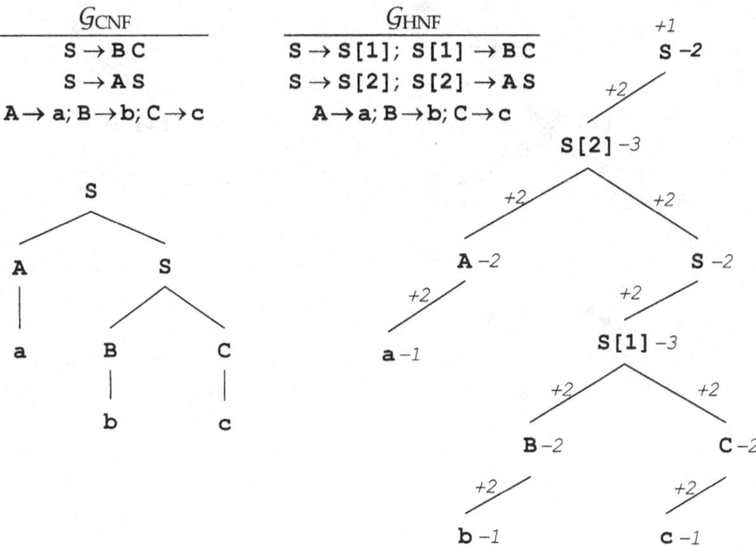

We can illustrate the operation of the harmonic grammar $\mathcal{G}_{\text{H}}$ with our running example, $\mathcal{G}_1$. The corresponding HNF grammar fragment given above is $\mathcal{G}_{\text{HNF}} \equiv$ {**A** → **A[1]**, **A[1]** → **B C**, **A** → **A[2]**, **A[2]** → **D E**, **F** → **F[1]**, **F[1]** → **B E**}. To avoid extraneous complications from adding a start node above and terminal nodes below, suppose that both **A** and **F** are valid start symbols and that **B**, **C**, **D**, **E** are terminal nodes. Then the corresponding harmonic grammar $\mathcal{G}_{\text{H}}$ assigns to the ill-formed tree [$_{\mathbf{A}}$ **B E**] the Harmony –4, since, according to $\mathcal{G}_{\text{HNF}}$, **B** and **E** are both missing a legal parent and **A** is missing two legal children. Introducing a subcategorized version of **A** helps, but not enough: [$_{\mathbf{A}}$ [$_{\mathbf{A[1]}}$ [**B E**]]] and [$_{\mathbf{A}}$ [$_{\mathbf{A[2]}}$ [**B E**]]] both have H = –2 since in each, one terminal node is missing a legal parent (**E** and **B**, respectively), and the **A[i]** node is missing the corresponding legal child. The correct parse of **B E**, [$_{\mathbf{F}}$ [$_{\mathbf{F[1]}}$ [**B E**]]], has H = 0 because no node is missing a valid parent or child.

This technique can be generalized from context-free to unrestricted (Type 0) formal languages, which are equivalent to Turing machines in the languages they generate (e.g., Hopcroft and Ullman 1979; recall Box 6:1). The *i*th production rule in an unrestricted grammar has the general form

$$R_i : \Gamma_1\Gamma_2\cdots\Gamma_{n_i} \rightarrow \Lambda_1\Lambda_2\cdots\Lambda_{m_i},$$

where each Γ_k and Λ_j is a terminal or nonterminal symbol. In the equivalent HNF grammar, R_i is replaced by the two rules

Figure 2. Connection weights: Context-free languages

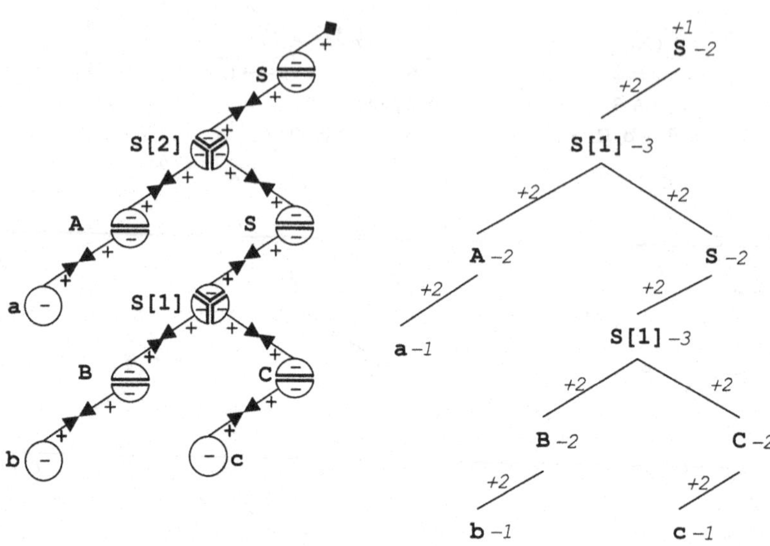

$$R_i' : \Gamma_1\Gamma_2\cdots\Gamma_{n_i} \rightarrow \mathbf{R[i]}$$

and

$$R_i'' : \mathbf{R[i]} \rightarrow \Lambda_1\Lambda_2\cdots\Lambda_{m_i},$$

introducing new nonterminal symbols **R[i]**.

Generalizing HNF to Type 0 grammars is not problematic, nor is expressing the HNF rewrite rules as HG soft rules. The challenge concerns the underlying data structure. While context-free derivations can be perspicuously represented by a tree, derivations with unrestricted rewrite rules are much less constrained. The data structure employed here is not as elegant as one would like; there may be better ones to replace it.

Figure 3 shows a simple derivation with unrestricted rewrite rules and its HNF counterpart. The data structure is a rendering of the derivation with a few conventions. The first (top) line is a new symbol *start*. The next line is a string of symbols; this is a **string line**. The next line is a **rule line**, which can host at most one **rule symbol R[i]**. String lines and rule lines alternate until the final line, which contains the new symbol *end*.

The rule symbol node **R[i]** can link to n_i consecutive nodes in the string line previous to (above) it; this node can have up to n_i 'parents'. This **R[i]** node can also link to m_i contiguous symbols in the line following it: up to m_i 'children'. Aside from

Figure 2

Figure 3. Harmony for unrestricted (Type 0) rewrite rules

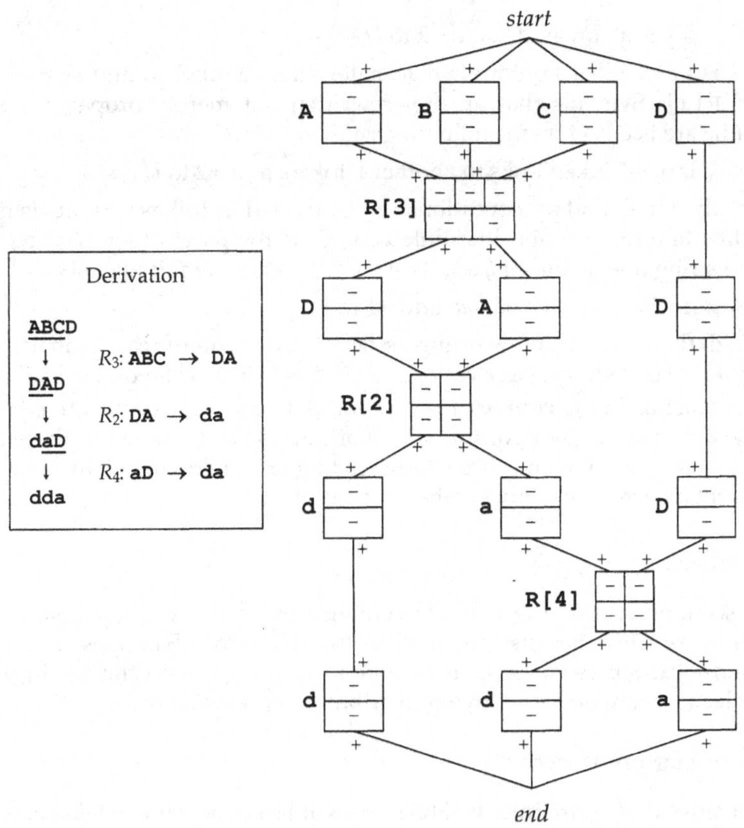

the new rule symbols **R[i]**, all other symbols can link to one previous and one following node; the previous node can be either the rule node in the previous rule line (if there is such a node) or a symbol in the previous string line. Likewise, the link to the following node can be to either the following rule line or the following string line. Links cannot cross.

The strategy for designing HG rules used in the context-free case applies to the new data structure as well, as shown in Figure 3. In the notation of the rewrite rules above, the soft rules in the harmonic grammar are then

If the kth parent of **R[i]** is Γ_k, add +2 to H

and

If Λ_k is the kth child of **R[i]**, add +2 to H.

There are also the rules

$R_{\mathbf{R[i]}}$: If $\mathbf{R}[i]$ is at any node, add $-(n_i + m_i)$ to H

and

R_Γ: If Γ is at any node, add -2 to H.

Here, Γ is an original nonterminal **A** or terminal symbol **a**: any symbol but a rule symbol **R[i]**. Symbols that are not rewritten but merely propagated to the next string line are licensed by the following rule:

R_{Faith}: If one Γ token links to another Γ token, add +2 to H.

Finally, the boundary conditions can be treated as follows. Symbols in the initial string line link to *start*, and that link 'counts' as the parent they require; symbols in the final string line link to *end*, and that counts as their required child:

R_{edge}: If Γ links to *start* or *end*, add +1 to H.

If desired, the R_{edge} rules rewarding association of nonterminal symbols to *end* could be omitted, thus requiring derivations to terminate in a string of terminal symbols.

Now just as in the context-free case, all derivations have negative Harmony except those that are legal according to the original Type 0 grammar: these have $H = 0$. Only by having legal connections to preceding and following elements can the Harmony debt incurred by every symbol be paid off.

2 Parsing

In this section, we discuss the implementation in a local connectionist network of an HG parser for CFLs. Because much of the formalism in ICS applies equally to distributed and local representations, it is hoped that progress on the local case will ultimately lead to networks employing distributed representations.

2.1 Grammar preprocessing

The penalties that figure into the HG rules will be connection weights and unit biases in a connectionist network that parses the grammar. The relation between the grammar and the network is established by two grammar transformations. The first ensures that the Unique Branching Condition of harmonic normal form is upheld; it was already illustrated in Section 1.

A grammar $\mathcal{G} = (V, \Sigma, R, \mathbf{S})$ is defined by four components: V is the set of all grammar symbols, Σ the subset of V that are terminal symbols, R the set of rules, and $\mathbf{S}$ the start symbol. Terminal symbols will be denoted with lowercase letters, and nonterminals with uppercase. For a nonterminal symbol **X**, *branchingRHS*(**X**) is the set of 'branching **X** rules' **X** → **A B** with **X** on the left-hand side and more than one symbol on the right-hand side. |*branchingRHS*(**X**)|, the size of the set *branchingRHS*(**X**), is the number of branching **X** rules.

Figure 3

(5) *Def.* $\mathcal{T}_{\text{HNF}}$ transform

Let $\mathcal{G} = (V, \Sigma, R, \mathbf{S})$ be a CFG in CNF. The HNF transform $\mathcal{T}_{\text{HNF}}$ of $\mathcal{G}$ is a new grammar $\mathcal{G}' = \mathcal{T}_{\text{HNF}}(\mathcal{G}) = (V', \Sigma', R', \mathbf{S}')$ where for each nonterminal **A** that appears in n branching $\mathcal{G}$-rules in R of the form $\mathbf{A} \rightarrow \mathbf{B}\ \mathbf{C}$, each such rule is replaced by two new $\mathcal{G}'$-rules in R' having the forms $\mathbf{A} \rightarrow \mathbf{A[i]}$ and $\mathbf{A[i]} \rightarrow \mathbf{B}\,\mathbf{C}$, containing a new nonterminal symbol $\mathbf{A[i]}$ not in V, with $\mathbf{i} = \mathbf{1}, \mathbf{2}, \ldots, n$. Call the set of new nonterminals that appear in these additional rules *bracket*(V'). The transformed set V' is the union of *bracket*(V'), the old nonterminals $\mathbf{X} \in V - \Sigma$ such that $|$*branchingRHS*$(\mathbf{X})| = 0$, and the old terminals Σ. The new Σ' and $\mathbf{S}'$ are the same as the original Σ and $\mathbf{S}$.

If a symbol is an element of the set *bracket*(V'), it is called **bracketed**; otherwise, it is **unbracketed**.

This first transform $\mathcal{T}_{\text{HNF}}$ essentially adds annotations to $\mathcal{G}$ showing exactly which rule is applied at each branch point in a derivation.

The second transformation adds information about string *positions* to every rule, and restricts the grammar to describing only sentences of a certain maximum length. Since this maximum can be arbitrarily large, it seems reasonable to maintain that CFGs for infinite languages are described in the limit (see Charniak and Santos 1987).

The annotation of string positions enables grammar symbols to directly serve as parser items. An **item** $\mathbf{B}_{jm}$ (or $\mathbf{B}_{j,m}$) is an assertion about the input string that means 'there is a constituent of type **B** that spans sentence positions j to m'. An item $\mathbf{A}_{jkm}$ (or $\mathbf{A}_{j,k,m}$) means 'there is a constituent of type **A** spanning sentence positions j to m, and this constituent consists of two contiguous, nonoverlapping subconstituents, the first ending at position k'. (If $k = m$, there is no second constituent.) **Itemification** of rules is the transformation defined in (6)–(7).

(6) *Definition.* Itemification of a binary rule

The itemification of a binary context-free rule $\mathbf{A} \rightarrow \mathbf{B}\ \mathbf{C}$ to a sentence length ℓ is the set of rules given by the schema $\mathbf{A}_{jkm} \rightarrow \mathbf{B}_{jk}\,\mathbf{C}_{km}$ for all $j, k, m = 0, 1, \ldots, \ell$ such that $j < k \leq m$.

(7) *Definition.* Itemification of a unary rule

The itemification of a unary context-free rule $\mathbf{A} \rightarrow \mathbf{B}$ to a sentence length ℓ is the set of rules given by the schema $\mathbf{A}_{jm} \rightarrow \mathbf{B}_{jkm}$ for all $j, k, m = 0, 1, \ldots, \ell$ such that $j < k \leq m$.

This second transform $\mathcal{T}_{\text{item}}$ annotates each symbol with the edge positions of the terminal symbols it spans.

Grammars that result from combining both transformations $\mathcal{T}_{\text{HNF}}$ and $\mathcal{T}_{\text{item}}$ include complex symbols of the form $\mathbf{A[i]}_{jkm}$. These symbols express the assertion that there is an **A**-type constituent spanning sentence positions j to m that was derived via the ith **A**-rule, and the left child's yield stops at position k. In this way, k plays the role of a pointer that identifies a bracketed parent's children. (Since the single rule expanding a bracketed symbol has the form $\mathbf{A[i]} \rightarrow \mathbf{B}\ \mathbf{C}$, if the assertion of the annotated symbol $\mathtt{A[i]}_{jkm}$ holds, then the two children of this node must be $\mathtt{B}_{jk}$ and $\mathtt{C}_{km}$.)

(8) *Definition.* Itemification of a grammar

Let $\mathcal{G} = (V, \Sigma, R, S)$ be a CFG in CNF. The itemification of $\mathcal{G}$ carried out for a sentence length ℓ is a grammar $\mathcal{G}'' = \mathcal{T}_{\text{item}}(\mathcal{G}, \ell) = (V'', \Sigma'', R'', S'')$ with the following properties:

a. Σ'' contains $\ell - 1$ symbols labeled $\mathbf{v}_{j,j+1}$ (where $j = 0, 1, \ldots, \ell-1$) for each terminal symbol $\mathbf{v}$ in Σ. (Terminal symbols extend only from j to the next position $j+1$.)

b. S'' is a new start symbol labeled $\mathbf{S}_{0\ell}$ (i.e., an S that spans the entire string).

c. R'' contains the itemification of each rule r in R.

d. V'' consists of all the symbols appearing in S'', R'', and Σ''.

Itemification ensures that children are directly adjacent, and in the correct order. For example (neglecting ks for a moment), a grammar can never contain a rule such as $\mathbf{X}_{13} \rightarrow \mathbf{Y}_{13}\ \mathbf{Z}_{23}$ where $\mathbf{Z}$'s yield—the string spanning positions 2 through 3—is enveloped by $\mathbf{Y}$'s yield; nor can it contain $\mathbf{X}_{14} \rightarrow \mathbf{Y}_{12}\ \mathbf{Z}_{34}$ where there is a gap (from 2 to 3) separating the two sister constituents $\mathbf{Y}$, $\mathbf{Z}$.

It is also convenient to define the width of two-index itemified symbols $\mathbf{X}_{ij}$ from V'' as $width(\mathbf{X}_{ij}) = j - i$.

We now show that a grammatical parse tree of the grammar $\mathcal{T}_{\text{item}}(\mathcal{G}')$ can always be converted into a legal parse tree on $\mathcal{G}'$, and that a valid parse of $\mathcal{T}_{\text{HNF}}(\mathcal{G})$ can be transformed into a licit parse of $\mathcal{G}$.

Given a grammar $\mathcal{G}$, following Nijholt 1980, Chap. 2, take a (potential) *parse* to be a pair consisting of a terminal string v and a string of rule numbers $\boldsymbol{\pi}$. (The intent of using indexed rules is solely to provide a way of unambiguously referring to particular grammar rules.) The **proper parse relation** on $\mathcal{G}$ is the set of all such pairs in which the rules referred to in the rule-number string $\boldsymbol{\pi}$ actually derive the given terminal string v from the start symbol; any such pair will be called a **proper parse.**[4] A **partial parse homomorphism** $\mathcal{F}$ is then a pair of maps: one, f_{symb}, from terminal strings of a source grammar $\overline{\mathcal{G}}$ to terminal strings in the target grammar $\mathcal{G}$, and the other, f_{rule}, from rule-number strings in $\overline{\mathcal{G}}$ to rule-number strings in $\mathcal{G}$. To qualify as a homomorphism, if $(\overline{\mathbf{v}}, \overline{\boldsymbol{\pi}})$ is a proper $\overline{\mathcal{G}}$-parse, then $(f_{\text{symb}}(\overline{\mathbf{v}}), f_{\text{rule}}(\overline{\boldsymbol{\pi}}))$ must be a proper $\mathcal{G}$-parse. Thus, every valid $\overline{\mathcal{G}}$-parse can be mapped to a valid $\mathcal{G}$-parse by the homomorphism $\mathcal{F} \equiv (f_{\text{symb}}, f_{\text{rule}})$.

A partial parse homomorphism $\mathcal{F}$ is a **cover** if it is surjective: each parse in its range is the value of some parse in the domain. In this case, every valid $\mathcal{G}$-parse can be recovered from some valid $\overline{\mathcal{G}}$-parse via $\mathcal{F} = (f_{\text{symb}}, f_{\text{rule}})$.

[4] Should it be ambiguous at some stage of derivation which nonterminal symbol $\mathbf{X}$ to expand by the next-numbered rule $\mathbf{X} \rightarrow \cdots$, a convention can be adopted, for example, requiring the leftmost $\mathbf{X}$ to be expanded by the next rule. There is no loss of generality with respect to generating parses of nonterminal strings.

Figure 3

Restricting consideration to terminal strings having length no more than ℓ, we now see how covers can be defined between $\mathcal{G}'' \equiv \mathcal{T}_{\text{item}}(\mathcal{G}', \ell)$ and $\mathcal{G}'$, and between $\mathcal{G}' \equiv \mathcal{T}_{\text{HNF}}(\mathcal{G})$ and $\mathcal{G}$: given a parse on a transformed grammar, partial parse homomorphisms $\mathcal{F}_{\text{item}}(\ell)$ and $\mathcal{F}_{\text{HNF}}$ are the inverse mappings that, given a parse on a transformed grammar, supply the corresponding parse on the untransformed grammar—essentially undoing the work of their namesakes. The basic idea is that both transformations only annotate the original symbols and rules, rather than deleting or altering them, so their effects can be undone after the parsing is completed, essentially by simply discarding the annotations. This is spelled out in (9).

(9) Recovering parses on $\mathcal{G}$

a. $\mathcal{F}_{\text{HNF}}$: a partial parse homomorphism from $\mathcal{G}' \equiv \mathcal{T}_{\text{HNF}}(\mathcal{G})$ to $\mathcal{G}$, defined by

i. Mapping f_{symb} on terminal strings

✦ the identity map (v mapped to v)

ii. Mapping f_{rule} on rule strings

f_{rule} applied to a string of rule numbers is the concatenation of the results of applying f_{r0} to each number in the string; f_{r0} is defined by

✦ the number of a rule **A** → **a** in $\mathcal{G}'$ is mapped to the number of the same rule in $\mathcal{G}$;

✦ the number of a rule **A[*i*]** → **B C** in $\mathcal{G}'$ is mapped to the number of the corresponding rule **A** → **B C** in $\mathcal{G}$;

✦ the number of a rule **A**→**A[*i*]** in $\mathcal{G}'$ is mapped to the empty string.

b. $\mathcal{F}_{\text{item}}(\ell)$: a partial parse homomorphism from $\mathcal{G}'' \equiv \mathcal{T}_{\text{item}}(\mathcal{G}', \ell)$ to $\mathcal{G}'$ defined by

i. Mapping f'_{symb} on terminal strings

f'_{symb} applied to a string of terminal symbols is the concatenation of the results of applying f'_{s0} to each symbol in the string; f'_{s0} is defined by

✦ a terminal $\mathbf{v}_{j,j+1}$ is mapped to **v**, for all terminal positions j.

ii. Mapping f'_{rule} on rule strings

f'_{rule} applied to a string of rule numbers is the concatenation of the results of applying f'_{r0} to each number in the string; f'_{r0} is defined by:

✦ the number of a rule $\mathbf{A}_{jkm} \rightarrow \mathbf{B}_{jk}\,\mathbf{C}_{km}$ in $\mathcal{G}''$ is mapped to the number of the corresponding rule **A** → **B C** in $\mathcal{G}$;

✦ the number of a rule $\mathbf{A}_{jm} \rightarrow \mathbf{B}_{jkm}$ in $\mathcal{G}''$ is mapped to the number of **A** → **B** in $\mathcal{G}$.

Proof sketch that $\mathcal{F}_{\text{HNF}}$ and $\mathcal{F}_{\text{item}}$ are in fact partial parse homomorphisms. To show that $\mathcal{F}_{\text{HNF}}(\mathcal{G})$ is a homomorphism, we need to show that, given any proper parse (v′, π′) on $\mathcal{G}' \equiv \mathcal{T}_{\text{HNF}}(\mathcal{G})$, (v, π) is a legal parse of $\mathcal{G}$, where v ≡ f_{symb}(v′) = v′ and π ≡ f_{rule}(π′). Consider a particular $\mathcal{G}'$-rule *r*′ numbered π′, one number in the string of rule numbers π′. Since $\mathcal{G}' \equiv \mathcal{T}_{\text{HNF}}(\mathcal{G})$, *r*′ is either a unary rule of the form **A** → **a** or **A** → **A[*i*]** or a binary rule of the form **A[i]** → **B C**. Since π′ is a legal derivation, which must terminate in terminal symbols, each **A[i]** generated during the derivation must later be eliminated, necessarily by a rule **A[i]** → **A B**. A bracketed symbol can only be generated by a rule **A** → **A[i]**, so the derivation must previously have generated an **A** in the same string location as the **A[i]** (unary rules do not affect string position). The net effect of these two $\mathcal{G}'$-rules **A** → **A[i]** and **A[i]** → **B C** is equivalent to the effect of the $\mathcal{G}$-rule **A** → **B C**. Thus, $\mathcal{F}_{HNF}(\mathcal{G})$'s eliminating the number of **A** → **A[i]** and replacing the number of **A[i]** → **A B** in π′ by the number of **A** → **B C** to produce π means that after the application of the branching rule, the strings generated by π′ and π will be in the same state at the location of this **A/A[i]** symbol: since the **A** must have been previously generated in π′, we can be sure that the rule **A** → **B C** can apply in π. And $\mathcal{F}_{HNF}(\mathcal{G})$'s replacing the number of a rule **A** → **a** in $\mathcal{G}'$ by the number of the same rule in $\mathcal{G}$ also ensures that the two derivations π′ and π will be in the same state at the location of the **A** when this rule applies. Thus, since π′ derives v′ = v, π must derive v also; if (v′, π′) is a proper parse on $\mathcal{G}'$, then (v, π) is a proper parse on $\mathcal{G}$.

To show that $\mathcal{F}_{HNF}(\mathcal{G})$ is a cover, we need to show that, given any parse (v, π) on $\mathcal{G}$, there is some parse (v′, π′) on $\mathcal{G}' \equiv \mathcal{T}_{HNF}(\mathcal{G})$ such that $\mathcal{F}_{HNF}$ maps (v′, π′) to (v, π). Since the terminal string homomorphism part of $\mathcal{F}_{HNF}$ is the identity, all terminal strings are their own source and target: we have v′ = v. Now consider any parse π on $\mathcal{G}$; we construct the needed π′. π is a sequence of rule numbers, where each rule is a CNF rule **A** → **a** or **A** → **B C**. A unary rule **A** → **a** is mapped to itself under $\mathcal{T}_{HNF}$, so we just replace the number of any such rule in π with the number of the same rule as a rule of $\mathcal{G}'$ in order to define π′. If an element in π is the number of a binary rule **A** → **B C**, then we replace it with a pair of numbers (n_1, n_2). The second member of the pair, n_2, is the number of the rule **A[i]** → **B C** in $\mathcal{G}'$: there must be exactly one value of **i** for which this rule exists, by the definition of $\mathcal{T}_{HNF}$. The first member of the pair, n_1, is the number of the rule **A** → **A[i]** in $\mathcal{G}'$, for the same value of **i**; this rule too must exist. Now making all these replacements of numbers in π gives a string π′ of rule numbers for $\mathcal{G}'$. Because the number of the rule **A** → **B C** in $\mathcal{G}$ has been replaced by the pair of numbers for **A** → **A[i]**, **A[i]** → **B C** in $\mathcal{G}'$, it must be that π′ derives a legal $\mathcal{G}'$-parse of v′. Clearly, by construction, $\mathcal{F}_{HNF}(\mathcal{G})$ maps π′ to π.

A similar argument shows that $\mathcal{F}_{item}(\ell)$ is a cover, where the length of the terminal string is less than or equal to ℓ. Rather than subcategorization annotation as in $\mathcal{T}_{HNF}$ (where **A** becomes **A[i]**), here we have terminal-string-span annotation (where **A** becomes $\mathbf{A}_{jk}$); but there is still a direct correspondence between annotated and unannotated parses—ignoring all the position indices in π′ directly gives π.

Finally, let the **parent set** of a grammar symbol Γ be the set of all nonterminals that appear on the left-hand side in rules that include Γ on the right-hand side.

(10) *Definition.* Parent set

Let $\mathcal{G} = (V, \Sigma, R, \mathbf{S})$ be a CFG and let $\gamma_0, \gamma_1 \in V^*$ be strings of symbols in V (possibly empty). Then the set of all possible parents of a nonterminal element $\mathbf{X} \in V - \Sigma$ is

$$parents(\mathbf{X}, \mathcal{G}) \equiv \{\mathbf{P} : \exists\, \gamma_0, \gamma_1 \in V^* \text{ such that } [\mathbf{P} \rightarrow \gamma_0\, \mathbf{X}\, \gamma_1] \in R\}.$$

Every CFG with a finite number of rules has a **maximal parent multiplicity** $p_{max}(\mathcal{G})$, the highest number of possible parents for any symbol. $p_{max}(\mathcal{G})$ will usually be abbreviated p.

Figure 3

All these concepts and definitions will be used to completely specify the parsing network in Section 2.3.

2.2 Example

As an example, consider the ambiguous grammar in (11)

(11) A simple ambiguous grammar $\mathcal{G}_0$

a. **S → A B**

b. **A → A A**

where **S** is the start symbol. We follow Nijholt 1990 in assuming that preterminal rules such as **A → v** do not play a role and parsing may begin at the nonterminals. On this grammar, the input sequence **AAAB** is ambiguous between an analysis where the leftmost pair of **A**s form a constituent [[[**AA**] **A**] **B**] and one where the rightmost pair of **A**s form one [[**A** [**AA**]] **B**]. Either analysis is compatible with a correct parse.

To build a parser for this grammar for sentences of length $\ell = 4$, the grammar is first transformed by $\mathcal{T}_{HNF}$. Even though this grammar $\mathcal{G}_0$ is already in HNF, $\mathcal{T}_{HNF}$ here serves to explicitly encode the unary/binary status of each rule via the bracketed nonterminals.

(12) $\mathcal{G}_0' \equiv \mathcal{T}_{HNF}(\mathcal{G}_0)$: HNF of $\mathcal{G}_0$

a. **A → A[1]**

b. **A[1] → A A**

c. **S → S[1]**

d. **S[1] → A B**

Next, itemification is performed, resulting in a larger grammar in which all possible rule applications have been annotated with string position indices for every possible location at which they could be applied.

(13) $\mathcal{G}_0'' \equiv \mathcal{T}_{item}(\mathcal{G}_0')$: Itemification of $\mathcal{G}_0'$

a. **A → A[1]** is replaced by

i. $\mathbf{A}_{02}$ → $\mathbf{A[1]}_{012}$

ii. $\mathbf{A}_{02}$ → $\mathbf{A[1]}_{022}$

iii. $\mathbf{A}_{03}$ → $\mathbf{A[1]}_{013}$

iv. $\mathbf{A}_{03}$ → $\mathbf{A[1]}_{023}$

⋮

b. **A[1] → A A** is replaced by

i. $\mathbf{A[1]}_{012}$ → $\mathbf{A}_{01}$ $\mathbf{A}_{12}$

ii. $\mathbf{A[1]}_{013}$ → $\mathbf{A}_{01}$ $\mathbf{A}_{13}$

iii. $\mathbf{A[1]}_{023}$ → $\mathbf{A}_{02}$ $\mathbf{A}_{23}$

⋮

c. `S → S[1]` is replaced by
   i. $\mathtt{S}_{02} \rightarrow \mathtt{S[1]}_{012}$
   ii. $\mathtt{S}_{02} \rightarrow \mathtt{S[1]}_{022}$
   iii. $\mathtt{S}_{03} \rightarrow \mathtt{S[1]}_{013}$
   ⋮

d. `S[1] → A B` is replaced by
   i. $\mathtt{S[1]}_{012} \rightarrow \mathtt{A}_{01}\ \mathtt{B}_{12}$
   ii. $\mathtt{S[1]}_{013} \rightarrow \mathtt{A}_{01}\ \mathtt{B}_{13}$
   iii. $\mathtt{S[1]}_{023} \rightarrow \mathtt{A}_{02}\ \mathtt{B}_{23}$
   ⋮

After both the $\mathcal{T}_{\text{HNF}}$ and $\mathcal{T}_{\text{item}}$ transforms of $\mathcal{G}_0$, there are 54 symbols in the final grammar $\mathcal{G}_0''$.

2.3 Hopfield network

The parsing network contains one unit for each symbol in the doubly transformed grammar $\mathcal{G}''$. It is a Hopfield network with units whose states take on the values 0 and 1. The network will be constructed to parse the grammar $\mathcal{G}'' \equiv \mathcal{T}_{\text{item}}(\mathcal{T}_{\text{HNF}}(\mathcal{G}),\ell) = (V'', \Sigma'', R'', \mathbf{S}'')$ with maximal parent multiplicity $p = p_{\max}(\mathcal{G}'')$. The unit activations are a_α, $\alpha = 1, 2, \ldots, |V''|$; these are linear threshold units (Section 9:3.1.3). That is, they update themselves according to the transition rule

$$\text{(14)} \quad \mathrm{a}_\alpha \rightarrow \begin{cases} 0 & \text{if } \sum_\beta \mathrm{W}_{\alpha\beta}\mathrm{a}_\beta + \mathrm{b}_\alpha < 0 \\ 1 & \text{otherwise} \end{cases},$$

where $\mathrm{W}_{\alpha\beta}$ are the connection weights, and b_α the biases, to be defined below. NB: The activation value a_α is 1, not 0, when the input to α from other units $\Sigma_\beta \mathrm{W}_{\alpha\beta}\mathrm{a}_\beta$ exactly cancels its bias b_α.

Let f_α denote the application of the transition rule to the αth threshold logic unit. Then a network update f_{network} is a sequential update of all units in a random sequence: $f_{\text{network}} = f_{\rho(|V''|)} \circ \cdots \circ f_{\rho(2)} \circ f_{\rho(1)}$, where ρ is a random permutation of 1, 2, …, $|V''|$.

W is a symmetric $|V''| \times |V''|$ weight matrix indexed by grammar symbols; for example, one element might be $\mathrm{W}_{\mathtt{A[1]}_{023},\mathtt{S[1]}_{135}}$. A weight is only nonzero if its connection links a unit for a bracketed symbol with a unit for an unbracketed symbol; for example, $\mathrm{W}_{\mathtt{S}_{03},\mathtt{S[1]}_{023}} \neq 0$. (See Figure 4.) The quantitative values of the weights are given in (15).

(15) Connection weights

a. If there is a binary rule $\alpha \rightarrow \beta\ \gamma$ or $\alpha \rightarrow \gamma\ \beta$, then the weight between units α and β is 1.

Figure 3

b. If there is a unary rule $\alpha \to \beta$, then the weight between units α and β is the same as the maximal parent multiplicity, p.

c. Otherwise, the weight is zero.

So for the example grammar $\mathcal{G}_0$ (11), $W_{\texttt{S[1]}_{023},\texttt{B}_{23}} = 1$ from (15a) and (13d.iii), and $W_{\texttt{A}_{03},\texttt{A[1]}_{013}} = p$ from (15b) and (13a.iii).

The vector of $|V''|$ biases is **b**; its components are all negative. Component b_α is set to one of three possible values.

(16) Biases

a. If α = $\boldsymbol{S}_{0\ell}$, the unbracketed start symbol of width = ℓ, then $b_\alpha = -1$; if α is not a start symbol, then ...

b. if α is bracketed, then $b_\alpha = -(p + 2)$; otherwise ...

c. α is unbracketed and $b_\alpha = -(p + 1)$.

Thus, for $\mathcal{G}_0$, $b_{\texttt{S[1]}_{023}} = -(p+2)$ and $b_{\texttt{A}_{14}} = -(p+1)$.

These weights and biases reflect the kinds of input that bracketed and unbracketed units need in order to be correctly supported by units representing parents above them and units representing children below them.

(17) Bracketed units (Figure 4A)

By the Unique Branching Condition, these units have valence three.[5] They receive input from exactly one (unbracketed) parent (e.g., $\texttt{S}_{jm} \to \texttt{S[i]}_{jkm}$) and exactly two (unbracketed) children ($\texttt{S[i]}_{jkm} \to \texttt{A}_{jk}\ \texttt{B}_{km}$). If all three of these neighbors are in the 1 state, then the net input is $p+1+1$, representing, respectively, the contributions from the parent and each child. This exactly balances the bias $-(p + 2)$ and ensures the bracketed unit will be active. Bracketed units that are on are guaranteed to have correct parents and children on.

(18) Unbracketed units (Figure 4B)

These units can be connected to as many as p parents (all of them bracketed). Even if all possible parents are in the 1 state, an unbracketed unit's $-(p + 1)$ bias ensures that it can be in the 1 state itself only when supported by at least one bracketed child. Unbracketed units that are on are guaranteed to have at least one correct child on (but not necessarily a parent).

By construction, **W** is symmetric (if two symbols are in a parent-child relationship, they are also in a child-parent relationship), and **W** has zeros along the diagonal (no symbol is in a parent-child relationship with itself). Therefore, the results on convergence of Hopfield networks (Hopfield 1982; Section 9:3.1.1 here) are applicable. The dynamics reaches a Harmony maximum, at which point there is no Harmony change: $\Delta H = 0$. At this point, $\mathbf{a}^{\text{stable}} = f_{\text{network}}(\mathbf{a}^{\text{stable}})$.

During the network's operation, only the states of units associated with symbols of width greater than one may change. Width-1 units, specifying the input to be

[5] As defined in the proof of (4), the **valence** of a node (or link) is just the number of links (or nodes) attached to it in a legal tree.

parsed, are clamped to fixed values.

Note that unbracketed units will turn off only if all units representing their (bracketed) child options are off. Bracketed units will switch off if any of their neighbors switch off. The basic arrangement, depicted in Figure 4, is repeated throughout the entire network.

Figure 4. Parser connectivity

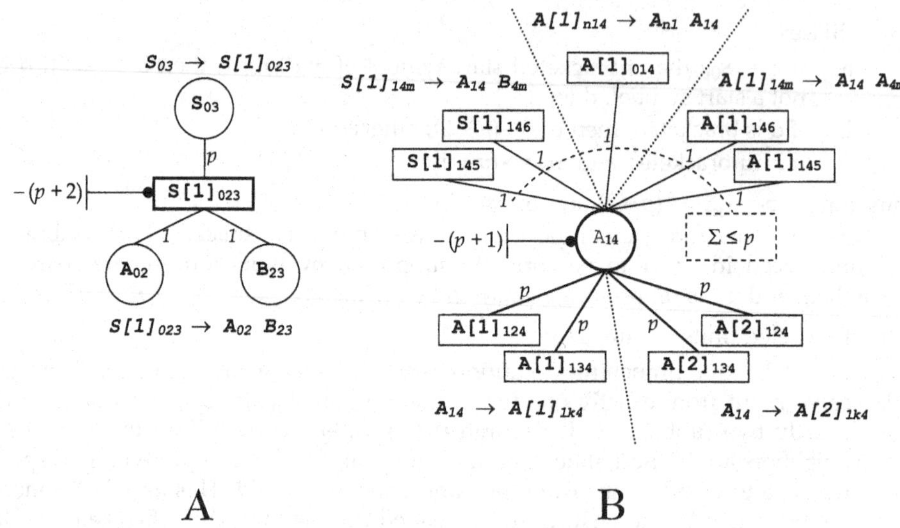

The parsing network computes a **shared packed forest** (Tomita 1986): for every constituent in each grammatical parse of the input, the corresponding unit is active in the output, and every active unit in the output corresponds to such a constituent.

(19) *Theorem.* Correctness

Let $\mathbf{a}^{\text{stable}}$ be a stable state of a Hopfield network constructed as above to parse $\mathcal{G}'' \equiv \mathcal{T}_{\text{item}}(\mathcal{T}_{\text{HNF}}(\mathcal{G}), \ell) = (V'', \Sigma'', R'', \mathbf{S}'')$, with initial state $\mathbf{a}^0$ determined by the input string $\text{v} = \mathbf{v}_{0,1}\mathbf{v}_{1,2}\cdots\mathbf{v}_{\ell-1,\ell}$ in the following way:

a. If a width-1 symbol $\text{v}_{j,j+1}$ is contained in the input, the corresponding unit has activity 1 in the initial state.

b. If a width-1 symbol $\text{v}_{j,j+1}$ is not contained in the input, the corresponding unit has activity 0 in the initial state.

c. All other units in the initial state have activity 1.

Then, if in the final state $\mathbf{a}^{\text{stable}}$ the unit for the width-ℓ start symbol $\mathbf{S}_{0\ell}$ has activity 1, the set of active units $\{\alpha : a_\alpha = 1\}$ determines a shared packed forest of v-parses on $\mathcal{G}$. Otherwise, the parser has rejected v.

Figure 4

Proof sketch. We must show that if a unit representing a start symbol spanning the entire input is in the active−1−state in $\mathbf{a}^{\text{stable}}$, then all trees determined by sequences of choices about which activated bracketed child-units to move to from activated unbracketed parent-units, going from the root to the leaves, are correct parses of v.

If a unit representing an unbracketed start symbol spanning the entire input is in the 1 state, it must be because its −1 bias has been counterbalanced by activation from at least one (bracketed) child, since by definition start symbols have no parents.

Select one of these bracketed children that are in the 1 state. Since it is bracketed, being on implies a full and correct set of neighbors in the 1 state. Two of these neighbors are (unbracketed) children. Each of these must have at least one active (bracketed) child: otherwise, as an unbracketed unit, it would be inactive.

Continue by selecting arbitrarily from among the activated bracketed children at each successive unbracketed unit. This selected unit must be part of a correct parse in virtue of a grammar rule, or it would not be activated. Eventually, because the network is finite, this selecting and traversing must end at clamped, unbracketed units of width 1.

Each selection of a bracketed unit from the perspective of an unbracketed parent is an unpacking of one choice that has been packed in the shared packed parse forest. The representation is shared because no symbol is represented more than once.

Since all of the active units are part of some correct parse corresponding to some sequence of bracketed-rule selections, for each such correct parse there must be a sequence $\pi = \pi_0, \pi_1, \ldots, \pi_n$ of rules that each describe one piece of local tree structure. Since the above argument did not depend on which bracketed-rule unit was selected at each point, each sequence of selections results in a correct parse and each resulting π stands in a proper parse relation with $\mathbf{v}$ on $\mathcal{G}'' \equiv \mathcal{T}_{\text{item}}(\mathcal{T}_{\text{HNF}}(\mathcal{G}),\ell)$. The proper parse relation on $\mathcal{G}$ is $\mathcal{F}_{\text{HNF}} \circ \mathcal{F}_{\text{item}}(\text{v}, \pi)$: the result of undoing the two transformations that led from $\mathcal{G}$ to the final grammar actually instantiated in the network.

(20) Completeness and the initial state

Suppose an initial state $\mathbf{a}^0$ includes a set of active units sufficient to describe a parse of v. Then that parse will be represented in the final state.

Proof. The parser's operation can only switch bracketed units $\alpha \in \mathit{bracket}(V'')$ in the 1 state into the 0 state, and not the other way around, because $\mathbf{W}$ is constructed so that α has exactly three nonzero incoming weights, and their sum is $(p + 2)$. These nonzero weights are exactly those for α's two unique children and unique parent. α's bias has also been constructed to be exactly $-(p+2)$. So given that α is on, it must be that all of α's neighbors are on and that they are licensed by the grammar. But bracketed units in the 1 state with *correct* parents and children do not change their state. So if all correct parents and children from a parse are active in the initial state, and no bracketed units can switch off, then all correct parents and children must still be on in the stable state.

2.4 Example

Returning to the simple ambiguous grammar $\mathcal{G}_0$ of Section 2.2, the corresponding network has 54 units, one for each symbol in the transformed grammar $\mathcal{G}_0''$. The network runs until it reaches a stable state, increasing Harmony at every transition. The Harmony values for one simulation run are shown in Figure 5.

Figure 5. Parsing as Harmony maximization

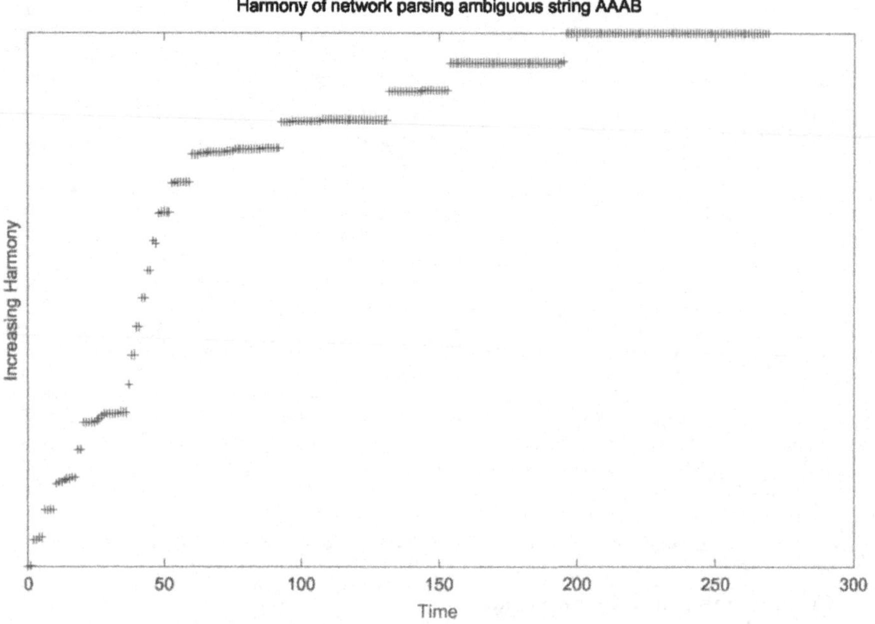

In the final state, the correct units are active: those representing the symbols $\mathbf{S}_{04}$, $\mathbf{S[1]}_{034}$, $\mathbf{A}_{03}$, $\mathbf{A[1]}_{013}$, $\mathbf{A[1]}_{023}$, $\mathbf{A}_{02}$, $\mathbf{A[1]}_{012}$, $\mathbf{A[1]}_{123}$, $\mathbf{A}_{13}$, $\mathbf{A}_{01}$, $\mathbf{A}_{12}$, $\mathbf{A}_{23}$, and $\mathbf{B}_{34}$ are all in the 1 state, and all others are in the 0 state. Since the start symbol $\mathbf{S}_{04}$ is activated, we can interpret the parse as having accepted **AAAB**. To determine the parses, we conceptually traverse downward from $\mathbf{S}_{04}$ to $\mathbf{S[1]}_{034}$, and then to $\mathbf{A}_{03}$ and $\mathbf{B}_{34}$. From $\mathbf{A}_{03}$, there is a choice of which of the two ambiguous parses to be taken. Both are represented by activated units, all of which are part of correct parses that figure into a shared packed parse forest. Selecting $\mathbf{A[1]}_{013}$ determines one parse, and selecting $\mathbf{A[1]}_{023}$ determines the other, just as in chart parsing.

2.5 Concluding remarks

One interesting property of this HG parser that distinguishes it from various other deterministic connectionist parsers (Fanty 1985; Nijholt 1990; Sikkel 1997) is the lack of central control over evaluation order. The formulation here is based on fixed points for randomly ordered, Harmony-increasing updates. Despite this apparent

Figure 5

freedom, the deactivation of unsupported units proceeds bottom-up, an order effect that emerges from the connectivity of the network.

Regarding future extensions, work by Hopfield (1984) suggests that the results for linear threshold units should extend straightforwardly to networks with continuous-valued units, while that of Stolcke (1989) points the way to more linguistically realistic unification-based grammars.

Also intriguing are connections to Optimality Theory (Prince and Smolensky 1993/2004). As in Optimality Theory, where all representational possibilities are said to come from *Gen*, the network parser described here starts from a state in which all possible constituents are represented. As processing moves forward, units representing constituents that lack support given the input string deactivate themselves. In this way, the parser acts as a filter that removes ungrammatical analyses from an initial universe of conceivable analyses. The parser is implementing constraints from a constraint set *Con* that contains the soft rules $\mathcal{G}_H$. However, because constraint interaction is numerical, strict domination need not necessarily hold: two or more violations of $R_{\mathbf{a}}$ can be just as bad as, or worse than, a single violation of $R_{\mathbf{A}}$ even though $R_{\mathbf{A}}$ dominates $R_{\mathbf{a}}$ in the sense of having greater numerical strength.

But while strict domination is not guaranteed by the architecture, the actual numerical values of weights in the parsing network have a tantalizing relation to strict domination. The weights in the network have two magnitudes: 1 and $p = p_{max}$, the maximal parent multiplicity. Why these two values? The answer lies in (18) and Figure 4B. A unit like $\mathbf{A}_{14}$ can have many parents, each capable of sending input 1 along its strength-1 connection to $\mathbf{A}_{14}$. (Since the overall scale of weights is arbitrary, we can without loss of generality set these weights to 1.) From $\mathcal{G}_0$, these parents derive rules like **S** → **A B**, which lead to $\mathcal{G}_0''$ rules like $\mathbf{S[1]}_{145} \to \mathbf{A}_{14}\ \mathbf{B}_{45}$. When the unit $\mathbf{A}_{14}$ receives input from an active parent—say, $\mathbf{S[1]}_{145}$—this amounts to satisfaction of a constraint we can call GOODPARENT. The other constraint, GOODCHILDREN, requires $\mathbf{A}_{14}$ to have an active child unit $\mathbf{A[i]}_{1k4}$; this relationship derives from the unary $\mathcal{G}'$ rules **A** → **A[i]**.

Now GOODPARENT can be satisfied as many as p times, leading to as many as p units of Harmony if $\mathbf{A}_{14}$ is active. Thus, the bias to the unit $\mathbf{A}_{14}$ must be more negative than $-p$ to ensure that activating $\mathbf{A}_{14}$ will produce negative Harmony if it has good parents but not good children, or equivalently, to ensure that $\mathbf{A}_{14}$ cannot get sufficient input from good parents alone to activate it. In our parser, this bias is set to $-(p + 1)$. Now to ensure that this bias can be overcome with one good child and one good parent—which is all the valence-2 symbol $\mathbf{A}_{14}$ requires in a valid parse—the weight to $\mathbf{A}_{14}$ from a child must be at least p, since a single parent only offers input 1. In our parser, the weight of this connection is indeed p.

It might be said that if we arbitrarily set the strength of GOODPARENT to 1, the strength of GOODCHILDREN must be at least p. This is exactly to ensure that a violation of GOODCHILDREN is so strong that it cannot possibly be overcome by satisfying GOODPARENT many times. In other words, strict domination has been ensured by the choice of weights: GOODCHILDREN ≫ GOODPARENT.

One source of the asymmetry between GOODCHILDREN and GOODPARENT is the directionality of the parser's task: the input provides constraints at the *bottom* of the tree, and these must percolate up from children to parents. The first units to deactivate from their initial active state must be those that require particular children in the input: the symbols absent in the input deny these units the children they need, and this constraint violation *GOODCHILDREN must be sufficiently serious that it cannot be overruled by the horde of good parents that all nodes have in the initial state, where all units are active except the symbols absent in the input. That is, the strict ranking GOODCHILDREN ≫ GOODPARENT is necessary in order for deactivation to spread bottom-up, from children to parents.

From this perspective at least, the connections in the parser do not appear to be simply an encoding of the grammar in a form independent of its use: they seem to be specialized for use in deactivation-driven bottom-up interpretation—as opposed, say, to activation-driven top-down generation. The *connectivity* of the network is transparently projected from the grammar, independently of any considerations of its use. But it may be necessary for the *strengths* of connections to be designed for a particular computational deployment of the grammar.

Figure 5

References

ROA = Rutgers Optimality Archive, http://roa.rutgers.edu

Charniak, E., and E. Santos. 1987. A connectionist context-free parser which is not context-free, but then it is not really connectionist either. In *Proceedings of the Cognitive Science Society 9.*

Fanty, M. 1985. Context-free parsing in connectionist networks. Technical report 174, Computer Science Department, University of Rochester.

Gazdar, G., E. Klein, G. Pullum, and I. Sag. 1985. *Generalized Phrase Structure Grammar.* Harvard University Press.

Hale, J., and P. Smolensky. 2001. A parser for harmonic context-free grammars. In *Proceedings of the Cognitive Science Society 23.*

Harrison, M. A. 1978. *Introduction to formal language theory.* Addison-Wesley.

Hopcroft, J. E., and J. D. Ullman. 1979. *Introduction to automata theory, languages, and computation.* Addison-Wesley.

Hopfield, J. J. 1982. Neural networks and physical systems with emergent collective computational abilities. *Proceedings of the National Academy of Sciences USA* 79, 2554–8.

Hopfield, J. J. 1984. Neurons with graded response have collective computational properties like those of two-state neurons. *Proceedings of the National Academy of Sciences USA* 81, 3088–92.

Nijholt, A. 1980. *Context-free grammars: Covers, normal forms and parsing.* Springer-Verlag.

Nijholt, A. 1990. Meta-parsing in neural networks. In *Proceedings of the 10th European Meeting on Cybernetics and Systems Research.*

Prince, A., and P. Smolensky. 1993/2004. *Optimality Theory: Constraint interaction in generative grammar.* Technical report, Rutgers University and University of Colorado at Boulder, 1993. ROA 537, 2002. Revised version published by Blackwell, 2004.

Sikkel, K. 1997. *Parsing schemata: A framework for specification and analysis of parsing algorithms.* Springer-Verlag.

Smolensky, P. 1993. Harmonic grammars for formal languages. In *Advances in neural information processing systems 5*, eds. S. Hanson, J. D. Cowan, and C. L. Giles. Morgan Kaufmann.

Stolcke, A. 1989. Unification as constraint satisfaction in structured connectionist networks. *Neural Computation* 1, 559–67.

Tomita, M. 1986. *Efficient parsing for natural language: A fast algorithm for practical systems.* Kluwer.

11

The Interaction of Syntax and Semantics: A Harmonic Grammar Account of Split Intransitivity

Géraldine Legendre, Yoshiro Miyata, and Paul Smolensky

Can the connectionist-derived description of grammatical knowledge embodied in the Harmonic Grammar (HG) formalism advance our understanding of linguistic phenomena that have proved problematic when this knowledge is described with symbolic, rule-based formalisms? In this chapter, we look at a basic component of syntactic structure, intransitive verbs. In many languages, intransitive verbs split into two classes that behave differently in select syntactic contexts. The split has clear semantic components, but capturing the complexity of the relations between semantic features and syntactic behavior is a major challenge in languages like French where the split actually differs from one context to another. This chapter reports a detailed study of French split intransitivity phenomena, arguing that HG provides a vehicle for expressing the semantic factors while accounting for the full syntactic complexity. This example allows us to illustrate how HG derives from a multilevel description of a single system: at the lower level, a network employing distributed representations, and at the higher level, a simpler network using local representations. A connectionist learning algorithm is used to extract from the French data numerical strengths for the HG constraints. These results contribute to link ③ of Figure 6 in Chapter 2's Integrated Connectionist/Symbolic Cognitive Architecture (ICS) map.

Contents

1 THE PROBLEM

1.1 Split intransitivity crosslinguistically

Of central importance in the interaction of syntax and semantics is the **argument structure** of verbs, which relates two types of roles: the **syntactic roles** of a verb's arguments in a sentence, and the **semantic roles** of those arguments' referents as participants in the described event (see Section 1:3.3).[1] Perhaps not surprisingly, given its central role in language, understanding argument structure has turned out to be a challenging problem, and attention has therefore often focused on the simplest case: events with a single participant described by intransitive verbs.

Intuitively, many intransitive verbs can be thought of as deriving from more basic transitive verbs in one of two ways: either of the two transitive verb's arguments can be eliminated. In the transitive sentence *Josh ate pasta,* we can omit the patient semantic role filled by *pasta,* getting the intransitive sentence *Josh ate.* Alternatively, in the transitive sentence *Karen rolled the ball,* we can delete the agent semantic role filled by *Karen* and get *the ball rolled.* While intransitive *eat* takes an agent as its single argument, intransitive *roll* takes a patient. In both cases, the single argument appears in the syntactic role of subject of the intransitive verb,[2] so the two verbs differ in the way they pair syntactic and semantic roles. Thus, with respect to argument structure, the class of intransitive verbs is not homogeneous, but **split**. Verbs like *eat* with agentive subjects are called **unergative**, and those like *roll* with patient subjects are called **unaccusative** (Perlmutter 1978); the phenomenon of split intransitivity is often referred to as 'unaccusativity'.

Split intransitivity would hardly be worth a great deal of thought if the characterization in the previous paragraph were truly accurate. In fact, however, the split among intransitive verbs is only partially correlated with the semantic agent/patient distinction; and since many intransitive verbs do not even have a transitive form, the conceptualization of the previous paragraph is also quite incomplete.

The crucial missing ingredient is the **syntactic** component of the split. For it's not just that the single argument of intransitive *roll* has **semantic** properties similar to those of the object of the corresponding transitive (i.e., filling the role of patient): it also bears syntactic similarities to an object, despite appearing as a subject.

Thus, it often happens that sentence constructions that allow objects but not subjects of transitives will also allow the arguments of unaccusative intransitives like *roll,*

[1] For example, the argument structure of the passive verb *was kissed* tells us that in the sentence *John was kissed by Mary,* the argument of *was kissed* filling the syntactic role of subject – *John* – plays the semantic role of *patient* in the correct semantic interpretation: the sentence describes an event in which John *receives* a kiss. The other argument of the verb, *Mary,* plays the semantic role of *agent,* characterized by volitional control over the event.

[2] This is true of many languages (like English and French), but not all; such variation is a primary topic of Chapter 15.

but not those of unergative intransitives like *eat*. One theoretical characterization of this difference is that for unaccusatives like *roll*, the single argument is a subject on the **surface level**, but at a **deep level** of representation, it is an object;[3] for unergatives like *eat*, however, the argument is a subject at both the surface and deep levels (Perlmutter 1978). Thus, the split is encoded syntactically in the **deep grammatical relation** of the argument: an object for unaccusatives, a subject for unergatives. For those syntactic constructions sensitive to deep grammatical relations, the argument of an unaccusative verb will behave like the object of a transitive verb, because at the deep level it *is* an object.

This syntactic approach to split intransitivity is schematically displayed in an early Government-Binding Theory form (Burzio 1986) in (1), which shows the two different syntactic roles in d(eep)-structure.

(1) A syntactically encoded unaccusative/unergative distinction

a. Transitive verb: $[_S$ NP $[_{VP}$ V NP]]

b. Unergative intransitive verb: $[_S$ NP $[_{VP}$ V]]

c. Unaccusative intransitive verb: $[_S$ $[_{VP}$ V NP]]

While transitive verbs take two noun phrase (NP) arguments, a subject and a direct object, unergative and unaccusative verbs take only one: a deep subject in the case of unergatives, a deep direct object in the case of unaccusatives.

The interrelation of the semantic and syntactic factors at play in split intransitivity is quite complex: Box 1 provides relevant background. The question is, can the kinds of interacting tendencies visible in this phenomenon be given a grammatical account with the help of Harmonic Grammar (HG)?

As an empirical testing ground in natural language for HG, there is much to recommend split intransitivity, particularly as manifest in French (Legendre, Miyata, and Smolensky 1990a, b, 1991; Smolensky, Legendre, and Miyata 1992): (i) Split intransitivity is a fundamental aspect of a central issue in syntax/semantics: argument structure, the relation between the syntactic roles of the arguments of verbs and the semantic roles of the event participants they designate. (ii) It is a phenomenon well studied by theoretical linguists (in particular, in French: Legendre 1986, 1989, 1992; Ruwet 1989; Labelle 1992; Cummins 1996). (iii) Traditional grammatical methods have failed to provide a completely satisfactory theory of split intransitivity, leaving opportunities for significant new contributions. (iv) The phenomenon sometimes exhibits strong, complex interactions of multiple simple constraints, each reflected in the data only as a "tendency"—it thus lends itself to one of the strengths of HG. (v) In addition to semantic factors, the phenomenon crucially involves syntactic structure (in our view), so it affords access to structural constraints, so central to grammar. (vi) The relevant syntactic distinction is, however, quite simple, and is accessible to initial work in a new syntactic framework.

[3] This parallels the sense in which, for a sentence like *the ball was rolled by Karen* in the passive voice, *the ball* is a subject on the surface, but an object at a deeper representational level. Passives and unaccusatives often exhibit similar syntactic behavior, contrasting with the active voice, *Karen rolled the ball.*

Box 1. Syntactic and semantic factors in verb-argument structure: Split intransitivity

In practically every language in which intransitive verbs have been carefully examined, it appears that they split into two classes, depending on whether their single argument behaves like the subject or like the direct object of a transitive verb. In some languages, the distinction among intransitive verbs is directly reflected in the morphological marking of the verb. In the Native American Siouan language Lakhóta, the two arguments of a transitive verb are directly encoded into the verb—**cross-referenced**—via a morpheme *X* corresponding to the subject and a morpheme *Y* corresponding to the direct object. Intransitive verbs contain a single morpheme corresponding to their single argument: for one class of verbs, the morpheme is *X*; for the other, *Y*. Verbs taking the *X* marking typically, but not always, have arguments that are agentive (i.e., volitional)—just as the subject of a transitive verb tends to be agentive. In contrast, the *Y*-taking verbs typically, but not always, have a nonagentive argument (Williamson 1979; Legendre and Rood 1992).[4]

In languages with impoverished inflectional morphology such as English and French, there is no immediately visible distinction among intransitive verbs; yet there are nearly always certain syntactic phenomena where a distinction is manifest. Such distinctions involve the **distributional properties** of different intransitive verbs: the pattern of syntactic contexts where they can and cannot be found. For example, French has a construction in which the main verb *croire* 'believe' occurs with a participial complement, corresponding to *I believe John gone.* In the French construction, with a transitive verb, only the direct object—not the subject—can appear after *croire.*[5] Mirroring this distinction, intransitive verbs split into two classes: a verb in the first class is acceptable in this construction (its argument has the same distribution as the direct object of a transitive verb, with respect to this construction at least); a verb in the second class is unacceptable in the *croire* construction (its argument behaves syntactically—that is, is distributed—like the subject of a transitive verb).[6]

The same distinction can be observed in a half-dozen other syntactic constructions in French (Legendre 1986, 1989, 1992). Typically, as in the *croire* case, the construction is acceptable when applied to the direct object but not to the subject of a transitive verb. The intransitive verbs are then seen to be split into two classes by the

[4] Examples illustrating the Lakhóta cross-referencing system (Legendre and Rood 1992):

	active	*stative*	*active intrans.*	*stative intrans.*	*transitive*
'I'	wa-	ma-	wa-psíča	ma-xwá	ma-yá-tke 'you kill me'
'you'	ya-	ni	'I jumped'	'I am sleepy'	I(stative)-you(active)-kill

[5] For example, *je croyais le pont détruit par une bombe* 'I believed the bridge [to be] destroyed by a bomb' is grammatical but **je croyais la bombe détruit le pont* 'I believed the bomb [to have] destroyed the bridge' is ungrammatical (*détruire* is strictly transitive). '*' marks an ungrammatical sentence.

[6] For example, *je croyais le pont effondré* 'I believed the bridge [to have] collapsed' is grammatical, but **je croyais le pont explosé* 'I believed the bridge [to have] exploded' is ungrammatical (*s'effondrer* and *exploser* are strictly intransitive). The reflexive marker *s'* that is obligatory in infinitive *s'effondrer* may not appear when embedded under *croire.* This is an additional constraint we may ignore here.

construction. Some intransitive verbs, called **unaccusative**, are acceptable in the construction; that is, their single argument behaves like the direct object of a transitive verb. Other intransitive verbs, called **unergative**, are unacceptable in the construction; their single argument behaves like the subject of a transitive verb. The construction itself is a **diagnostic test for unaccusativity**.

A variety of theoretical approaches have shed light on split intransitivity phenomena. Some analysts have emphasized the parallel described in the previous paragraph between the split among intransitives in diagnostic contexts and the corresponding split in behavior of the subject and direct object of transitives. They propose a **deep syntactic distinction**, claiming in essence that the argument structure of unaccusative intransitive verbs requires the argument to be a deep direct object, rather than a deep subject, which is required for unergative intransitives (Perlmutter 1978, 1983, 1989; Rosen 1984; Burzio 1986).

In such treatments, having a deep direct object argument is often claimed to be a necessary condition for an intransitive verb to be well formed in a given diagnostic (e.g., *croire*) construction. If a deep object were sufficient for well-formedness, each verb in a language would behave uniformly across all diagnostic contexts: all verbs with deep objects would be good in all contexts, and all with deep subjects bad. But this is not the case. The problem of **unaccusativity mismatches** is that different constructions do not split the intransitive verbs in exactly the same way. In addition to deep grammatical function, the acceptability of a diagnostic sentence is often sensitive to semantic properties—both of the intransitive verb and of its argument (Legendre 1989; Levin and Rappaport 1989; Van Valin 1990; Zaenen 1993; Levin and Rappaport Hovav 1995). The effects of the semantic factors differ from one diagnostic context to another—this is one reason that different diagnostics produce different splits. Thus, the deep syntactic approach must incorporate an explicit account of the interacting semantic factors if it is to give a complete account of the phenomena, including the complex pattern of mismatches.

The semantic factors that crosslinguistically appear to influence well-formedness in diagnostic contexts for unaccusativity include the animacy of the referent and whether the action is volitional (or agentive). Most important, though, are **aspectual** factors. The aspectual properties of a verb pertain to how the event it describes unfolds in time; for example, a verb is **telic** if the event has a definitive endpoint (*leave*), **stative** if it describes an enduring property (*love*), and **progressivizable** if it describes an ongoing activity (*live*). Largely aspectual criteria define a widely employed verb classification system that often correlates with unaccusativity. These **Aktionsart classes** (Vendler 1967; Dowty 1991) are as follows:

State verbs. Enduring property: *exist, stink, resemble, love, be clever*

Activity verbs. Enduring action: *run, sit, look, eat, rotate*

Achievement verbs. Change of state: *freeze, explode, begin, receive, collapse*

Accomplishment verbs. Change of state resulting from action: *destroy, boil, see, build, kill*

Box 1

These brief descriptions of each class are extremely crude; classifying a verb—or more generally, determining its aspectual properties—is actually a very complex matter involving a battery of diagnostic tests.[7]

The strong relations between a verb's semantic/aspectual properties and its status relative to the unergative/unaccusative distinction motivate another line of work that attempts to establish that the semantic/aspectual factors alone can provide a complete account, and that a deep syntactic distinction is unnecessary (e.g., Van Valin 1990; Dowty 1991; Zaenen 1993). This controversy cannot be separated from such central and far-reaching issues as whether syntactic representations do in fact have multiple levels. But whatever account ultimately emerges, it must cope with the great complexity of the interaction between semantic and syntactic factors that underlie split intransitivity. It is the rich syntax-semantics interaction that is the focus of the HG approach developed in this chapter.

1.2 Split intransitivity in French

Syntactically, the unaccusative/unergative distinction is motivated by the cross-linguistic fact that in certain syntactic contexts in which a verb may be embedded, the intransitive verbs of one class are acceptable while those of the other class are not. These syntactic environments are called **diagnostic contexts** (or **tests**) **for unaccusativity**; we will simply call them 'contexts' or 'tests'. An example from French from Legendre 1986, object raising (OR),[8] is illustrated in (2).

(2) Object raising with *faire*

a. **Une souris** est facile à faire ***tuer*** à un gros chat.
A mouse is easy to make a fat cat ***kill***.

b. ***Un gros chat** est facile à faire ***tuer*** une souris.
A fat cat is easy to make ***kill*** a mouse.

c. **Une souris** est facile à faire ***mourir***.
A mouse is easy to make ***die***.

d. ***Une souris** est facile à faire ***courir***.
A mouse is easy to make ***run***.

Each diagnostic context can be viewed as a sentence frame with two slots, typographically identified in (2): an **argument** slot for an NP that is an argument of the verb filling the ***predicate*** slot. French (but not English) OR exemplifies the following

[7] For example, one diagnostic for progressivity is the ability of a verb *V* to appear in the progressive: in English, *he is V-ing*, in French, *il est en train de V*.

[8] The term 'object raising' refers to the raising in (2a) of *une souris* 'a mouse' to the higher clause *une souris est facile …* 'a mouse is easy …' from the embedded or lower clause *faire tuer [une souris] à un gros chat* 'to make a fat cat kill [a mouse]'. This raising of the object of *faire tuer* is what distinguishes the OR construction from the alternative *il est facile de faire tuer une souris à un gros chat* 'it is easy to make a fat cat kill a mouse'; a dummy subject *il* 'it' is the subject of the higher clause, and *une souris* remains in the lower clause. (For more discussion, see Legendre 1986.)

characteristic property of diagnostic contexts: when a transitive verb is inserted in the predicate slot, the acceptability of the sentence depends on whether the argument slot is filled by the deep subject or the deep direct object of the verb. In (2a), an acceptable sentence results when the direct object of *tuer* 'kill'—*une souris* 'a mouse'—appears in the argument slot, but in (2b) an unacceptable sentence results when the subject appears instead—*un gros chat* 'a fat cat'. Paralleling this contrast between transitive subject and direct object is a contrast in the behavior of two classes of intransitive verbs. The sole argument of *mourir* 'die' is acceptable in the argument slot (2c), while the argument of *courir* 'run' is not (2d). Since the argument of *mourir* is acceptable, like the direct object of *tuer*, it is classified as unaccusative; since the argument of *courir* is unacceptable, like the subject of *tuer*, it is classified as unergative.

Diagnostic contexts vary crosslinguistically, although they are often shared between closely related languages such as French and Italian. In English, it turns out, diagnostic contexts for unaccusativity are few in number,[9] but this is by no means the case crosslinguistically. The subject of much recent research in syntax and semantics because they reveal basic properties of verbs, unaccusativity contexts are crosslinguistically a rich source of interesting patterns. Of central concern is the problem of **unaccusativity mismatches**, which are of two general types. First, across languages, synonymous verbs may be unaccusative in some languages and unergative in others (see Chapter 20). What is relevant here, however, are the language-internal mismatches: the existence of intransitive verbs that behave unaccusatively in some contexts and unergatively in others.

A good language in which to study language-internal unaccusativity mismatches is French. Legendre (1989) identifies 10 diagnostic contexts in French and argues that a necessary and sufficient condition for identifying a verb as unaccusative is that it behave unaccusatively in at least one of them. These contexts display a highly complex pattern of mismatches. It is a subset of these data for which we provide an HG account in this chapter. For this initial study, we selected, out of the 10 diagnostic contexts, the 4 that identify the largest numbers of unaccusative verbs. These 4 contexts are indicated in Table 1; the first is OR, illustrated in (2).[10]

[9] One English diagnostic context, according to Levin and Rappaport (1989; Levin and Rappaport Hovav 1995), is the **resultative** construction. Under the resultative reading 'the door was shut as a result of rolling', the sentence *the door rolled shut* is acceptable, while under the corresponding reading 'Sara was exhausted as a result of working', **Sara worked exhausted* is unacceptable. This parallels the contrast with transitive verbs between *Sara wiped the table clean* ('the table was clean as a result of wiping') and **Sara wiped the table exhausted* ('Sara was exhausted as a result of wiping the table'). The argument of intransitive *roll* behaves like the direct object of *wipe*, while the argument of *work* behaves like the subject of *wipe*: *roll* is unaccusative while *work* is unergative.

[10] The remaining three tests distinguish unaccusative and unergative verbs as follows. For the *croire* construction (CR), a sentence is grammatical or not depending on whether the verb of the embedded clause *la souris déjà morte* 'the mouse already dead' is unaccusative or unergative. The crucial verb *mourir* 'die' appears in the participial form *morte* 'dead'. The participial absolute (PA) employs an adjunct clause *la souris enfin morte* 'the mouse finally [having] died', adjoined to a main clause *le chat s'endormit au coin du feu* 'the cat fell asleep by the fire', providing additional information relevant to the event described; the crucial verb *mourir* again appears in the participial form *morte*. The reduced relative (RR) construction is the reduced counterpart of *la souris qui est morte hier à été trouvée* ...'the mouse that died

Table 1. French diagnostic contexts for unaccusativity

Context	French example	English gloss
Object raising (OR)	**Une souris** est facile à faire *mourir*.	**A mouse** is easy to make ***die***.
Croire 'believe' (CR)	Je croyais **la souris** déjà *morte*.	I believed **the mouse** already ***dead***.
Participial absolute (PA)	**La souris** enfin *morte*, le chat s'endormit au coin du feu.	**The mouse** finally [having] ***died***, the cat fell asleep by the fire.
Reduced relative (RR)	**La souris** *morte* hier a été trouvée à moitié dévorée.	**The mouse** [who] ***died*** yesterday was found half eaten.

Focusing on mismatches, several studies have argued that unaccusativity phenomena can be accounted for on purely semantic grounds by assuming that each diagnostic context involves a simple semantic restriction such as a hard constraint on the value of some semantic feature. Two examples, from Italian and Dutch, are described in (3).

(3) Semantic theories of split intransitivity

a. According to Van Valin (1990), auxiliary selection[11] in Italian is sensitive only to the aspectual classification of verbs proposed in Vendler 1967 and elaborated upon in Dowty 1979 (Box 1)—state, achievement, and accomplishment verbs select 'be' while activity verbs select 'have'—and to account for these data, the structural unergative/unaccusative distinction employed in Rosen 1984 and Perlmutter 1989 is therefore unnecessary.

b. Zaenen (1993) argues that auxiliary selection in Dutch is sensitive only to telicity[12] while impersonal passivization[13] in Dutch is sensitive only to volitionality of the argument—and that a nonsemantically based structural unergative/unaccusative distinction, as argued for in the Perlmutter 1978 account of these data, is again unnecessary.

The semantic/aspectual approach may be sufficient to characterize certain Italian and

yesterday was found ...', which has a full relative clause introduced by *qui* 'that'. This construction is featured in Bever's (1970) famous 'garden path' sentence: *the horse raced past the barn fell* (see Section 2:8 and Chapter 19).

[11] Verbs in many languages split according to whether they **select** the auxiliary *have* or *be* in constructions corresponding to *he has lied* versus *he is come*. Italian and Dutch have such a past tense construction, but the verbs selecting *be* in the two languages are not the same. For intransitive verbs, selecting *be* is one of the most-discussed putative tests for unaccusativity, especially in Romance languages. See Chapter 20.

[12] Recall that a **telic** verb describes an event with a definitive temporal endpoint (Box 1).

[13] Corresponding to a canonical passive like *many scones were eaten*, there exists in many languages the equivalent of *there is eaten many scones*, with a dummy subject: this is the **impersonal passive**. In Dutch, with a volitional argument as in *de kinderen lachen altijd* 'the children always laugh', there is a (roughly synonymous) impersonal passive form *er wordt altijd door de kinderen gelachen* 'it is always laughed by the children'. But with a nonvolitional argument, while *de kinderen groeien altijd erg snel* 'the children always grow very fast' is fine, the impersonal passive form is unacceptable: **er wordt altiijd door de kinderen erg snel gegroeid* 'it is always grown very fast by the children' (Rosen 1984, 59).

Dutch unaccusativity phenomena that had previously been analyzed in syntactic terms (but see Chapter 20). However, our data show that semantic/aspectual distinctions cannot *by themselves* characterize the French phenomena identified as syntactic diagnostics for unaccusativity in Table 1—at least, the simple semantic restrictions that have been proposed for other languages clearly do not work for French (Legendre 1992).[14]

Tables 2 and 3 suggest some of the difficulties. Table 2 illustrates that for each semantic/aspectual property, one can find a number of acceptable and unacceptable examples of OR in French. This is true of the other diagnostics as well.

Table 2. Semantic properties and the object raising unaccusativity test

Semantic/aspectual property (see Box 1)	**Object raising**			
	Acceptable		**Unacceptable**	
Accomplishment verb	s'asseoir	'sit down'	aller	'go'
Achievement verb	fondre	'melt'	s'écraser	'crash'
Activity verb	pleurer	'cry'	jouer	'play'
State verb	s'évanouir	'faint'	être	'be'
Telic verb	s'asseoir	'sit down'	aller	'go'
Atelic verb	fondre	'melt'	boire	'drink'
Volitional argument	s'asseoir	'sit down'	aller	'go'
Nonvolitional argument	sécher	'dry'	exister	'exist'
Animate argument	s'asseoir	'sit down'	aller	'go'
Inanimate argument	sécher	'dry'	s'écraser	'crash'

On the other hand, while they are not sufficient by themselves to provide simple semantic hard constraints to account for the data (Table 3), the argument features volitionality (VO) and animacy (AN), and the predicate features telicity (TE) and progressivizability (PR), show strong tendencies to influence acceptability in diagnostic contexts (Legendre 1992). These tendencies are implicit in Table 4, which displays the basic data set with which we are concerned in this chapter. The four features VO, AN, TE, and PR are the semantic/aspectual properties we employ in our account.

[14] More specifically, a number of the claims in Van Valin 1990 have been tested, with results such as these: his account is silent concerning approximately 70% of our data, since those verbs fall outside his verb classification based on the Aktionsart classes (Box 1); the putatively universal tendency of activity verbs to behave unergatively is indeed fairly well respected in French, but the other Aktionsart classes show only weak tendencies; and the claimed tendencies for the aspectual property telicity are observed only moderately, in one direction. Testing a proposal in Dowty 1979, it was discovered, for example, that the claim that atelicity and agentivity together "definitely" entail unergative behavior is fairly well corroborated, but the claim that telicity and nonagentivity together entail unaccusative behavior is not well respected. An adequate treatment of these proposals and others is well beyond the scope of this chapter, especially since our results show that the phenomena are much more complex than has been suggested in the literature, including Van Valin 1990 and Zaenen 1993 (see Legendre 1992 for further discussion).

Table 3. Semantic properties and unaccusativity tests

Predicate		Argument		Predicate		Tests			
		AN	VO	TE	PR	OR	CR	PA	RR
Unaccusatives									
fondre	'melt'	–	–	–	+	+	+	+	+
s'évanouir	'faint'	+	–	+	+	+	+	+	+
partir	'leave'	+	+	+	+	?	+	+	+
sortir	'go out'	+	+	+	?	+?	+	+	+
Unergatives									
travailler	'work'	+	+	–	+	–	–	–	–
méditer	'meditate'	+	+	–	+	–	–	–	–
éternuer	'sneeze'	+	–	–	–	?	–	–	–
empirer	'worsen'	–	–	+	+	–?	–	–	–

Our first descriptive goal is to account for the acceptability judgments exhibited in Table 4. In this table, each row gives the acceptability values for four sentences, differing in the syntactic construction employed: these are the diagnostic contexts given in Table 1. The symbols '+', '+?', '?', '–?', and '–' respectively denote 'acceptable', 'marginally acceptable', 'of indeterminate acceptability', 'marginally unacceptable', and 'unacceptable'. (The judgments are those of several mutually consistent informants, one of whom is Legendre.) At the right end of each row is the identity of the embedded intransitive verb or predicate; it is preceded by the values of the four semantic/aspectual features (in the order VO, AN, TE, PR) characterizing the verb and its argument. The rows are sorted, roughly from most unergative to most unaccusative behavior. Table 4 contains 190 rows (argument-predicate pairs) involving 143 different predicates (intransitive verbs), with a range of semantically appropriate arguments. This constitutes acceptability judgments for $190 \times 4 = 760$ different sentence types.

All the components of a sentence's structural description that are relevant to our analysis are summarized in (4) and Table 5 (the last column is for use below in Section 3). The deep grammatical relation (**DGR**) of the argument (subject or object) is 'hidden' structure assigned by the grammar.

(4) The basic data set

a. A total of 760 sentence types

b. s = context + **argument** + ***predicate*** + [deep grammatical relation] (typeface conventions of Table 1)

Accounting for the French data appears to require combining syntactic and semantic restrictions in a complex way. We will argue that this capability is just what

Table 4. The basic data set

OR	CR	PA	RR	Feats.	Predicate	OR	CR	PA	RR	Feats.	Predicate	OR	CR	PA	RR	Feats.	Predicate
−	−	−	−	−−−+	sévir	−	+	+	+	++−−?	se réfugier	+	−	−	−	++++	réagir
−	−	−	−	−−−+	résister	−	+	+	+	+++−	surgir	+	−	−	−	++++	céder
−	−	−	−	−−−+	persister	−?	−	−	−	−−−?	subsister	+	+?	+?	+?	−−−+	se modifier
−	−	−	−	−−−+	continuer	−?	−	−	−	−−−+	empirer	+	+?	+?	+?	−−++	dissiper
−	−	−	−	−−+−	ouvrir sur	−?	−	−	−	++−+	sourire	+	+?	+	+?	−−−+	peler
−	−	−	−	−+−−	exister	−?	−	−	−	++−+	ronchonner	+	+?	+	+	−−−+	vieillir
−	−	−	−	−+−+	souffrir	−?	−	−	−	++−+	exploser	+	+	−	+?	−−++	pâlir
−	−	−	−	−+−+	persévérer	−?	−	−	−	++++	changer d'avis	+	+	+?	+?	−−−+	se disperser
−	−	−	−	+−−+	marcher	−?	−	−	−	++++	s'esquiver	+	+	+?	+?	−+++	changer
−	−	−	−	++−−	survivre	−?	−?	?	?	++++	s'enfuir	+	+	+?	+	−−−+	pousser
−	−	−	−	++−−	succéder	−?	+?	−	+?	−+−−?	peler	+	+	+?	+	−−+−	éclater
−	−	−	−	++−−	subsister	−?	+?	+	+	++++	venir	+	+	+	+	−−−+?	jaillir
−	−	−	−	++−−	régner	−?	+	−	+?	?+++	pâlir	+	+	+	+	−−−+?	exploser
−	−	−	−	++−−	persister	−?	+	−	+	−+−+	grandir	+	+	+	+	−−−+	tomber
−	−	−	−	++−−	mendier	−?	+	+	+	−−−+	se retirer	+	+	+	+	−−−+	sombrer
−	−	−	−	++−−	être	−?	+	+	+	−−++	s'ouvrir	+	+	+	+	−−−+	sécher
−	−	−	−	++−−	(dés)obéir	−?	+	+	+	−+−+	geler	+	+	+	+	−−−+	s'agrandir
−	−	−	−	++−−	cesser	−?	+	+	+	−++−	parvenir	+	+	+	+	−−−+	rouiller
−	−	−	−	++−−?	déambuler	−?	+	+	+	++−+	se retirer	+	+	+	+	−−−+	rôtir
−	−	−	−	++−?	exagérer	?	−	−	−	++−−	éternuer	+	+	+	+	−−−+	ralentir
−	−	−	−	++−+	travailler	?	−	−	−	++++	reculer	+	+	+	+	−−−+	paraître
−	−	−	−	++−+	téléphoner	?	+	+	+	−+−+	vieillir	+	+	+	+	−−−+	noircir
−	−	−	−	++−+	souffler	?	+	+	+	−+−+	brunir	+	+	+	+	−−−+	monter
−	−	−	−	+−+−	sévir	?	+	+	+	−++−	naître	+	+	+	+	−−−+	mariner
−	−	−	−	++−+	sautiller	?	+	+	+	−+++	guérir	+	+	+	+	−−−+	geler
−	−	−	−	++−+	rouspéter	?	+	+	+	++−+	monter	+	+	+	+	−−−+	fondre
−	−	−	−	++−+	rêver	?	+	+	+	++−+	descendre	+	+	+	+	−−−+	fermer
−	−	−	−	++−+	résister	?	+	+	+	+++−	entrer	+	+	+	+	−−−+	disparaître
−	−	−	−	++−+	répondre	?	+	+	+	+++−	arriver	+	+	+	+	−−−+	descendre
−	−	−	−	++−+	réfléchir	?	+	+	+	+++−	apparaître sur scène	+	+	+	+	−−−+	cuire
−	−	−	−	++−+	ralentir	?	+	+	+	++++	partir	+	+	+	+	−−−+	cristalliser
−	−	−	−	++−+	penser	+?	−	−	−	−−−+	durer	+	+	+	+	−−−+	brunir
−	−	−	−	++−+	parler	+?	−	−	−	+++?	capituler	+	+	+	+	−−−+	brûler
−	−	−	−	++−+	mentir	+?	−	−	−	−+−+?	rougir	+	+	+	+	−−−+	bouillir
−	−	−	−	++−+	méditer	+?	−	−	−	−+−+?	parler sous la torture	+	+	+	+	−−−+	baisser
−	−	−	−	++−+	jouer	+?	−	−	−	+++−	trébucher	+	+	+	+	−−−+	augmenter
−	−	−	−	++−+	jongler	+?	+?	+	+?	−−++	s'éloigner	+	+	+	+	−−+−	entrer
−	−	−	−	++−+	insister	+?	+?	+	+?	++−+	s'éloigner	+	+	+	+	−−+−	apparaître
−	−	−	−	++−+	hésiter	+?	+	+	+?	−−−+	surgir	+	+	+	+	−−+?	sauter
−	−	−	−	++−+	gémir	+?	+	+	+	−−−+	sortir	+	+	+	+	−−++?	arriver
−	−	−	−	++−+	errer	+?	+	+	+	−−+−	venir	+	+	+	+	−−++	s´éteindre
−	−	−	−	++−+	danser	+?	+	+	+	−−++	s'effacer	+	+	+	+	−−++	s'envoler
−	−	−	−	++−+	continuer	+?	+	+	+	−++−	tomber	+	+	+	+	−−++	se casser
−	−	−	−	++−+	cogner	+?	+	+	+	++−−	disparaître	+	+	+	+	−−++	se briser
−	−	−	−	++−+	circuler	+?	+	+	+	++−?	se dissimuler	+	+	+	+	−−++	parvenir
−	−	−	−	++−+	agir	+?	+	+	+	++−+	sombrer	+	+	+	+	−−++	partir
−	−	−	−	++++	sauter	+?	+	+	+	+++??	se blottir	+	+	+	+	−−++	naître
−	−	−	−	++++	renoncer	+?	+	+	+	+++?+?	se recroqueviller	+	+	+	+	−−++	guérir
−	−	−	−	++−+	trottiner	+?	+	+	+	+++?	sortir	+	+	+	+	−−++	éclore
−	−	−	−	−+−−	durer	+?	+	+	+	++++	s'exiler	+	+	+	+	−−++	cicatriser
−	−	−	−	−+−−	boiter	+	−	−	−	−−−+	souffler	+	+	+	+	−−++	changer
−	−	−	−	−+−−	bégayer	+	−	−	−	−−−+	régner	+	+	+	+	−−++	casser
−	−	−	−	−+−−?	baisser	+	−	−	−	−−−+	reculer	+	+	+	+	++−+	se réunir
−	−	−	−	++−−	balbutier	+	−	−	−	−−−+	courir	+	+	+	+	++++	se noyer
−	−	−	−	++−+	flâner	+	−	−	−	−−−+	couler	+	+	+	+	−+−+	grossir
−	−	−	−	++−+	courir	+	−	−	−	−−−+	circuler	+	+	+	+	−+++	s'évanouir
−	−	−	−	+++−	aller	+	−	−	−	−−−+	cesser	+	+	+	+	−+++	mourir
−	−	−	−	+++−?	courir	+	−	−	−	−+−+	tousser	+	+	+	+	++−+	se décourager
−	−	−	+	−−−−	rester	+	−	−	−	−+−+	régresser	+	+	+	+	++−+	se cacher
−	?	+?	?	++−−	tomber	+	−	−	−	−+−+	pleurer	+	+	+	+	++++	s'évader
−	+	+	+	−+−−	décéder	+	−	−	−	−+−+	marcher	+	+	+	+	++++	se disperser
−	+	+	+	−++−	périr	+	−	−	−	++−+	se taire	+	+	+	+	++++	s'asseoir
−	+	+	+	++−−	s'effacer	+	−	−	−	++−+	se saoûler						
−	+	+	+	++−−	rester	+	−	−	−	++−+	rire						

Features: Semantic/aspectual features, ordered: Argument: VOlitional ANimate; Predicate: TElic PRogressivizable
Tests: OR (object raising); CR (*croire* 'believe' construction); PA (participial absolute); RR (reduced relative)

Table 5. HNet encoding of the basic data set

S component	Description	HNet
Context	No internal structure; label only: OR, CR, PA, RR	4 input units
Argument	Two semantic features: ±AN, ±VO	2 input units
Predicate	Two aspectual features: ±TE, ±PR [predicate *F*]	2 input units
	Identity: *agir*, ... [predicate *ID*]	143 input units
Hidden structure	Deep grammatical relation: 1 (subject) or 2 (direct object)[15]	2 hidden units
Grammaticality	Graded between 0 and 1; discretized to +, +?, ?, –?, –	1 output unit

HG offers. Replacing the all-or-none categories and constraints used in purely symbolic accounts with soft constraints that formalize the semantic and syntactic tendencies evidenced in the data allows the HG account to achieve a degree of coverage of unaccusativity data, including a complex pattern of mismatches, that to our knowledge is unparalleled in the existing literature. At the same time, the new approach readily addresses two aspects of this problem that are quite difficult to capture naturally in a hard-constraint formalism.

(5) Gradedness of split intransitivity

a. *The graded character of the unaccusative/unergative categories.* Some intransitive French verbs behave unaccusatively in 6 of the 10 contexts, others in 4, and still others in only 1.[16] Clearly the condition proposed in Legendre 1989—an intransitive verb is unaccusative if and only if it behaves unaccusatively in at least one diagnostic context—is failing to capture the fact that "some verbs are more unaccusative than others," an aspect of the phenomenon that is formally expressed in and crucial to our HG account.

b. *The graded character of the acceptability judgments in diagnostic contexts.* Our account formally predicts not only the polarity of acceptability judgments, but also their strength. While we admit that the accuracy of our account in predicting judgment strengths can stand improvement, it is nonetheless a virtue of the HG approach that it makes precise, falsifiable predictions about gradations of acceptability.

[15] The notations '1' and '2' are taken from Relational Grammar (e.g., Perlmutter 1983; Rosen 1984), a grammar formalism in which much of the foundational research on unaccusativity was conducted; this framework will appear again below.

[16] It is striking that the verbs that are commonly assumed to be prototypical unaccusatives because of their semantic properties actually behave unaccusatively in the fewest diagnostic contexts. While *exister* 'exist' and *être* 'be' are strong examples of patient-taking verbs, *exister* behaves unaccusatively in only one context and *être* in only two.

2 A Harmonic Grammar account

In this section, we give a high-level description of an HG account of French split intransitivity. In the next section, we derive this account from assumptions about its connectionist realization.

2.1 Review of Harmonic Grammar

In its most intuitive form, the central idea of HG is to replace 'hard' constraints on well-formedness of the form (6a) with 'soft' constraints of the form (6b).

(6) Hard versus soft constraints

a. Condition *X* must never be violated in well-formed structures.

b. If condition *X* is violated, then the Harmony of the structure is diminished by H_X.

The differences between the old and new types of syntactic and lexical constraints in French are illustrated in (7) and (8), respectively.

(7) Syntactic constraints on DGRs

a. In the *croire* construction, the argument of the embedded verb can never be a deep subject (DGR = 1) in a well-formed sentence.

b. In the *croire* construction, if the argument of the embedded verb is a deep subject, then the well-formedness of the sentence is diminished by $H_{CR,1}$ (= 5.0).

(8) Lexical constraints on DGRs

a. The argument of *fondre* 'melt' must not be a deep subject.

b. If the argument of *fondre* is a deep subject, then the well-formedness of the sentence is diminished by $H_{fondre,1}$ (= 4.5).

The constraints are combined to predict the acceptability of a given sentence as in (9). (Explanation follows.)

(9) Harmony evaluation

a. $H = H_{nonstructural} + H_{structural}$

b. $H_{nonstructural}$ = sum of contributions from all applicable nonstructural constraints in grammar

c. $H_{structural}$ = maximum of H_1 and H_2

d. H_1/H_2 = sum of contributions from all applicable structural constraints in the grammar and lexicon, given assignment of DGR 1/2 (subject/object)

e. **Harmonic structural assignment**: The grammar and lexicon assign to an input *s* the structural description that maximizes total Harmony, *H*.

f. Grammaticality is a monotonically increasing function *f* of *H*,[17] such that

[17] That is, as *H* increases, grammaticality increases.

i. $H < 0$: ungrammatical ('−'),
ii. $H > 0$: grammatical ('+'),
iii. $H = 0$: marginal ('?').

A sentence's well-formedness, measured by the quantity H, consists of two parts, the **nonstructural Harmony** $H_{\text{nonstructural}}$ and the **structural Harmony** $H_{\text{structural}}$, which are simply added together numerically (9a). Each applicable nonstructural rule contributes a certain numerical value; the sum of these numbers is the nonstructural Harmony, which can be positive or negative (9b). The structural Harmony is a bit more complex, because the structural constraints refer to the DGR of the argument, which is of course not given by the input sentence directly: it must be assigned by the grammar, as follows. First, hypothesize that the DGR to be assigned is 2; then add up all the contributions of the applicable structural constraints, getting a number H_2 (9d). Then hypothesize that the DGR to be assigned is 1, and repeat, computing H_1. If H_2 is greater than H_1, then the grammar assigns DGR 2 to the argument, and the structural Harmony is H_2 (9c). Otherwise, the grammar assigns DGR 1 to the argument, and the structural Harmony is H_1. This means of assigning DGRs is a simple special case of the most fundamental principle of HG, expressed in (9e).[18] Finally, the acceptability of a sentence is computed from the total Harmony H. Qualitatively, this is described in (9f); the function f that provides the quantitative relation is a detail to be discussed below.

The general principle (9e) enables highly context-dependent structural assignments. In our HG account of unaccusativity, for example, the DGR assigned to the argument of the embedded predicate is sensitive to the syntactic construction in which it is embedded and the semantic features of the argument, as well as the aspectual features of the predicate and the identity of the predicate; the verb contributes a preference or bias for the DGR assigned to its arguments, but this is merely one of several factors all of which determine the Harmony-maximizing choice of DGR.

[18] It is interesting to note that HG involves a kind of numerical counting that Dowty also invokes in his account (Dowty 1991). His framework centers on prototypes for agent and patient that are each characterized by a list of properties or implications: a participant in an event is assigned the role of agent or patient (an important element of his account of unaccusativity, as well as many other phenomena) in such a way as to *maximize the number of correct implications.* This is analogous to the way an argument of a verb is assigned a role in our HG account—indeed, HG could be used to formalize Dowty's account as a collection of soft constraints such as 'If a volitional argument is assigned the role agent, add 1 to the well-formedness of the structure'. Generally, in HG, the number appearing in such a soft rule need not be 1; rather, it is a quantity specifying the strength of the implication 'agent ⇒ volitional' relative to other interacting soft constraints. Dowty in fact explicitly suggests that such relative weighting might be desired within his framework (p. 574). The formalism of HG systematically integrates numerical weighting with structural constraints. Thus, the form of computation employed in our HG account of unaccusativity, and even the content of many of the constraints, constitutes in many respects a systematic formalization of Dowty's account. It should be noted, however, that Dowty intends 'argument selection' to refer to generalizations concerning possible argument structures. In order to reflect this aspect of Dowty's analysis, the soft constraints that we take to define the well-formedness of structural descriptions of sentences would have to be reinterpreted as defining the well-formedness not of entire sentences but of argument structures in the lexicon.

2.2 The constraints

In our account of the data in Table 4, the grammar consists of 32 simple, general constraints. In addition, the lexicon contributes an unergative/unaccusative bias for each of the 143 verbs. The constraints are outlined in (10) and explained below.

(10) Grammatical constraints: 32

Structural constraints: 8

a. Context and DGR: 4
   i. The *croire* construction "strongly prefers" the argument of the embedded predicate to be a deep direct object.
   ii. If the context is CR and the DGR is 2, add 5.0 to the well-formedness.
   iii. CR & 2 ⇒ +5.0
   iv. *(CR & 1)
   v. [CR & 1 ⇒ −5.0]

b. Argument and DGR: 2
   i. Animate arguments "strongly prefer" to be deep subjects.
   ii. If the argument is +AN and the DGR is 2, add −4.4 to the well-formedness.
   iii. +AN & 2 ⇒ −4.4
   iv. [−AN & 2 ⇒ 0]

c. Predicate$_F$ and DGR: 2
   i. Telic predicates "prefer" their arguments to be deep direct objects.
   ii. +TE & 2 ⇒ +2.7

Nonstructural constraints: 24

d. Context and argument: 8
   CR & +AN ⇒ +5.1

e. Context and predicate$_F$: 8
   CR & +TE ⇒ +1.2

f. Predicate$_F$ and argument: 4
   +TE & +AN ⇒ +6.8

g. Context: 4
   CR ⇒ −10.6

The grammatical constraints consist of 8 structural and 24 nonstructural constraints. The structural constraints refer to the DGR borne by the argument of the embedded predicate: 4 of these constraints refer to the context, 2 to the semantic features of the argument (ANimacy, VOlitionality), and 2 to the aspectual features of the predicate (TElicity, PROgressivity).

One structural constraint referring to the syntactic context is given in four notations in (10a). In words, the constraint is loosely stated in (10a.i). The vague phrase "strongly prefers" is made precise in (10a.ii). (On the arbitrarily chosen scale of Harmony defined below, the minimal difference in well-formedness between completely acceptable and completely unacceptable sentences is about 3 units. Note that (10a.i–ii) restate (7a–b).) (10a.ii) is expressed more compactly in (10a.iii), which we will take to be the standard notation. This constraint can also be regarded as a soft version of the well-formedness filter in (10a.iv); the corresponding constraint appearing in our HG account, (10a.v), could also be viewed as a quantified markedness condition (recall Chapter 4).

In our account, for each structural constraint referring to 2-hood, like (10a.iii), there is a **mirror constraint**, like (10a.v), that refers to 1-hood, containing a numerical constant that is the negative of the constant appearing in the corresponding 2-hood constraint. (In the counts of constraints, we have not counted mirror constraints, which, as we will show, need never be explicitly used in grammatical computation.)[19] The other three structural constraints referring to contexts involve replacing CR with OR, PA, and RR, with each constraint having its own numerical parameter. (The differences across contexts of these and other context-sensitive constraints are what makes unaccusative mismatches possible.)

The remaining types of grammatical constraints are illustrated in (10b–g). An example of a structural constraint referring to the semantic features of the argument is given in (10b.i–iii), using three notations, parallel with (10a.i–iii). As indicated in (10b.iv), all our constraints referring to features apply only to the + value; features with value − do not contribute to the computation of well-formedness.

The other structural constraints that are central to the syntactic analysis of unaccusativity correspond in our account to the 143 lexical constraints stating the preferences of individual lexical items for the DGR of their argument. An example is illustrated in two notations in (11a). This lexical constraint, stated loosely in English in (11a), is stated more precisely using our standard notation in (11a.ii) (see also (8)). Note that this constraint says that, independent of its aspectual features, *fondre* 'melt' strongly prefers a 2; in our account, *fondre* is **structurally unaccusative**. By contrast, *éternuer* 'sneeze' is **structurally unergative**, as expressed in (11b.i–ii). There is one such constraint for each of the 143 predicates we consider.

[19] There is no loss of generality in assuming that the Harmony penalty of a structural constraint referring to DGR 1 is of equal magnitude and opposite sign relative to the corresponding constraint referring to DGR 2: 'mirror constraints. Suppose we start with a pair of such corresponding constraints referring to DGR 1 and 2, with Harmony penalties H_1 and H_2. Now change the penalties to $H_1' \equiv ½(H_1 - H_2)$, $H_2' \equiv ½(H_2 - H_1)$, and let $H_0 \equiv ½(H_1 + H_2)$. Clearly, now $H_1' = -H_2'$. Notice that $H_1' = H_1 - H_0$ and $H_2' = H_2 - H_0$. So in the modified grammar, the Harmony values contributed by these constraints are the same as before, but shifted down by H_0. But adding a constant to the Harmony values of all structures has no effect on determining which maximize Harmony. Now we can add H_0 to the Harmony penalty for each of the diagnostic contexts: $H_C' \equiv H_C + H_0$. Since every sentence instantiates exactly one context, this will just add H_0 to the total Harmony of every network state, canceling the Harmony shift resulting from the transition from $H_{1/2}$ to $H_{1/2}'$. Now not only relative but also absolute Harmony values with the mirror constraints ($H_{1/2}'$, H_C') are the same as for the original Harmony penalties ($H_{1/2}$, H_C).

(11) Lexical constraints: 143

Structural constraints on predicate$_{id}$ and DGR

a. Unaccusative bias

i. *Fondre* "strongly prefers" its argument to be a deep direct object.

ii. *fondre* & 2 ⇒ +4.5

b. Unergative bias

i. *Eternuer* "strongly prefers" its argument to be a deep subject.

ii. *éternuer* & 2 ⇒ −3.4

3 The Connectionist Realization

In this section, the HG account described in the previous section is formally derived from lower-level connectionist hypotheses. At the same time, we show how this account may be realized in connectionist networks; this allows automatic computation of the levels of grammaticality assigned by the grammar to the 760 sentences making up our basic data set (Table 4). More importantly, these networks enable automatic computation of the particular numerical strengths of the soft constraints defining a particular harmonic grammar.

3.1 The networks

In total, we will describe three connectionist networks for realizing HG. The first is the fundamental one, providing the most literal description, at the lowest level: we call it **LNet**. Next, we show how LNet can be redescribed, at a higher level of description; this description is *also* a network description: **HNet**. Since HNet and LNet are higher- and lower-level descriptions of the same system, the Harmony of a given linguistic representation is the same whether computed with the LNet or the HNet description. The final network we describe is different from HNet, but closely connected to it; it is called **NHet'**. Whereas the Harmony of a linguistic representation **s** in HNet is a distributed quantity, spread, as it were, over all the connections in HNet, in the new network, this same value—the Harmony of **s** in HNet—is localized in the activation of a single output unit. This makes it possible to train HNet' relatively easily, finding a set of weights that can be immediately converted to a set of weights for HNet such that the Harmony of **s** in HNet is the correct one to fit the observed acceptability level of the sentence that **s** represents. HNet' is just a convenient adaptation of HNet that makes it easier to fit the Harmony function to the data. The result is a set of automatically computed numbers that define the strengths of the HG constraints in the account of French split intransitivity presented in the previous section.

3.1.1 LNet

The fundamental ICS assumptions relevant to this analysis are synopsized in (12):

(12) Assumptions relating connectionist and symbolic descriptions of the harmonic grammar for French split intransitivity

a. Symbolic structural descriptions of sentences are approximate higher-level descriptions of the patterns of activity in a connectionist network LNet realizing the mental representations of those sentences. In particular, the argument of an intransitive verb fills, among other roles, either the structural role of deep subject or that of deep direct object (DGR 1 or 2, respectively).

b. In particular, these patterns of activity can be approximated as tensor product representations based on a filler/role decomposition exemplified as follows for the vector **s** realizing the mental representation of the object raising (OR) sentence *une souris est facile à faire mourir* 'a mouse is easy to make die' (assuming the grammar assigns DGR 2 to the argument *une souris*):

$$\mathbf{s} = \mathbf{OR} \otimes \mathbf{r}_{\text{Context}} + \mathbf{mourir} \otimes \mathbf{r}_{\text{Pred}} + \mathbf{une\_souris} \otimes \mathbf{r}_{\text{Arg}} + \mathbf{2} \otimes \mathbf{r}_{\text{Struc}}$$
$$\equiv \mathbf{C} + \mathbf{P} + \mathbf{A} + \mathbf{S}.$$

That is, the vector representing a sentence can be approximated as the sum of four vectors, each of which represents a kind of constituent that is appropriate for the particular data under study: an argument A, a context C, a predicate P, and a **hidden** structural variable (DGR) S (either 1 or 2). These four constituents are the bindings—differing from sentence to sentence—of the roles $\{r_{\text{Context}}, r_{\text{Pred}}, r_{\text{Arg}}, r_{\text{Struc}}\}$. One way of instantiating these roles in a symbolic analysis is illustrated in Figure 1, which shows the structural description of this sentence in the analysis of Legendre 1986, employing the Relational Grammar syntactic framework (Perlmutter 1983; Figure 1 omits the labels of the grammatical relations other than the relevant one).

The relational network of Figure 1 represents a complex syntactic structure built upon a clause in which *mourir* 'die' is the predicate and *une souris* 'a mouse' is an argument bearing DGR 2: direct object. This clause ('a mouse die') is denoted by the lowest dot in Figure 1, with two arcs connecting it to *mourir* and *une souris*. This clause is embedded as an argument of a larger clause represented by the middle dot of Figure 1 ('make a mouse die'); the predicate of this clause is *faire* 'make'. In this **union** clause, *mourir* and *une souris* are themselves absorbed directly as arguments: the clause node has arcs to both of them as well as to *faire*.[20] Finally, this clause is in turn the argument of the outermost clause, with *est facile* 'is easy' as its predicate ('to make a mouse die is easy'). In this outer clause, *une souris* is **raised** to become itself an argument of *est facile*: 'a mouse is easy to make die'. The surface form of the sentence is

[20] The Relational Grammar notion of **clause union** (Aissen and Perlmutter 1983; Gibson and Raposo 1986) describes situations in which two clauses merge into one: in this clause, the two verbs form a single unit. This unity is revealed for example in the placement of an object pronoun that immediately precedes the verb of which it is an argument. In *il **la** fait casser* 'he makes it break', the object pronoun ***la*** refers to the argument of *casser* but does not immediately precede it; instead, it immediately precedes *fait casser* 'make break', which functions like a single verb. (Compare the union *fait casser* with nonunion *va casser* 'will break' in *il va **la** casser* 'he will break it': here, ***la*** occupies its normal position immediately before the verb *casser* of which it is an argument.)

then *une souris est facile à faire mourir.*

Figure 1. Filler/role decomposition: Object raising

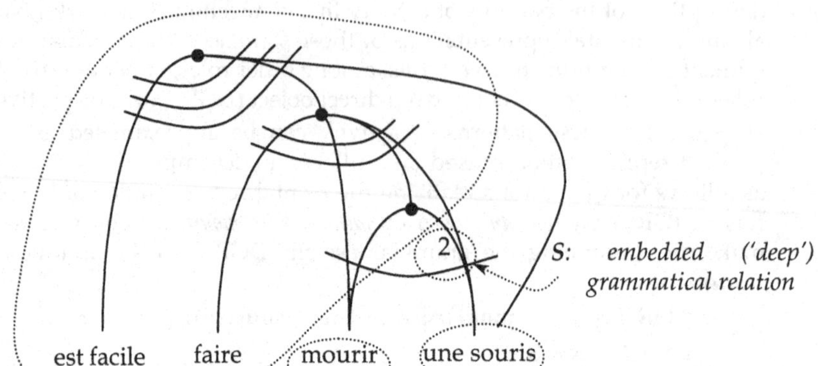

It is a virtue of HG that we need not further spell out LNet beyond specifying the representational structure (12b) and requiring that the equations governing activation flow be among the many that maximize Harmony (Chapter 9)—in other words, that the architecture be that of a **harmonic network** (Chapter 6 (11)). In particular, we need not specify vectors representing the individual fillers and roles. In the most general case, these vectors may be presumed to be fully distributed, giving rise to a representation of sentences in which each connectionist processing unit is part of the representation of every constituent. It will not matter to our analysis, however, whether this fully distributed case, or a more localized special case, obtains.

There is no particular point in drawing a picture of LNet; we need only imagine a large network (like those of Figures 4:3 and 8:5) that hosts a mental representation of the sentence as a pattern of activity that is the sum of four constituent patterns (each of which may well involve activation over the entire network), according to (12). Three constituents of this vector – the argument, context, and predicate – are specified in the input: the surface word string of a given sentence. The fourth constituent – the structural feature – is not given in the input; it is hidden and must be computed by the network through activation spread to maximize Harmony.

Following (9f), the degree of grammaticality of a sentence **s** with network realization **s** is taken to be $f(H)$, where H is the Harmony of this activation pattern, and f is some monotonically increasing function (i.e., the higher H, the more grammatical). As an implementational detail, we choose f to be the logistic function:

(13) $f(H) = \dfrac{1}{1+e^{-H}}$.

The values of $f(H)$ run from 0 (large negative H, highly ill formed) to 1 (large positive H, highly well formed); intermediate values correspond to intermediate levels of grammaticality.

In LNet, grammaticality is a distributed property; there is no "output unit" giving the network's grammaticality evaluation. As always, the Harmony value determining the grammaticality is a sum over all connections in the network, $H \equiv \Sigma_{\alpha\beta}\, a_\alpha W_{\alpha\beta} a_\beta$ (Section 6:1).

Why assume the filler/role decomposition of (12b) in Figure 1? Because it is the simplest imaginable decomposition of a linguistically well-motivated structure (Legendre 1986). The success of the consequent account provides some evidence in favor of this very simple assumption. It should be made clear, however, that the HG framework permits assuming a different filler/role decomposition of the sentences, and following it through to a correspondingly different higher-level analysis.

3.1.2 HNet

It is time to invoke the fundamental formal results underlying HG, as stated in Chapter 6 (15a) and (19). LNet is specified as a harmonic network (Chapter 6 (11)); it is therefore subject to the theorem stated in Chapter 6 (12), repeated as (14).

(14) Harmony Maximization Theorem

In harmonic networks, at each moment of processing, the Harmony of the total activation vector increases (or stays the same). Furthermore, for a very wide set of activation functions, the activation settles to a final vector that maximizes $H(\mathbf{a})$, among the vectors $\mathbf{a}$ that are completions of the input $\mathbf{i}$.

LNet is specified as subserving grammatical analysis, so the principle stated in Chapter 6 (19), repeated as (15), applies.

(15) $\text{Fun}_{\text{ICS}}(H,\text{HC})$

Given an input symbolic structure I, the harmonic grammar assigns to I the output symbolic structure ('parse') $\mathbf{s}$ with maximum Harmony, among those that are completions of I. The higher the Harmony value of this parse structure $\mathbf{s}$, the more well formed the grammar judges the input.

The representations in LNet are specified as tensor product representations, so the principle stated in Chapter 6 (15a), repeated as (16), applies.

(16) $\text{Wf}_{\text{ICS}}(\text{HC})$: Harmonic Grammar Soft-Constraint Theorem

Suppose $\mathbf{a}$ is a tensor product vector realizing a symbolic structure $\mathbf{s}$ with constituents $\{\mathbf{c}_i\}$, according to $\text{Rep}_{\text{ICS}}(\text{HC})$.

The Harmony of this representation is

$$H(\mathbf{s}) \equiv H(\mathbf{a}) = \Sigma_{i \le j}\, H(\mathbf{c}_i, \mathbf{c}_j),$$

where $H(\mathbf{c}_i, \mathbf{c}_j)$ – the Harmony resulting from the co-occurrence of $\mathbf{c}_i$ and $\mathbf{c}_j$ in the same structure – is a constant for all **s**.

Now combining this general form of the Harmony function with the assumptions specific to this account of French split intransitivity (12), we get (17).

(17) The acceptability of a sentence **s** consisting of the context C, the predicate P, and the argument A is

$$\text{grammaticality}(s) = f[\max_S H(\mathbf{C} + \mathbf{P} + \mathbf{A} + \mathbf{S})].$$

Here $\max_S$ denotes the maximal value achieved by letting S range over the two possible DGRs, 1 and 2, and

$$H(\mathbf{C} + \mathbf{P} + \mathbf{A} + \mathbf{S}) = H_C + H_P + H_A + H_S + H_{C,P} + H_{C,A} + H_{C,S} + H_{P,A} + H_{P,S} + H_{A,S}.$$

(For compactness, a term in (16) such as $H(C, P)$ will here be written as $H_{C,P}$.) This expression includes all possible Harmony terms that are first and second order in the four constituents C, P, A, and S.

Now this equation for H involves a prohibitively large number of higher-level parameters H_i and $H_{i,j}$ – an excess of soft rules. We eliminate a great many of these parameters by appealing to a number of linguistically motivated assumptions.

(18) Linguistically motivated assumptions concerning Harmony terms

a. $H_P = const$: All predicates in the sentences used are equally well formed internally.

b. $H_A = const$: All arguments in the sentences used are equally well formed internally.

c. $H_S = const$: The grammar has no intrinsic (context-independent) preference between deep subjects and deep direct objects.[21]

d. $H_{C,A} = H_{C,\text{VO}} + H_{C,\text{AN}}$: The grammatical restrictions imposed by the diagnostic context on the argument depend only on general semantic features of the argument; we take these features to be VO (volitionality) and AN (animacy).

e. $H_{P,A} = H_{\text{TE,VO}} + H_{\text{TE,AN}} + H_{\text{PR,VO}} + H_{\text{PR,AN}}$: For semantically appropriate arguments, a predicate can only express preference for general semantic features of its argument (again, VO and AN) and these preferences can depend only on general semantic features of the predicate (specifically, TE (telicity) and PR (progressivity)).

f. $H_{A,S} = H_{\text{VO},S} + H_{\text{AN},S}$: Concerning semantics, the grammatical preferences for assigning DGR 1 or 2 to the argument can depend only on its general semantic features (VO, AN).

g. $H_{C,P} = H_{C,\text{TE}} + H_{C,\text{PR}}$: The grammatical restrictions placed by a diagnostic context on the predicate can depend only on general semantic features of the predicate (not, e.g., on specific verbs); we take these features to be TE

[21] This assumption does not actually constrain the grammar. If we add $\pm x$ to each of the four values $H_{C,S}$, the result is identical to adding a soft rule 'Don't have DGR 1' with strength $\pm x$.

and PR.[22]

h. $H_{C,S}$: The grammatical restrictions on the diagnostic context can depend on the DGR (1 or 2) of the argument.

i. $H_{P,S}$: The lexical entry for an individual predicate can include a structural preference for the DGR of its argument.

Adopting these assumptions, and dropping H_P, H_A, and H_S because they do not vary across sentences (18a–c), we can rewrite the Harmony function as follows:

(19) $$H(\mathrm{C} + \mathrm{P} + \mathrm{A} + \mathrm{S}) = H_C + [H_{C,TE} + H_{C,PR}] + [H_{C,VO} + H_{C,AN}] + H_{C,S} + [H_{TE,VO} + H_{TE,AN} + H_{PR,VO} + H_{PR,AN}] + H_{P,S} + [H_{VO,S} + H_{AN,S}].$$

The key next step is to recognize this as the Harmony function of another network, HNet, illustrated in Figure 2. There are symmetric connections between the units of this network; they are depicted as L-shaped lines linking two units with a dot at the corner denoting the weight on the connection. The nonzero connections in this network have their weight dots in the rectangles of Figure 2 with labels such as $\mathrm{H}_{\mathrm{C,A}}$; in this rectangle are the weights for all the connections between C (context) and A (argument) units. One such connection is shown, linking the OR diagnostic context unit with the AN argument-feature unit. One connection is shown for each rectangular block of weights. There is one weight for each term in the Harmony function (19).

HNet uses a local representation, with a single input unit for each context, argument feature, structural feature, predicate feature, and individual predicate; these input units are indicated in the last column of Table 5. In addition, there are two **hidden units, 1** and **2**, which are local representations for the DGR assigned by the grammar. So the representation in HNet of a sentence consists of one active context unit (it has activity 1; the others, 0); active units for the features characterizing the argument (VO, AN) and predicate (TE, PR); one active predicate ID unit, identifying exactly which predicate appears in the sentence; and finally one active **structure unit**, either **1** or **2**, depending on the DGR assigned by the grammar to the argument in this sentence.

Each **unit** in HNet corresponds to a *pattern* in LNet. HNet is a higher-level network that is **isoharmonic**[23] to LNet: the Harmony values of corresponding states in the two networks are the same. An example is presented in (20).

(20) An example

a. Suppose the argument is animate [+AN] and the predicate is telic [+TE] (as in *une souris est facile à faire mourir* 'a mouse is easy to make die').

b. The realization in HNet of just these two features of the sentence is simply the activity (value 1) of the AN and TE units: $a_{AN} = 1 = a_{TE}$.

c. The Harmony contribution of this feature pair is $a_{TE} \cdot W_{TE,AN} \cdot a_{AN} =$

[22] This constraint is particularly important since without it, every pair of context and individual predicate would have its own free parameter, giving rise to 572 parameters of this type alone—with only 760 data points to fix the parameters.

[23] This apt term is due to Alan Prince (personal communication).

$1 \cdot W_{TE,AN} \cdot 1 = W_{TE,AN}$, the weight of the connection between the AN and TE units. (This weight is represented in Figure 2 by the dot in the H_{PA} rectangle at the corner of the "L" connection between these two units.) This weight is set to the Harmony penalty $H_{TE,AN}$ assessed by the soft constraint 'A telic predicate must not have an animate argument'.

d. The same state described at the lower level is, in accord with (12b), a pattern of activity in LNet given by $\mathbf{a} = \mathbf{TE} \otimes \mathbf{r}_{Pred} + \mathbf{AN} \otimes \mathbf{r}_{Arg}$, where **TE** is a filler vector realizing the feature [+TE], **AN** is a filler vector realizing [+AN], and $\mathbf{r}_{Pred}$ and $\mathbf{r}_{Arg}$ are the role vectors for the predicate and the argument.

e. The contributions of **a** to the Harmony of LNet are the appropriate terms $H(\mathbf{c}_i, \mathbf{c}_j)$ in (16)—that is, $H_{P,A}$ of (18e), specifically, the term $H_{TE,AN}$.

f. Since the weight $W_{TE,AN}$ of HNet equals $H_{TE,AN}$, the same contribution is made by the realizations of the pair of features [+TE] and [+AN] in both HNet and LNet.

g. For the entire sentence, the Harmony is the sum of the contributions of all the pairs of 'constituents' (16); since what we've said about [+TE] and [+AN] holds of any pair of constituents (e.g., features), adding together all the pairwise Harmony contributions must give the same total Harmony in both LNet and HNet.

HNet can be used to compute grammaticality as follows. A given sentence is represented over the input units. We activate whichever of the hidden units gives the greatest Harmony; this can be achieved by having the two units compete so that the unit with the greater net input wins. The net input to each hidden unit is precisely the contribution to the total Harmony that this hidden unit would make if it were to have activation value 1 (Chapter 6 (9)). The hidden units are thus a little **winner-take-all** group in which the winning unit has activation value 1, and the other unit, 0. There is a strong inhibitory connection between the two hidden units, which entails that the maximum Harmony pattern will have essentially zero activation on the hidden unit with less input.[24]

Given an activity pattern in HNet, we compute the Harmony H of the representation using the standard expression in (21) (Chapter 6 (4)):

(21) Wf_{PDP}

The Harmony of an activation vector **a** is defined to be

$$H(\mathbf{a}) = \Sigma_{\alpha\beta} H_{\alpha,\beta} = \Sigma_{\alpha\beta}\, a_\alpha W_{\alpha\beta} a_\beta = \mathbf{a}^{\mathrm{T}} \cdot \mathbf{W} \cdot \mathbf{a}.$$

In HNet, the variables H_α and $H_{\alpha,\beta}$ now play the roles of the weights $W_{\alpha\beta}$. Putting this value H into f, we get the grammaticality $f(H)$, following (9f).

The weights in this network are the Harmony values H_α and $H_{\alpha,\beta}$ of (17); from

[24] The Harmony of a state with hidden unit activations a_1, a_2 is $H = a_1\iota_1 + a_2\iota_2 - \lambda a_1 a_2$, where ι_1, ι_2 are the inputs to the two hidden units, and $-\lambda$ is the weight of the inhibitory connection between them. If the hidden unit activations are limited to the range [0, 1], as $\lambda \rightarrow \infty$, the maximum of H is achieved when $a_1 = 1$, $a_2 = 0$, if $\iota_1 > \iota_2$, and the reverse if $\iota_1 < \iota_2$.

the point of view of the original lower-level network LNet, each of these weights represents the aggregate Harmony of a set of weights and activity vectors, as spelled out in Chapter 6 (15d). We'd like to work backward from the data to infer what these aggregate values must be in order to produce the observed well-formedness pattern, but training all the weights (i.e., Harmony values that are distributed throughout this network) is not straightforward. A few simple modifications in the network, though, will fix this.

Figure 2. HNet

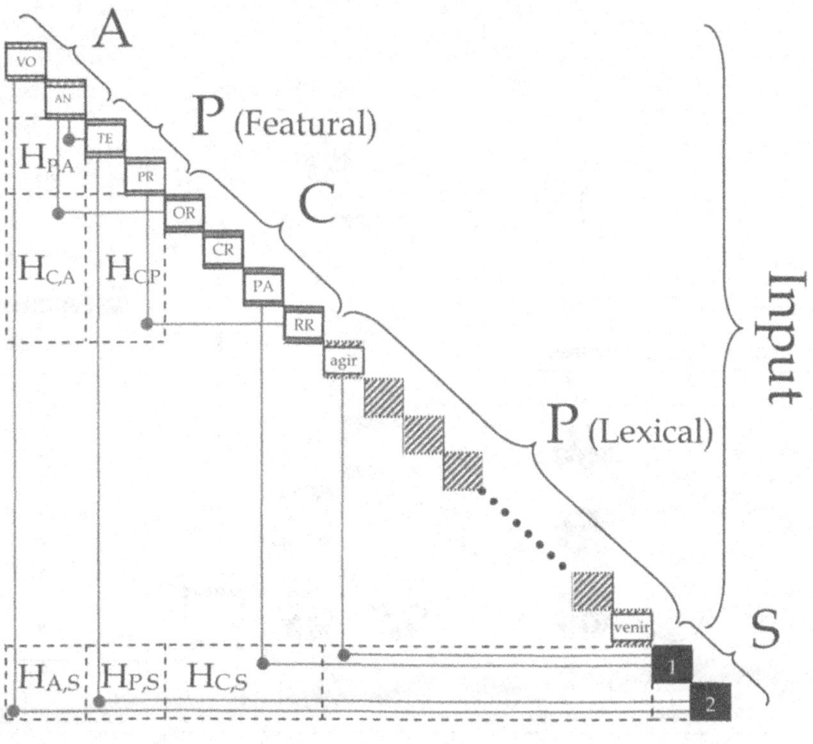

3.1.3 HNet′

To enable standard connectionist supervised learning from the data, we now create a network HNet′ that is precisely equivalent to HNet, but possesses a single output unit *O* that explicitly computes acceptability. HNet′ is a feed-forward network; activation flows unidirectionally from the input units to *O*.

The new network HNet′ is shown in Figure 3. Its input units are the same as those of HNet. A sentence is given to the network by appropriately setting the activities of the input units: the context unit corresponding to the appropriate syntactic construction (test) is given activity 1, the other three context units are given activity 0; among the 143 predicate-identity units, the one corresponding to the appropriate embedded predicate is given activity 1 and the others activity 0; for the two argument (VO, AN) and two predicate (TE, PR) feature units, the unit for each feature is given a numerical activity value encoding that feature's value: 1 for +, 0 for −, and .3, .5, and .7 for −?, ?, and +?, respectively.

Figure 3. HNet′

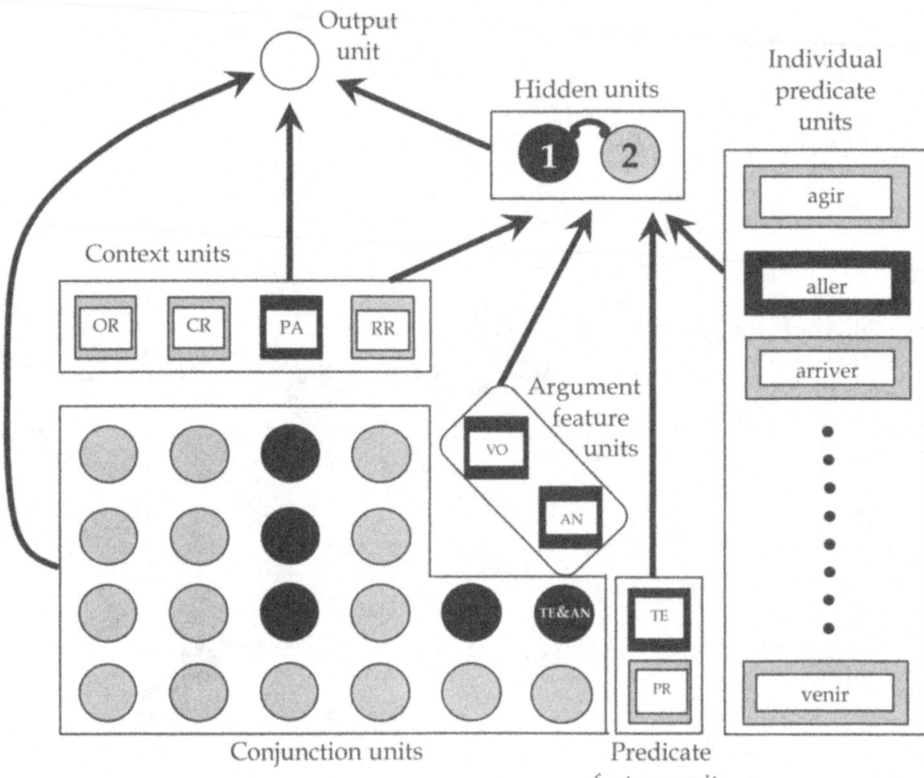

In addition to the input units, HNet′ contains a single output unit *O*. This output unit will explicitly represent the grammaticality of the input sentence; its activation value ranges between 0 (most ungrammatical) and 1 (most grammatical). *O* is a nonlinear unit that uses *f* (13) to transform its net input to its activation value; thus, according to (17), its activation value will be exactly the grammaticality level, provided we can arrange for its net input to be the Harmony *H* of the pattern in HNet representing the sentence, with the correct DGR assigned to maximize Harmony.

The main trick in achieving this is illustrated in Figure 4. We replace the connection between input units α and β of HNet, carrying weight $H_{\alpha,\beta}$, by a **conjunction unit** $c_{\alpha,\beta}$ whose activity is the product $a_\alpha a_\beta$; we then connect $c_{\alpha,\beta}$ to O with a connection of strength $H_{\alpha,\beta}$. Then the contribution to O's net input coming from $c_{\alpha,\beta}$ is $(a_\alpha a_\beta)H_{\alpha,\beta}$, which is just the amount of Harmony in HNet contributed by the original connection between α and β (21). Thus, the total net input to O from all the conjunction units is just $H_{\text{nonstructural}}$ (9b), the component of the Harmony that does not depend on the structural variable, the DGR of the argument.[25]

Figure 4. From HNet to HNet′

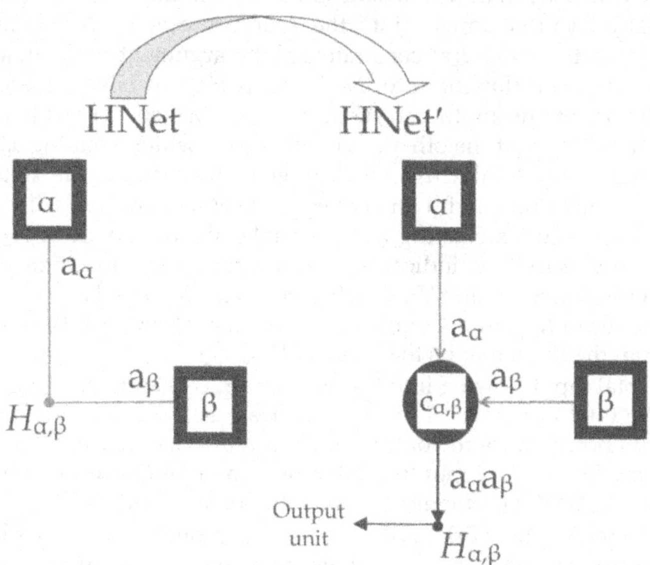

For example, in Figure 3 the unit $c_{\text{TE,AN}}$ for the conjunction of TE and AN is explicitly labeled **TE&AN**. The activation value of **TE&AN** is the numerical product of the activations of the **TE** and **AN** units; if both TE and AN are +, the corresponding units have activity 1 and so does **TE&AN**; if either TE or AN is −, the activity of **TE&AN** will be 0. If both TE and AN are +, **TE&AN** will have activity 1 and will contribute to the net input of the output unit O the quantity $1 \cdot H_{\text{TE,AN}}$, because its connection to O has strength $H_{\text{TE,AN}}$. Thus, this conjunction unit contributes an amount of input to O equal to the contribution to the Harmony of HNet resulting from having both AN and TE present in the sentence. A connection of strength +6.8 from the **TE&AN** unit to O implements

[25] The first-order Harmony terms in (19) constitute H_{context}; their contributions to the Harmony computation in HNet′ are achieved by connecting the context unit for context C (e.g., OR) directly to the output unit O, with weight equal to H_C. Thus, the net input that the context units provide to O is exactly H_C, where C is the diagnostic context instantiated by the current input sentence.

the soft constraint written as '+TE & +AN ⇒ +6.8' in (10f).

So far, the net input to O equals $H_{\text{nonstructural}}$. In order to provide the other Harmony contribution, $H_{\text{structural}}$, we need the two hidden units, labeled **1** and **2**: if the network decides to activate unit **1** (or **2**), that implements the grammar's assignment of DGR 1 (or 2) to the argument. Now in defining HNet′, the trick of replacing HNet connections with conjunction units should *not* be applied to the connections to the hidden units; these connections just stay as in HNet. Thus, in HNet′, as in HNet, the connection between an input unit α and hidden unit **2** is $H_{\alpha,2}$. If the element that α represents, say, the context CR, is present in the sentence, that input unit has activity 1 and so the activation it sends to unit **2** is $1 \cdot H_{\text{CR},2}$; this is exactly the contribution to the structural Harmony that CR would contribute if the DGR assigned were 2.[26] Thus, the total activation flowing into the **2** unit is exactly the Harmony H_2 that would result from the structural constraints if the argument were assigned DGR 2. Similarly, the activation flowing into the **1** unit is H_1.[27] In HNet′, these two hidden units mutually inhibit one another in such a way that whichever hidden unit receives more activation will inhibit the other's activation to 0, while retaining as its own activation level exactly the total activation it receives from the input units (i.e., HNet′ contains linear hidden units with an activity floor of 0 connected with strong mutually inhibitory connections creating a winner-take-all subnet). So if $H_2 > H_1$, unit **1** will be inhibited to activity 0, indicating that the grammar has assigned DGR 2, and unit **2** will have activation value H_2, which is $H_{\text{structural}}$ (9c). In HNet′, each hidden unit is connected to the output unit O with a connection of strength 1; thus, the activation flowing up from the hidden units to O will be $H_{\text{structural}}$.

Now the total input flowing into the output unit O is equal to $H_{\text{nonstructural}} + H_{\text{structural}}$, that is, the total Harmony H of the sentence s as it would be realized in HNet. And, as already noted, since the output unit computes its activation by applying the logistic function f to its net input, the activation value of O is exactly the grammaticality assigned to s by the harmonic grammar embodied in HNet.[28]

The feed-forward network HNet′ we have just defined can now be trained by an appropriately modified form of the standard connectionist supervised learning algorithm, back-propagation (Rumelhart, Hinton, and Williams 1986).[29] During train-

[26] Thus, the soft constraint 'CR & 2 ⇒ +5.0' (10a.iii) is implemented by a connection of strength +5.0 from the **CR** unit to the **2** unit.

[27] Actually, H_1 is simply the negative of H_2, because the Harmony contributions of the constraints involving DGR 1 are exactly the negative of those involving DGR 2: see (10) and the discussion of mirror constraints. Thus, rather than separately computing H_1 and H_2 to see which is larger, we can simply compute, say, H_2. If it is positive, DGR 2 is assigned and $H_{\text{structural}} = H_2$; if it is negative, DGR 1 is assigned and $H_{\text{structural}} = -H_2$.

[28] To fully specify LNet, the winner-take-all character of the HNet′ hidden layer needs a distributed, lower-level realization; this is currently an open problem.

[29] The algorithm performs gradient descent (with momentum) on the squared error between the output and the target averaged across all the 760 sentences of Table 4. For the weights to the hidden units, the winning hidden unit is first allowed to change its incoming weights, and the weights to the other hidden unit are then constrained to be the negative of the winner's weights. For the weight changes to the winning unit, the standard back-propagation rule can be used, as it can on all the connections from conjunctive units to the output unit O.

ing, 'supervision' consists in supplying each sentence in the basic data set of Table 4 together with the informants' acceptability judgment of the sentence, that is, 'correct' values for O (with the five acceptability levels −/−?/?/+?/+ arbitrarily quantified to 0.1/0.3/0.5/0.7/0.9).

The particular values of the 175 independent numerical parameters that appear in the soft constraints of our HG account of French split intransitivity were computed in just this fashion: they correspond exactly to the 175 free connection weights in HNet′ (143 lexical constraints, 32 grammatical constraints).

Note that the "learning" in HNet′ is not a plausible model of language acquisition; for one thing, negative as well as positive data concerning acceptability are crucial. "Learning" in HNet′ is purely a computational procedure for parameter fitting, a formal trick for automating a (particularly nasty) part of the job of the harmonic grammarian: determining the numerical constants H_X in the soft constraints (6b). An ultimate model of real language acquisition may well operate at the lower level, in LNet, and may not be formally describable at the higher level of HNet′ (see Chapters 21 and 23 for related discussion).

3.2 Methodological summary

The method of HG exemplified above can be summarized as the following series of steps:

(22) The Harmonic Grammar method

a. Choose a linguistically informed filler/role decomposition for the structures whose well-formedness is to be accounted for.

b. Postulate a lower-level model LNet using a tensor product realization of these structures, via the filler/role decomposition.

c. Take the formula (21) for the Harmony of LNet in terms of its weights and activities, and change variables ...

d. ... to get a formula (16) for the Harmony as a function of the constituents of the structure realized. This function involves aggregated Harmony values indexed by pairs of constituents; treat these values as independent high-level variables.

e. Prune the number of these variables by appealing to linguistically moti-

That is, for each training example, the weight change for any direct connection to O from β is modified by $\Delta W_{O\beta} = \varepsilon\, \delta_O\, a_\beta$, where ε is the learning rate; a_β is the activation value of β; and the **error** $\delta_O = (t_O - a_O)\, g$, where t_O is the teacher-supplied target activation value for the correct acceptability value, a_O is the actual activation value of O, and g is a scaling factor ($= f'(\iota_O) = a_O\,[1 - a_O]$, the derivative of f given the input ι_O that O receives). For the winning hidden unit γ, the error propagated back from O is the same as for O itself, since the connection weight between γ and O is $W_{O\gamma} \equiv 1$: $\delta_\gamma = \delta_O$. Then the change to any weight going into γ from an input unit β is also $\Delta W_{\gamma\beta} = \varepsilon\, \delta_\gamma\, a_\beta$. In addition, "momentum" was used. To each ΔW_t at time t is added $\varepsilon'\, \Delta W_{t-1}$ to smooth the learning trajectory by effectively performing a running average over time; ε' is the momentum magnitude.

Note that the assumption that higher-level variables are independent (Chapter 6 (34b)) is relevant here, since the training procedure incorporates no constraints between weights other than that between mirror constraints.

vated restrictions, ensuring that the set of data points is large relative to the number of variables.

f. Embody the resulting Harmony function as a local connectionist network HNet whose connection strengths are the high-level Harmony variables.

g. Create HNet′ by adding to the input units of HNet an output unit, which explicitly computes the HNet Harmony (and corresponding grammaticality value) by means of additional conjunctive units and winner-take-all linear hidden units.

h. Train HNet′ using a connectionist supervised learning algorithm, for example, the version of back-propagation appropriate for the architecture of HNet′.

i. Interpret HNet′ as embodying soft grammatical and lexical constraints.

j. Analyze these constraints for new insight into the original linguistic problem.

It is to this last step that we now turn.

4 Analyzing the Account

The method developed above automatically computes numerical strengths for a given set of soft constraints. This method involves parameters (e.g., initial values, learning rates) that can influence the outcome of the automatic process: multiple sets of constraint strengths can be computed, depending on these parameters, and each set of strengths constitutes a different harmonic grammar. In this discussion, we will identify a particular harmonic grammar with the network HNet′ that implements it.

4.1 Empirical adequacy

As the performance measure, we count two kinds of errors the network makes after training. The network makes a **major error** when its output and the correct (or **target**) value are of opposite polarity—that is, when the output was + or +? and the correct value was − or −?, or vice versa. The network makes a **minor error** if the discretized value of the output differs at all from the target (e.g., output +, target +?). We will almost exclusively discuss major errors here.

The network tends to be quite close to a solution in fewer than 1,000 iterations through the training sentences and the number of major and minor errors changes little afterward, but the training is always continued for 5,000 iterations.

The network's performance varies slightly depending on a few learning parameters. In our initial study, the best network made 2 major errors and 64 minor errors over the 760 sentences.[30] The worst network made 9 major and 120 minor errors. Despite these variations, the solutions displayed the following consistencies.

[30] A more elaborate learning procedure (utilizing line search to find the lexical rule strengths (11)) can reduce the number of major errors to 0, with 30 minor errors.

4.2 Consistency

Errors. The major errors made by alternative networks (grammars) turn out to define a striking hierarchy: if Account 1 makes more errors than Account 2, then the sentences on which Account 1 errs are a strict superset of those on which Account 2 errs. That is, there is a well-defined notion of one sentence being "more difficult to account for" (more "exceptional" perhaps) than other sentences; more successful accounts correctly account for more difficult sentences.

Structural biases of individual verbs. We can compare, across different accounts, the lexical constraints that specify whether a given intransitive verb prefers the DGR of its argument to be 1 (unergative bias) or 2 (unaccusative bias), and how strongly. A high degree of consistency is observed.

Grammaticality patterns. By numerically varying the unergative/unaccusative structural bias of the verb, it is possible to compute which grammaticality patterns across contexts are possible for a novel predicate-argument pair with given features. For example, the numerical constraints of a particular harmonic grammar may entail that any predicate-argument pair with the features +TE, −VO, and +AN will always be grammatical in the contexts CR and RR. The different networks make somewhat different predictions of this sort, but overall they are quite consistent.

Strong, conflicting constraints. The networks always seemed to achieve their performance by striking a delicate balance among the weights. For example, in a typical case, in order to fully turn on the output unit by providing it a net input of +1.5, a network uses 10 positive contributions adding up to 34.5 and 9 negative contributions adding up to −33.0. As a result, the output can be completely flipped by the change of a single input feature (thus changing the violation status of a small number of constraints).

4.3 Comprehensibility

Our account of unaccusativity in French copes with a large and complex set of data, but at a price: the account itself is very difficult to understand. This is a problem endemic to connectionism, and a primary topic of Chapter 22. While our HG account seems quite complex when compared to other linguistic accounts of unaccusativity, it is in fact quite simple and comprehensible relative to most connectionist models. The account's explanation of even the simplest cases involves the interplay of 29 numbers; for detailed discussion of several particular verbs, see Smolensky, Legendre, and Miyata 1992, App. A.

4.4 Necessity of semantic and syntactic features

The variables used in this account—the features VO, AN, TE, and PR, and the hidden variable we interpret as a DGR—are all implicated in previous semantic and syntactic accounts of unaccusativity in general, as well as analyses of the particular French data. It is possible, especially given the power of soft constraints, that an HG account of these data could be worked out using only a subset of these variables. Indeed, a purely syntactic account would invoke only the DGR, and a purely semantic account would omit this hidden variable altogether. These hypotheses can be tested by following the same procedure that led to the account presented above (including connectionist learning), with some subset of the variables excluded. Tests of this sort have been performed, employing an improved connectionist learning algorithm capable of finding a harmonic grammar that accounts correctly for all 760 sentences.[31] Deleting one of the four semantic features produces errors ranging from 2 (for AN) to 16 (for VO). Deleting two of the four semantic features leads to roughly 20 errors (depending on which features were excluded). Deleting the hidden variable (interpreted as a DGR) produces about 100 errors.

4.5 Generality

The extensibility (or generalizability) of the HG account was tested as follows. We performed connectionist training using 536 sentences involving 67 verbs, getting a set of 67 lexical constraints for those verbs and a set of grammatical soft constraints that do not refer to individual lexical items. We then asked: without changing these grammatical soft constraints, can we accommodate 20 new verbs by an appropriate choice of one lexical constraint for each of them? Of the 80 new sentences involving these new verbs (in the four unaccusativity tests), 78 could be correctly accounted for.

Furthermore, by examining the numerical strengths of the grammatical constraints of alternative HG accounts of the basic data, it can be determined that collectively they imply that a certain pattern of grammaticality across the various contexts is impossible for any intransitive verb in French—regardless of the strength and orientation (unergative vs. unaccusative) of its preference for the DGR of its argument. The prediction is that −VO, +AN, +TE predications cannot fail all the unaccusativity tests—in fact, they must pass the CR and RR tests specifically. This prediction is in fact verified, on the basis of a large, nearly exhaustive list of French intransitive verbs. And the feature combination −VO, +AN, +TE—a nonvolitional, animate participant in an event with an inherent endpoint—turns out to characterize a set of verbs that are quite robustly unaccusative, both within French and crosslinguistically. (Examples in the training corpus include *mourir* 'die', *naître* 'be born', *s'évanouir* 'faint', *vieillir* 'grow old'. Such verbs are often called **change-of-state** verbs.)

4.6 Extending the account

In the basic data set (Table 4), the syntactic contexts are all unaccusativity tests: all are constructions in which unaccusatives but not unergatives are, ideally, grammatical. We can extend this data set to include a fifth syntactic context with the opposite orientation: it is an unergativity test in which, idealizing, only unergatives are gram-

[31] See Footnote 30.

matical.[32] Using the same HG approach as that described above for the four contexts (adding in HNet and HNet' a fifth context unit, and the corresponding conjunctive units and connections), it is possible to train a network that correctly accounts for the acceptability judgments of all but 3 of the 885 sentences involving 143 intransitive verbs in five syntactic constructions (Smolensky, Legendre, and Miyata 1992).

A more comprehensive HG approach to French unaccusativity, based on a study of 8,393 sentences involving 225 transitive verbs and 183 intransitive verbs in 11 syntactic contexts, is described in Legendre, Miyata, and Smolensky 1991. This approach handles embedded *transitive* verbs as well as intransitives, and, using a much more complex network architecture, explicitly treats the argument of an intransitive as either the subject or direct object of a transitive—whichever produces maximum Harmony in a given syntactic context. Furthermore, rather than allowing each individual verb to have an arbitrary preference for the DGR of its argument, as in the earlier account, connectionist learning is used to automatically extract from the data a small number of predicate 'features' that—like telicity and progressivity in the earlier account—serve to determine each verb's preference for the DGR (and semantic properties) of its argument. One version of this account (using six learned predicate features) correctly accounts for the acceptability judgments of all but 104 of the 8,393 sentences. Of the 3,608 sentences with intransitives, the focus of the study, all but 14 are correctly accounted for. Statistical cluster analysis of the learned features reveals some provocative connections to aspectual properties.

5 Conclusion

Much previous research on unaccusativity debates whether a semantic- or a syntactic-based formalism is best. We believe that a grammar formalism is needed that can effectively combine both syntactic and semantic constraints, and that HG can deliver this. The formalism must allow the interaction between syntactic and semantic constraints to be quite intense—HG, a high-level formalization of connectionist constraint interaction, seems to provide this. Unaccusativity phenomena provide a difficult challenge to the theory of grammar: they demand a formalism that provides a way to state the relevant universal *tendencies*, both syntactic and semantic, without making them hard requirements, since they are far from absolutely respected. But a true formalism is needed, one that doesn't just state vague tendencies, but makes precise predictions, decisively adjudicating between frequently conflicting universal tendencies. HG provides this: it allows the content of the grammar to consist entirely in those constraints defining the universal tendencies, with numerical strengths doing all the work of mediating the strong interactions between the often conflicting

[32] The pronoun *on* has come to completely replace *nous* 'we' in the spoken register of contemporary French. While *on* can always be interpreted as 'we', in a restricted class of cases it can also be interpreted as the indefinite 'one' (someone). The restriction is that the DGR of *on* must be 1 (Legendre 1990). The verb *aller* 'go' requires DGR 2, so *on est allé au cinéma* cannot mean 'someone went to the movies'; instead, it must mean 'we went ...'. In contrast, the verb *téléphoner* 'call' requires DGR 1, so *on a téléphoné* is ambiguous between 'someone called' and 'we called'.

demands of these constraints. And the precision with which strong constraint interaction is handled is such that HG even assigns different **degrees** of grammaticality, along a continuum from maximally ill formed to maximally well formed. Deploying only substantive semantic and syntactic properties that have been argued within linguistic theory to bear on explaining unaccusativity phenomena, HG accounts for complex patterns better than any previous approach. The complexity of the account does, however, present a significant challenge to the analyst.

References

Aissen, J., and D. M. Perlmutter. 1983. Clause reduction in Spanish. In *Studies in Relational Grammar 1*, ed. D. M. Perlmutter. University of Chicago Press.

Bever, T. G. 1970. The cognitive basis for linguistic structures. In *Cognition and the development of language*, ed. J. R. Hayes. Wiley.

Burzio, L. 1986. *Italian syntax: A government-binding approach.* Reidel.

Cummins, S. 1996. Meaning and mapping. Ph.D. diss., University of Toronto.

Dowty, D. 1979. *Word meaning and Montague Grammar.* Reidel.

Dowty, D. 1991. Thematic proto-roles and argument selection. *Language* 67, 547–619.

Gibson, J., and E. Raposo. 1986. Clause union, the Stratal Uniqueness Law and the chômeur relation. *Natural Language and Linguistic Theory* 4, 295–331.

Labelle, M. 1992. Change of state and valency. *Journal of Linguistics* 28, 375–414.

Legendre, G. 1986. Object raising in French: A unified account. *Natural Language and Linguistic Theory* 4, 137–84.

Legendre, G. 1989. Unaccusativity in French. *Lingua* 79, 95–164.

Legendre, G. 1990. French impersonal constructions. *Natural Language and Linguistic Theory* 8, 81–128.

Legendre, G. 1992. Split intransitivity: A reply to Van Valin 1990. Technical report ICS-TR-92-3, Institute of Cognitive Science, University of Colorado.

Legendre, G., Y. Miyata, and P. Smolensky. 1990a. Can connectionism contribute to syntax? Harmonic Grammar, with an application. In *Proceedings of the Chicago Linguistic Society 26.*

Legendre, G., Y. Miyata, and P. Smolensky. 1990b. Harmonic Grammar—a formal multi-level connectionist theory of linguistic well-formedness: An application. In *Proceedings of the Cognitive Science Society 12.*

Legendre, G., Y. Miyata, and P. Smolensky. 1991. Unifying syntactic and semantic approaches to unaccusativity: A connectionist approach. In *Proceedings of the Berkeley Linguistics Society 7.*

Legendre, G., and D. S. Rood. 1992. On the interaction of grammar components in Lakhóta: Evidence from split intransitivity. In *Proceedings of the Berkeley Linguistics Society 18.*

Levin, B., and M. Rappaport. 1989. An approach to unaccusative mismatches. In *Proceedings of the North East Linguistic Society 19.*

Levin, B., and M. Rappaport Hovav. 1995. *Unaccusativity: At the syntax-lexical semantics interface.* MIT Press.

Perlmutter, D. M. 1978. Impersonal passives and the Unaccusative Hypothesis. In *Proceedings of the Berkeley Linguistics Society 4.*

Perlmutter, D. M., ed. 1983. *Studies in Relational Grammar 1.* University of Chicago Press.

Perlmutter, D. M. 1989. Multiattachment and the Unaccusative Hypothesis: The perfect auxiliary in Italian. *Probus* 1, 63–119.

Rosen, C. 1984. The interface between semantic roles and initial grammatical relations. In *Studies in Relational Grammar* 2, eds. D. M. Perlmutter and C. Rosen. University of Chicago Press.

Rumelhart, D. E., G. E. Hinton, and R. J. Williams. 1986. Learning internal representations by error propagation. In *Parallel distributed processing: Explorations in the microstructure of cognition.* Vol. 1, *Foundations,* D. E. Rumelhart, J. L. McClelland, and the PDP Research Group. MIT Press.

Smolensky, P., G. Legendre, and Y. Miyata. 1992. Principles for an integrated connectionist/symbolic theory of higher cognition. Technical report CU-CS-600-92, Computer Science Department, and 92–8, Institute of Cognitive Science, University of Colorado at Boulder.

Van Valin, R. D. 1990. Semantic parameters of split intransitivity. *Language* 66, 221–60.

Vendler, Z. 1967. Verbs and time. In *Linguistics and philosophy.* Cornell University Press.

Williamson, J. S. 1979. Patient marking in Lakhóta and the Unaccusative Hypothesis. In *Proceedings of the Chicago Linguistic Society 15.*

Zaenen, A. 1993. Unaccusativity in Dutch: Integrating syntax and lexical semantics. In *Semantics and the lexicon*, ed. J. Pustejovsky. Kluwer.

12

Optimality Theory: The Structure, Use, and Acquisition of Grammatical Knowledge

Paul Smolensky, Géraldine Legendre, and Bruce Tesar

The final principle of the Integrated Connectionist/Symbolic Cognitive Architecture (ICS), P_4: OT, identifies the architecture of the human language faculty as that of Optimality Theory (Prince and Smolensky 1993/2004). P_4 is elaborated here into a comprehensive series of principles that articulate the internal structure of OT; these principles are illustrated for both phonology and syntax. The original formulation of the theory is extended to incorporate interpretation as well as generation. Computational issues in the use and acquisition of OT grammars are also discussed. Finally, frequently asked questions concerning explanation in OT are addressed. In the ICS map of Chapter 2, this chapter contributes to ③ of Figure 5 and to the top portion of Figure 9. It provides the theory that is applied in all chapters of Part III.

Section 4 is based on an article that appeared in Japanese translation in *Gengo* (Smolensky 2001), and in English in *Phonological Studies* (Smolensky 2002).

Contents

Harmony provides the Integrated Connectionist/Symbolic Cognitive Architecture (ICS) an important bridge between the lower-level description of the human language faculty as a connectionist network and the higher-level description of the same system as a symbolic grammar. Conceptually, it is natural that Harmony, a measure of connectionist well-formedness, be linked to grammatical well-formedness. Technically, however, there is a crucial divergence: connectionist well-formedness is, of course, a matter of numerical computation, as in Harmonic Grammar (HG); but in grammatical computation, numbers can play no role. The fundamental empirical generalization that *grammars can't count* is discussed in Section 20:1.2.1.1. The point here is that this generalization suggests we seek a kind of well-formedness computation that is like Harmony maximization in HG, but with no numerical arithmetic. The simplest way that a set of conflicting well-formedness criteria can interact nonnumerically to produce a preference ordering of competing outcomes is by strict priority ranking: in determining the relative Harmony of *O* and *O′*, the most important constraint decides, unless that constraint evaluates *O* and *O′* as equal, in which case the decision is passed to the next-most-important constraint, where the process begins again. The relative priority of constraints—their relative rank in a constraint hierarchy—completely determines harmonic evaluation: no numerical computation is involved.[1]

When Prince and Smolensky examined this simplest possibility within phonology, they found that, despite the seeming rigidity of the evaluation scheme, interesting patterns of well-formedness emerge. Most importantly, *empirically sound* patterns emerge. When their previous numerical, HG account of stress patterns was reexamined, it turned out that the empirically adequate numerical strengths had a special property: each constraint was stronger than all the weaker constraints combined. Observed crosslinguistic variation in stress patterns was well modeled by reranking constraints in strict domination hierarchies, but numerical weighting predicted the existence of empirically unacceptable stress systems. Thus Optimality Theory (OT) was created. The principle of strict domination of universal well-formedness constraints is stated as the final ICS principle, P_4: OT.

The relation between HG and OT involves a number of subtleties; its discussion is postponed until Chapter 20, after OT has been further developed in this and subsequent chapters. Until then, we pursue the line of research defined by OT in its own terms, to see where it leads.

What is a grammar? No consensus has arisen in the cognitive science community on the answer to this seemingly simple question. The question is important because one of the central constituencies of cognitive science, the linguistics community, concerns

[1] In economic choice theory, a preference function in which different factors interact by strict domination is called **lexicographic**: it orders options 'alphabetically', where the first 'letter' of an option is its evaluation by the top-ranked constraint, its second 'letter' is the evaluation by the next constraint, and so forth (Kreps 1988, 24; Prince and Smolensky 1993/2004, Fn. 20).

itself to a large extent with the development of a satisfactory theory of grammar. What this theory is a theory of—what it is *about*—matters greatly for determining its proper role in the overall theory of cognition that cognitive science seeks to develop. The question has immediate relevance to the discussion in this chapter, which presents a theory of grammar: Optimality Theory (Prince and Smolensky 1993/2004).

The view has been expressed on more than a few occasions that the grammar of a language $\mathcal{L}$ is a description of the sentences or words that make up the grand corpus of all expressions uttered, written, or signed by speakers of $\mathcal{L}$. A grammar is useful, on this view, for defining the *problem* to which a theory of the human language capacity must provide a solution.

The robustness of this view is rather curious, given its explicit, complete, insistent, consistent, and continual rejection by such leading figures in modern grammatical theory as Noam Chomsky. Here is one example, of perhaps literally hundreds, that may be found in Chomsky's writings. In this quotation from a lecture series for a general audience, Chomsky states the defining questions of linguistics, questions concerning **grammar**, which, he asserts, simply refers to *knowledge of language*.

(1) The defining questions of generative linguistics

"1. What is the system of knowledge?
2. How does this system of knowledge arise in the mind/brain?
3. How is this knowledge put to use?
4. What are the physical mechanisms that serve as the material basis for this system of knowledge and for the use of this knowledge?" (Chomsky 1988, 3)

These are truly great questions—few cognitive scientists could deny that. What is more controversial is whether the pursuit of a theory of grammar, as practiced by generative linguists following the Chomskyan program, is profitably viewed as directed toward actually answering these questions. Linguistic research within the Chomskyan **Principles-and-Parameters** framework (e.g., Chomsky 1981) is so heavily focused on Chomsky's first question that it is not easy to discern a central role for research more explicitly directed toward answering the other three.[2] This exclusivity may readily be rationalized by the convictions that (i) the latter three questions cannot be profitably pursued until the first has been answered satisfactorily, and (ii) generative linguistics has not yet achieved this—as must be expected of a science so young.

Such modesty on the part of this community of linguists about the progress they have achieved on their crucial first question may be admirable, and may even be

[2] There is indeed an important group of researchers studying acquisition and processing from a Principles-and-Parameters perspective (see, e.g., Hyams 1986; Wexler and Manzini 1987; Berwick, Abney, and Tenny 1991; Lust, Hermon, and Kornfilt 1994; Lust, Suñer, and Whitman 1994; Clahsen 1999; Crain and Lillo-Martin 1999; Jackendoff 2002). But since the size of this group is extremely small relative to the overwhelming majority of linguists exclusively addressing the first question, it seems appropriate to describe the Principles-and-Parameters community as 'heavily focused' on it.

merited (although we think not). But the rest of cognitive science proceeds despite its youthfully incomplete understanding. It seems worth seriously exploring the possibility that the insights linguistics can currently contribute concerning the first question can—even at this early stage—effectively inform contemporary research directly aimed at answering the other three questions. Viewed in the context of a cognitive science of which linguistics is only one part, it would indeed seem essential to examine whether, to enable the active pursuit of answers to Chomsky's last three questions, it is possible to constructively integrate current insights from the theory of grammar with current understanding of the use, acquisition, and neural realization of knowledge, understanding that can be gleaned from cognitive psychology, developmental psychology, neuroscience, and computation theory. And indeed several generative linguistic traditions—including Lexical-Functional Grammar (Bresnan 1982, 2001), Head-Driven and Generalized Phrase Structure Grammar (Gazdar et al. 1985; Pollard and Sag 1987, 1991), Categorial Grammar (Steedman 2000), and others—have been developed in which computational considerations play a central role.

While Chomsky has of course contributed enormously to creating the modern science of cognition, he is not the first to articulate the view that grammatical theory must play a central role in the general cognitive science of language. An antecedent directly relevant to OT is Roman Jakobson (1941/1968; 1962; see Section 4:2), who identified a unifying linguistic concept—markedness—and actively pursued its use in connecting the phenomena central to linguistic theory with those of the other cognitive disciplines.

OT can usefully be viewed as a descendant of markedness theory, with markedness itself formalized as (negative) Harmony (Chapters 4 and 14).[3] As anticipated by Jakobson's program, OT has served as a theory of grammar that addresses not only the central data of generative linguistics, but also the data of other cognitive disciplines.

This chapter introduces OT in the general context of Chomsky's four central questions (1). OT's contribution to the explicit pursuit of the last three questions is the topic of five chapters in Part III of the book: Chapters 17 (acquisition of phonological knowledge), 18 (acquisition of syntactic knowledge), 19 (use of syntactic knowledge), 20 (neural realization of grammatical knowledge, computational focus), and 21 (neural realization of the acquisition of grammatical knowledge, biological focus). But as with all generative theories of grammar, the developments and applications of OT have first and foremost been centered in theoretical linguistics. OT seeks to provide the same general types of answers to the same types of questions as other generative theories. Hence, most of this chapter is devoted to showing how OT answers the formal part of Chomsky's first question, which we might phrase: what is the functional architecture in which our knowledge of language resides? Thus, OT will be introduced in the context of the data and explanatory objectives of generative grammar (the compatibility of these objectives with a connectionist-based cognitive architec-

[3] Harmony combines markedness with another crucial notion, faithfulness; see (45k).

ture is the topic of Chapter 22). In Part III of the book, a few applications of OT within core linguistic theory are presented: Chapters 13–14 (phonological theory) and 15–16 (syntactic theory). Many more examples are electronically available from the Rutgers Optimality Archive (http://roa.rutgers.edu); see also the collections Beckman, Walsh Dickey, and Urbanczyk 1995; Barbosa et al. 1998; Hermans and van Oostendorp 1999; Dekkers, van der Leeuw, and van de Weijer 2000; Legendre, Vikner, and Grimshaw 2001; Lombardi 2001; Sells 2001; Coetzee, Carpenter, and de Lacy 2002; Blutner and Zeevat 2003; Féry and van de Vijver 2003; Holt 2003; McCarthy 2004.

OT characterizes grammatical knowledge as a system of universal violable constraints on well-formed linguistic combinations, ranked into a language-particular hierarchy. In this chapter, we present the theory in detail, beginning in Section 1 with the perspective of theoretical linguistics, question (1.1). In Section 2, we turn to the perspective of computational linguistics and briefly discuss the problem of computing grammatical (optimal) forms in OT, question (1.3). In Section 3, we consider the problem of learning the ranking of constraints that individuates the grammar of a particular language, question (1.2). Neural realization of OT knowledge, question (1.4), is taken up in Chapters 20 and 21. In Section 4 of this chapter, we consider some frequently asked "questions" about the explanatory value of OT.

We propose to formulate the objective of tightly integrating linguistic theory with the rest of the cognitive science of language as in (2); the four subparts correspond to Chomsky's four questions.

(2) Goals for a strongly grammar-centered cognitive science of language

a. **Inherent typology.** A grammatical formalism $\mathcal{G}$ in which language-particular grammatical analysis consists in identifying the interaction of universal principles that formally determine a typology of possible human grammars; inherent in any analysis of some phenomenon Φ in some language $\mathcal{L}$ is a theory of Φ in all the world's languages.

b. **General processing theory.** A general theory $\mathcal{P}$ for computing the generation and interpretation functions determined by any $\mathcal{G}$-grammar; inserting a particular grammar G into $\mathcal{P}$ directly yields algorithms for processing with G.

c. **General learning theory.** A general theory $\mathcal{L}$ for acquiring an individual grammar within any typology $\mathcal{T}$ of $\mathcal{G}$-grammars; inserting into $\mathcal{L}$ the particular set of universal principles determining $\mathcal{T}$ directly yields learning algorithms for finding any target grammar G in $\mathcal{T}$ on the basis of positive data from the language determined by G.

d. **General theory of neural (genetic) realization.** A general theory $\mathcal{N}$ for realizing the universal principles of a $\mathcal{G}$-typology $\mathcal{T}$ in a neural network; inserting the particular principles of $\mathcal{T}$ into $\mathcal{N}$ directly yields a network $\mathcal{N}$ that can be configured to realize any grammar G in $\mathcal{T}$ (i.e., compute the functions determined by G) and can learn this configuration on the basis of positive data from the language determined by G. Also, a general theory

$\mathcal{M}$ for encoding the universal principles of any $\mathcal{G}$-typology $\mathcal{T}$ in a genome $\mathcal{M}$ that governs the growth and operation of the neural networks of $\mathcal{N}$.

This chapter points to results suggesting that OT can enable significant progress toward these goals; later chapters furnish some of this evidence.

The characterization of OT presented here is essentially that developed in Prince and Smolensky 1993/2004, but it incorporates fundamental insights of the Correspondence Theory of faithfulness developed in McCarthy and Prince 1995. Correspondence Theory is now standard in phonology, although somewhat less so (or less explicitly so) in syntax. The presentation here extends the original formulation of OT to include linguistic interpretation as well as linguistic generation (Wilson 1995, 2001a; Smolensky 1996a, c, 1998; Zeevat 2000; Blutner 2001; Hendriks and de Hoop 2001); this is nonstandard. Two running examples are employed, one from phonology (syllable structure), the other from syntax (the distribution of clausal subjects). The plan for introducing the key concepts of OT is summarized in (3).

(3) Presentation of OT principles

a. Linguistic representations: structural descriptions (Section 1.1)
b. Candidates in generation and interpretation (Section 1.2)
c. Harmony and competition (Section 1.3)
d. Violable constraints (Section 1.4)
e. Harmonic ordering; optimality (Section 1.5)
f. Universality; factorial typology; Richness of the Base (Section 1.6)
g. Lexicon optimization (Section 1.7)

Section 1.8 further characterizes OT's constraints, and Section 1.9 summarizes some claims for OT's contributions to theoretical linguistics, especially phonology.

The most basic major feature of OT is that it is a *framework for stating theories of linguistic phenomena;* it is not itself such a theory. OT is a theory of the *structure of universal grammar,* not of its *content.* In this sense, OT is comparable to a theory claiming that knowledge of language consists in a set of symbol-manipulating rules, applied in a specified order, or a theory asserting that knowledge consists in a set of weights in a connectionist network. Specific theories of, say, knowledge of phonological stress would propose particular rules, or a particular network with particular weights—or, for OT, a particular set of constraints.

An OT grammar is a theory concerning the universal content of some part of our knowledge of language, a theory instantiating the structure that OT hypothesizes as the functional architecture of the language faculty. To present the principles defining OT itself, it is necessary to illustrate its highly general principles by discussing particular linguistic theories that have been developed within the OT framework. The running examples below from phonology and syntax—or even the entire population of which they are a tiny sample—must not be confused with OT itself. The principles defining OT that we now present characterize the various elements of any grammar—the *form* of the grammar; each actual OT theory of some grammatical phenomenon will instantiate these elements in concrete terms in its own characteristic way.

1 Principles of Optimality Theory: OT in Theoretical Linguistics

1.1 Structural descriptions

Fundamentally, the job of a grammar is to link linguistic forms and their meanings. Within the symbolic theory of cognition, as laid out in Section 1:3, this is done by the **combinatorial strategy**: parts of linguistic forms are related to parts of meanings, and wholes derive their meanings from their parts and the way these parts are combined. For this purpose, the decomposition of linguistic structures into their parts—**parsing**—must be done properly, and grammars define what the correct decompositions are. These decompositions are the **structural descriptions** that are the central objects of grammatical theory. The most fundamental aspect of specifying a grammar is defining the universe of potential structural descriptions; we will call this universe $\mathcal{U}$.

Generalizing somewhat the conception in McCarthy and Prince 1995, we will take the structural descriptions employed in OT to have three complex parts; we will call these an **interpretation**, an **expression**, and a **correspondence relation** between the interpretation and the expression. Within the expression is a substructure called the **overt part**, or **surface form**, of the expression. This conception is stated in (4); it will be exemplified first within syntax, and then within phonology.

(4) Universe of structural descriptions: $\mathcal{U}$

a. A particular grammatical theory specifies a universe of structural descriptions S, each of which has the form $(I, E, \mathfrak{R})$, where
   i. I is an interpretation,
   ii. E is an expression,
   iii. $\mathfrak{R}$ is a correspondence relation between I and E.

b. Within each expression E is an overt part, written *overt*(E); this is the portion of E that is directly available to the hearer.

To repeat, OT is not a theory of what the structural descriptions are. OT is a theory asserting that structural descriptions have the very general form described in (4). A particular OT theory of, say, syllables, must hypothesize particular structural descriptions of syllables that instantiate $\mathcal{U}$; the syllable theory we discuss below is merely one of many ways that this can be (and has been) done within the OT framework. That the architecture of OT does have important implications for the nature of structural descriptions in a specific grammar module—the organization of phonological features—is a main point of Chapter 14.

1.1.1 Syntax

An example syntactic structural description is given in (5b). (Box 1, p. 466, provides an introduction to the concepts and terminology used here.)

(5) A single structural description *S* (syntax): *he has sung*

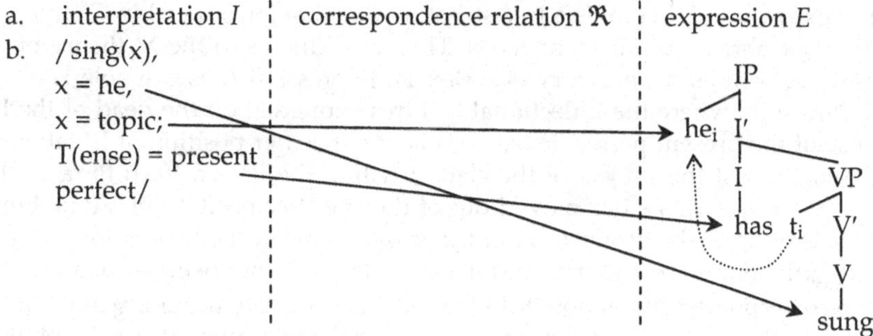

c. /sing^1(x^2), x = topic, x = he; T^3 = present perfect/; [$_{IP}$ he$^2{}_i$ has^3 [t$_i$ sung^1]]

This structural description comes from one of the two running examples we will use through much of this chapter: the theory of clausal subjects proposed in Grimshaw and Samek-Lodovici 1995 (see also Samek-Lodovici 1996; Grimshaw and Samek-Lodovici 1998). We will refer to this theory here as **GSL**.

To repeat one last time, OT itself asserts only that grammars concern structural descriptions of the general form (4); it is not the OT framework but rather the particular OT theory, GSL, which asserts that clauses have the particular structural descriptions illustrated in (5). While the structural descriptions of GSL inherit a number of their properties from structural descriptions posited within the Government-Binding (GB) approach to syntax (Chomsky 1981), this is far from true of all OT work in syntax. The OT syntax papers collected in Legendre, Vikner, and Grimshaw 2001 include syntactic theories with structural descriptions that derive from several other generative syntactic traditions.[4] And even within the present book, Chapter 15 presents an early mapping-theory-style analysis—where structural descriptions are simply explicit mappings between semantic and surface syntactic roles—and Chapter 16 another GB-style theory that differs in significant respects from GSL. In general, OT analyses (in both syntax and phonology) are not developed in a vacuum; they build on insights gained from previous analyses of many linguistic phenomena. And like previous research, OT analyses adopt a great diversity of assumptions concerning the nature of structural descriptions and the constraints governing them.

In the example (5b), the interpretation *I*—which we delimit with slashes '/'—is a proposition asserting that *x* has sung, where *x* is masculine singular (the referent of

[4] These include mapping theory (Gerdts 1993), minimalism (Chomsky 1995), and Lexical-Functional Grammar (LFG; Bresnan 1982, 2001). Indeed, Sells 2001 contains many papers in the rapidly developing OT-LFG theory of syntax (Bresnan 1996, 2000).

he) and *x* is the current discourse topic. More generally, in GSL, an interpretation is "a lexical head with a mapping of its argument structure into other lexical heads, plus a tense specification ... as in Grimshaw (1993). ... [The interpretation] also specifies which arguments are foci, and which arguments are co-referent with the topic" (Grimshaw and Samek-Lodovici 1995, 590).

The expression *E* in (5b) is a tree structure like that introduced in Chapter 1 (7): a nested set of phrases of different types. This tree adheres to the X′ theory of phrase structure, as well as trace theory (see Box 1). Expression *E* as a whole is an Inflectional Phrase IP, where the inflectional features expressed on the head of the IP, *has*, are those of the present perfect tense; *he* is in the specifier position of IP (abbreviated SpecIP), making it the subject of the clause; within the IP is a Verb Phrase VP with head *sung*. The subject he_i has moved out of the specifier position of VP (abbreviated SpecVP), leaving a silent trace t_i behind. The overt part of the expression is the string *he has sung*; the phrase boundaries and the silent trace are not overt—not audible.

The correspondence relation $\Re$ in (5b) connects the predicate *sing* in the interpretation *I* with the main verb *sung* in the expression *E*, the argument *x* in *I* with the subject *he* of *E*, and the tense features [present perfect] of *I* with the inflectional head of *E*, *has*.

In (5c), the same structural description denoted by (5b) is expressed much more compactly, with brackets denoting major phrase boundaries in *E* and matching superscript numerals showing the correspondence $\Re$.

The expression given in (5) is one of many candidates for expressing the interpretation *I* = /sing(x), x = topic, x = he; T = present perfect/; in a language other than English, a different expression may be the one designated as correct by the grammar.[5] Several examples are given in (6); the one discussed above is (6b).

(6) Candidate expressions *E* for the interpretation

I ≡ /sing(x), x = topic, x = he; T = present perfect/

a. $[_{IP}$ has [sung]]

b. $[_{IP}$ he_i has [t_i sung]]

c. $[_{IP}$ has [[t_i sung] he_i]]

d. $[_{IP}$ it has [[t_i sung] he_i]]

The four candidates in (6) will appear several times below and will be consistently labeled *a–d* as in (6). Expression (6a) is a clause with no subject: the highest projection of the verb, labeled IP, has no specifier position.[6] Expression (6b), as already discussed, has *he* in SpecIP, coindexed with a trace in SpecVP. The **chain** formed by he_i and t_i is a representation of the movement of *he* from the position

[5] As discussed in Section 1.6, the sets of all potential interpretations and all potential expressions are each universal: the same in every language. So even distinctions made in other languages but not in English must be taken into account.
[6] The expressions of GSL are X′ structures (see Box 1) employing the notion of **extended projection** (Grimshaw 1991).

marked by *t*. Expression (6c) has no SpecIP position; *he* is right-adjoined to VP, co-indexed with a trace in SpecVP. Expression (6d) is the same, but with an expletive (meaningless) subject in SpecIP.

Where the optimal correspondences are obvious, as here, they will usually not be explicitly represented in candidates. In the candidates (6), the correspondences intended are analogous to those made explicit in (5c). In candidate (6a), the argument element *x* of the interpretation *I* has no correspondent in the expression *E;* and in candidate (6d), the element *it* of E has no correspondent in *I*.

1.1.2 Phonology

As in syntax, in phonology a structural description consists of an interpretation *I*, an expression *E*, and a correspondence relation ℜ between them. In phonology, an expression *E* is a symbol structure much like the tree used in the syntactic expression above. (See Box 2, p. 473, for a brief introduction to phonological representations.) The interpretation *I* is rather different, however: it is a structure built from the lexical forms of morphemes that are combining to form a word or phrase. An example is given in (7).

(7) A single structural description *S* (phonology): *churches*

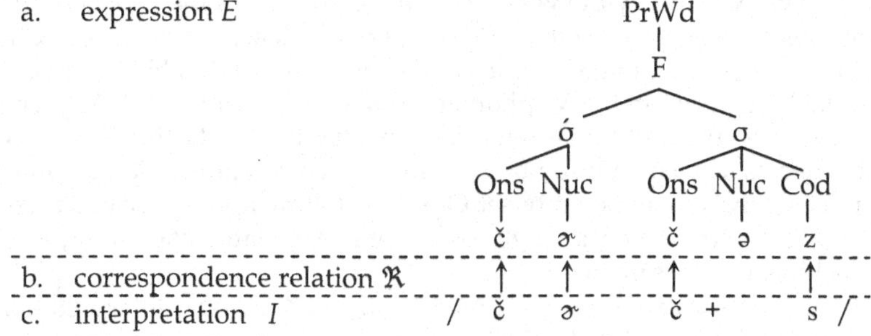

In (7), the lexical items constituting the interpretation are the noun stem *church* and the plural morpheme *-s*. The phonological forms of these morphemes stored in the lexicon—their **underlying forms**—are /čɚč/ and /s/, where *č* and *ɚ* represent the segments—speech sound units—spelled *ch* and *ur* in *church*, and the slashes '/' systematically delimit underlying forms. The expression as a whole is a **prosodic word** PrWd, containing a metrical **foot** F, in turn containing a stressed syllable σ́ followed by an unstressed syllable σ. The stressed syllable consists of a consonant-vowel—CV—sequence, the C (*č*) filling the role of syllable **onset**, the V (*ɚ*) filling the role of syllable **nucleus**. The second syllable has the form CVC, with the final C (*z*) filling the role of syllable **coda**. The overt part of this expression is the sound sequence [čɚ́.čəz], the pronunciation of *churches* (the '.' denotes a syllable boundary, which is at least sometimes overtly realized—for example, via the exact timing of the segments; Turk 1994).

The correspondence relation in (7) relates segments of the interpretation (*č, ɚ, č, s*) to their pronunciations in the expression. Note that the final segment /s/ in the interpretation (which we assume here to be the lexically stored underlying form of the plural morpheme) corresponds to a [z] in the expression: that is the final sound in *churches,* written *s* but pronounced *z.* And there is a segment in the expression, the **schwa** [ə], that corresponds to no segment of the interpretation: it is a weak vowel inserted—**epenthesized**—between the final [č] of *church* and the [z] of the plural morpheme, to improve the sound sequence ("improve" being given a formal definition in OT, as we will show). In this case, the epenthetic vowel is actually represented in the written form (by *e*); the context-sensitive presence or absence of epenthetic segments is, however, often not reflected orthographically (e.g., the *e* in the written form *faded* does correlate with an epenthetic *ə* in its pronunciation, but that in *faked* does not).

The phonological running example we will use in this chapter (and in numerous subsequent chapters) is actually a simplified system in which the differences between consonants are abstracted away, all consonants being simply denoted C, and all vowels, V. Sound sequences are represented as strings of Cs and Vs; for example, the pronunciation of *churches* is abstracted to [CVCVC] and its interpretation, to /CVC+C/. Here, we will focus on the parsing of sound sequences into syllables, largely ignoring the higher levels of phonological structure such as the foot and prosodic word. The OT CV theory of syllabification we will use is the **Basic CV Syllable Theory**. This theory was proposed in Prince and Smolensky 1993/2004, Chap. 6, which is reprinted here as Chapter 13; it builds upon a considerable body of earlier work on syllable theory and CV phonology (e.g., Clements and Keyser 1983; Vennemann 1988; see the additional references in Chapter 13). In this simplified theory, a syllable necessarily contains a nucleus **Nuc**, which contains a single vowel; preceding the nucleus there may be an onset **Ons**, and following the nucleus there may be a coda **Cod**, each containing a single consonant. A syllable containing a coda is **closed**; one lacking a coda is **open.**

In the Basic CV Syllable Theory—which we'll call **CVT**—an interpretation is a string of Cs and Vs, for example, /VCVC/. An expression is a parse of the string into syllables; three notations for such expressions are illustrated in (8).

(8) Candidate parses of /VCVC/ = /$V^1C^2V^3C^4$/ into syllables

a. .V.CVC. = [$_\sigma$V] [$_\sigma$CVC] = [$_\sigma V^1$] [$_\sigma C^1V^3C^4$]
b. ⟨V⟩.CV.⟨C⟩ = V [$_\sigma$CV] C = [$_\sigma C^2V^3$]
c. ⟨V⟩.CV.C□́. = V [$_\sigma$CV] [$_\sigma$C □́] = [$_\sigma C^2V^3$] [$_\sigma C^4V$]
d. .□V.CV.⟨C⟩ = [$_\sigma$□V] [$_\sigma$CV] C = [$_\sigma CV^1$] [$_\sigma C^2V^3$]

Expression (8a) is an onsetless open syllable followed by an onsetted closed syllable. With '.' marking syllable boundaries, this is represented as '.V.CVC.' in the simplest notation, which is the one used in Prince and Smolensky 1993/2004 (our Chapter 13). The second notation more explicitly represents the constituents: '[$_\sigma$V] [$_\sigma$CVC]'. The third notation, introduced in McCarthy and Prince 1995 and considered standard today, explicitly shows the correspondence between the segments in *I* and *E*. (Under Correspondence Theory, other correspondences for .V.CVC. are also possible—for example, $.V^1.C^4V^3C^1.$, according to which the two Cs have been interchanged. For our purposes, only the 'sensible' correspondences shown in (8) need be considered, since the other correspondences will in the end never be selected by any grammar.)

Expression (8b) contains only an onsetted open syllable. The initial V and final C of the interpretation are excluded from—not parsed into—syllable structure, as notated by the angle brackets '⟨ ⟩'. These segments exemplify **underparsing**: they are not phonetically realized, so (8b) is 'pronounced' simply as .CV.—as clearly indicated in the third notation, '$[_\sigma C^2V^3]$'. .CV. is the **overt form** contained in (8b), however it may be notated.

Expression (8c) consists of a pair of onsetted open syllables, in which the nucleus of the second syllable is not in correspondence with—or **filled by**—a segment of the interpretation. This empty nucleus, which is notated □́, exemplifies **overparsing**. (In general, in this notation, the acute accent marks the syllable nucleus.) The phonetic interpretation of this empty nucleus is an epenthetic vowel, like the [ə] in *churches* (7). Thus, (8c) is pronounced—has as its overt form—.CV.CV. . As in (8b), the initial V of the interpretation is unparsed in (8c).

Expression (8d) also consists of a pair of onsetted open syllables (with overt form .CV.CV.), but this time it is the onset of the first syllable that is unfilled (notated □—phonetically, an epenthetic consonant); the final C is unparsed, hence unpronounced.

1.1.3 Summary

(9) summarizes the discussion so far, filling in a few more details concerning structural descriptions; these details will be relevant to later chapters, but not to this one.

(9) Structural descriptions in OT phonology and syntax

A structural description *S* is a triple: an interpretation *I*, an expression *E*, and a correspondence relation $\mathfrak{R}$ between them.

a. In phonology (7),
   i. an interpretation is set of underlying phonological forms of morphemes, appropriately structured (e.g., by concatenation);
   ii. an expression is a sequence of segments, structured into phonological constituents (e.g, syllables) and decomposed into distinctive features;
   iii. a correspondence relation links segments of the interpretation with segments of the expression.
b. In syntax (5),
   i. an interpretation is a discourse/semantic structure, a logical form containing predicates and their arguments,[7] as well as the information or

[7] For the study of information questions in Chapter 16, the logical form part of the interpretation will also include question operators and variables.

discourse status of elements (such as topic or new information);

ii. an expression is a sequence of words structured into syntactic constituents (phrases), possibly containing chains linking elements in their surface position with ('movement') traces in other positions;

iii. a correspondence relation connects the entities of the interpretation—for example, predicates, arguments, operators, variables—with the elements that express them in the syntactic expression.

Box 1. The X′ Theory of phrase structure

A **declarative** sentence (or statement) is a unit of speech whose meaning (**semantic interpretation**) is an event as mentally represented. A **phrase** is a subunit of a sentence composed of a sequence of words. In the simple declarative sentence *boys play games*, the word *boys* can be elaborated to the sequence *teenage American boys* or *the boys down the street; play games* can be replaced by *often play games*. This **substitution test** shows that the sentence *boys play games* is made up of two main **constituent** phrases: [*boys*] [*play games*]. Applying the substitution test further to the phrase *play games*—elaborating it to *play truly violent games*—reveals that this phrase can be decomposed further into two (sub)phrases, [*play*] [*truly violent games*]. Thus, the **phrase structure** of *boys play games* is [[*boys*] [*play* [*games*]]].

A phrase can be substituted for another of the same **syntactic category**. The phrase *teenage American boys* is about boys. We say that *boys* is the **head** of the phrase. The syntactic category of *boys* is noun (N); hence, the phrase it heads is of category Noun Phrase (NP). An NP consists minimally of its obligatory part, a head N. The optional words that precede the head *boys* in the phrase *teenage American boys* express properties of the head; they are (adjective) **modifiers** of the head. Similarly, *play games, often play*, and *play* are Verb Phrases (VPs) whose head is the verb (V) *play*. Generally, NPs correspond to the participants of an event and the VP corresponds to the event type, such as activity (*play games*) or property (*is tired*).

The theory of phrase structure known as **X′** (read 'X-bar') **Theory** (Chomsky 1970; Jackendoff 1977) hypothesizes that all phrases (NPs, VPs, etc.) have the same basic structure, the **X′ schema:** [$_{XP}$ Specifier [$_{X'}$ Head Complement]]. A general head is denoted **X**; a noun head is N. The **complement** is a participant in a complex that is set up by the head—for example, *games* in the phrase *play games*. The head and the complement form a constituent called the **intermediate projection**, written **X′** (e.g., if the head is a verb, the head and complement together make up a V′—"V-bar"—phrase). The **specifier**, written **SpecXP**, delimits the relevant instance(s) of the head—for example, the **determiner (D)** *the* in *the boy down the street*, or *ten* in *ten boys*, or *a* in *a boy*. A convenient way to visually represent relations between a head X, its intermediate projection X′, and its **maximal projection** XP is via the tree diagram given in (1). Moreover, word order can be read off the structure directly.

(1) Simple declarative sentence

[$_{XP}$ Specifier [$_{X'}$ Head Complement]] = [$_{VP}$ *boys* [$_{V'}$ *play games*]]

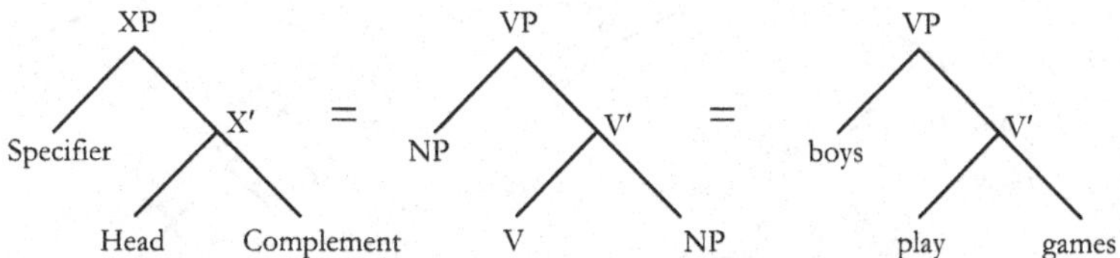

In this sentence, *boys* is an NP and thus according to X′ Theory it consists of a specifier, a head, and a complement—it so happens that the specifier and complement are empty. The intermediate projection N′ is as always present, so the full structure is as shown in the left tree of (2). The right tree employs a standard abbreviation in which a triangle stands in for further internal phrase structure.

(2) Abbreviating X′ structure

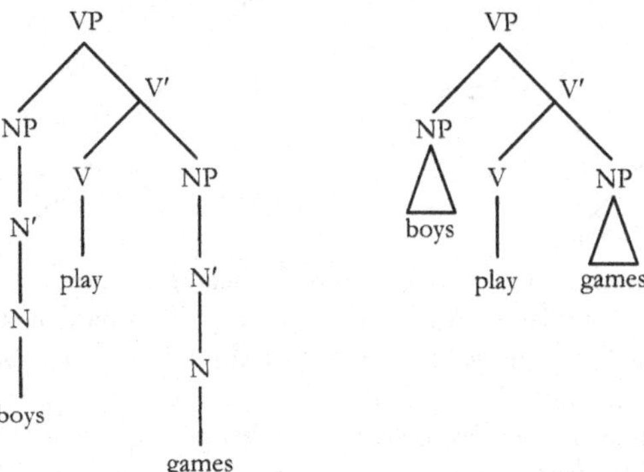

The NP *boys* can be elaborated to an NP of any internal complexity. An example is the NP represented in (3), *those boys down the street,* where the head is *boys*, the specifier is *those*, and the complement is the Prepositional Phrase (PP) *down the street.* Such NPs are termed **complex NPs**. In (3), the dotted, dashed and solid lines identify the individual X′ templates that are combined in this example.

Play games can be replaced by *always play games*, to give *boys always play games.* Hence, *always play games* must be of the same syntactic category as *play games*, namely, V′. The adverb *always* is **adjoined** (attached) to *play games*, with no effect on the category. The structure is shown in (4).

A sentence denoting a single, simple event is a **clause**. A sentence denoting a complex event typically consists of several clauses, one embedded inside (or 'under') another. In a sentence there is generally one clause for each **lexical** verb (verbs such as *play*, *sing*, *love*, in contrast to **auxiliary** verbs such as those boldfaced in ***has** played* and ***were** sung*).

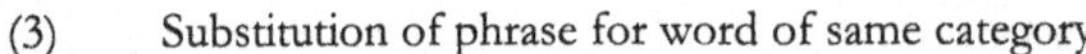

(3) Substitution of phrase for word of same category

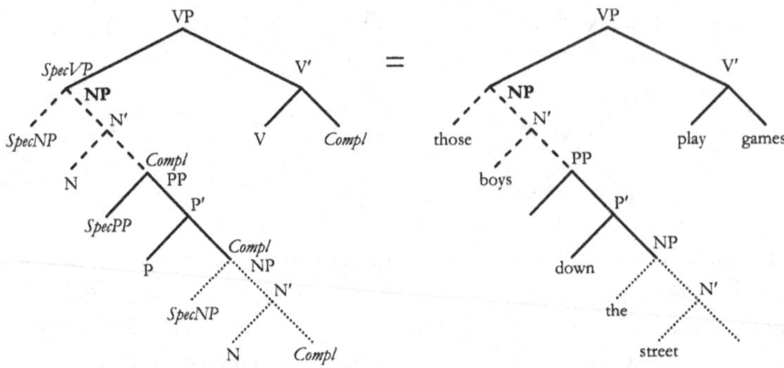

(4) Adjunction of an adverb

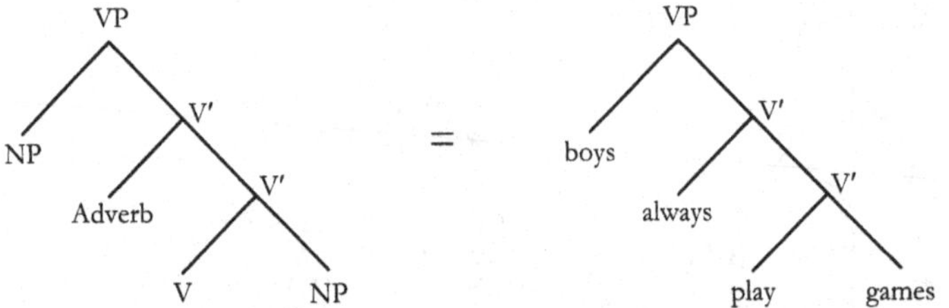

The **phrase structure** of a sentence is hidden from the hearer, as there are few direct phonetic cues to phrase boundaries. An example of the role of hidden structure comes from cases of **structural ambiguity**. The sentence *I watched the boy with binoculars* is ambiguous between two readings. One is that the speaker is using binoculars to watch the boy; the other is that the boy has binoculars in his possession. The PP *with binoculars* modifies *watched* in the first interpretation, but *the boy* in the second. Accordingly, the two readings correspond to two different phrase structures. In the first phrase structure (left tree of (5)), the PP *with binoculars* is adjoined to VP; in the second (right tree), the PP is a complement of the head noun *boy*, forming a complex NP.

Other properties of a clause can be superimposed on phrase structures like (1)–(5). These include characterizing NPs in terms of their structural relation to V. The specifier of the VP in (1) (*boys*) is the **subject** of *play*; the complement (*games*) is the **direct object** of *play*. These are **grammatical functions** (also called **grammatical relations** or **syntactic roles**); others include **indirect object** (*to Mary*) and **oblique** (a cover term for **locative** phrases like *in Baltimore*, **temporal** phrases like *at noon*, **manner** phrases like *with a hammer*, etc.). The **arguments** of *play* are the two NPs in subject and direct object position. Other verbs may take fewer or more arguments: *give* takes an indirect object as well as a direct object and subject, while *laugh* takes only a subject.

(5) Ambiguity of phrase structure

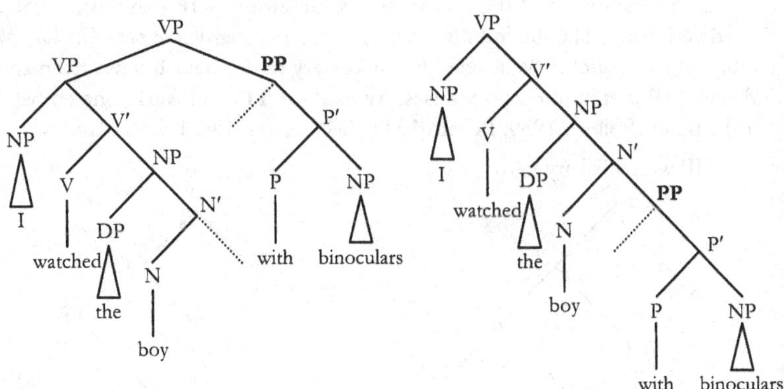

The relative **salience** of phrases within a sentence can also be superimposed onto phrase structures. In *boys play games*, the VP is *play games*; this denotes a property or a **predicate** (which holds of an individual *x* if and only if *x* plays games). This property is asserted to hold of *boys*, which plays a distinguished role in the sentence: it is the **topic**—what the sentence is about. Now it might be argued that *boys play games* asserts something about games (they are played by boys), and something about playing (it is something boys do with games). But the meaning of a sentence has cognitive structure. *Boys play games* denotes an assertion about boys: *boys* denotes the **figure**, and *play games* the **ground**; the referent of *boys* is accorded the greatest salience. Once a new topic like *boys* is introduced in the discourse, subsequent mentions of its referent often take the shape of a **pronoun** like *they*. Pronouns are NPs that have no intrinsic referent; they take their referent from the referent of a previously mentioned NP. Ambiguous expressions like pronouns are preferentially interpreted as referring to the most salient entity in the discourse: in *boys play games; they are silly*, the pronoun *they* refers to the boys, not the games. The subject position is the preferred location for the topic. A topic-referring element conveys **old**—previously stated—**information**. Within a clause, a topic-referring element is typically opposed to the **focus**, which conveys **new information** (e.g., *silly* above).

In the phrase structures (1)–(3), the entire clause *boys play games* is analyzed as a VP. Its subject *boys* occupies SpecVP, expressing the close semantic relationship between the V and its arguments. A more usual analysis treats the VP and the clause as a whole as having different heads. The **periphrastic** verbal form *have played* consists of the auxiliary verb *have* plus the past participle *played*, as in *boys have played games*: (6) shows an analysis of this sentence in which *played* heads VP, while *have* heads the clause as a whole. *Have* is **finite**—it marks the tense of the clause, and *have*, rather than *played*, is the verb that must agree with the subject (**George have played games*). In other words, *have* is the verb that is **inflected** for tense and **agreement features** such as number (singular/plural). The category of *have* is thus called **I** ('I', often also written 'INFL', abbreviates 'inflection'), and the clause here is therefore an **IP** (Chomsky 1986). Uninflected verb forms like the infinitive *to play* or the past participle *played* in *have played* are usually called **nonfinite.** (Whenever it is necessary to distinguish tense from agreement inflection, IP is split into two phrases, **TenseP** (or **TP**) and **AgrP**, one embedded under the other (Pollock 1989; Belletti 1990). See Section 18:3.1 for examples.)

(6) IP with auxiliary verb

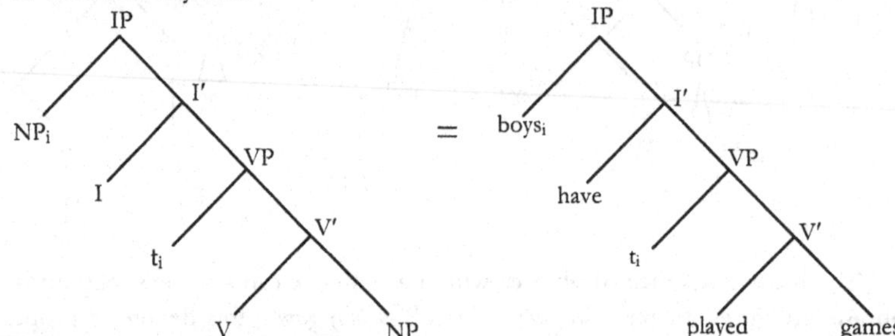

We are now faced with the challenge of reconciling, on the one hand, the close semantic relationship between the V *played* and its argument NP *boys*, and on the other hand, the actual position of the NP—before the auxiliary. What we need is a means of connecting two positions (SpecIP and SpecVP), for example, an abstract **chain** with two members that are **coindexed** (assigned the same arbitrary subscript or index, such as *i*): $boys_i$ in SpecIP and an empty placeholder in SpecVP called a **trace,** t_i. Coindexation is a formal device denoting a **dependency** relation between elements. Here, this relation has several facets. For example, in the event described, the role of *boys* is determined by *play*: this role is the one filled by any NP in the specifier of a VP headed by *play*. Figuratively, the role *play* assigns to its subject gets assigned to t_i, which then shares it with $boys_i$ in virtue of the dependency marked by their coindexation. Also, the presence of *boys* in SpecIP prevents the presence of another NP in SpecVP: **boys have girls played games* is not possible. The silent trace t_i 'fills' SpecVP, leaving no place for another NP like *girls*; and this silent filler's existence is in turn dependent on the presence of the coindexed NP $boys_i$.

In the chain consisting of the two coindexed NPs $boys_i$ and t_i, $boys_i$ is the **head** and t_i the **tail** of the chain. Such a chain is often conceived as being formed by **movement**: $boys_i$ 'starts out' in SpecVP (tail) and then 'moves' to SpecIP (head), leaving the trace t_i behind. Whether an element *x* can perform a given movement typically depends on what material *x* would 'pass over' in moving from its original **base** position to its **landing site**. Movement will be discussed further in Chapter 16.

Returning now to our original sentence, *boys play games:* like *boys have played games,* this sentence involves tense and agreement; but instead of being associated with the auxiliary *have*, these are now associated with the main (lexical) verb *play*. (The present tense in *play* is revealed by the contrasting past tense in *boys played games*; the agreement property of *play* is revealed by the contrasting **Dick play games*, unacceptable because of the failure of *play* to agree with the singular number of its subject.) In conformity to the analysis (6) (and putting aside other aspects of English), *boys play games* can be analyzed with *play* as an I head. The structure is shown in (7). As before, there is a chain with head *boys*$_i$ in SpecIP and tail t_i in SpecVP; the upper arrow shows this movement. But now in addition, the verb has moved from the head of VP to the head of IP, the position where tense marking and subject agreement occur, creating a second chain consisting of head *play*$_k$ coindexed with tail t_k.

(7) IP without auxiliary

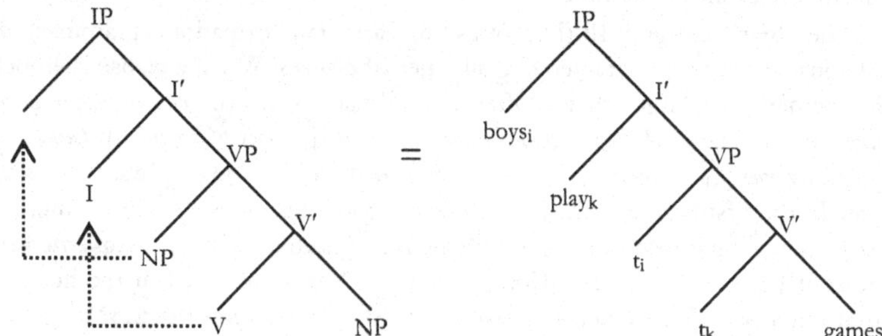

This theoretical step is actually quite significant (and controversial). It is one thing to posit a tree position I for an overt auxiliary verb *have* as in (6); it is another to posit this position when there is no auxiliary as in (7). There is no audible difference between the IP tree (7) and the VP tree (1). The argument given above, that *play* must be located in I rather than in V because it carries tense and agreement just like the auxiliary *have*, takes information traditionally seen as residing in the **morphology**—the internal structure of words—and encodes it in the syntax. The head I contributes only **functional features** like [past] and [singular]: I is a **functional head**, as opposed to N and V, which are **lexical heads** that contribute all the featural information present in the lexical entry of a noun or verb. Sometimes the functional features of I manifest themselves as an independent word—an auxiliary verb, like *have* in (6). Other times the functional features of I are expressed as an inflection (e.g., a suffix) on the main verb, which, like *play* in (7), has moved from V to I "in order to get the functional features" in some sense.

Whether an inflected main verb like *play* should be analyzed as moving from V to I (7) or as simply remaining in V (1) must ultimately be decided by the different empirical predictions these analyses make; this is not the place to review and assess the empirical evidence. But it is worth pointing out a metatheoretical tension at play here. On the one hand, the I analysis for *play* promotes **uniformity**: the tree structure for a simple sentence is the same whether the particular tense and agreement features being expressed happen to call for a separate auxiliary verb or merely inflection on the main verb. On the other hand, the I analysis clearly posits considerably more structure and movement. In much OT syntax (e.g., Chapter 18), economy constraints of the *STRUCTURE family provide pressure (within the grammar itself) to minimize structure, favoring the simple VP analysis (1); in the tradition defined by Chomsky's work, notions of theoretical simplicity dependent on uniformity of structure provide pressure (at the metatheoretical level) favoring the more complex IP analysis (7) (Chomsky 1986; cf. the 'fallacy of uniformity', Prince 1993). Positing the position I into which a main verb moves in the absence of an auxiliary takes the theory down a path that ultimately leads to proposals for some 30 functional heads present in every sentence (Cinque 1999, 106). Ultimately, the difference in complexity of the analysis of *boys play games* without or with functional heads is no small matter. See Chapter 18 for other relevant discussion.

The phrasal category IP (known as S in early transformational grammar) turns out to be insufficient for characterizing all types of clauses. When a clause is embedded as an argument of a larger clause, often a word such as *that* or *because* appears to introduce the embedded clause: *everyone knows* [$_{XP}$ ***that*** [$_{IP}$ *boys play games*]]; *teenage American boys play games* [$_{XP}$ ***because*** [$_{IP}$ *they are easily bored*]]. What type of phrase XP is involved here? In the first example, the clause *boys play games* becomes the complement of *know*; *that* prepares the clause to be a complement and is thus called a **complementizer**. The phrase it heads is therefore a Complementizer Phrase or **CP**. But the head of CP is often not a complementizer. A question of the type *what will they play?* is typically analyzed as a CP in which C houses the auxiliary *will*. To form a question from [$_{IP}$ *they will* [$_{VP}$ *play games*]], *will* moves from I up to C. The question word or ***wh*-phrase** *what* is analyzed as starting in the location of *games* and moving up to SpecCP, as shown in (8). See Chapter 16 for extensive discussion.

(8) Complementizer Phrases with complementizer or *wh*-phrase

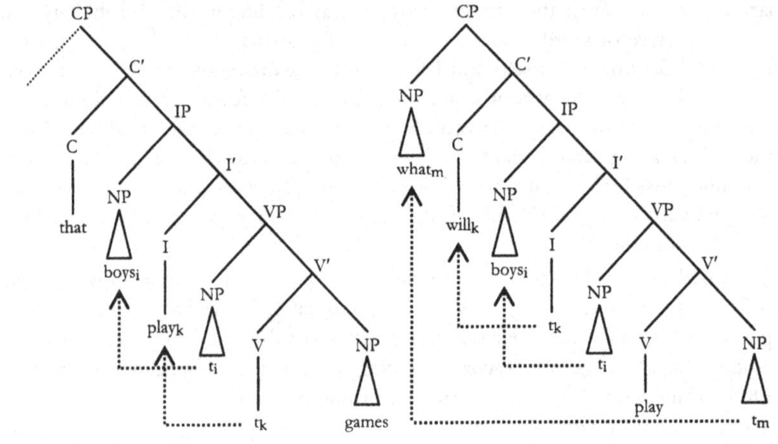

Box 2. Rudiments of phonological theory

Why does English have words like *belfry* but not **fbrlei* or **rbelfi* or **rilefb*? (As usual, * marks impossible forms.) Why are both *feet* and *fee* possible, but not both *fit* and **fi* (*fit* without the *t*)? Why *sibilant* but not **bilantsib*? By addressing these questions briefly, we can introduce several key concepts of phonological theory in a specific context. (See, for example, Hammond 1999 for full exposition and details.) A systematic presentation of the theory follows.

A word is a sequence of legal *syllables*—**fbrlei* is not. A syllable is a sequence of three sound groups: a series of consonants forming an **onset**, a series of vowels or vowel-like consonants forming the syllable **nucleus**, and finally a series of consonants forming a **coda**. An English onset cannot contain four consonants, so there is no possible first syllable with which **fbrlei* can begin. This problem does not afflict **rbelfi*, which might consist of two syllables *rbel* and *fi*. But while English syllables are not prohibited from having two-consonant onsets, not all consonant pairs are possible: *rb* is not. Similarly, while two-consonant codas are not forbidden in general, *fb* is not a possible coda, so there is no syllable with which **rilefb* can end. The set of possible English words is enormously restricted by the requirement that a word be a sequence of legal syllables.

As for **fi*, it is simply too short or **light** to be an English word: excepting a few function words like *the*, an English word must have at least two units of **weight**. The unit of weight is the **mora** **μ**. Now *feet*, *fee*, and *fit* all contain (at least) two moras: the long vowel in *feet* and *fee* has weight 2μ in virtue of being long; the short vowel in *fit* has only one mora, but the coda consonant *t* contributes the necessary second mora. **fi* weighs in at only 1μ.

Finally, unlike *sibilant*, **bilantsib* has no possible **stress pattern**. Spelled *bil*, the second syllable of *sibilant* is actually pronounced *bl̩*: the vowel-like consonant *l̩* (marked with ' ̩ ') is the syllable nucleus. Similarly, orthographic *lant* is pronounced *ln̩t*, with nucleus *n̩*. Syllables with nuclear consonants like *l̩* and *n̩* cannot bear stress. **bilantsib* denotes *bl̩.ln̩t.síb*; the stress must fall on the final syllable, marked with '´'. Now while each of these three syllables (separated by '.') is individually possible, this sequence is not. Denoting stressed and unstressed syllables respectively by σ́ and σ, the stress patterns of *sibilant* and **bilantsib* are σ́σσ and σσσ́, respectively. Possible stress patterns in English are governed by several requirements. Syllables are grouped into **feet**, which consist of either [σ́] or [σ́σ]. It is possible for an isolated syllable of an English word to not be part of a foot, but two adjacent syllables cannot both be unfooted. Thus, the stress pattern σ́σσ is possible, footed as [σ́σ]σ, but σσσ́ is impossible: neither of the first two syllables can be parsed into a legal foot, [σ́] or [σ́σ].

Virtually all of the generalizations invoked in these explanations are not specific to English: they are evident, in one form or another, in the phonologies of many other languages. By giving precise accounts of the sound patterns of specific languages, phonological theory strives to identify the universal explanatory principles of phonological knowledge that underlie detailed language-particular analyses.

Universal phonology

The phonological component of universal grammar is characterized by many cross-cutting generalizations. These generalizations concern the internal properties of speech sounds and the ways they are assembled into linguistic expressions in the languages of the world. Particularly important are the entities the generalizations refer to, such as codas, moras, syllables, feet: these are the **constituents** making up the **combinatorial structure** of phonological expressions. Many phonological generalizations have been shown to be active in the knowledge of speakers; for example, speakers are known to manipulate newly encountered forms in conformity with these generalizations.[8] Thus, the constituent structure of phonological expressions is hypothesized to characterize the mental representations actually subserving human speech.

The fundamental generalizations of phonological theory are not immediately observable on the surface of natural language. This is formally explained as follows in OT. Phonological generalizations are the surface reflex of **universal constraints** on what constitutes a well-formed sound structure, and these constraints are highly conflicting in their demands. Thus, the surface sound patterns of a language are the result of competing requirements, and many of the constraints generating these patterns are not strong enough to impose themselves without exception across the language. Furthermore, since the strength of constraints varies across languages, even if a constraint should happen to be strong enough to hold exceptionlessly on the surface in one language, the same is not expected to be true in other languages though they are nonetheless shaped to some degree by that constraint.

Descriptively, then, the sound patterns of a language can be understood as a series of approximations of greater and greater complexity, achieving successively better accuracy and completeness. Each approximation incorporates additional, more specialized constraints. This box sketches a first-order approximation of phonological theory, a more or less mainstream view shared by most phonologists working within OT.

Prosodic structure

A natural language expression is a sequence of well-formed **phonological words**, each of which is composed of a sequence of well-formed **syllables**. The syllables of a word must group together to make well-formed **metrical feet** that characterize the prominence or **prosodic** structure of the word. Each foot contains a relatively prominent (or strong, or **stressed**) syllable and perhaps also a nonprominent (weak, unstressed) syllable. A phonological word contains a maximally prominent foot, the strong syllable of which provides the word with its **primary stress**. The feet of a word are subject to a number of constraints, the relative strengths of which define the **stress system** of the language. A foot with its strong syllable on the left is called **trochaic**; on the right,

[8] Several examples pertaining to the case taken up in Box 14:1, Finnish vowel harmony, are discussed in Campbell 1980. Here the generalizations concern the vowels of a word, which must agree or 'harmonize' in certain properties. Vowels in foreign words are often actively modified by speakers to create harmony.

iambic. The stress system of a given language typically requires all feet to be either trochaic or iambic.[9]

The notion of 'prominence' involved in stress systems is one internal to the cognitive system characterized by phonological theory. Speakers are generally conscious of the relative prominence of the constituents of expressions, and generally consistent in their judgments. But it is difficult, perhaps impossible, to identify prominence by readily measurable properties of the acoustic signal—just as it is difficult or impossible to identify a noun by measuring low-level acoustic signals, or, for that matter, to identify a goose by measuring low-level optical signals, even though our minds continually identify such abstractions from low-level sensory input signals. Phonological prominence is correlated with physical energy, but only roughly.

Syllables

In a given language, to first approximation, a well-formed syllable comprises a sequence of segments constituting a well-formed **onset**, followed by a sequence of segments constituting a well-formed **nucleus**, followed by a sequence of segments constituting a well-formed **coda**. Each of these three syllable positions is limited to a certain number of segments: in many languages, this limit is one; in others, two; in a relatively small number of languages, more than two are allowed. When multiple segments are allowed in a syllable position, the permissible sequences are limited by the **phonotactic constraints** of the language (English allows onset *sp*, but not *ps*; French allows both: *spécial, psycho*). In a number of languages, the maximum number of segments possible in the coda is zero; in most languages, the set of segments allowed in well-formed codas is limited by stringent **coda conditions**. Syllables lacking codas are **open**, those with codas are **closed**. A long vowel or double consonant (called a **geminate**) typically acts like two identical segments for the purposes of syllable structure.

A given language typically has an upper limit on a syllable's prominence level: for example, a long vowel may be allowed in an open syllable, but only a short vowel may be permitted in a syllable with a coda. A second vowel in the nucleus, or a coda consonant, contributes one unit of syllable **weight**, a **mora**; the first vowel also contributes a mora. Syllables with one mora are **light**, those with two are **heavy**; **super-heavy** syllables, with more than two moras, are often ill formed. The portion of the syllable that contributes to the weight of a syllable is the **rime**: the nucleus and the coda together; onsets have no weight.

To form a well-formed word, syllables and feet often need to coordinate, so that a syllable of high prominence—a heavy syllable—falls in the prominent foot position. The **Weight-to-Stress Principle** (WSP; Prince 1990) requires that a heavy syllable be stressed.

[9] English feet are trochaic, as in *(sí.bḷ)lṇt*, where parentheses enclose a foot. Choctaw (a Muskogean language of Oklahoma and Mississippi) illustrates a typical iambic foot pattern in such words as *(li.tí:)(ha.tók)* 'it was dirty' and *(sa.lí:)(ti.há:)(tók)* 'I was dirty', where ':' marks long vowels, and the vowel length alternation between *lití:ha* and *lí:tihá*: 'dirty' shows the effect of vowel lengthening in stressed syllables (Hayes 1994, 210).

Segments

For the purpose of characterizing the **distribution** of segments—which segments are allowed in which positions—segments are grouped into many cross-cutting classes. In English, in the position (or **environment**) *s_aı* the stops {*t k p*} are permitted (*sty, sky, spy*), whereas the stops {t^h k^h p^h} are not; in the position *_aı*, just the reverse is true (*tie, chi* [χ], *pie*). The latter segments are the **aspirated stops**; they are said to share the **distinctive feature** [+aspirated], denoted '*h*'.[10] A distinctive feature identifies a class of segments with similar distributional properties. The feature [+aspirated], like most features, has a **phonetic correlate**, a physical property (or cluster of properties): the "puff of air" that accompanies the release of the closure forming the consonant, or the concomitant burst of acoustic noise. Phonetic correlates can be articulatory or perceptual. But the identification of the distinctive features of a language's segment inventory is *not* a phonetic issue: it is entirely internal to phonology, determined by the segment classes defined by the sound patterns of the language.[11] Mistaking phonological features for phonetic properties is an easy but dangerous error to make.

Using **IPA** (International Phonetic Alphabet) symbols, (1) identifies several features that distinguish the different **sonority** classes. Sonorant segments are [+sonorant] while obstruent segments are [−sonorant], continuant segments are [+continuant], nasal segments are [+nasal], and so on. Like [±aspirated], [±voiced] is a feature correlated to articulation in the glottis: it is a **laryngeal** feature. The true abstractness of phonological features is illustrated by voicing, for while the value [−voiced] is commonly conceived in terms of the number of milliseconds separating the release of the oral closure and the onset of the glottal pulses defining phonation (or 'voicing'), in fact the perception of a stop as voiced is at least as sensitive to the absence of aspiration and the slight shortening of a preceding vowel (see Lisker 1957 and other references in Kingston and Diehl 1995).

Another important class of phonological features are those of **place**. The primary phonetic correlates here concern the location of the tongue and other vocal articulators during the formation of the segment. For vowels, the place features are correlated with the tongue body position, [±high] and [±low], [±front] and [±back]; the tongue root, [±advanced tongue root] = [±ATR]; and the lips, [±rounded]. For consonants, they are correlated with the location of the primary oral constriction and the articulator forming that constriction: for the tongue tip, [coronal]; the tongue body, [dorsal]; the tongue root, [pharyngeal]; the lips, [labial].

[10] Fundamental to much phonological theorizing is the notion of **phoneme**. In English, *t* and t^h are two variants of a single underlying phoneme: which pronunciation appears is determined by the context (as in ***staı*** 'sty' vs. ***t^haı*** 'tie'). In Thai, however, *t* and t^h represent different phonemes. Both can appear in the same environment; for example, ***taı*** and ***t^haı*** are different possible Thai words. In phonemic theories, phonemes are the building blocks for lexical entries. But the notion of phoneme is inessential in OT, and the subtleties inherent in it will be put aside here. A phoneme is essentially a class of similar, distributionally related segments; individual segments themselves suffice in OT.

[11] A phonological theory is said to be **natural**—as opposed to **abstract**—to the extent that the features it posits have strong phonetic correlates and the rules it proposes have identifiable **phonetic motivation**, such as decreasing articulatory or perceptual difficulty.

Box 2

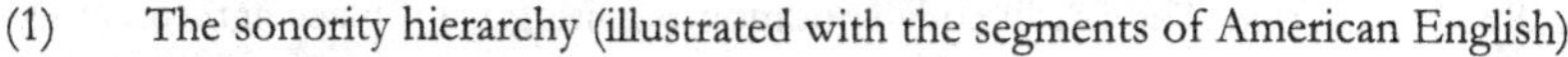
(1) The sonority hierarchy (illustrated with the segments of American English)

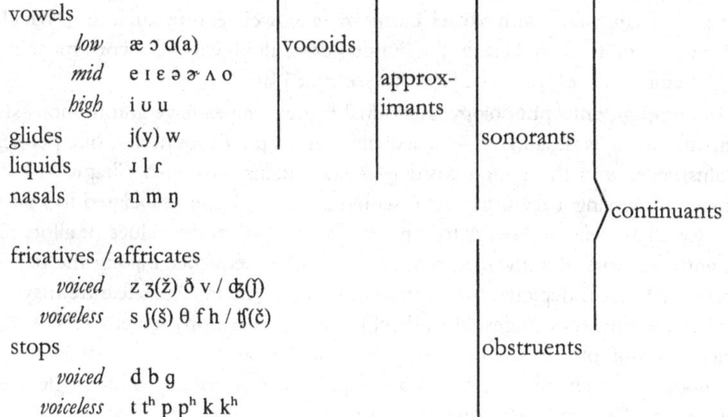

æ cat, ɔ **caught**, ɑ(a) cot, e Kate, ɪ kit, ɛ keg, ə catastrophe, ɚ **curt**, ʌ cut, o coat, i parakeet, ʊ **cook**, u coot

j(y) you, ɹ rye, ɾ atom, ŋ **sing**, ʒ(ž) **azure**, ð **this**, ʤ(ǰ) **gin**, ʃ(š) **shy**, θ **thigh**, ʧ(č) **chin**, g gone, t/p/k stint/**spin**/**skin**, tʰ/pʰ/kʰ tin/pin/kin

As an example of a phonological constraint dependent on place, in English, additional segments can be piled on the end of a word, after the final syllable, but these sounds must always be [coronal]: *arms*, *armed*, *fifth*, *twelfths*. In the Australian language Lardil, the coda constraint is heavily sensitive to place: a coda consonant may only be a consonant with [coronal] place or a nasal with the same place as the following consonant (see Prince and Smolensky 1993/2004, Chap. 7 and references cited there). (This **nasal place agreement** constraint plays a central role in Chapter 17.)

Features

A phonological feature is not merely a property shared by segments with common distributional patterns; some generalizations target features independently of the segments that express them. Features that function autonomously from segments are called **autosegments. Tone** is a feature of vowels phonetically correlated with pitch or fundamental frequency, modulated by the tension of the vocal folds. We can let H, M, D, and L stand for [high], [mid-high], [mid], and [low] values for this feature, and let a_H designate the vowel *a* with tone H. Consider Vata (Ivory Coast) verbs in the perfective aspect (completed action, glossed with the past tense). The generalization uniting them is that the tone L appears at the end of the word—but this tone is expressed differently from word to word. In some words, L is expressed on its own, single vowel (a_H la_L 'you carried'); in certain other words, L shares a vowel with a preceding tone (la_{HL} 'called'); in still other words, L is expressed over multiple consecutive final vowels (kla_L le_L 'grabbed with'). (See Kaye 1989, 81–98 for a basic introduction.)

Many features function autonomously in this fashion, although often not as dramatically as does tone. The Lardil coda condition requiring nasal place agreement essentially demands that a single place feature be expressed on two consonants (the first a nasal). In languages with **vowel harmony**, a vowel feature such as [+back] is expressed over multiple vowels; in the limiting case, all vowels of a word must express a single feature, either [+back] or [−back] (see Box 14:1).

In **autosegmental phonology**, individual feature values have autonomous status. A segmental string is designated by a sequence of abstract **root nodes**, one per segment; (9) illustrates, with the Lango word *gódì* 'mountains' (see also Chapter 14 (54)). A segment expressing a feature is represented as a root node **associated** to that feature value via an **association line**. A root node is associated to the values of all its features. The autosegments of a given feature are temporally sequenced along the **tier** for that feature; each tier is depicted by a dotted horizontal line in (9). A feature may be associated to multiple root nodes, like [+back] in a back-harmony system, or [+ATR] in (9). Sometimes multiple consecutive values of a single feature are associated with a single root node, as when multiple tones are expressed sequentially on a single vowel—a **contour tone**, like the falling tone of Vata la_{HL} 'called'.[12]

A single tone (or other autosegmental feature) can be associated to—expressed by—several segments. For a series of tones to be analyzed as multiple tones, there must be a contour at the juncture of the tones—a change from one tonal value to another; this is the **Obligatory Contour Principle (OCP)** (Leben 1973; Goldsmith 1976; McCarthy 1979, 1981, 1986). Thus, the OCP asserts that when consecutive segments express the same tonal value, they must be analyzed as sharing a single tone feature. When two identical tones come together, as in a word root and an ending, often one changes to a different tone, so that two autonomous tones are maintained, to satisfy the OCP.

(9) Autosegmental representation of *gódì*

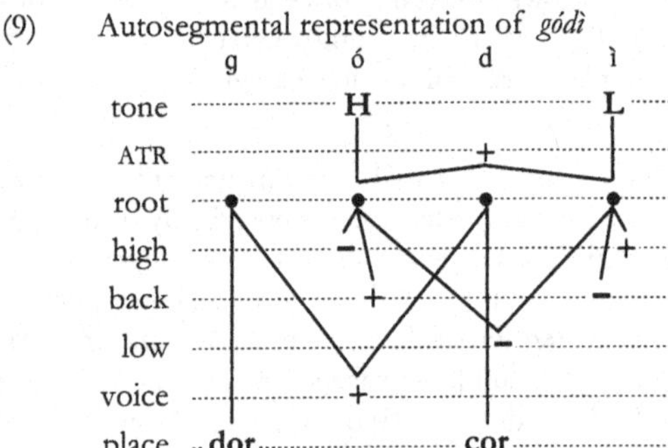

A binary feature [f] defines an **opposition** between linguistic forms with the two alternate values [+f] and [−f]. *t* and *d* illustrate the opposition of [±voice]. The Prague School linguists (Trubetzkoy 1939/1969; Jakobson 1941/1968, 1962) studied such

[12] The customary notations for single H and L tones on a vowel *a* are *á* and *à*, respectively; falling and rising contour tones are correspondingly written *â* and *ǎ* (e.g., see (9)).

oppositions across many languages, concluding that typically there is a universal asymmetry between the two members of an opposition, one being consistently 'preferred' to the other. The dispreferred member was called the **marked** pole of the opposition; the other, **unmarked.** In our example, *d* is marked relative to *t.* The senses in which marked structures are 'dispreferred' span the full spectrum of language phenomena: marked elements are prone to be omitted from the phonological inventories of the world's languages; marked elements in underlying forms are prone to be modified by the phonology so that in the surface form the unmarked element appears instead; in environments where one member of an opposition is prohibited, it is the marked member; when present in a language, marked elements are typically less frequent than their unmarked counterparts; children acquiring language acquire the marked member of an opposition later than the unmarked; aphasic patients are prone to lose marked structures while retaining unmarked ones.

In OT, marked elements are dispreferred because they violate **markedness constraints** (like 'A [–sonorant] segment must be [–voice]', a constraint violated by *d* but satisfied by *t*). Often, phonetic motivations can be found for markedness constraints: the marked pole is articulatorily or perceptually more difficult. But as with phonological features, the question of which elements are marked is properly the purview of phonology, not phonetics: marked elements are those that are phonologically dispreferred in the above senses, whether or not some underlying phonetic correlate of 'difficulty' can be identified.

Underlying and surface forms

The pronounced forms of speech—**surface forms**—express meanings. The phonological system mediates between two other linguistic systems: the **lexicon/morphology** and the **phonetics.** In the former system, the minimal meaningful units of language—**morphemes**—are stored in a mental lexicon, including their sound structure; and in this system, morphological knowledge is used to combine morphemes to produce the **underlying forms** of words and phrases. For *scones,* this is /skon+s/, a **stem** for the morpheme *scone,* with stored lexical sound structure /skon/, and a **suffix** /-s/, the stored lexical sound structure of the plural morpheme. The underlying form of a word provides the raw material from which the phonology computes the surface form, which specifies the actual pronunciation of the word. The surface form—also called the **phonetic form**—is interpreted by the phonetic system. The phonetics connects physical variables with the abstract representations over which phonology computes. The perceptual component of the phonetics converts acoustic stimuli to abstract phonological surface representations; the articulatory component of the phonetics converts such representations to motor plans for driving the physical articulators that produce speech.

In OT, the phonological grammar contains two classes of constraints, each responsible for the needs of one of the systems with which phonology connects or **interfaces:** the lexicon and the phonetics. To a certain degree, phonetic forms are designed by the phonology to avoid marked structure—that is, to satisfy markedness constraints. Functionally, this can be seen as pressure for pronounced forms to be efficiently articulable and effectively perceivable: markedness constraints are serving the demands of the phonetic interface. But phonetic forms must also be designed to enable the hearer to recover the morphemes—and hence the meaning—being expressed. This is achieved in the phonology by **faithfulness constraints**, which demand that the phonetic form equal the stored lexical form that the hearer can recognize; these constraints serve the needs of the lexical interface of phonology.

The lexical representation of a word or phrase is a structure built from **underlying representations** of morphemes in the lexicon. For *scones*, this is /skon+s/. The requirements of the lexical system are encoded in faithfulness constraints, which, if fully satisfied, would ensure that the pronounced form was identical to the lexical form: [skons]. But conflicting with faithfulness is a markedness constraint requiring that coda consonants agree in voicing; this constraint dominates, yielding the actual pronunciation [skonz].

Morphological systems

The sound structures of morphemes in the lexicon can take a variety of forms, and can be combined with one another in several ways. In **concatenative morphology**, the most familiar system, the underlying form of a morpheme is a sequence of segments, which combine by concatenation: one follows the other in a sequence, as in /skon+s/. Vata (above) illustrates a variant: the stored lexical form of the perfective morpheme is simply the tone L.

In **root-and-pattern morphology**, a morpheme may be a sequence of segments, as in concatenative morphology, but alternatively it may be a pattern or **template**. The Arabic word *kuttib* 'was made to write' is the combination of the root morpheme /ktb/ 'write', the grammatical morpheme /ui/ 'passive voice', and the templatic morpheme CVCCVC 'causative'; the segmental morphemes are used to fill in the template (see, e.g., Kenstowicz 1993, 396ff., for an introduction). Note that the root /ktb/ is a sequence of consonants that only becomes pronounceable when it is mapped to a template, along with another morpheme's vowels, which interdigitate between the root consonants.

Similarly, a **reduplicative morpheme** is often a template (e.g., CV) that appears to the left or right of (or sometimes inside) a **base** morpheme, the segments of the base being copied to fill in the template. Thus, in the Australian language Mangarayi, adding the reduplicative morpheme marking the plural to *baraŋali* 'father-in-law' yields ***bar**araŋali*; to *jimgan* 'knowledgeable person', ***jimg**imgan* (see McCarthy and Prince 1993b, 121, for an OT analysis).

1.2 Grammars specify functions; candidates from *Gen* and *Int*

Consider an interpretation I_0 and an expression E_0. The set of potential or **candidate** expressions of I_0 and the set of potential interpretations of E_0 are delimited by the universe of structural descriptions, $\mathcal{U}$. Specifically, the set of all potential expressions of a particular interpretation I_0 is the set of all structural descriptions $S = (I_0, E, \mathfrak{R})$ in $\mathcal{U}$—where S contains the particular interpretation I_0, and E and $\mathfrak{R}$ are any expression and correspondence relation that, together with I_0, yield a structural description in $\mathcal{U}$. This set is called *Gen*(I_0). *Gen* is the function that 'generates' all potential structural descriptions of an interpretation; it was introduced in Prince and Smolensky 1993/2004.

Analogously, the set of all potential interpretations of a particular expression E_0 is the set of all structural descriptions $S = (I, E_0, \mathfrak{R})$ in $\mathcal{U}$—where S contains the particular expression E_0, and I and $\mathfrak{R}$ are any interpretation and correspondence relation that, together with E_0, yield a structural description in $\mathcal{U}$. This set will be called *Int*(E_0). *Int* is the function that 'generates' all potential structural descriptions for interpreting E_0; it was introduced implicitly in Smolensky 1996c and explicitly in Smolensky 1996a, 1998 (see also Wilson 1995, 2001a; Boersma 1998; Hendriks and de Hoop 2001; Blutner and Zeevat 2003).

This characterization of the basic functions subserved by a grammar is laid out in (10)–(11).

(10) Candidate sets: *Gen* and *Int*

a. A structural universe comprises

i. a **universe of interpretations** $\mathcal{U}_I$: a set of structures I;

ii. a **universe of expressions** $\mathcal{U}_E$: a set of structures E; for each E there is a substructure $O = overt(E)$ called the **overt part** of E;

iii. for each $I \in \mathcal{U}_I$ and $E \in \mathcal{U}_E$, a **universe of correspondence relations** $\mathcal{U}_\mathfrak{R}(I, E)$, each member of which is a relation $\mathfrak{R}$ between the elements constituting the structure I and those constituting E; and

iv. a **universe of structural descriptions** $\mathcal{U}_S$: a collection of triples $S = (I, E, \mathfrak{R})$ where $I \in \mathcal{U}_I$, $E \in \mathcal{U}_E$, and $\mathfrak{R} \in \mathcal{U}_\mathfrak{R}(I, E)$; S is 'an expression of I' as well as 'an interpretation of E' and 'an interpretation of $O = overt(E)$'.

b. The functions *Gen*, *Int*, and *Int'* are defined by

i. $Gen(I_0) \equiv \{S \in \mathcal{U}_S \mid \exists E \in \mathcal{U}_E, \mathfrak{R} \in \mathcal{U}_\mathfrak{R}(I, E) \text{ such that } S = (I_0, E, \mathfrak{R})\}$;

ii. $Int(E_0) \equiv \{S \in \mathcal{U}_S \mid \exists I \in \mathcal{U}_I, \mathfrak{R} \in \mathcal{U}_\mathfrak{R}(I, E) \text{ such that } S = (I, E_0, \mathfrak{R})\}$;

iii. $Int'(O_0) \equiv \{S \in \mathcal{U}_S \mid \exists I \in \mathcal{U}_I, E \in \mathcal{U}_E, \mathfrak{R} \in \mathcal{U}_\mathfrak{R}(I, E) \text{ such that } S = (I, E, \mathfrak{R}) \text{ and } overt(E) = O_0\}$.

c. Candidates

i. *Gen*(I_0) is the set of **candidate expressions** of the interpretation I_0.

ii. *Int*(E_0) is the set of **candidate interpretations** of the expression E_0.

iii. *Int'*(O_0) is the set of **candidate interpretations** of the overt structure O_0.

(11) Grammar-determined production and comprehension functions: f_{prod}, f_{comp}

a. A grammar specifies a **production** (or **generation**) **function** f_{prod} and **comprehension** (or **interpretation**) **functions** f_{comp}, f'_{comp}, where

i. $f_{\text{prod}}(I_0) \subset Gen(I_0)$;
ii. $f_{\text{comp}}(E_0) \subset Int(E_0)$;
iii. $f'_{\text{comp}}(O_0) \subset Int'(O_0)$.

b. Grammatical structures
i. If $S = (I_0, E, \mathfrak{R}) \in f_{\text{prod}}(I_0)$, then S is a **grammatical expression** of the interpretation I_0.
ii. If $S = (I, E_0, \mathfrak{R}) \in f_{\text{comp}}(E_0)$, then S is a **grammatical interpretation** of the expression E_0.
iii. If $S = (I, E, \mathfrak{R}) \in f'_{\text{comp}}(O_0)$, then S is a **grammatical structural description** of the overt structure $O_0 = overt(E)$.

c. The **(expression) language** specified by a grammar is the set $\mathcal{L}$ of expressions in the outputs of the function f_{prod}: $\mathcal{L} \equiv \{E_0 \mid \exists I_0 \in \mathcal{U}_I, \mathfrak{R}_0 \in \mathcal{U}_{\mathfrak{R}}$ such that $f_{\text{prod}}(I_0) = (I_0, E_0, \mathfrak{R}_0)\}$.

Note that (11) asserts that it is the responsibility of the grammar to *specify* production and comprehension functions, not to *compute* them. That is, the grammar provides an account of production and comprehension at a **functional** level (what Marr (1982) called the 'computational' level), not the algorithmic or implementational levels—the grammar need not describe human language *processes*. These dicey matters are taken up at length in Chapter 23.

To see how *Gen* works (10), consider first CVT. For any interpretation I_0—a string of segments affiliated with various morphemes—the candidate structural descriptions in *Gen*(I_0) consist of all possible parses of the segment string into syllables, including the possible over- and underparsing structures exemplified in (8). The four candidates with /VCVC/ in (8) merely illustrate the full set *Gen*(/VCVC/). Since the possibilities of overparsing are literally unlimited, *Gen*(/VCVC/) in fact contains an infinite number of candidates.

For the syntactic interpretation $I_0 \equiv$ /sing(x), .../ given in (6), *Gen*(I_0) includes the four X′ structures (6a–d), along with others, such as the entirely empty **null parse,** ∅. Note that each structural description of I_0 in *Gen*(I_0) includes I_0 itself as a subpart, along with the X′ expression. As in phonology, *Gen*(I_0) includes candidates employing under- and overparsing. Output (6a), [$_{\text{IP}}$ has [sung]], displays underparsing: an element of the interpretation, *x*, has no correspondent in the expression. The null parse ∅ underparses the entire interpretation: the expression is completely devoid of content. Output (6d), [$_{\text{IP}}$ it has [[t$_i$ sung] he$_i$]], exhibits overparsing: an element of the expression, *it*, has no correspondent in the interpretation.

The production and comprehension functions take different types of input: production takes an interpretation; comprehension, an expression. Thus, neither the interpretation nor the expression can be called 'the input' without potential confusion. We have therefore avoided using this term, which was employed in Prince and Smolensky 1993/2004 and standardly in the OT literature since; 'the input' *I* in OT refers to what we have called the interpretation *I*. This reflects the fact that OT, like theoretical linguistics in general, focuses heavily on the production function f_{prod}; indeed, in the OT literature f_{prod} is typically taken to *be* 'the grammar'. There are a number of good reasons for the asymmetric treatment of production and comprehension, one of the most basic being this: crosslinguistically, while the set of expressions for which an interpretation is demanded varies widely, the set of interpretations for which languages may be expected to provide expressions is plausibly universal. Thus, the inputs I to f_{prod} are universal in a sense in which the inputs E to f_{comp} are not. The specification of a function f must pick out an output for any input f receives, but f says nothing about how to "pick" its input. In generative grammar, the language-particular patterns we seek to understand are patterns among expressions, so it is the production function that will tell us how these patterns emerge from a relatively language-independent base of expressions. For the study of universal grammar, f_{prod} provides a considerably better foundation than does f_{comp}. Thus, it is f_{prod} that defines 'the language' specified by the grammar (11c).

In the rest of this chapter, and in the other chapters of this book, the common practice will be followed: the interpretation and the expression will normally be referred to as the 'input' and 'output', respectively; thus, except where explicitly noted, these terms should be construed as appropriate for f_{prod}.[13]

[13] Although the story takes us rather far afield into linguistic theory, it is worthwhile pointing out a major motivation for the rather idiosyncratic conception of OT presented here—where both production and comprehension functions are specified by a single grammar. Such a formulation holds the promise of formalizing a range of types of explanations based on a loose notion of **recoverability**. Take an interpretation I and feed it to f_{prod} to produce an expression E; now take E (or its overt part O) and feed it in turn to f_{comp} to yield an interpretation I'. If $I' = I$, we can say that the interpretation I is *recoverable* from the expression E: if the speaker utters E, the hearer will correctly interpret it as I. Now it is possible to formalize the notion "deletion under recoverability," which would eliminate constraints like DROPTOP (18e) (roughly, 'Topics should not be expressed'). Such constraints identify particular contexts (like referring to the topic) and demand minimal structure there. They miss the generalization that the contexts in which reduction is favored are often just those in which the information omitted can be filled in "by default." Consider DROPTOP. To interpret an unexpressed argument, choose the least marked referent: the topic. There is no need to express the argument overtly because the least marked interpretation already interprets an argument as referring to the topic, unless that is inconsistent with the overtly expressed information. The generic constraints of the family *STRUC oppose all structure: the idea is to arrange the optimization architecture so that these constraints will prevail, leading to expressions in which information is omitted, wherever that information will be filled in in the optimal interpretation. This requires a general OT architecture in which the grammatical expression E of an interpretation I can be sensitive to whether E enables I to be recovered. Such an architecture employs some kind of **bidirectional optimization**, which appropriately couples the separate optimizations defining f_{prod} and f_{comp} (12d). The first such architecture was developed by Wilson (1995, 2001a): anaphors, in which certain features are 'dropped', are grammatical if and only if the correct binder can be recovered. Smolensky (1998) develops a different bidirectional architecture for the study of **ineffability**—where some meanings cannot be recovered from *any* expression. It is argued that within a uniform OT architecture, basic differences between syntax and phonology explain why ineffability arises systematically in syntax but not phonology, yielding the impression that syntactic but not phonological constraints are inviolable. Smolensky and Wilson (2000) develop another double-optimization theory of recoverability that accounts for a wide range of variability in recoverability-related phenomena in phonology, syntax, and semantics. Buchwald et al. (2002) propose a bidirectional optimization account of pragmatic interactions between the discourse prominence levels of arguments, their syntactic roles, and their degree of reduction (pronominalization). See also Boersma 1998; Zeevat 2000; Blutner 2001; Hendriks and de Hoop 2001.

1.3 Harmonic ordering: *H-eval* and competition

Among the candidate structural descriptions in $Gen(I_0)$, f_{prod} picks the one(s) providing a well-formed parse of the interpretation I_0. How does the grammar determine this selection? This is the point at which the central innovation of OT enters.

(12) Competition: *H-eval*

a. Informally: the grammatical expression of an interpretation I_0 is the candidate parse in $Gen(I_0)$ that is the "best," or 'least marked', or **most harmonic**, or **optimal**.

b. More formally: an OT grammar determines a function ***H-eval*** that compares the relative **Harmony** of any pair of structural descriptions. If one structural description, S', has higher Harmony than another, S, then we write

$S' \succ S$ (equivalently, $S \prec S'$).

If *H-eval* assigns the same Harmony to S' and S, we write

$S' \approx S$.

For every pair of structural descriptions $S', S \in \mathcal{U}$, *H-eval* must declare that exactly one of the following holds:

$S' \approx S$,
$S' \succ S$, or
$S' \prec S$.

The order $\succ$ is called the **harmonic ordering** of structural descriptions.

c. Given a set of candidate structural descriptions $\mathcal{S}$, the set of **most harmonic** or **optimal** candidates of $\mathcal{S}$ is

$opt[\mathcal{S}] \equiv \{S \in \mathcal{S} \mid \nexists S' \in \mathcal{S} \text{ such that } S' \succ S\}$.

d. The production and comprehension functions select the optimal candidate(s)

i. $f_{prod}(I_0) \equiv opt[Gen(I_0)]$,
ii. $f_{comp}(E_0) \equiv opt[Int(E_0)]$,
iii. $f'_{comp}(O_0) \equiv opt[Int'(O_0)]$.

The optimization defining f_{prod} is the 'standard' optimization employed in all OT work, the **production-directed** or **expressive optimization**; this is to be contrasted with the **comprehension-directed** or **interpretive optimization** defining f_{comp} (and f'_{comp}).

1.4 Violable constraints: *Con*, Markedness, and Faithfulness

How does *H-eval* determine the relative Harmony of two structural descriptions?

(13) ***Con***

H-eval compares two candidate structural descriptions via a set of well-formedness constraints: *Con*. The constraints in *Con* evaluate a candidate in parallel (i.e., all constraints apply simultaneously).[14] Given a candidate, each constraint assesses a list of **marks**, where each mark corresponds to one violation of the constraint. The collection of all marks assessed a candidate parse *S* is denoted *marks*(*S*). A mark assessed by a constraint $\mathbb{C}$ is denoted $*\mathbb{C}$. A parse *S* is more harmonic—or less marked—than a parse *S′* with respect to $\mathbb{C}$ if and only if $\mathbb{C}$ assesses more marks to *S′* than to *S*; this is written

$S \succ_{\mathbb{C}} S'$.

(OT recognizes the notions more and less marked, but not absolute numerical degrees of markedness. That is, only the relations > and < are defined for the sizes of mark sets; within OT, it is not possible to perform arithmetic operations such as addition and multiplication with such lists, nor even to test whether a set of marks contains one member.)[15]

(14) **MARKEDNESS and FAITHFULNESS**

The well-formedness constraints in *Con* are of two types. Given a structural description $S = (I, E, \mathfrak{R})$, the constraints of the markedness family, collectively called 'MARKEDNESS' (or sometimes 'MARK'), evaluate only the expression *E*, assessing the inherent well-formedness of the structural properties of *E*. Constraints of the faithfulness family, collectively called 'FAITHFULNESS' (or some-

[14] For those familiar with the multilevel structural descriptions typical of phonology and syntax, it is worth mentioning that as originally formulated in Prince and Smolensky 1993/2004, OT makes no commitment concerning the number of levels found within structural descriptions. A particular substantive OT theory might employ structural descriptions that comprise multiple levels, such as lexical and postlexical levels in phonology, or d- and s-structure in syntax. An OT theory might even use derivations as structural descriptions: a series of partial representations leading up to the final surface representation. Prince and Smolensky 1993/2004 defines **Harmonic Serialism** as a deployment of OT in which an impoverished initial representation is taken as input to the grammar, and the optimal output is a representation only somewhat more complete than the input (see (60)). This optimal output is then treated as the input for a second round of optimization, producing a second output still more complete than the first. This continues until no further changes are possible. An extensive analysis of syllabification under Harmonic Serialism is presented in Prince and Smolensky 1993/2004. At each serial step, one bit of structure is added: a new syllable, a syllable onset, an epenthesized segment, and so on. See McCarthy 1999a for important discussion. In phonology, other works employing multilevel structural descriptions in OT include McCarthy and Prince 1993b; Black 1993; Kiparsky, to appear (see also **Harmonic Phonology**, Goldsmith 1993). In syntax, the pros and cons of harmonic-derivational theories along minimalist lines are discussed in, among other works, Legendre, Smolensky, and Wilson 1998; Heck and Müller 2000; Müller 2002, 2003; Hale and Legendre, 2004 (see also Section 16:5.3). Most OT work, however, has studied only single-level structural descriptions; this is the conception behind the formulation presented here.

[15] The ultimate responsibility of a constraint $\mathbb{C}$ is to harmonically order candidates, to define a total order $\succ_{\mathbb{C}}$. An alternative formulation of OT developed by Wilson (2000, 2001b) results from weakening this assumption to allow **targeted constraints**, which define only a *partial* order on the candidate set: a targeted constraint has the additional option of asserting nothing about the relative Harmony of two structures *S* and *S′* (this is entirely different from asserting that they are equally harmonic, $S \approx S'$). A targeted constraint can "target" a kind of "repair." For example, a constraint that says $\sim X_{[+voi,-son]}]_\sigma\sim \succ \sim X_{[-voi,-son]}]_\sigma\sim$ but says nothing about the relative Harmony of any other pairs of strings can make optimal devoicing of obstruents in codas, but not, say, epenthesis that avoids the coda: the latter would require the relation $\sim X_{[+voi,-son]}]_\sigma[\sim \succ \sim]_\sigma[X_{[-voi,-son}\sim$, which this constraint does not provide. In general, a targeted constraint prefers to *S* only those instances of *S′* most similar to *S*.

times 'FAITH'), evaluate only the correspondence relation $\mathfrak{R}$, penalizing all deviations from one-to-one (or **faithful**) parsing.[16]

To illustrate first with our running phonological example, the CVT constraints from Prince and Smolensky 1993/2004 (Chapter 13 here) are given in (15).

(15) Basic CV Syllable Theory constraints evaluating $S = (I, E, \mathfrak{R})$

Markedness[17]

a. **ONSET** Each syllable in E has an onset.

b. **NOCODA** Each syllable in E does *not* have a coda.

Faithfulness: Parse/Fill Theory

c. **PARSE** Each segment in I (the underlying form) corresponds under $\mathfrak{R}$ to a segment in E that is parsed into a syllable position (Ons, Nuc, or Cod).

d. **FILL**^{Nuc} The nucleus position of each syllable in E is filled with a segment that corresponds under $\mathfrak{R}$ to an underlying segment in I.

e. **FILL**^{Ons} The onset position of each syllable in E, if present, is filled with a segment that corresponds under $\mathfrak{R}$ to an underlying segment in I.

These constraints can be illustrated with the candidate outputs in (8). The marks incurred by these candidates are summarized in (16).

(16) Constraint tableau for $\mathcal{L}_1$

Candidates	ONSET	NOCODA	FILL^{Nuc}	PARSE	FILL^{Ons}
/VCVC/→					
d. .□V.CV.⟨C⟩				*	*
b. ⟨V⟩.CV.⟨C⟩				* *	
c. ⟨V⟩.CV.C□́.			*	*	
a. .V.CVC.	*	*			

This is an OT **constraint tableau**, introduced here in Chapter 4. The competing candidates are shown in the left column. Heading the other columns are the constraints; constraint violations—marks—are indicated with '*', one for each violation.

Candidate (16a) = .V.CVC. violates ONSET in its first syllable and NOCODA in its second; the remaining constraints are satisfied. The single mark that ONSET assesses .V.CVC. is denoted *ONSET. This candidate is a faithful parse: it involves neither underparsing nor overparsing and therefore satisfies the faithfulness constraints PARSE and FILL. By contrast, the unfaithful parse (16b) = ⟨V⟩.CV.⟨C⟩ violates PARSE, twice: the initial and final underlying segments have no syllabified correspondents. This tableau will be further explained below.

16 For a recently proposed alternative, see McCarthy 2002a.

17 'ONSET' and 'NOCODA' are the more readable names from McCarthy and Prince 1993b for the constraints 'ONS' and '–COD' of Prince and Smolensky 1993/2004.

The PARSE/FILL Theory of (15) was the first formalization of faithfulness in OT, proposed in Prince and Smolensky 1991a, 1993/2004. In an important development, an alternative conception of faithfulness was proposed in McCarthy and Prince 1995; this has become the dominant approach. The new model introduced the correspondence relation ℜ that we have incorporated into the present exposition. In the Correspondence Theory of faithfulness, PARSE and FILL are replaced respectively by the constraints MAX and DEP; these and other basic constraints of FAITHFULNESS are defined in (17). The term 'unit' is used to refer to the elements that stand in correspondence under ℜ. In phonology, these units are usually segments, but sometimes subsegmental features or suprasegmental structures like syllables. In syntax, correspondence is often not made explicit, and it varies considerably depending on the type of syntactic structures employed. However, the relevant units are the types of elements shown to be in correspondence in the example (5): in *I*, predicates, arguments, functional features, and so on; in *E*, heads, specifiers, functional features, and so on.

(17) FAITHFULNESS—Correspondence Theory, evaluating $S = (I, E, \Re)$

a. **MAX** Every unit in *I* stands in correspondence with at least one unit of *E* (expression is **max**imal).

b. **DEP** Every unit in *E* stands in correspondence with at least one unit of *I* (an expression unit is a **dep**endent of an interpretation unit).

c. **IDENT[φ]** Elements in correspondence have identical values of feature [φ]. (A syntactic example is PARSE-*wh* (Chapter 16), requiring correspondents to bear identical values of [±wh]. Currently, the term 'PARSE' is often used for a range of faithfulness constraints in syntax.)

d. **INTEGRITY** Every unit in *I* stands in correspondence with at most one unit of *E* (an interpretation unit is not 'split up' in the expression).

e. **UNIFORMITY** Every unit in *E* stands in correspondence with at most one unit of *I* (an expression unit does not express multiple interpretation units).

f. **LINEARITY** Given a pair of units *i*, *i'* in *I* and a pair *e*, *e'* in *E* with *i* corresponding to *e*, and *i'* to *e'*, linear order is preserved by ℜ: *i* precedes *i'* if and only if *e* precedes *e'*. (In phonology: the linear order of segments is not altered—no **metathesis**. In syntax, an analogous constraint is PARSE-SCOPE of Legendre, Smolensky, and Wilson 1998 (partially reprinted in Chapter 16): if an operator *Op* in *I* has scope over an element *x* of *I* (Section 1:3.2), and each has a correspondent in *E*, then the correspondent of *Op* has scope over the correspondent of *x*.)

g. **X-ANCHOR** (X = Left or Right) A unit at the *X*-edge of *I* has a correspondent at the *X*-edge of *E*.[18]

The strict decomposition of *Con* into MARKEDNESS and FAITHFULNESS as defined in (14) is not truly a principle of OT, and some proposed constraints do not fall into either family. But the class of MARKEDNESS/FAITHFULNESS theories plays such a central role in OT theory and practice that it is appropriate to regard (14) as a fundamental principle adopted in most OT work.

The GSL constraints (Grimshaw and Samek-Lodovici 1995, 590)—reworded to conform to the present exposition and simplified somewhat—are given in (18).

(18) Constraints of the GSL theory of subjects, evaluating $S = (I, E, \mathfrak{R})$

Markedness

a. **SUBJ** **Subject.** In *E*, the subject position of a clause must be filled.

b. **ALFOC** **Align Focus.** In *E*, the left edge of a focused constituent is aligned with the right edge of a maximal projection XP.

Faithfulness

c. **PARSE** (MAX) A unit of *I* has a correspondent in *E*.

d. **FULLINT** **Full Interpretation.** (DEP) A unit of *E* has a correspondent in *I*.

e. **DROPTOP** **Drop Topic.** Arguments in *I* referring to the topic have no correspondent in *E*.[19]

These constraints can be illustrated with the candidate outputs in (6), as shown in (19). (In all candidates, ALFOC is vacuously satisfied, because *I* ≡ /sing(x), x = topic, x = he; Tense = PresPerf/ has no focus.)

[18] In phonology, this constraint requires that morpheme edges be preserved, which may be functionally motivated by the requirement that the hearer parse the speech stream into morphemes, that is, locate morpheme edges. It is unclear whether ANCHOR has an instantiation in syntax. In phonology, the segmental vocabulary in which both *I* and *E* are stated means they share a notion of linear order, so it makes sense to connect edgemostness in the two structures. In syntax, *E* possesses a notion of linear order, but it is not clear that this is true of *I*. Adopting a less literal reading of ANCHOR, an 'edgemost' element of *I* might be the element most extreme on an abstract scale that is expressed in *E* through linear order. For example, TOP-FIRST (Costa 2001, 176) requires the topic in *I* to stand at the left edge of a sentence *E*. If topicality is a scale, 'the topic' in this constraint refers to the element at one extreme of the scale. In fact, if topicality is represented with the forward-looking centers list Cf of Centering Theory (Grosz, Joshi, and Weinstein 1995; Walker, Joshi, and Prince 1998), 'the topic' is essentially the preferred center, Cp; this is the leftmost list member, and TOP-FIRST is quite literally LEFT-ANCHOR (Buchwald et al. 2002).

[19] This would seem to be a kind of *anti*-MAX constraint, not consistent with FAITHFULNESS in rewarding identity between *I* and *E*. See Footnote 13. It may, however, be appropriate to consider DROPTOP as analogous to the type of constraint required in phonology to account for **subtractive** morphology, where a morpheme is expressed not by presence but by absence of phonetic material (Horwood 2001; Kurisu 2002). (Something like the [informal] or perhaps [affectionate] morpheme that induces the truncation of *Mary* to *Mare*; see Benua 1995, 1997.) However it is to be formalized, the intuition is that to be *faithful* to the demands of such a morpheme is to *omit* material that would otherwise be present. It is of course the real essence of *faithfulness* that FAITHFULNESS must ultimately capture; formalization in terms of strict identity under correspondence may need to be replaced by something less rigid even for phonology, just as it must immediately be for syntax.

(19) Constraint violations in GSL

/sing(x), x=topic, x=he; T=PresPerf/	PARSE	SUBJ	FULLINT	DROPTOP	ALFOC
b. $[_{IP}$ he_i has $[t_i$ sung]]				*	
d. $[_{IP}$ it has $[[t_i$ sung] $he_i]]$			*	*	
c. $[_{IP}$ has $[[t_i$ sung] $he_i]]$		*		*	
a. $[_{IP}$ has [sung]]	*	*			

In candidate (19a), the argument *x* in *I* has no correspondent in *E*, violating PARSE. In (19c), there is no subject—or there is a **null subject**—in violation of SUBJ: there is no filled specifier of IP, the subject position. In (19d), the element *it* in *E* has no correspondent in *I*: *it* doesn't contribute to the interpretation, in violation of FULLINT. (This is the **dummy** or **expletive** *it* that appears in English *it has rained*—in order to satisfy SUBJ, according to GSL. Recall Section 4:1.) And (19b) violates DROPTOP because the topical element *x* does have a correspondent (*he*) in *E*.

We have interpreted PARSE and FULLINT as members of the faithfulness family of constraints: they are analogous to PARSE and FILL of CVT. Because it evaluates $\mathfrak{R}$ rather than *E*, we have also interpreted DROPTOP as a kind of faithfulness constraint, albeit an odd one: it demands that an element *not* have a correspondent. Faithfulness is a rather straightforward matter in phonology, because the interpretation and the expression are framed in basically the same vocabulary—segments; FAITHFULNESS simply demands one-to-one mapping of segments under $\mathfrak{R}$. But in OT syntax, interpretations are discourse/semantic structures and expressions are syntactic structures; these vocabularies diverge in many ways, and so the status of FAITHFULNESS is more complex and controversial (see Chapter 16 for extensive discussion).

Section 1.8 discusses the general structure of *Con* in more detail; we postpone that discussion until after presentation of all OT principles.

1.5 Optimality, harmonic ordering, and constraint ranking

The production function f_{prod} assigns to any interpretation *I* its grammatical structural description(s): the parse(s) that *H-eval* assigns maximum Harmony, via the constraints of *Con* (12d). For a single constraint $\mathbb{C}$, it is unambiguous which structural descriptions are preferred: those that have no (or the fewest possible) violations of $\mathbb{C}$. But there are multiple constraints in *Con*, and no guarantee that they will all agree on which parse is best. When constraints disagree on which structural descriptions are best, they are said to **conflict**. The more general the constraints, the larger the set of parses on which they conflict; and in OT, where constraints are typically highly general, conflict is rampant.

Such conflict is evident in the examples discussed above. Among the candidates in (16), for example, the parse of /VCVC/ that best satisfies PARSE is (16a), .V.CVC.; but this is the parse that is worst according to ONSET. No candidate at all—even considering the infinitely many others not shown in (16)—is evaluated as best with respect to all the constraints. And the same conclusion holds for the syntax example shown in (19). The parse of the interpretation *I* judged best by DROPTOP is (19a): [$_{IP}$ [$_{VP}$ has sung]]. But this parse is judged worst by PARSE and SUBJ. The grammar needs a basis for resolving these ubiquitous constraint conflicts.

OT gives a precise and restrictive theory of how constraint conflict is resolved. In a given language, different constraints are assigned different priority levels or strengths; this is termed **constraint ranking**. When a choice must be made between satisfying one constraint or another, the stronger must take priority. The result is that the weaker will be violated in a grammatical structural description.

(20) Constraint ranking

a. Each grammar **ranks** the *Con* constraints in a **strict domination hierarchy**.

b. When one constraint $\mathbb{C}_1$ dominates another constraint $\mathbb{C}_2$ in the hierarchy, the relation is denoted $\mathbb{C}_1 \gg \mathbb{C}_2$. The ranking defining a grammar is total: the hierarchy determines the relative dominance of every constraint pair:

$$\mathbb{C}_1 \gg \mathbb{C}_2 \gg \cdots \gg \mathbb{C}_N.$$

c. A grammar's constraint ranking induces a harmonic ordering $\succ$ of all structural descriptions: this **harmonic ordering of forms** defines *H-eval*. *H-eval* compares two structural descriptions S' and S by identifying the highest-ranked constraint $\mathbb{C}_K$ with respect to which S' and S are not equally harmonic (i.e., for which $S' \not\approx_{\mathbb{C}_K} S$). If S is the candidate that is more harmonic with respect to $\mathbb{C}_K$ (i.e., $S \succ_{\mathbb{C}_K} S'$), then S is more harmonic with respect to the grammar as a whole (i.e., more harmonic with respect to the entire constraint hierarchy): $S \succ S'$.

For a given interpretation I_0, $f_{\text{prod}}(I_0)$ is the set of maximum-Harmony parses in $Gen(I_0)$. When can this set contain more than one parse—when can more than one parse in a candidate set be optimal? Since a grammar is a total ranking of the constraints in *Con*, there is only one possible way that two competing candidates can be simultaneously optimal: they must have identical constraint violations (otherwise, there would be a highest-ranked constraint on which they differed, and this would pick one of the candidates as more harmonic). Two candidates that are assessed exactly the same marks by all the constraints cannot be distinguished on the basis of *any* constraint ranking and will always be equally harmonic. If two (or more) candidates have equal Harmony, and both are more harmonic than all the other candidates, then the two candidates are both optimal, with the interpretation of free alternation. In practice, it is quite rare for $f_{\text{prod}}(I_0)$ to contain more than one parse, because *Con* is generally sufficiently rich and fine-grained that two different parses cannot equally violate *all* constraints.

Note that the harmonic evaluation of structural descriptions is entirely relativized to candidate sets; no significance is attached to the absolute number or distribution of constraint violations assessed to a candidate. A candidate with 1,500 constraint violations is thereby no less grammatical provided it satisfies the ranked constraints better than any of its competitors. And an optimal candidate in one candidate set $Gen(I_1)$ – a grammatical form – will often be less harmonic than a suboptimal candidate in another candidate set $Gen(I_2)$ – an ungrammatical form.[20]

It is also the case that, within a single candidate set, the harmonic ordering of the suboptimal candidates is of no grammatical significance: in particular, it cannot support a sensible notion of 'degrees of grammaticality'. For a simple but dramatic example, consider a ranking in which the FILL constraints are lowest ranked. When forced, epenthesis of consonants and vowels will be optimal; /VCCV/ will surface as .□V.C□́.CV. What are the next-most-harmonic candidates after the optimal one? These will be the ones that violate the lowest-ranked constraints – the FILL constraints. Now p_1 ≡ .□V.C□́.CV.□□́. epenthesizes a gratuitous final syllable, but the resulting violations of FILL are low ranked, so this parse p_1 is more harmonic than, say, p_2 ≡ ⟨V⟩.C□́.CV., where the initial V is deleted, incurring a higher-ranked violation of PARSE. Now in fact, the higher-Harmony parse p_1 is never optimal, in any language – it violates Theorem (30) of Chapter 13. However, the lower-Harmony parse p_2 is clearly optimal in a language that ranks PARSE beneath FILL^{Ons} – for example, $\mathcal{L}_2$ (28). Next, notice that not only is it more harmonic to gratuitously epenthesize one syllable (p_1) than to delete the initial V (p_2), it is also more harmonic to gratuitously epenthesize 42 syllables than to delete the initial V – thanks to strict domination. If we were to assert that more harmonic means more well formed in a gradient theory of well-formedness, we would derive the absurd conclusion that epenthesizing *any* number of syllables produces an output that is more well formed than p_2.

A formulation of harmonic ordering that is often useful involves **mark cancellation**, an operation that must be applied separately to *pairs* of candidates. Consider a pair of competing candidates S' and S, with corresponding lists of violation marks *marks(S')* and *marks(S)*. Mark cancellation applies to this pair of lists of marks: it cancels violation marks in common to the two lists. Thus, if a constraint $\mathbb{C}_K$ assesses one or more marks $*\mathbb{C}_K$ to both *marks(S')* and *marks(S)*, an instance of $*\mathbb{C}_K$ is removed from each list, and the process is repeated until at most one of the lists still contains a mark $*\mathbb{C}_K$. (Note that if S' and S are equally marked with respect to $\mathbb{C}_K$, the two lists contain equally many marks $*\mathbb{C}_K$, and all occurrences of $*\mathbb{C}_K$ are eventually removed.) Denote the resulting lists of **uncanceled marks** by $marks^{\times}(S')$ and $marks^{\times}(S)$. If a mark $*\mathbb{C}_K$

[20] For example, assuming the constraints to be listed in domination order in tableau (16), for the input /VCVC/ the grammatical form is (d), .□V.CV.⟨C⟩. Joining two copies of this input with a CV in the middle gives the input I_1 ≡ /VCVCCVVCVC/, whose optimal parse must be two copies of (d) with a .CV. in between: S_{opt} ≡ .□V.CV.⟨C⟩.CV.□V.CV.⟨C⟩. Then $marks(S_{opt})$ = {*FILL^{Ons} *FILL^{Ons} *PARSE *PARSE}. Now consider the input /CV/. Since the optimal parse is just the perfect syllable .CV., it follows that S_{subopt} ≡ ⟨C⟩.□V. is suboptimal; but $marks(S_{subopt})$ = {*FILL^{Ons} *PARSE}. So clearly $S_{subopt} \succ S_{opt}$. The four violations committed by S_{opt} are forced: they can (and indeed must) occur in an optimal parse. The two violations of S_{subopt} are gratuitous; no higher-ranked constraints force them. But the notion 'forced violation' is inherently comparative: a violation is forced if and only if no *alternative* is better. Thus, for deep reasons rooted in the logic of violable constraints – minimal violation (24), essentially – it is not possible to conceive of the grammatical forms as all those with a Harmony that exceeds some threshold; it must be relative, not absolute, Harmony that defines grammaticality.

remains in the uncanceled mark list of S', then S' is more marked with respect to $\mathbb{C}_K$. If the highest-ranked constraint assessing an uncanceled mark has a mark in $marks^{\times}(S')$, then $S' \prec S$: this is the characterization of harmonic ordering $\prec$ in terms of mark cancellation. In other words:

(21) Cancellation/Domination Lemma

Let S_1 and S_2 be two candidates, with mark lists in which cancellation has been performed. Then $S_1 \succ S_2$ if and only if every one of S_1's uncanceled marks is dominated by an uncanceled mark of S_2.

This is due to Prince and Smolensky 1993/2004, Chap. 8 (see Box 13:1 (8)).

Mark cancellation is indicated by 'crossing out the marks' in the tableau in (22): one mark *PARSE cancels between the candidates (d) and (b) of (16), and one uncanceled mark *PARSE remains in $marks^{\times}$(b). (23) is another representation of (22), illustrating the **comparative tableau** introduced in Prince 2000 (see Prince 2002a). In each row of such a tableau, two candidates are compared, notated '$S_1 \sim S_2$'. For each constraint $\mathbb{C}$ (column), a 'W' indicates that the first, S_1, 'wins' with respect to $\mathbb{C}$; 'L' indicates that S_1 'loses'; and a blank means that $\mathbb{C}$ rates them equally.

(22) Mark cancellation

Candidates	ONSET	NOCODA	FILL^{Nuc}	PARSE	FILL^{Ons}
d. .□V.CV.⟨C⟩				~~*~~	*
b. ⟨V⟩.CV.⟨C⟩				~~*~~ *	

(23) Comparative tableau

/VCVC/ →	ONSET	NOCODA	FILL^{Nuc}	PARSE	FILL^{Ons}
.□V.CV.⟨C⟩ ~ ⟨V⟩.CV.⟨C⟩				W	L

Defining grammaticality via harmonic ordering has an important consequence:

(24) **Minimal Violation**

The grammatical candidate violates the constraints minimally, with respect to the constraint ranking.

The constraints of *Con* are violable: they are potentially violated in well-formed structures. Such violation is minimal, however, in the following sense. Suppose S is the grammatical parse of an interpretation I_0, and suppose S violates a constraint $\mathbb{C}$ to some degree. Then any parse of I_0 that violates $\mathbb{C}$ to a lesser degree than S will violate to a greater degree than S some constraint $\mathbb{C}'$ that is higher ranked than $\mathbb{C}$.

Harmonic ordering can be illustrated with CVT by reexamining the tableau in (16), reproduced as (26), under the assumption that the constraint hierarchy for a language $\mathcal{L}_1$ is that given in (25).

(25) Constraint hierarchy for $\mathcal{L}_1$

ONSET $\gg$ NOCODA $\gg$ FILL^{Nuc} $\gg$ PARSE $\gg$ FILL^{Ons}

(26) Constraint tableau for $\mathcal{L}_1$

Candidates	ONSET	NOCODA	FILL^Nuc	PARSE	FILL^Ons
/VCVC/→					
d. ☞ .□V.CV.⟨C⟩				⊛	⊛
b. ⟨V⟩.CV.⟨C⟩				* *!	
c. ⟨V⟩.CV.C□́.			*!	*	
a. .V.CVC.	*!	*			

The constraints (and their columns) are ordered in (26) left to right, reflecting the hierarchy in (25). The candidates in this tableau have been listed in harmonic order, from highest to lowest Harmony; the optimal candidate is marked manually.[21] Starting at the bottom of the tableau, (a) ≺ (c) can be verified as follows. The first step is to cancel common marks: here, there are none. The next step is to determine which candidate has the worst uncanceled mark (i.e., which most violates the highest-ranked constraint that distinguishes them): it is (a), which violates ONSET. Therefore, (a) is the less harmonic.

To determine that (c) ≺ (b), we first cancel the common mark *PARSE; (c) then earns the worst remaining mark of the two, *FILL^{Nuc}. When we compare (b) with (d), one *PARSE mark cancels, leaving *marks*$^{\times}$(b) = {*PARSE} and *marks*$^{\times}$(d) = {*FILL^{Ons}}. The worst mark is the uncanceled *PARSE incurred by (b), so (b) ≺ (d).

The tableau (26) is annotated in the standard way: '!' in the row for a suboptimal candidate S_{subopt} identifies the mark causing S_{subopt} to lose out to the optimal form S_{opt} (this is a violation of the highest-ranked constraint $\mathbb{C}$ that distinguishes S_{subopt} from S_{opt}; $\mathbb{C}$ necessarily disfavors S_{subopt}). Shaded cells for suboptimal candidates are not relevant to optimality computation because the candidate has already been eliminated; shaded cells for the optimal candidate are not relevant because no further competitors remain. (Such shading, while standard, is not often used in this book.) A nonstandard convention deployed sometimes in this book is to use '⊛' to indicate the marks incurred by the optimal candidate; this is shown in (26).

$\mathcal{L}_1$ is a language in which all syllables have the overt form .CV.: onsets are required, codas are forbidden. In the case of problematic inputs such as /VCVC/ where a faithful parse into CV syllables is not possible, this language uses overparsing (of consonants) to provide missing onsets for vowels, and underparsing (of consonants) to avoid codas (it is the language denoted $\Sigma^{CV}_{ep,del}$ in Prince and Smolensky 1993/2004; see Section 13:2.2.2 of this book).

Exchanging the two FILL constraints in $\mathcal{L}_1$ gives the grammar $\mathcal{L}_2$:

(27) Constraint hierarchy for $\mathcal{L}_2$

ONSET ≫ NOCODA ≫ FILL^{Ons} ≫ PARSE ≫ FILL^{Nuc}

[21] Determining that this candidate is optimal requires demonstrating that it is more harmonic than *any* of the infinitely many competing candidates: see Footnote 36 and (62).

Now the tableau corresponding to (27) becomes (28); the columns have been reordered to reflect the constraint reranking, and the candidates have been reordered to reflect the new harmonic ordering.

(28) Constraint tableau for $\mathcal{L}_2$

Candidates	ONSET	NOCODA	FILL^{Ons}	PARSE	FILL^{Nuc}
/VCVC/→					
c. ☞ ⟨V⟩.CV.C□́.				*	*
b. ⟨V⟩.CV.⟨C⟩				* *!	
d. .□V.CV.⟨C⟩			*!	*	
a. .V.CVC.	*!	*			

Like syllables in $\mathcal{L}_1$, all syllables in $\mathcal{L}_2$ are CV; /VCVC/ gets syllabified differently, however. In $\mathcal{L}_2$, underparsing (of vowels) is used to avoid onsetless syllables, and overparsing (of vowels) to avoid codas ($\mathcal{L}_2$ is the language $\Sigma^{CV}_{del,ep}$ of Prince and Smolensky 1993/2004; see Section 13:2.2.2).

The relation between the CV languages $\mathcal{L}_1$ and $\mathcal{L}_2$ illustrates a central principle of OT: the grammars of different languages differ in their ranking of the constraints in *Con*. This is the topic of the next subsection.

To illustrate the principles developed in this subsection within syntax, we return to the GSL theory. To begin, mark cancellation is illustrated in (29).

(29) Mark cancellation

/sing(x), x=topic, x=he; T=PresPerf/	PARSE	SUBJ	FULLINT	DROPTOP	ALFOC
b. ☞ [$_{IP}$ he$_i$ has [t$_i$ sung]]				~~*~~	
c. [$_{IP}$ has [[t$_i$ sung] he$_i$]]		*!		~~*~~	

Harmonic ordering can be illustrated with GSL by reexamining the tableau in (19), reproduced here as (31), under the assumption that the universal constraints are ranked by a particular grammar of a language $\mathcal{L}'_1$ with the ranking given in (30). (This is a language like English with respect to the distribution of subjects.)

(30) Constraint hierarchy for (English-like) $\mathcal{L}'_1$

PARSE ≫ SUBJ ≫ FULLINT ≫ DROPTOP ≫ ALFOC

As always in tableaux, the constraints are ordered in (31) left to right, reflecting the hierarchy in (30). The candidates in this tableau have been listed in harmonic order, from highest to lowest Harmony. Starting at the bottom of the tableau, we can verify that (a) ≺ (c) as follows. The first step is to cancel common marks: here, *SUBJ. Then (c) and (a) have uncanceled marks *marks'*(c) = {*DROPTOP} and *marks*$^{\times}$(a) = {*PARSE}; since PARSE ≫ DROPTOP in $\mathcal{L}'_1$, (a) is less harmonic. Next we verify that (c) ≺ (d): the sole uncanceled mark of (c), *SUBJ, is assessed by a constraint that is higher ranked in

$\mathcal{L}'_1$ than that assessing the uncanceled mark of (d), FULLINT. Finally, (d) ≺ (b) holds because (d) has an uncanceled mark while (b) does not.

(31) Constraint tableau for (English-like) $\mathcal{L}'_1$

/sing(x), x=topic, x=he; T=PresPerf/	PARSE	SUBJ	FULLINT	DROPTOP	ALFOC
b. ☞ [$_{IP}$ he$_i$ has [t$_i$ sung]]				*	
d. [$_{IP}$ it has [[t$_i$ sung] he$_i$]]			*!	*	
c. [$_{IP}$ has [[t$_i$ sung] he$_i$]]		*!		*	
a. [$_{IP}$ has [sung]]	*!	*			

As shown in the tableau in (31), $\mathcal{L}'_1$ is a language in which unfocused topic-referring subjects are parsed into subject position (SpecIP). This English-like behavior changes to Italian-like behavior when PARSE and SUBJ are lowered to their positions in the hierarchy defining language $\mathcal{L}'_2$.

(32) Constraint hierarchy for (Italian-like) $\mathcal{L}'_2$

FULLINT ≫ DROPTOP ≫ PARSE ≫ ALFOC ≫ SUBJ

As tableau (33) shows, now an unfocused topic-referring subject is not parsed:

(33) Constraint tableau for (Italian-like) $\mathcal{L}'_2$

/sing(x), x=topic, x=he; T=PresPerf/	FULLINT	DROPTOP	PARSE	ALFOC	SUBJ
a. ☞ [$_{IP}$ has [sung]]			*		*
b. [$_{IP}$ he$_i$ has [t$_i$ sung]]		*!			
c. [$_{IP}$ has [[t$_i$ sung] he$_i$]]		*!			*
d. [$_{IP}$ it has [[t$_i$ sung] he$_i$]]	*!	*			

1.6 Universality, factorial typology, and Richness of the Base

In the previous subsection, we illustrated a central OT principle: grammars are related by reranking. The strongest version of this principle is given in (34).

(34) Typology by reranking

Systematic crosslinguistic variation is due entirely to differences in language-specific rankings of the constraints in *Con*, which are universal. Analysis of the optimal forms arising from all possible total rankings of *Con* gives the typology of possible human languages. Universal grammar may impose restrictions on the possible rankings of *Con*.

So, for example, analysis of all rankings of the CVT constraints reveals a typology of basic CV syllable structures that explains Jakobson's typological generalizations

(Jakobson 1962; Clements and Keyser 1983); see Chapter 13. In this typology, licit syllables may have required or optional onsets, and, independently, forbidden or optional codas.

Similarly, analysis of all rankings of the GSL constraints derives an empirically sound typology of subject distribution, relating the presence or absence of topical subjects, the presence or absence of expletive subjects, and the pre- or postverbal positioning of focused subjects (see Grimshaw and Samek-Lodovici 1995, 1998; Samek-Lodovici 1996).

The simplest interpretation of the universality of *Con* (34) is that the constraints are innately specified, but that is not required by the theory itself. OT only requires that *Con* be universal; how this arises is not in the purview of the theory itself (for some discussion of constraint innateness, see Chapter 21).

In (35a–b), we elaborate (34), and in (35c), we introduce a closely related principle.

(35) Universality

a. The universe of possible linguistic structures $\mathcal{U}$ (4), the functions *Gen* and *Int* that produce sets of competing candidates (10), and the constraints *Con* (13) are all universal: literally the same in all languages. All systematic crosslinguistic grammatical differences between languages arise from differences in constraint ranking.

b. **Factorial typology**. Except as restricted by universal constraint rankings implementing markedness hierarchies (41), every constraint ranking defines a possible language. The typology of all possible human grammars is formally specified by exactly the factorial ranking possibilities of *Con*.

c. **Richness of the Base**. The space of possible interpretations—inputs to the production function f_{prod}—is universal. All systematic language-particular restrictions on what is grammatical must arise from the constraint ranking defining the grammar: there are no systematic language-particular restrictions on inputs (Prince and Smolensky 1993/2004, Sec. 9.3).

(The banned restrictions on inputs alluded to in (35c)—for example, **morpheme structure constraints**—play an essential role in rule-based grammars (see, e.g., Kenstowicz and Kisseberth 1979, 424–36.)) Richness of the Base is key in defining grammaticality within OT.

(36) Grammaticality and Richness of the Base

a. For a traditional rewrite-rule grammar, an ungrammatical overt form is, by definition, one the grammar cannot assign a parse to. In OT, however, every overt form is assigned a parse by the interpretation function f_{comp} defined by the grammar.

b. In OT, a structure is **ungrammatical** if and only if, no matter the input, it is never found in the output of the production function f_{prod}. (The production function **filters out** any ungrammatical structures that may be (implicitly) present in the input.)

Richness of the Base insists that systematic differences in the inventories of expressions *E* across languages must arise from differences in constraint rankings, not differences in allowable interpretations *I*. In phonology, we normally consider *I*s that consist of morphemes drawn from the lexicon of a language. As discussed in the next subsection, in OT, a lexicon is a 'random' sample from the inventory of possible inputs: all *systematic* properties of the lexicon must arise indirectly from the grammar, which delimits the inventory from which the lexicon is drawn. There are no morpheme structure constraints on phonological inputs, no lexical parameter that determines whether a language has a null subject (Italian-like $\mathcal{L}'_2$). In language $\mathcal{L}_1$, all syllables have the form .CV. not because the possible *inputs* are restricted ahead of time to consist only of forms with strict CV alternation, but because the grammar so restricts the *outputs*. Richness of the Base extends this style of explanation to all inventory phenomena. If any language lacks a particular structure, it is because any input containing the structure will have, as its optimal candidate, a structural description with an output that does not contain that structure: in the optimal candidate, it will always have been changed into something else.

It often happens that a structural configuration X is guaranteed to be suboptimal in *every* ranking; this entails that X is universally banned from all languages. Often, this arises when a candidate containing X incurs a set of marks that is a strict superset of the marks incurred by a competitor *X'*: X incurs all the marks that *X'* does, plus additional marks. In this case, no matter the ranking, X will be less harmonic than *X'*. Here, X is said to be **harmonically bounded** by *X'* (Samek-Lodovici 1992; Prince and Smolensky 1993/2004, Sec. 9.1.1; Legendre, Raymond, and Smolensky 1993; Samek-Lodovici and Prince 1999, 2002). (As an example, with respect to the GSL constraints shown in (19), candidates (c) and (d) are both harmonically bounded by (b); for this input, it is predicted that forms (c) and (d) will not be grammatical in any language.)

Chapter 17 provides an intuitive exposition of Richness of the Base, explores some of its theoretical consequences, and describes attempts to experimentally test these predictions in infants. What follows is a somewhat more formal discussion of this rather subtle principle.

1.7 Lexicon optimization

In our CV language $\mathcal{L}_1$, if the lexical form of some morpheme *M* is abstractly I_M = /$V^1C^2V^3C^4$/, then *M* is expressed as E_M = .$CV^1.C^2V^3$. Why, in this case, is the underlying lexical form of *M* not simply $I_M' \equiv$ /$C^0V^1C^2V^3$/? Then no epenthesis or deletion would be needed: the optimal surface form would be completely faithful to the underlying form.

This question—call it *Q*—has three answers that require consideration. The first answer (abbreviated) is: because it so happens that when *M* is preceded by a consonant-final prefix, no C^0 appears; and when *M* is followed by a vowel-initial suffix, C^4

appears.[22] (In reality, of course, this answer applies to a less ethereal realm than that of Cs and Vs. We can think of the Cs and Vs here, distinguished by superscripts, as standing in for actual segments distinguished by their features; perhaps $C^0 = t$, $V^1 = i$, etc.) This answer might be dubbed 'paradigmatically motivated disparity' between underlying and surface forms ('paradigmatic' referring to the role of *M*'s multiple instantiation with various prefixes and suffixes across its **paradigm**). While C^0 may be visible, and C^4 invisible, when *M* appears alone, the reverse is true when *M* appears in other forms of its paradigm. This is the essential locus of underlying/surface disparity.

Suppose now there is no paradigmatic motivation for disparity, no forms in which *M* appears as anything but .CV.CV. Now, two answers to our question *Q* arise. One—the second answer to *Q*—is that the underlying form of *M* can be I_M because it just doesn't matter. That is, it might as well have been I_M', but it just happens (for a particular speaker, say) to be I_M. What is crucial is the grammar. That is what ensures that I_M surfaces as .CV.CV.; the lexical form of *M* is only important to the extent that, together with the grammar of $\mathcal{L}_1$, it produces the correct expression. From this perspective, Richness of the Base can be understood as the requirement that the speaker may posit *any underlying form*. Again, what is critical is the *grammar*. The fact that surface forms in $\mathcal{L}_1$ always have strictly CV syllables cannot be due to a stipulated ban on underlying forms with other structures, like I_M = /VCVC/. Rather, surface forms have strictly CV syllables because the grammar actively ensures—via unfaithfulness—that this will be true for *any* underlying form.

The third answer to *Q* is that absent paradigmatic motivation for a disparity between underlying and surface forms, the underlying form of *M isn't* surface-disparate I_M—it is surface-faithful I_M'. This might seem to be inconsistent with Richness of the Base, but in fact a more subtle interpretation of this principle is possible. The crucial element in this interpretation is **lexicon optimization**, due to Prince and Smolensky 1993/2004, Chap. 9.

(37) Lexicon optimization

When multiple underlying forms yield the same surface form (in all paradigmatic contexts), the form selected for inclusion in the lexicon is the one yielding highest Harmony.

If there is a possible underlying form I_0 for *M* that is faithfully parsed by its optimal surface form, then I_0 will be selected by the lexicon optimization principle.[23] Other

[22] The example of French *petit* 'small' in Sections 4:2 and 22:4.2 illustrates this sort of behavior for C^4.

[23] This argument assumes a MARKEDNESS/FAITHFULNESS grammar. Prince and Smolensky (1993/2004, Chap. 9) show that lexicon optimization can also lead to underlying forms that are minimally rather than maximally specified: if a constraint prohibiting underlying material exists and is high ranked—namely, *SPECIFICATION, or simply *SPEC. Clearly, *SPEC is neither a markedness nor a faithfulness constraint, under our definitions. But even if *SPEC exists, it cannot be visible in the standard operation of the grammar, f_{prod}, since all competitors share a common underlying form, hence equally violate *SPEC. *SPEC clearly matters for lexicon optimization, however, and also for f_{comp}, where alternative interpretations compete; *SPEC favors minimal interpretations generally, including minimal

possible underlying forms have the same markedness violations as I_0, since they have the same surface form and since markedness constraints, by definition, inspect only the surface form; but only I_0 has no faithfulness violations, rendering it the most harmonic alternative. In our example, I_0, the selected underlying form for M, is $I_M{}' =$ /CVCV/.

Under lexicon optimization, surface regularities—such as 'No CC or VV sequences': strict CV syllabification—get pushed back into the lexicon, giving rise to restrictions on underlying forms. This is *not* inconsistent with Richness of the Base, since these 'restrictions' are entirely determined by the grammar.

This somewhat subtle point can be brought out with the help of (38).

(38) Lexicon optimization and lexical regularities

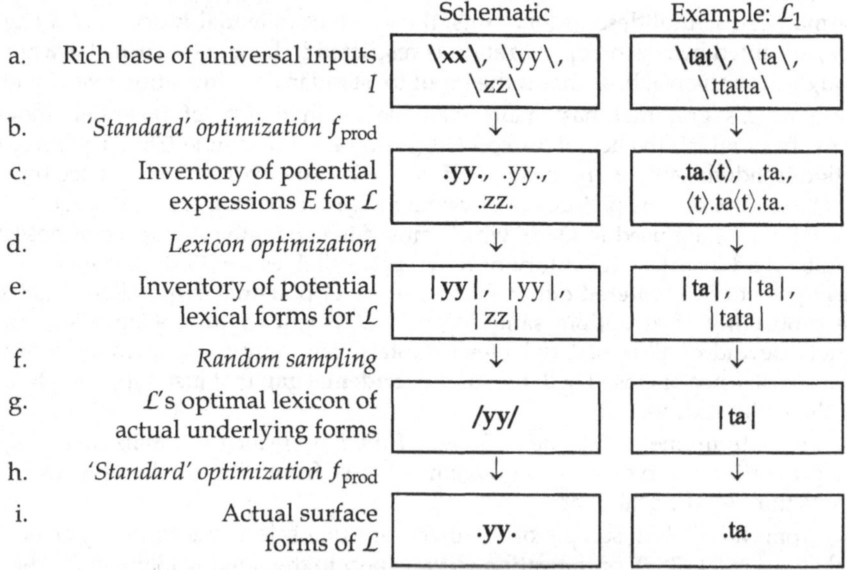

The content of representations is here simplified to schematic 'xx, yy, zz'; the one to watch is 'xx', in boldface. In this discussion only, we are distinguishing interpretations with different status by the ad hoc delimiters \xx\ and |xx| as well as the conventional /xx/.

The analytic starting point is the universal set of all potential input forms: the rich, universal base $\mathcal{U}_I$ of interpretations in the universe of structural descriptions $\mathcal{U}$ (4). In (38a), the input forms of the universal base are schematically designated \xx\; in phonological theory, we can think of these as \tat\, \ta\, and so on. Next, in row (38b), this universal input base is filtered by 'standard' (expressive) optimization f_{prod}

underlying forms.

(12d) with respect to the constraint hierarchy of a particular language $\mathcal{L}$. The example $\mathcal{L}_1$ (25) is illustrated, with Cs and Vs replaced by segments *t* and *a*. At this stage, there is great neutralization of contrasts: only a highly restricted subset of the contrasts available in the universal input set surface in any given language. In the syllable structure example $\mathcal{L}_1$, the open/closed syllable contrast neutralizes to the unmarked (open) case: the input \tat\ surfaces as .ta.⟨t⟩, phonetically equivalent to the output .ta. of another input, \ta\. Filtering the universal rich base through $\mathcal{L}$'s constraint hierarchy gives the inventory of potential expressions for $\mathcal{L}$ (38c).

Next, lexicon optimization applies (38d), selecting for each distinct potential surface form .yy. of $\mathcal{L}$ an optimal lexical entry |yy|. Assuming no paradigmatic motivation for underlying/surface disparity, for the surface form .ta. the selected underlying form is what we will write as |ta|. In fact, \tat\ also surfaces as .ta., but lexicon optimization does not produce |tat|: it is **occulted** by |ta|, which yields a higher-Harmony structural description. Thus, the space of potential lexical *underlying forms* (38e) admitted by lexicon optimization is restricted in language-particular ways, even though the universal base that is the input to 'standard' optimization (38b) is not.

Now $\mathcal{L}$'s grammar has made available an inventory of potential underlying forms from which the actual lexicon (38g) is a random sample (38f). The force of the notion 'random sample' here is this. If we look at the words of $\mathcal{L}$ and see only open syllables, then on this picture, this systematic property of $\mathcal{L}$ can only arise from one place: the ranking used in (38b), which must filter the universal space of possible inputs to yield a surface inventory of only open syllables .xx. (38c). For if closed syllables have not been filtered out of the inventory of potential expressions *E* (38c), then the probability of a random sampling of that inventory producing a lexicon completely devoid of all closed syllables is fantastically minute. Such an account would treat the absence of closed syllables as an **accidental gap** that just happened to permeate the entire lexicon.

The bottom line is this: the Richness of the Base principle entails that all systematic properties observed in a language must arise from filtering the universal base of inputs through the grammar.

From the random sample of the inventory that selects the forms /yy/ of the actual lexicon of $\mathcal{L}$ (38g), optimization with respect to the ranking (38h) yields the actual surface forms .yy. of the language (38i). This last step, from actual lexical underlying form to actual surface form, gets a lot of attention during the development of OT analyses. Yet it would be a serious mistake to regard this last step in the story as the only, or even the primary, locus of explanation. In fact, the focus of OT explanation is more properly the *first* step (38b), where a rich base of universally available surface forms is transformed to a language-particular inventory. The subsequent steps in (38) are needed to connect this explanatory focal point with the empirical data provided by actual forms of the language, but the role of these steps is in most theoretical respects secondary.

This discussion has been principally aimed at phonology, where the set of 'interpretations'—underlying forms—is in the most literal sense highly arbitrary and language specific. The conclusion, however, is that the explanatory action is actually independent of the arbitrariness of a language's lexicon: it resides in the initial filtering (38b) of the universal base. This is to a large extent immediately the situation in syntax, where predicate-argument structure interpretations are not heavily language particular (with respect to syntactically relevant features).[24] But one explanatory strategy popular in recent syntactic theory is to locate explanation of crosslinguistic variation precisely in the purported arbitrariness of the functional lexicon. In an OT theory of syntax, as in any theory in the OT framework, the lexicon is not an independent site of variation: any apparent lexical variation is explained as a *consequence* of differences in the rankings defining language-particular grammars. (For one simple example, see the discussion of resumptive pronouns in Legendre, Smolensky, and Wilson 1998, Sec. 5.1; other examples are identified in the overview of Legendre, Vikner, and Grimshaw 2001. See also (69) below.)

1.8 The structure of *Con*

The universal constraint set *Con* has considerable structure. In the interests of conciseness, a quick, partial summary is given in (39)–(44).

1.8.1 Constraint schemata

In OT, general schematic forms for constraints play a central role in both faithfulness theory (39) and markedness theory (40).

(39) FAITHFULNESS

The correspondence constraints of (17) are schemata. For example, MAX(*X*) pertains to the correspondence relations of units of type *X*; IDENT[φ] inspects feature [φ]. There are multiple classes of correspondence relations:

a. *I–E* correspondence, discussed in (17): correspondence between interpretation *I* and expression *E* (standardly called '**IO**' correspondence, for 'input/output' correspondence: McCarthy and Prince 1995)

b. *E*-internal correspondence: in phonology, for example, between segments in the base of a word and the 'copies' of those segments in a reduplicative affix (called '**BR**' correspondence, for 'base-reduplicant' correspondence: McCarthy and Prince 1993b); in syntax, for example, between elements of c-structure and f-structure in LFG representations[25]

[24] The syntactically relevant information in a predicate-argument structure comprises the embedding of arguments within one another, the semantic roles assigned to various arguments, their discourse properties (such as topicality), their tense and agreement features, and so on. These elements and their possible combinations—the interpretations in syntax—are relatively uniform across languages, relative to the entirely arbitrary combinations of phonological features that make up the lexical items serving as interpretations in phonology.

[25] In LFG, a structural description is a phrase structure—a **constituent-** or **c-structure**—paired with the assignments of grammatical functions to constituents—a **functional-** or **f-structure**. Constituents in the

c. *E–E* correspondence: in phonology, between instances of the same morpheme in different words (called '**OO**' correspondence, for 'output-output' correspondence: Burzio 1994; Benua 1995)

(40) MARKEDNESS

a. ***X**: No *X* (where *X* is a type of element in a representation)—the ***STRUCTURE** constraint family

b. ***Y/*X**: No *X* as a constituent of *Y*

c. ***[φ, ψ]**: No coincidence of features [φ] and [ψ] (e.g., within the same segment)

d. **ALIGN(X_1, D_1, X_2, D_2)**: The D_1-edge (D_1 = Left or Right) of every *X* must coincide with the D_2-edge of some X_2 (McCarthy and Prince 1993a)[26]

1.8.2 Universal markedness hierarchies

Universal markedness hierarchies are used in the following ways (among others):

(41) **Markedness scales** (Prince and Smolensky 1993/2004, Chap. 9)

Universal markedness hierarchies encode a scale of relative markedness of values along a single dimension. For example, for place of articulation,

*[lab] $\gg_{UG}$ *[cor]

requires that this relative ranking obtain in every hierarchy admitted by universal grammar; this asserts that [labial] place is (universally) more marked than [coronal] place—in other words, that [labial] is the marked pole of the [labial]–[coronal] dimension of variation.

(42) **Prominence Alignment**: ⊗ (Prince and Smolensky 1993/2004, Secs. 5.1, 8.2)

Universal markedness hierarchies encode the compatibility between two dimensions *d*, *d'*.

The operation of Prominence Alignment yields rankings asserting that elements at the most prominent pole of the *d* dimension are less marked when they are also at the most prominent pole of the *d'* dimension, and likewise for the least prominent pole. For example, if *d* is the syllable position dimension Nucleus-Onset, with Nucleus the prominent pole, and *d'* is the dimension of inherent phonetic prominence (energy) called **sonority** (Box 2), the Prominence

c-structure component of a structural description are in correspondence with constituents in the f-structure.

[26] Under the name EDGEMOST, one of the first uses of ALIGN constraints was to define a prefix (or suffix) as a morpheme subject to a left- (or right-) edgemost requirement (McCarthy and Prince 1993b; Prince and Smolensky 1993/2004). EDGEMOST constraints, like all ALIGN constraints, are gradiently violable: they register a stronger degree of violation the more material intervenes between the two aligned edges. Thus, when dominated by other constraints, they can position a prefix near but not at the left edge of a domain. EDGEMOST constraints have thus proved to have much explanatory power with respect to the difficult problem of clitic placement: clitics (as well as other functional morphemes) are analyzed as affixes to phrases rather than words (Anderson 1993, 1996, 2000; Legendre 1998, 1999, 2000a, b, c, d, 2001); they are positioned, like all affixes, by ALIGN/EDGEMOST constraints.

Box 2

Alignment of *d* and *d'* is a universal ranking entailing that the least-marked Nucleus is a segment of highest sonority (e.g., *a*), and the least-marked Onset is a segment of lowest sonority (e.g., *t*); see Chapter 13.[27]

Sonority ⊗ syllable structure Prominence Alignment:
Binary prominence scale (syllable structure): Nuc > Ons
Aligned prominence scale (sonority): $a > i > \cdots > d > t$
Universal constraint hierarchies from alignment:[28]

$$\text{*Nuc}/t \gg_{\text{UG}} \text{*Nuc}/d \gg_{\text{UG}} \cdots \gg_{\text{UG}} \text{*Nuc}/i \gg_{\text{UG}} \text{*Nuc}/a$$
$$\text{*Ons}/a \gg_{\text{UG}} \text{*Ons}/i \gg_{\text{UG}} \cdots \gg_{\text{UG}} \text{*Ons}/d \gg_{\text{UG}} \text{*Ons}/t$$

The process also yields universal markedness orderings of structures, the **Harmonic Alignment** of the scales. For the sonority example:

$$\text{Nuc}/a \succ_{\text{UG}} \text{Nuc}/i \succ_{\text{UG}} \cdots \succ_{\text{UG}} \text{Nuc}/d \succ_{\text{UG}} \text{Nuc}/t$$
$$\text{Ons}/t \succ_{\text{UG}} \text{Ons}/d \succ_{\text{UG}} \cdots \succ_{\text{UG}} \text{Ons}/i \succ_{\text{UG}} \text{Ons}/a$$

1.8.3 Local constraint conjunction

In Chapter 14, I argue that OT must include the following operation:

(43) Local conjunction of constraints: $\&_{\mathfrak{D}}$ (Smolensky 1993, 1995, 1997; cf. Hewitt and Crowhurst 1996)

a. A constraint $\mathbb{C}$ in *Con* may be the **local conjunction** of two simpler constraints in *Con*, $\mathbb{A}$ and $\mathbb{B}$: if $\mathbb{C} = \mathbb{A} \&_{\mathfrak{D}} \mathbb{B}$, then $\mathbb{C}$ is violated whenever $\mathbb{A}$ and $\mathbb{B}$ are both violated within a common domain $\mathfrak{D}$.

b. $\mathbb{C}$ may be viewed as implementing the **conjunctive interaction** of A and B.

c. Universally, the conjunction dominates its conjuncts:

$$\mathbb{A} \&_{\mathfrak{D}} \mathbb{B} \gg \{\mathbb{A}, \mathbb{B}\}.$$

d. The **self-conjunction** of $\mathbb{C}$ with domain $\mathfrak{D}$, $\mathbb{C}^2$, is violated whenever there are two distinct violations of $\mathbb{C}$ within a single domain $\mathfrak{D}$. Higher powers $\mathbb{C}^3$, $\mathbb{C}^4$, … are defined recursively. Universally, $\mathbb{C}^n \gg \mathbb{C}^{n-1}$, giving rise to the universal **power hierarchy** over $\mathbb{C}$:

[27] In Chapter 15, case prominence is aligned with thematic role and with discourse prominence. Aissen (2003) analyzes differential object marking via alignment of grammatical function (subject > object) with animacy (human > animate > inanimate) and with definiteness (pronouns > ⋯ > nonspecific indefinites). See references in Aissen 2003 for Prominence Alignment analyses of "voice and subject choice; word order, the syntax of pronouns, nominal-internal structure, the distribution of null pronouns, agreement, and case" (p. 440).

[28] It may be appropriate to omit the lowest-ranked constraint in each hierarchy, expressing the view that *t* is *not* marked at all as an onset, and likewise *a* as a nucleus. When the aligned dimension—the sonority scale in the text example—is binary, this is especially convenient as it reduces a hierarchy of two constraints to a single constraint. For instance, if the sonority scale were just *a* > *t* or, better, V > C, the two lowest constraints in the hierarchies would be *Nuc/V and *Ons/C. If these are omitted, what remains are the two constraints *Nuc/C and *Ons/V. These two are precisely the constraints assumed in the CVT (see Chapter 13 (9)–(10); see also Footnotes 14:30, 14:37, and 14:40).

$$\cdots \gg \mathbb{C}^3 \gg \mathbb{C}^2 \gg \mathbb{C}.$$

(44) Local conjunction respects universal markedness hierarchies (Smolensky 1993; Spaelti 1997; Itô and Mester 1998; Aissen 1999)

If a universal markedness hierarchy

$$\mathbb{A} \gg_{UG} \mathbb{B} \gg_{UG} \cdots \gg_{UG} \mathbb{D}$$

is locally conjoined with a constraint $\mathbb{C}$, the resulting constraints are also universally ranked:[29]

$$\mathbb{A} \,\&\, \mathbb{C} \gg_{UG} \mathbb{B} \,\&\, \mathbb{C} \gg_{UG} \cdots \gg_{UG} \mathbb{D} \,\&\, \mathbb{C}.$$

Universal markedness hierarchies and local conjunction are primary topics of Chapter 14. LOCALITY is formalized as a power hierarchy in the sentence-processing research of Chapter 19, as is MINLINK in the theoretical syntax work of Chapter 16.

Prince (1997) argues that the OT architecture itself imposes **endogenous constraints** on the form of a possible OT constraint. Types of effects that arise through OT constraint *interaction* are ipso facto not appropriate for inclusion within a single constraint. A constraint of the form "*A* except when *B*" is unacceptable because its effect can be achieved by ranking simpler constraints that independently govern *A* or *B*. "*C* must be minimal" is likewise an unacceptable OT constraint since its effect can arise from competition among candidates under a constraint prohibiting *C*. "Except ..." clauses and minimality requirements emerge naturally from constraint interaction in OT; they therefore should not be compiled into a single, unnecessarily complex constraint. And finally, it is unacceptable for an individual constraint to be formulated in terms of comparisons that are properly the province of optimality computation, *H-eval*. This is a central point of Chapter 16: the work done in other theories by constraints requiring that dependencies be "as local as possible" is shown to arise in OT syntax from the interaction of constraints that individually involve no comparison, no use of the formally murky locution "as possible."

1.9 Optimality Theory's contributions to linguistic theory

This is not the place to attempt a comprehensive evaluation of OT's contributions to theoretical linguistics. For syntax, such evaluation may be premature, and for phonology, the depth and breadth of critical analysis required would go far beyond the scope of this book (for an excellent comprehensive yet concise overview of many OT results to date, with numerous literature citations, see McCarthy 2002b; for critical reviews, see Ritter 2000 and references cited therein). The summary in (45) is intended merely to convey—certainly not defend—the types of claims of significant explanatory progress that are made in the OT literature, especially concerning pho-

[29] A reason not to omit the lowest-ranked constraint $\mathbb{C}_{low}$ of a hierarchy $\mathcal{H}$ resulting from Prominence Alignment (see Footnote 28) is that when conjoined with some $\mathbb{C}$, the constraint $\mathbb{C}\&\mathbb{C}_{low}$ is often useful for marking $\mathbb{C}$-violators even if they are only $\mathbb{C}_{low}$-violators on $\mathcal{H}$. See Footnotes 14:30, 14:37, and 14:40.

nology (see also Prince and Smolensky 2003).

(45) OT contributions to the explanatory power of phonological theory

a. Process versus product: Conspiracies

In the very first volume of *Linguistic Inquiry,* Kisseberth (1970) observed that within a language's phonology, rule systems often 'conspire' to bring about an end result: different rules apply different operations to different structures in order to bring about a common outcome. Kisseberth showed, for example, that in the Native American language Yawelmani Yokuts, several rules involving different conditions and operations (including deletion and epenthesis) all have a functionally unified result: in contemporary terms, conformity to the language's syllable template. In OT terms, the conspiracies' results are structures that satisfy constraints which would otherwise have been violated. Not just within a language, but crucially, across languages, these constraints provide a unifying explanation of disparate 'processes'. In a wide range of linguistic phenomena, what is universal are not the rules, but the constraints satisfied by the *outcomes* of the rules—it is in the ultimate *products,* not the *processes* that create them, that universal principles are found. (See McCarthy 2002b on 'homogeneity of target/heterogeneity of process'.)

b. The duplication problem

The conspirators in rule-based analyses sometimes consist of a rule from the grammar and a rule (or 'condition') from the lexicon: for example, a rule may require a rather complex formulation to prevent it from creating *X*, which just happens to be the same structure that is banned from the lexicon by a separate mechanism. In OT, Richness of the Base asserts that apparent restrictions on the lexicon are actually the product of the grammar itself: a single highly ranked markedness constraint *X does the work of duplicated rules, ensuring both that lexical items will not contain *X* and that when surface forms differ from underlying forms, the 'process' involved will never create *X* (see the discussion of closed syllables in Sections 1.6–1.7). This problem is noted in Goldsmith 1976, 107, N. 16; Kenstowicz and Kisseberth 1977, 1979, 427–36.

c. Explaining 'do unless/except' patterns

In part as a response to the conspiracy problem, rule-based theories have sometimes supplemented rules with inviolable constraints: 'repair rules' are 'triggered' when a constraint is violated, or are 'blocked' when applying them would create a violation. But rules and constraints do not prove such good bedfellows. The concept of violable constraint allows the work of both rules and constraints to be done within a single, formally simple, homogeneous architecture. The notion of constraint ranking immediately explains the pervasiveness of empirical generalizations of the inelegant form "*A* is true, except when *B* applies," or in the procedural vernacular,

"Do α, except when β holds" (or "Do α, unless that creates γ"). These arise in OT from constraints that just say 'No γ'—when these conflict, ranking leads to patterns of violation descriptively appearing as "except" clauses (see Prince and Smolensky 1993/2004, Chaps. 3–4 for phonology; Speas 1997 for syntax).

d. Rule-ordering paradoxes
Two generalizations that can each be encoded as rules can sometimes not be ordered with respect to one another without producing incorrect results. The effect of simultaneous rule application, or repeated rule application, required by such cases is the immediate consequence of parallel evaluation of constraints in OT.[30] On the flip side, rule ordering provides an elegant analysis of many **phonological opacity** phenomena, which are difficult to analyze with parallel evaluation; see (61) (also McCarthy 2002b, 163–78 and references cited therein).

e. Analytic typology; restrictiveness; 'tendencies' formalized
The wide range of phonological phenomena observed crosslinguistically requires a correspondingly wide range of rules, a small proportion of which are present in any one language's grammar. It proves very difficult to find a restrictive metalanguage that allows this wide range of rules to be expressed, without also predicting the existence of many unwanted rules. Given the nonuniversality of rules—point (45a)—rule-based analysis of individual languages is not tightly coupled to typological theories delineating the possible and impossible types of crosslinguistic variation. Typological generalizations often have the form "Languages tend to have property *P*," with many exceptions; these do not combine well with formal rule-based computation. But in OT, language-particular analysis is inseparable from typological analysis. The elements used to construct one language's grammar are all and only the elements that can be used to con-

[30] An example from Prince and Smolensky 1993/2004, Chap. 3, concerns the Polynesian language Tongan (for another example, see the very end of Chapter 7 of that work). In Tongan, heavy syllables—of the form CVV—are always stressed, as in *.húu.* 'go in' (with accent marking stress, periods marking syllable edges). Thus, it would appear that rules of syllabification must precede rules of stress, so that the stress rules can identify the heavy syllables. But the situation is complicated by the requirement that main stress fall on the penultimate vowel. In /huu+fi/, stress must fall on the second *u*, but that is only possible if the syllabification is *.hu.ú.fi.* (for in the syllable *.huu.*, stress cannot fall on the second 'half' of the nucleus; it must be stressed *.húu.*). And indeed the correct syllabification *is* *.hu.ú.fi.* 'open officially'—despite the fact that CVV is syllabified .CVV., not .CV.V., elsewhere in the language. But this means that syllabification must *follow* the main stress rules, for it is only this stress that prevents the otherwise obligatory syllabification *.húu.*. Thus, syllabification can neither precede nor follow stress. Now rules are an extremely flexible device, and rule-ordering problems can usually be worked around: for example, rules can be applied cyclically, so syllabification and stress cycle back and forth, each preceding *and* following the other; or later rules can undo the effect of earlier rules, so stress rules can break up syllables constructed previously. Here the claim is simply that the most *insightful* analysis is one where syllabification and stress principles apply simultaneously: as ranked violable constraints (with the main-stress constraint ALIGN dominating the syllable structure constraint ONSET violated by the syllabification *.hu.ú.fi.*).

Box 2

struct every other language's grammar. Since these elements are variably ranked, violable constraints, they immediately explain the character of typological generalizations, from within an entirely formal framework. (The analyses of syllabification, grammatical voice, and unaccusativity in Chapters 13, 15, and 20 are illustrative examples.)

f. The subordination spectrum in broad typological generalizations
OT allows typological generalizations to be understood (and formally treated) simply as the effects of conflicts among universal pressures, varying crosslinguistically only in their relative priorities. It becomes possible to perceive a very broad crosslinguistic generalization pattern—the **subordination spectrum**—that is completely entailed by the simple statement '$\mathbb{C} \in$ *Con*': in some languages (where $\mathbb{C}$ is highly ranked), $\mathbb{C}$-violating structures *M* will be absent entirely; in other languages (where $\mathbb{C}$ is less highly ranked), *M* will be limited to a special context (where $\mathbb{C}$'s violation is forced by one of the few constraints that outrank it); in still other languages (as $\mathbb{C}$ is ranked lower and lower), *M* will appear in more and more contexts (as more conflicting constraints outrank $\mathbb{C}$) (Smolensky 1999; Prince and Smolensky 2003).

g. Formal theory of markedness
The structures *M* appearing in the typological generalizations of the previous paragraph were central to the Prague School of linguistics in the 1930s; such dispreferred structures *M* were said to be **marked** (e.g., Trubetzkoy 1939/1969; Jakobson 1962; Battistella 1990, 1996). While markedness was shown to be a pervasive organizing force in grammar, as the basis of a formal theory it is problematic, because the principles characterize 'tendencies', as previously discussed. Identifying marked structures as those that violate a universal constraint in an OT architecture permits much of the substantive linguistic insight of markedness theory to play a central role in a formal grammatical theory. Jakobson sought to explain the universal syllable structure typology from the markedness of closed syllables; [31] the constraint NoCoda, formalized within the OT architecture, can be used to formally derive this typology (Chapter 13). The development of OT shows that it is critical to enrich markedness theory in fundamental ways if it is to function formally: see (45i–k) below.

h. Implicational typological universals
An important typological pattern is that characterized by **implicational universals**, which assert that if a language has elements at one pole *M* of a structural dimension *d*, then that language will also have elements at the opposing pole *U*.[32] In this case, *M* is the marked pole, *U* the unmarked

[31] See Footnote 33.
[32] See, for example, Greenberg 1978b. Some implicational universals concern entire inventories, rather than individual structures; for example, the first of the 40 implicational universals in Greenberg 1978a

pole of dimension *d*. In the example of (41), *d* is place of articulation, and *M* and *U* are labial and coronal place, respectively. OT explains such an implicational universal as the consequence of a markedness constraint or universal markedness hierarchy that is better satisfied by *U*- than by *M*-expressions. For place of articulation, this is achieved in (41) via the universal hierarchy *[lab] $\gg_{\text{UG}}$ *[cor]. *M*-structures will in general surface in a language $\mathcal{L}$ because *M*-inputs are forced to surface faithfully by a faithfulness constraint $\mathbb{F}$ that (in $\mathcal{L}$) outranks the highest-ranked markedness constraint $\mathbb{C}$ violated by *M*. It then follows that a *U*-input must surface faithfully, since its highest markedness violation is lower ranked than that of *M*. As an example, for a [lab] input segment to surface faithfully, $\mathbb{F} \equiv$ ID[place] must outrank *[lab]; this entails that $\mathbb{F}$ outranks *[cor], so a [cor] input must also surface faithfully. Thus is derived the implication that if a language has labial consonants, it must also have coronal consonants. Implicational universals result directly from the same basic OT mechanisms needed for language-internal analysis (Prince and Smolensky 1993/2004, Chap. 9; see Chapter 14).

i. Competition as a formal grammatical mechanism
One enrichment of markedness theory contributed by OT—consonant with parallel developments in syntactic theory (Barbosa et al. 1998)—is the formalization of **competition** as a central grammatical mechanism. For a grammar to formally define as well formed a structure that is "as unmarked as possible" in some respect, it is necessary for alternatives to explicitly compete: these alternatives determine which degrees of markedness are "possible."

j. Multidimensional markedness
A unitary constraint hierarchy allows OT to solve the critical problem of comparing two structures when one is more marked on one linguistic dimension, and the other is more marked on another. Crucial is OT's recognition that this integration of multiple markedness dimensions is language particular, even though the markedness dimensions individually are universal. (For examples, recall the syntactic dimensions evaluated by SUBJ and FULLINT in (18).)

k. Faithfulness theory
When are marked structures grammatical? Here, a major innovation of OT, FAITHFULNESS, is crucial. Phonological representations serve two masters: the phonetic interface, for which MARKEDNESS favors felicitous structures, and the lexical interface, for which FAITHFULNESS favors adherence to fixed lexical forms (Box 2). Grammar turns centrally on the eternal con-

(based on a survey of 104 languages) is "For [word-] initial and final [consonant cluster] systems, if x is the number of sequences of length m and y is the number of sequences of length n and $m > n$, and p is the number of consonant phonemes, then $x/p^m \le y/p^n$" (pp. 248–9; i.e., the proportion of all clusters that are legal in a language decreases with the size of the cluster).

flict between MARKEDNESS and FAITHFULNESS: the OT notion of Harmony combines both MARKEDNESS and FAITHFULNESS in a single scale along which conflicts are resolved. Since it tells only half the story, MARKEDNESS cannot suffice for a grammatical theory.

FAITHFULNESS has been greatly elaborated since the original proposal, shedding new light on many phenomena. Some key developments, beyond Correspondence Theory (McCarthy and Prince 1995) and the early use of Base-Reduplicant Faithfulness for reduplication in McCarthy and Prince 1993b, are Positional Faithfulness (Beckman 1997); Output-Output Faithfulness (Burzio 1994; Benua 1995); and Sympathy Theory (McCarthy 1999b), employing faithfulness to suboptimal candidates.

l. Acquisition
The Jakobsonian program of using markedness to unify linguistic universals, language-particular alternations, and child language[33] is advanced by OT research in which the same markedness constraints governing adult inventories and phonologies also drive child phonology. OT research on acquisition of phonology and syntax are the topics of Chapters 17 and 18 (see also Davidson and Legendre 2003; Legendre et al. 2004).

m. Learnability theory
The difficult 'logical problem of language learnability' (Baker 1979), long regarded as central to linguistic explanation (e.g, Chomsky 1965, 25–7), has yielded considerably to analysis under OT; this is discussed below in Section 3.

n. The phonology/phonetics interface
Like typological universals and markedness theory, generalizations from phonetics often bear on phonology in the form of tendencies. Formalized within OT as violable constraints, phonetic factors can be more directly integrated into phonology (see Flemming 2001; Gussenhoven and Kager 2001; Hayes, Kirchner, and Steriade 2004 and the references cited therein).

o. Pan-grammatical theorems
Independently of the content of the constraints and representations that define a particular OT grammar, the general formal properties that OT imposes on all grammars have sufficiently rich structure to enable the proof of interesting theorems that apply equally to any OT grammar, phonological or syntactic. Examples are Pāṇini's theorem concerning the in-

[33] Relating to the markedness of syllable coda: "During the babbling period in the infant's development, many of the uttered syllables consist of a vocalic sound succeeded by a consonantal articulation. … As soon as the child moves from his babbling activities to the first acquisition of conventional speech, he at once clings to the model 'consonant plus vowel'. The sounds assume a phonemic value and thus need to be correctly identified by the listener, and since the best graspable clue in discerning consonants is their transition to the following vowels, the sequence 'consonant plus vowel' proves to be the optimal sequence, and therefore it is the only universal variety of the syllable pattern" (Jakobson 1941/1968, 24–5).

teraction between general and specific constraints (Prince and Smolensky 1993/2004 , Chap. 5; Prince 1999), characterizations of universally possible optima in terms of a finite candidate set (Samek-Lodovici and Prince 1999), the formal logic of deducing rankings from data (Prince 2002a, b), and the **harmonic completeness** of grammatical inventories (Prince and Smolensky 1993/2004, Chaps. 8, 9 and Chapter 14 here).

2 THE GRAMMAR-PROCESSING PROBLEM

In the remaining sections of this chapter, we pass from aspects of OT internal to linguistic theory to other aspects central to the cognitive science of language. We begin with processing. The general problem is defined in (46).

(46) Processing

An OT processing theory provides algorithms for computing the production and comprehension functions f_{prod} and f_{comp}—optimization algorithms that, at least to some level of approximation or idealization, compute maximum-Harmony linguistic representations. Human linguistic **performance** is to be modeled by the performance characteristics of these algorithms—such as the resources (time, memory, ...) they require for different inputs, and the errors they make, relative to the exact **competence** functions the grammar defines.

Ultimately, the ICS cognitive architecture needs solutions to this problem in the form of processing algorithms that are realized in connectionist computation. Results relevant to this problem are presented in Chapters 8, 10, 20, and 21; Chapters 22–23 discuss foundational questions concerning the relation between OT grammars and connectionist computation.[34]

Empirically oriented studies of two representative processing domains are presented in this book: phonological production (Chapter 17) and syntactic comprehension (Chapter 19).

With respect to phonological production, as Yip (1993) observed early on, OT is particularly useful for the study of loanword (and second language) phonology because the same grammar needed for the native language—a complete ranking of the universal constraints *Con*—necessarily yields an output for *any* input, even one derived from a foreign form illegal in the native language. Davidson (2001) experimentally examined adult English-speakers' production of inputs with initial consonant clusters that are illegal in English, to see whether the outputs could be understood as arising from an OT grammar. These experiments revealed 'hidden rankings' among constraints all of which are unviolated with native English inputs. These rankings separate illegal clusters into increasingly ill-formed strata, directly analogous to the native-to-foreign stratification of the Japanese lexicon given an OT analysis by Itô and

[34] For an implementation of OT processing and learning in ACT-R, a hybrid connectionist/symbolic production-system-based architecture (Anderson and Lebiere 1998), see Misker and Anderson 2003.

Mester (1995). This work is presented in Chapter 17.

In regard to syntactic comprehension, Gibson and Broihier (1998) point out that OT is well suited to the study of incremental, real-time sentence processing because the same grammar that yields a well-formed parsed output for a complete input sentence necessarily also produces an output for an incomplete input consisting of the first *n* words of a sentence. Such an output is not a well-formed sentence, but is nonetheless the optimal parse—the best the grammar can do with the fragmentary input. Chapter 19 shows how a significant body of experimental results concerning the relative processing difficulty of varying sentence types follows from the natural principle that difficulties arise when the structure that is optimal for the first *n* words must be restructured to become optimal for the first $n + 1$ words. Results concerning English follow from a proposed partial grammar employing only constraints that are well motivated by standard syntactic competence theory: no special 'processing heuristics' are needed. For example, other theories posit a 'late closure heuristic' in which the human parser prefers to attach a new word in such a way as to minimize the number of phrases that are thereby 'closed off' (Frazier 1978): this is not a principle of grammar, but a putative rule of thumb employed by the parser when it is forced to make decisions midsentence, before all relevant information has been received. But in the OT analysis, effects of this heuristic follow instead from a principle of grammar, Kayne's (1994) Linear Correspondence Axiom, construed as a violable constraint.[35] In addition, the OT analysis predicts a crosslinguistic typology of patterns of preferences for prepositional phrase attachment sites; this typology follows from the reranking of independently motivated (competence-theoretic) syntactic constraints. This work pursues the possibility that under OT, the human sentence processor is simply applying its competence theory grammar incrementally: no separate principles for parsing per se are involved. (For general discussion of competence and performance theories, see Chapter 23.)

In addition to *empirical* questions addressing human performance in the psycholinguistics lab, *formal* questions concerning computational linguistics within OT loom large in the study of the use of OT grammars. One question that comes up repeatedly about the computation of optimal forms in OT concerns infinity. In the CVT, and quite typically in OT phonology, at least, *Gen*(*I*) contains an infinite number of candidate structural descriptions of each interpretation *I*. The question is, in the face of this infinity, is the theory well defined?

Of course, the overwhelming majority of formal systems in mathematics—all of them rigorously well defined—involve an infinity of structures; the mere fact of infinity means only that the most primitive conceivable method for studying the system, listing all the possibilities and checking each one, is infeasible. But even in finite

[35] The Linear Correspondence Axiom states that if α c-commands β but β does not c-command α, then α must precede β in the linear ordering of phrases in the sentence. For an introduction to the notion c-command, see Box 16:3. See also LOCALITY in Section 19:1.

cases, this method is commonly infeasible anyway, so finiteness is neither necessary nor sufficient for feasibility.

In order for an OT grammar to be well defined, it must be formally determinate, for any input, which structure is optimal. The necessary formal definitions are respectively provided and demonstrated in Prince and Smolensky 1993/2004, Chap. 5 and App. To show that a given structure is the optimal parse of *I*, we need to prove that none of the (infinitely many) other parses in *Gen*(*I*) has higher Harmony. A general technique for such demonstration, the Method of Mark Eliminability (Prince and Smolensky 1993/2004, Sec. 7.3), proceeds by showing that every attempt to avoid the marks incurred by the putatively optimal output leads to alternatives that incur worse marks.[36]

Thus, the infinite candidate set has a perfectly well-defined optimum (or set of optima, if multiple outputs incur exactly the same, optimal set of marks). Yet it might still be the case that the task of actually computing the optimal candidate cannot be performed efficiently; optimization problems in general are computationally complex (Garey and Johnson 1979; see also Aarts, Korst, and Zwietering 1996). But as Tesar (1994, 1995a, b, 1996) has shown, computational feasibility is not a problem either, at least in the general cases studied to date. One reason is that the infinity of candidates derives from the unbounded potential for empty structure. But empty structure is always penalized by constraints of the FILL family: these militate against empty syllable positions in phonology (FILL^{Ons}, FILL^{Nuc}), empty head positions in syntax (OBLIGATORY-HEADS of Grimshaw 1993, 1997; Grimshaw and Samek-Lodovici 1995), uninterpretable elements (FULLINT), and the like. *Optimal* structures may have empty structure, violating FILL, only when that is necessary to avoid violating higher-ranking constraints. This will not be the case for unbounded quantities of empty structure. It follows that each finite input will only have a finite number of structural descriptions that are potentially optimal, under some constraint ranking. Thus, a parser constructing an optimal parse of a given input *I* need only have access to a finite part of the infinite space *Gen*(*I*).

The parsing algorithms developed by Tesar construct optimal parses from increasingly large portions of the input, requiring an amount of computational time and storage space that grows with the size of the input only as fast as for parsers of conventional, rewrite-rule grammars of corresponding complexity. The structure in the space of candidates allows for efficient computation of optimal parses, even though the grammar's specification of well-formedness makes reference to an infinite set of parses.

In the remainder of this section, we summarize some of the formal results proven to date concerning the tractability of computing optimal forms in OT; they constitute

[36] This can be briefly illustrated in reference to optimal candidate (d) of (16). Here, avoiding the mark *PARSE of (d) entails violating higher-ranked NOCODA (as in candidate (a)), and avoiding the mark *FILL^{Ons} of (d) entails violating either ONSET (as in (a)) or PARSE (as in (b)), both of which are higher ranked than FILL^{Ons}. This proves that among the infinitely many candidates in *Gen* (/VCVC/), none is more harmonic than candidate (d).

a solid foundation for developing a formal theory of computing with OT grammars. These theorems unfortunately require a technical base that is infeasible to develop here.

(47) *Theorem* (Tesar 1994, 1995a, b, 1996). Suppose
   a. *Gen* parses a string of input symbols into structures specified via a context-free grammar, and
   b. *Con* constraints meet a tree locality condition and penalize empty structure.

   Then a given dynamic programming algorithm is
   c. left to right,
   d. general (*any* such *Gen*, *Con*),
   e. guaranteed to find the optimal outputs, and
   f. as efficient as parsers for context-free conventional (rewrite-rule) grammars.

(48) *Theorem* (Ellison 1994). Suppose
   a. *Gen*(*I*) is representable as a (nondeterministic) finite-state transducer (particular to *I*) mapping the input string to a set of output candidates, and
   b. *Con* constraints are reducible to multiply-violable binary constraints each representable as a finite-state transducer mapping an output candidate to a sequence of violation marks.

   Then composing the *Gen*(*I*) and rank-sequenced constraint-transducers yields a transducer that
   c. directly maps *I* to its optimal output(s) and
   d. can be efficiently pruned by dynamic programming.

(49) *Theorem* (Frank and Satta 1998; see also Karttunen 1998). Suppose
   a. *Gen* is representable as a (nondeterministic) finite-state transducer mapping an input string to a set of output candidates, and
   b. *Con* has the property that the set of structures incurring *n* violations of each constraint is generable by a finite-state machine, and *n* can be finitely bounded for each constraint.

   Then the mapping from inputs to optimal outputs has the complexity of a finite-state transducer.

(50) *Theorem* (Frank and Satta 1998, attributed to personal communications from Marcus Hiller (1996) and Paul Smolensky (1997)). If the *n* in (49b) is unbounded, then there are (extremely simple) OT grammars with computational complexity greater than that of any finite-state transducer.

(51) *Theorem* (Eisner 1997). Even under finite-state assumptions, the problem of computing the optimal output(s) given (*I*, *Con*)—any input and any possible constraint set—is NP-hard (see also Wareham 1998).

Thus, for *any* given OT system (*Gen*, *Con*) that meets certain finiteness conditions, there is an efficient algorithm for computing the optimal output(s) for any input, although there is no efficient single algorithm that computes optima for *all* such *Con*.

3 THE GRAMMAR-LEARNING PROBLEM

Much empirical research has employed OT to shed new light on language acquisition, mostly in phonology, but also in syntax (Chapter 18 analyzes early sentence production in French). To address one of OT's conceptual contributions in this area, consider early child phonology. Empirical research, in both the OT and rule-based frameworks, has tended to assume that young children's underlying forms are relatively faithful to the adult forms, even though these children's productions are massively unfaithful.[37] Under this view, however, the grammar that maps a child's underlying form to its surface form must make massive changes. In a rule-based theory, this requires children's grammars to have many phonological simplification rules that must then be 'lost' during acquisition; in effect, their grammars must start off very complex and become simpler. By contrast, the OT account posits a simple ranking as the child's initial state $\mathcal{H}_0$: MARKEDNESS dominates FAITHFULNESS—that is, all constraints of one type simply dominate all constraints of the other. During acquisition, the hierarchy becomes more complex in the sense that a complex pattern of interleaved markedness and faithfulness constraints develops. Experimental testing of the hypothesis that the infant grammar is $\mathcal{H}_0$ is a main topic of Chapter 17.

In addition to empirical questions addressing language acquisition, formal questions concerning language learnability and computationally adequate learning algorithms are central to understanding the origin of grammatical knowledge, in OT as in any other grammatical framework.

OT is quite clear about exactly what the learnability problem is. Since constraint ranking is language specific, at the very least a language learner must learn this from available data. Even if the learner were to have innate access to all universal elements of grammar, and access to all the covert elements in grammatical structural descriptions, learning the constraint ranking would be a highly nontrivial problem. We begin by formulating this problem, and then move on to expand the scope of the learning theory.

(52) The core learning problem for OT

Given:

The universal components of a particular OT grammar:

the set of possible inputs

[37] This seemingly odd hypothesis can be rendered logically coherent within OT. In the initial state $\mathcal{H}_0$, a single grammar yields both faithful perception—needed to acquire adult-like underlying forms—and massively unfaithful production. This perception/production gap is due to the contrast between production- and comprehension-directed optimization with grammars (Smolensky 1996c; see Section 4:4).

the function *Gen* generating the candidate outputs for any input
the constraints *Con* on well-formedness
Learning data in the form of full grammatical structural descriptions
Find:
A language-particular OT grammar consistent with all the given data: a ranking (or set of rankings) of the constraints in *Con*

The initial data for this learning problem are well-formed candidate structural descriptions; each consists of an input together with the output that is declared optimal by the target grammar. For example, the learner of the CV language $\mathcal{L}_1$ might have as an initial datum .□V.CV.⟨C⟩, candidate (d) of (16), the parse assigned to the input I = /VCVC/; the learner of the Italian-like language $\mathcal{L}'_2$ might have as an initial datum the input I = /sing(x), x = topic, x = he; T = pres perf/ together with its grammatical parse, p = [$_{IP}$ has [sung]] (33a).

Because OT is inherently comparative, the grammaticality of a structural description is determined not in isolation, but with respect to competing candidates. Therefore, the learner is not informed about the correct ranking by positive data in isolation; the role of the competing candidates must be addressed. This fact is not a liability, but an advantage. A comparative theory gives comparative structure to be exploited: each piece of positive evidence, a grammatical structural description, brings with it a body of **implicit negative evidence** in the form of the competing descriptions. Given access to *Gen* (which is universal) and the underlying form (contained in the given structural description), the learner has access to these competitors. Any competing candidate, along with the grammatical structure, forms a **data pair** informative about the correct ranking: the correct ranking must make the grammatical structure more harmonic than the ungrammatical competitor.

This can be stated more concretely in the context of our running example, the GSL theory. Suppose the learner receives a piece of explicit positive evidence such as the form p = /sing(x), x = topic, x = he; T = pres perf/, [$_{IP}$ has [sung]]. (Recall that in OT, a full structural description consists of an interpretation, an expression, and a correspondence between their elements. This example informs the learner that an unfocused, topic-referring subject is not overtly realized in the target language.) Now consider any other parse p' of the interpretation of p: I = /sing(x), x = topic, x = he; T = pres perf/; for example, the parse p' with expression [$_{IP}$ he$_i$ has [t$_i$ sung]]. In the general case, there are two possibilities. One is that the alternative parse p' has exactly the same marks as p, in which case p' has the same Harmony as p (no matter what the unknown ranking) and must be tied for optimality: p' too then is a grammatical parse of I. This case is unusual, but possible. In the overwhelming majority of cases, p' and p will not have identical marks. In this case, the harmonic ordering of forms (20c) determined by the unknown ranking will declare one more harmonic than the other; it must be p that is the more harmonic, since it is given as well-formed learning data and is thus optimal.

Thus, for each well-formed example p a learner receives, every other parse p' of the same input must be suboptimal, that is, ill formed—unless p' happens to have exactly the same marks as p. Thus, a single positive example, a parse p of an input I, conveys a body of implicit negative evidence: all the other parses p' in *Gen*(I) (with the exception of parses p' that the learner can recognize as tied for optimality with p in virtue of having identical marks).

In our GSL example, a learner given the positive datum p knows that, with respect to the unknown constraint hierarchy of the language being learned, the alternative parse of the same input, p', is less harmonic:

(53) for I = /sing(x), x = topic, x = he; T = pres perf/,
[$_{IP}$ he$_i$ has [t$_i$ sung]] $\prec$ [$_{IP}$ has [sung]].

Furthermore, corresponding harmonic comparisons must hold for every other parse p' in *Gen*(I).

Thus, each positive initial datum conveys a large amount of inferred comparative evidence of the form

(54) [suboptimal parse of input I: '*loser*']
$\prec$ [optimal parse of input I: '*winner*'].

Such pairs can drive a learning algorithm. Each pair carries the information that the constraints violated by the suboptimal parse *loser* must outrank those violated by the optimal parse *winner*.

This can be made precise using the characterization of optimality given in Section 1.5; (55) is the result.

(55) The Principle of Constraint Demotion
For any constraint ℂ assessing an uncanceled winner mark, if ℂ is not dominated by a constraint assessing an uncanceled loser mark, demote ℂ to immediately below the highest-ranked constraint assessing an uncanceled loser mark.

Constraint Demotion learning algorithms typically start with an initial state in which most of the universal constraints *Con* are unranked with respect to each other; in the simplest case, *all* are unranked, and they form one **stratum** of equally ranked constraints. (Strata are ranked relative to one another, forming **stratified hierarchies**.) In tableaux, when two adjacent constraints lie in the same stratum, a dotted line separates their columns. Then constraints are demoted following the Principle of Constraint Demotion in response to learning data. At each learning step, the current winner is indicated with '✓'; '☞' denotes the structure that is optimal according to the learner's current grammar, which may not be the same as the winner (the structure that is grammatical in the target language). The constraint violations of the winner, *marks*(*winner*), are distinguished by the symbol '⊛', as in (26). Depending on the precise form of the algorithm, a loser is chosen, and its marks in common with the winner are canceled. Constraints are demoted according to (55) and more learning data are then analyzed.[38]

To illustrate one demotion for the GSL theory, assume all the constraints of (18) are initially unranked, forming a single stratum. Then suppose the learner receives the form p above (the winner) and selects form p' above as the loser; these forms are shown in tableau (56). In this case, there are no common marks to cancel, so we proceed directly to constraint demotion. In order for p to be more harmonic than p', each mark of p (⊛) must be dominated by at least one mark (*) of p'. This is achieved by demoting the constraints that p violates, SUBJ and PARSE, beneath the constraint that p' violates, DROPTOP. After demotion, the constraint hierarchy now consists of two strata, with SUBJ and PARSE forming the lower stratum and the remaining constraints the higher stratum.

Given positive datum p, how is the corresponding implicitly negative datum p' required by Constraint Demotion chosen? In the **Error-Driven Constraint Demotion Algorithm** (Tesar 1998), the loser is chosen to be the optimal parse of the input I of p: the current grammar erroneously declares this to be optimal, instead of p'. It can be shown that this choice of p' will be informative for reranking if any candidate is; if the learner's current grammar correctly parses I as p (i.e., if $p' = p$), no learning can occur.

(56) Constraint Demotion for (Italian-like) $\mathcal{L}_2$

/sing(x), x = topic, x = he; T = pres perf/		SUBJ	DROP-TOP	AL-FOC	FULL-INT	PARSE	PARSE	SUBJ
p. ✓	[$_{IP}$ has [sung]]	⊛				⊛	⊛	⊛
p'.	[$_{IP}$ he$_i$ has [t$_i$ sung]]		*!					

(The first SUBJ and PARSE columns are shaded, with arrows demoting them to the rightmost PARSE and SUBJ columns.)

Having briefly described Constraint Demotion (**CD**), we now turn to its analysis. The following two theorems are proved in Tesar and Smolensky 1998.

(57) Correctness of Constraint Demotion

Starting with an arbitrary initial ranking of the constraints in *Con*, and applying CD to informative positive evidence as long as such exists, the process converges on a stratified hierarchy such that all totally ranked refinements of that hierarchy correctly account for the learning data.[39]

[38] The **Recursive Constraint Demotion** algorithm processes the complete set of learning data at once. An 'online' version of CD, which processes one learning datum at a time, is discussed below.

[39] That is, the learned grammar generates all the positive evidence. Different initial rankings may lead to different generalizations to unseen examples. If the learner is to generalize conservatively from the evidence, the initial state must have MARKEDNESS ranked above FAITHFULNESS (Smolensky 1996b), and reranking must be designed to preserve this initial configuration when possible. **Biased Constraint Demotion** (Prince and Tesar 2004) is a CD algorithm biased in favor of demoting faithfulness constraints as opposed to markedness constraints. Conservative generalization is important for learning phonotactics: the learner's grammar must rule out illegal segmental sequences even though explicit evidence of the illegality of these structures is absent (see Hayes 2004; Tesar and Prince, to appear).

(58) Data complexity of Constraint Demotion

The number of informative winner-loser pairs required for learning is at most $N(N-1)$, where N = number of constraints in *Con*.[40]

The significance of the **data complexity** result (58) is perhaps best illustrated by comparing it with the number of possible grammars. Given that a possible grammar is a total ranking of N constraints, the number of possible grammars is the number of possible total rankings, $N!$. This number grows very quickly as a function of the number of constraints N, and if the amount of data required for learning scaled with the number of possible total rankings, it would be cause for concern indeed. Fortunately, the data complexity of CD is quite reasonable in its scaling. In fact, it does not take many universal constraints to give a drastic difference between the data complexity of CD and the number of possible grammars. When $N = 10$, the CD data complexity is 45, while the number of total rankings is over 3.6 million. When $N = 20$, CD requires at most 190 informative examples to pick the correct grammar out of a space containing over 2 billion billion (2.43×10^{18}) possibilities. This reveals the restrictiveness of the structure imposed by OT on the space of grammars: a learner can efficiently home in on any target grammar, managing an explosively sized grammar space with quite modest data requirements by fully exploiting the inherent structure provided by strict domination.

It is important to note that the complexity result (58) gives an upper bound on the number of *informative positive examples* needed to learn a correct hierarchy. A positive example is **informative** if and only if the learner's current grammar erroneously declares it ungrammatical. Thus, (58) provides an upper limit to the number of *errors* that can be made during learning. The only way to delay the learner from arriving at a correct grammar is to withhold examples on which the current grammar is incorrect. And even in this case, the learner's performance remains correct on all data not withheld.

For the CD learner, every error made moves the grammar closer to a correct one. This is in clear contrast to trigger- or cue-based learners (Dresher and Kaye 1990; Gibson and Wexler 1994): these will continue to make errors for as long as it takes to receive a datum—a trigger or cue—with the special form needed to enable a learning step.

The number of grammars made available by a grammatical framework—a theory of universal grammar (UG)—is a truly crude measure of its explanatory power. A more significant measure is the degree to which the *structure* of UG allows rich grammars to be learned with realistically few positive examples. The rudimentary number-of-grammars measure may be the best one can do given a theory of UG that does not enable the better learnability measure to be determined. In OT, however, we do have a

[40] Eisner (2000) provides an efficient method of storing the data that reduces the complexity of Recursive CD from n^2 to n, and an algorithm that (like Recursive CD) treats all training data at once, but (like Error-Driven CD) calls a procedure that computes the optimal forms for an input given a constraint hierarchy. This algorithm finds a ranking in which all training examples are optimal in time proportional to n^2 times the number of examples.

quantitative and formally justified measure of learnability available in the $N(N-1)$ limit on the number of informative examples needed to solve the grammar-learning problem. And we can see precisely how large the discrepancy can be between the number of grammars made available by a UG and the efficiency of learning that its special structure enables.

This dramatic difference between the size of the OT grammar space and the number of informative examples needed to learn a grammar is due to the well-structured character of the space of fully ranked constraint hierarchies. It is useful to consider a set of parameters in the grammar space that suffice to specify the $N!$ grammars: these parameters state, for each pair of different constraints $\mathbb{C}_1$ and $\mathbb{C}_2$, which is dominant—that is, whether $\mathbb{C}_1 \gg \mathbb{C}_2$ or $\mathbb{C}_2 \gg \mathbb{C}_1$. There are in fact $N(N-1)/2$ such dominance parameters, half the maximum number of informative examples needed to learn a correct hierarchy. Efficient learning via CD is possible because the search space allows these dominance parameters to be unspecified (constraints can be unranked) and because evidence for adjusting these dominance parameters can be assessed independently (via the Principle of Constraint Demotion). A single adjustment may not irrevocably set a correct value for any dominance parameter, but each adjustment brings the hierarchy closer to the target, and eventually the adjustments are guaranteed to produce a correct set of parameter values. Note that what is independently adjustable here is not the substantive *content* of individual grammatical principles: it is the *interaction* of the principles, as determined by their relative rankings. This is an important point to which we return shortly.

We close this section by summarizing the OT learnability theory developed in Tesar and Smolensky 2000, including aspects that space considerations did not allow us to consider above. (For other approaches to learning in OT, see, for example, Hale and Reiss 1997; Pulleyblank and Turkel 1998; Tesar 1998b, 1999, 2000a, b, 2002; Hayes 1999, 2004; Prince and Tesar 1999, 2004; Alderete and Tesar 2002; Tesar et al. 2003; Tesar and Prince, to appear. For **gradual learning** in **Stochastic OT**, see Boersma 1998; Boersma and Hayes 2001. For statistical learning of a different probabilistic version of OT, see Goldwater and Johnson 2003.)

An OT grammar is a ranked set of violable constraints that defines a notion of relative Harmony of structural descriptions, the maximally harmonic or optimal structures being the grammatical ones. The consequences of constraint hierarchies for surface patterns can be quite subtle and often surprising. Remarkably different surface patterns can emerge from the reranking of the same set of universal constraints.

All this is integral to the explanatory power of OT as a linguistic theory, formally capturing the simultaneous diversity and uniformity of human languages. But it also raises concerns about learnability. If the relation between grammatical forms and grammars is so complex and opaque, how can a child cope?

Linguists working in OT are frequently faced with a hypothesized set of universal constraints and a collection of surface forms to which they have given hypothetical structural descriptions; the question then arises, is there a ranking of the constraints that yields the correct structures? Typically, this turns out to be a challenging question to answer. Of course, with even a modest number of constraints, the number of possible rankings is much too large to examine exhaustively.

So the starting point of the learning theory is the question, are there reliable, efficient means for finding a ranking of a given set of constraints that correctly yields a given set of grammatical structural descriptions? We have shown that the answer is yes, if the learner is given informative pairs of optimal structures with suboptimal competitors. For any set of such data pairs consistent with some unknown total ranking of the given constraints, CD finds a stratified hierarchy consistent with all the data pairs.

A key to these results is the implicit negative evidence that comes with each positive example: all the universally given competitors to each optimal structure (excluding any that may have identical constraint violations). These are guaranteed to be suboptimal and therefore ill formed. The pairs of optimal forms and suboptimal competitors are the basis of CD: the constraints violated by the optimal form are minimally demoted to lie below a constraint violated by the suboptimal form (excluding canceled marks).

Is it necessary that a 'teacher' provide informative suboptimal forms to the learner? Tesar (1998a) shows that the answer is no. Given a grammatical structural description as a learning datum, the learner can identify the input in the structural description, and compute the optimal parse of that input using the currently hypothesized hierarchy: that parse can be used as the suboptimal competitor, unless it is equal to the given parse, in which case the example is not informative—no learning can occur. This is Error-Driven CD.

Formal analysis shows that learning in all these cases is efficient, in the sense that the number of informative examples, or number of learning operations (demotions), is guaranteed to be no more than $N(N-1)$, where N is the number of constraints. This number grows quite modestly with N and is vastly less than the number of grammars, $N!$.

The most important next step addresses the question, must full structural descriptions of positive examples be provided to the learner?[41] The CD algorithms operate on constraint violations or marks, and these can be determined only from full structural descriptions. We have proposed that the learner, given only the overt part of grammatical structures, can compute the full structural description needed for CD by computing the parsing function f'_{comp} (12d): using the currently hypothesized grammar, the learner finds the maximum-Harmony structural description consistent with the overt form (and the currently hypothesized lexicon). Such parsing is a neces-

[41] Eisner (2000) shows that learning a ranking can become very costly computationally (NP-hard) when the training data do not include hidden structure. It is not clear that realistic restrictions on the type of hidden structure can decrease this complexity. Tractability therefore would seem to require some (unknown) restrictions on the constraint sets that a general learning algorithm is required to rank. An efficient learning algorithm for a given fixed set of constraints may however still exist.

sary part of the overall theory anyway, independent of learning, since grammar *users* must perform it when interpreting overt forms.

Coupling comprehension-directed optimization (f'_{comp}) to the CD solution to the problem of learning a grammar from full structural descriptions yields an algorithm we call **RIP/CD**,[42] a new member of the family of iterative model-based solutions to the general problem of learning hidden structure. In other learning domains, these solutions have been highly successful in both theory and practice; in OT, positive experimental results in the domain of acquiring stress are reported in Tesar 1997 and Tesar and Smolensky 2000.

A related, CD-based approach to the problem of learning from overt forms is embodied in an algorithm called the **Inconsistency Detection Learner** (Tesar 2000, 2004). This approach combines error-driven learning with Recursive CD (a version of CD that simultaneously processes multiple data forms) and takes advantage of the fact that Recursive CD can detect when a set of full structural descriptions are mutually inconsistent, that is, when no ranking exists in which each of the full structural descriptions is optimal. The learner uses this ability to test different possible assignments of structural descriptions to overt forms until it finds a set of structural descriptions that are consistent. Significant positive experimental results have also been achieved for this approach in the domain of metrical stress.

In the case of phonology acquisition, must the learner be provided with the lexicon of underlying forms (necessary for computing f_{comp}, as well as for constructing the inputs to production-directed optimization)? Tesar and Smolensky (1996, Sec. 9) propose that, as part of the same iterative process that is adapting the grammar to accommodate the structural descriptions produced by interpretive parsing (RIP/CD), the learner can incrementally learn the lexicon via *lexicon optimization at the level of the morphological paradigm*. At each stage of learning, the current grammar is used to find the underlying form for morphemes that yields the maximum-Harmony structural descriptions for paradigms. Tesar and Smolensky also provide a miniature example of how this can work in the face of phonological alternation.[43]

Taken as a whole, our OT learning theory constitutes a proposal for how a learner, provided with the universal elements of any OT UG system and the overt parts of forms grammatical with respect to some grammar admitted by that UG, could learn the grammar, the structural descriptions, and the lexicon. This proposal decomposes the problem into three subproblems: comprehension-directed optimization for interpreting overt forms, lexicon learning, and grammar learning. Work to date has produced formal results on the key grammar-learning subproblem.

How do these learnability considerations relate to OT work on actual acquisition? Smolensky (1996c), pursuing an insight from Alan Prince (personal communication,

[42] 'RIP' denotes Robust Interpretive Parsing, our customary name for f'_{comp}.
[43] See also Tesar et al. 2003 and Tesar and Prince, to appear concerning iterative learning of the grammar and lexicon via phonotactic learning through Biased Constraint Demotion (Footnote 39).

1993), considers the question of the initial state, and develops a 'subset'-type argument that uses Richness of the Base to show that, in general, FAITHFULNESS constraints must be low ranked in the initial state $\mathcal{H}_0$ if unmarked inventories are to be learnable. (This argument is sketched in Section 17:2.1.) It turns out that the concept of comprehension-directed optimization defining f_{comp} makes sense of the proposal that despite the relative poverty of their productions, children's inputs are essentially the correct adult forms (see Footnote 37). This connects a fundamental principle of OT and learnability considerations to two important assumptions underlying much OT research on phonological acquisition: initial low ranking of FAITHFULNESS and the hypothesis that children's inputs closely approximate the adult forms (Demuth 1995; Gnanadesikan 1995; Levelt 1995; Pater and Paradis 1996; Levelt and Van de Vijver 1998; Stemberger and Bernhardt 1998; Legendre et al. 2000a, b, 2001, 2002, 2004; Davidson and Legendre 2003; Kager, Pater, and Zonneveld 2004).

And finally, how does the emerging OT learning theory relate to linguistic explanation? In OT, constraint interaction is simultaneously the key to both linguistic explanation and learnability: constraint conflict, resolved by language-specific ranking, provides both the explanatory power of OT as a linguistic theory and the evidence learners need to deduce their target grammar.

How, exactly, is learnability enhanced by the structure imposed by a particular grammatical theory on the space of possible human grammars? The work summarized here provides evidence that OT's claims about the structure of UG have manifold implications for learning. The claim that constraints are universal entails that the learner could in principle use a given set of constraints to evaluate structural descriptions. The claim that grammatical structures are optimal, and grammars are total rankings of violable constraints, entails that with every piece of explicit positive evidence comes a mass of implicit negative evidence, and that constraints can be ranked so that those violated by explicit positive data are dominated by those violated by implicit negative data. The claim that grammars are evaluators of structural descriptions turns out to provide a uniform basis for computing the hidden structure in an expression when only its overt part is available, constructing a grammatical expression of a given interpretation, and deducing new underlying forms for insertion into the lexicon: these are merely three different directions of accessing the evaluative structure that is the grammar (Tesar and Smolensky 1996, Sec. 9). The claim of Richness of the Base connects the OT basis for adult typologies with fundamental hypotheses underlying acquisition research.

All these implications follow not from a particular OT theory of stress, or of phonology, but from the fundamental structure that OT claims to be inherent in all of grammar. Our learning algorithms derive from this general grammatical structure alone, and so apply to the learning of any OT grammar. At the same time, our algorithms are not generic search procedures, uninformed by grammatical theory. The special, characteristically linguistic structure imposed by OT on UG is sufficiently strong to allow the proof of learnability theorems stating that large spaces of possible

Box 2

grammars can be efficiently navigated to home in on a correct grammar.

4 Frequently Asked "Questions": Explanation in Optimality Theory

This section reviews several points raised in the chapter, recruiting them to address issues frequently raised by linguists. Many concern the nature of linguistic explanation under OT; others address wider cognitive issues such as the psychological reality of OT optimization. The nature of explanation in ICS more broadly is the primary topic of Chapter 23.

OT's mode of explanation departs significantly from strategies used previously in generative grammar. This creates exciting new possibilities for theoretical linguistics and, as we have been arguing, for the cognitive science of language more broadly. With OT's novel style of explanation comes a host of potential misconceptions, however, to which we now turn. In this section, we address 13 basic "questions" — most stated as challenges; these are frequently recited by those attempting to understand and evaluate the explanatory value of OT.

(59) **"OT says that the grammatical forms are those that optimally meet output constraints, so every word should surface as *ba* [*sic*]."**

This elementary misunderstanding was clearly addressed above. From its inception (Prince and Smolensky 1991a, b), OT has posited faithfulness constraints which demand that outputs be identical to inputs (Section 1.4). The diversity of outputs follows from the great diversity of possible inputs, which is universal. It is true that when all faithfulness constraints are ranked below all markedness constraints—forming the hierarchy denoted $\mathcal{H}_0$—only unmarked outputs may surface. This is not a failure of the theory, however. On the contrary, the hierarchy $\mathcal{H}_0$ is central in OT's theory of acquisition, as mentioned toward the end of Section 3.

(60) **"OT is an inadequate theory because syntax/phonology is derivational, and OT assumes it isn't."**

From the outset, OT has been formulated in both derivational and nonderivational or 'parallel' forms. Both variants are coherent expressions of the theory because the fundamental principle of OT is that representation$_n$ is the optimal representation in the candidate set generated by representation$_{n-1}$, where 'optimal' means 'best satisfies a ranked set of violable constraints'. The question of the structure of the set {representation$_n$, $n = 1, \ldots, ?$} is not directly related to optimality, and OT per se makes no assumptions about it. One possibility is that the representations involved constitute a derivation; this was formulated as **Harmonic Serialism** at the beginning of Prince and Smolensky 1993/2004 and illustrated with syllabification: "Serial Harmonic Syllabification (informal): Form the optimal syllable in the domain. Iterate until nothing more can be done" (Prince and Smolensky 1993/2004, (9)). (A detailed account of Berber syllabification employing Harmonic Serialism is provided in Prince and Smolensky

1993/2004: Sec. 5.2.3.3, Fn. 49. See also McCarthy 1999a.) Now it is true that "the great majority of the analyses presented in [OT] … use the parallel method of evaluation. … 'Harmonic Serialism' is worthy of exploration as well, and many hybrid theories can and should be imagined …" (Prince and Smolensky 1993/2004, Sec. 2.2); "it is important to keep in mind that the serial/parallel distinction pertains to *Gen* and not to the issue of harmonic evaluation per se. It is an empirical question of no little interest how *Gen* is to be construed, and one to which the answer will become clear only as the characteristics of harmonic evaluation emerge in the context of detailed, full-scale, depth-plumbing, scholarly, and responsible analyses" (Prince and Smolensky 1993/2004, Sec. 5.2.3.3).

It is true that parallel analyses in OT syntax and phonology have proved to have great explanatory value, and have strongly dominated OT research to date (indeed, the parallel conception has been implicitly adopted in the presentation here). But the power of parallel constraint evaluation is a *result* of OT research, not a stipulated assumption of the theory. And the parallel/serial issue remains a topic of some debate within both OT phonology (Clements 2000; McCarthy 2002b, 138–78) and OT syntax (e.g., Müller 1997).

(61) **"Opacity effects in phonology (like Hebrew spirantization) are not naturally accounted for in (parallel) OT and are not treated in the OT literature."**

Opacity effects, especially those in which a crucial intermediate stage of derivation is posited in rule-based derivational accounts, indeed pose a challenge to the parallel variant of OT (45d). Considerable research in OT has been directed to this challenge, and many broad classes of opacity effects have lent themselves to natural analyses within parallel OT, notably via the independently motivated notion of Output-Output Faithfulness (39c), which requires the expression of a morpheme in different words to be identical (e.g., Burzio 1994; Benua 1995). Another class of opacity effects has been analyzed with the independently motivated notion of local conjunction of constraints (Łubowicz 2002; (43) above). Other proposals have been explicitly formulated to address residual opacity cases, notably **Sympathy Theory** (McCarthy 1999b) and **Turbidity Theory** (Goldrick 2000). Sympathy Theory is an extension of faithfulness theory positing correspondence and hence faithfulness between the output of f_{prod} and a key suboptimal candidate. Turbidity Theory sees certain opacity effects as manifestations of representational divergence between the relations in the phonological structure determining pronunciation and those encoding the projection of abstract structure by elements of the input. In such turbid representations, unpronounced material is visible to constraints and can therefore affect pronounced material through constraint interaction, as has long been assumed in syntactic theory.

(62) **"Since *Gen* typically generates an infinite number of candidates, OT is psychologically impossible."**

It is the job of **competence theories** in linguistics to provide the most unified, perspicuous, and insightful accounts of UG. Such theories must not be confused with

performance theories in psycholinguistics, whose job is to describe the cognitive processes by which linguistic knowledge is deployed (46). It is an elementary fact of computer science that the most insightful characterization of a mathematical function—competence theory—can almost never be directly construed as an efficient algorithm—performance theory; this is especially true in the theory of optimization. (For extensive discussion of this point of view, see Chapter 23.)

Now the most insightful characterization of UG in OT employs a rich, infinite, universal base of possible interpretations and an infinite, universal set of possible expressions. Optimality can be *understood*—and results can be rigorously *proven*—in terms of constraints evaluating the entire set of candidates.[44] Optimality cannot be *computed* by an efficient algorithm that way. But since the early days of OT (Ellison 1994; Tesar 1994, 1995a, b) it has been known that efficient OT computation is possible, by provably correct algorithms that, for any particular input, explore only a finite part of the infinite candidate space, a part guaranteed to contain the optimal output (Section 2). The psychological relevance of such algorithms is unclear, but the computational relevance is unequivocal: infinite candidate spaces in OT are no obstacle to efficient optimization.

Finally, the optimization mode of computation of OT is inherited, according to ICS, from optimization at subsymbolic, connectionist levels. A connectionist network computes an optimal representation by navigating through a space of subsymbolic representations to ultimately construct the activation pattern that realizes an optimal symbolic structure. In no sense do such algorithms "generate alternative structures, evaluate them, and then pick the best." In general, the only symbolic structure ever realized by such an algorithm is the optimal one; at prior stages of computation, the algorithm constructs activation patterns that have no symbolic interpretation. (See the connectionist syllabification network of Chapter 20 for a concrete illustration.)

(63) **"OT is unexplanatory because you can make up any constraint you want; in OT, you just give up on seeking explanatory factors."**

It is a simple observation, but one frequently unappreciated in critiques of OT, that it is the job of *substantive theories* in linguistics to provide a restricted vocabulary over which constraints/rules/principles are to be stated. The OT *formal framework* is neutral on this issue; any inadequate restrictiveness of constraints/rules/principles is a failure of substantive theories, not of the formal framework. A theorist who believes that LFG/GB/minimalism provides the right limited vocabulary can employ the OT framework to develop accounts in which structural descriptions and constraints are formulated within that restricted vocabulary (for a variety of syntactic examples, see Legendre, Vikner, and Grimshaw 2001). This point was emphasized at the beginning of the chapter.

[44] In the large-scale empirical analysis presented in Prince and Smolensky 1993/2004, Chap. 7, deploying over 10 constraints and an infinite candidate set, over a half-dozen generalization patterns are rigorously proved to be consequences of the analysis.

Furthermore, stringent formal and empirical metaconstraints restrict the formulation of OT constraints. Formally, there is a strong pressure requiring constraints to be very simple, since linguistic explanation is to turn on the complexities arising through constraint *interaction*, not on complexities or subtleties within single constraints. Prince's 'endogenous constraints' (Section 1.8) restrict OT constraints in other important ways. The extremely challenging empirical requirements on the content of OT constraints is discussed under (65).

(64) **"Any framework that leads to the morass of constraints found in OT analyses in phonology can't possibly be explanatorily adequate."**

It is true that, compared with, say, the half-dozen constraints making up the core of GB, the multitude of constraints in OT phonology is overwhelming. But such a comparison makes little sense. If it's about anything at all, it's about the differences between generative phonology and generative syntax – it has nothing to say about OT. The only potentially relevant standard of comparison to OT phonology is *pre*-OT phonology. Which is more explanatory, the pre-OT panoply of rewrite rules, or the OT morass of constraints? One reason many phonologists have selected constraints over rewrite rules is that one constraint typically does the work of many rules. This fundamental insight was already formulated by Kisseberth (1970): multiple rules (within and especially across languages) typically 'conspire' to produce a common result in the output. *Output constraints are universal; rules are not* – see (45a). In addition, the majority of constraints in OT phonology fall within the small number of rather well-defined general classes discussed in Section 1.8.

(65) **"Stipulating a constraint ranking is as unexplanatory as stipulating an extrinsic rule ordering."**

In extrinsic rule-ordering "theory," there are virtually no restrictions on what rules can be proposed and no restrictions on rule ordering. By contrast, in OT, no constraint can be legitimately proposed without arguments for its universality. And a constraint ranking cannot be arbitrarily exploited either. The fundamental OT principle of factorial typology (35b) entails that the ranking $\mathbb{C}_1 \gg \mathbb{C}_2$ can only be exploited in the analysis of language $\mathcal{L}_1$ if the ranking $\mathbb{C}_2 \gg \mathbb{C}_1$ can be demonstrated in some other language $\mathcal{L}_2$ (or if it can be argued that $\mathbb{C}_1 \gg \mathbb{C}_2$ is a universal markedness scale, holding in every language). This is an extremely limiting explanatory restriction, a very heavy explanatory burden—and a vital part of the actual practice of OT. Examples too numerous to list may be found in the OT literature in both phonology and syntax.

This important conclusion bears repeating. *In OT, an account of* ***one*** *language is actually an account of* ***all*** *languages*: to propose a constraint ranking for a language is to claim that all rerankings of those constraints yield all and only the possible human languages (with respect to the grammar module under study, of course). This is the property dubbed 'inherent typology' in (2a). To compare this degree of analytic restrictiveness to extrinsic rule-ordering "theory" is ludicrous.

Box 2

(66) **"OT analyses are entirely circular: the only justification for a proposed ranking is exactly the data that the ranking is supposed to explain."**

This misses just the same point as (65). The true prediction of an OT analysis is typically not the data of a language: it is a universal typology. That a ranking of a proposed set of constraints generates the data of a language is merely a single observation on the road to showing how the patterns arising from all possible rankings of those constraints account for all and only the variation actually observed crosslinguistically.

But in fact even within a single language, there is explanatory power in a hierarchy that can, with a modest set of simple constraints and by a single ranking, consistently account for a relatively complex pattern of data. A set of constraints can be brought into conflict in a large number of ways, and if a single ranking correctly predicts the results of many such interactions, it has successfully explained a complex pattern as the consequence of a relatively small set of simple principles that generate complexity via the single, strongly restricted mechanism of interaction through strict domination.

(67) **"Reranking is a totally unconstrained theory of crosslinguistic variation, relative to the Principles-and-Parameters framework."**

OT provides a relatively strong characterization of crosslinguistic variation: the subordination spectrum (45f). Contrast this with a core characterization of the Principles-and-Parameters framework in which parameters turn a principle 'on' or 'off': this theory asserts that principles of grammar hold in all languages—except in those where they don't. And a theory that crosslinguistic variation arises from differences in the "lexical items" available for generating inputs to the grammar (e.g., the Minimalist Program's 'numeration') is only as restrictive as its formal definition of what constitutes a possible "lexical item" (e.g., exactly what abstract features are made available by UG?).

One critical measure of the strength of a theory's delimitation of crosslinguistic variation is the extent to which it enables efficient learning algorithms. Since Tesar and Smolensky 1993, it has been known that the limitations imposed by factorial typology enable efficient, provably correct learning algorithms when the learner is presented with full structural descriptions; optimization techniques have since been developed enabling the learner to work directly from overt data alone (Tesar and Smolensky 1996; Tesar 1997 et seq.). It is crucial that these learning procedures exploit *only the general characterization of crosslinguistic variation* provided by OT: they can be applied to any OT grammar, in phonology or syntax, regardless of the representations and constraints employed by a particular grammar. A *particular* Principles-and-Parameters theory (postulating specific substantive principles) may provide an explanatory account of a particular grammatical module. But as a *general* theory of possible modes of crosslinguistic variation, the 'Theory of Principles and Parameters' is really no theory at all. Its failure to restrict the space of possible UGs is evidenced by the lack of grammar-learning algorithms that exploit such general structure (Tesar and Smolensky 2000). This stands in stark contrast to the restrictiveness of OT.

(68) **"Reranking is essentially the same as parameters that turn on/off any constraint: burying the constraint at the bottom of the hierarchy turns it off, and putting it at the top of the hierarchy makes it inviolable."**

It is a crucial property of OT—evident in virtually every OT analysis in the literature—that a constraint that is undominated and unviolated in language $\mathcal{L}_1$ is dominated in another language $\mathcal{L}_2$, where it is violated, *but still active, emerging in environments in which no dominant constraint contravenes.* Constraints that are unviolated in one language are still crucial in another, even though violated there. The lowest-ranked constraint in Italian-like $\mathcal{L}'_2$ of GSL (33), SUBJ, is highly ranked and evident in English (31), yet roundly violated in Italian. But even in Italian, this lowest-ranked constraint is not 'turned off' at all. It forces clauses to have a subject, whenever the would-be subject does not bear topic or focus features; then higher-ranked DROPTOP and ALFOC are vacuously satisfied, and do not contravene lowly SUBJ, which imposes itself upon the optimal expression.[45]

Even the top-ranked constraint will be violated if there are no candidate outputs that satisfy it, and as we have just shown, even the lowest-ranked constraint will control the grammatical expression when doing so does not violate any higher-ranked constraints. OT's theory of crosslinguistic variation is not merely substantially *different* from turning constraints 'on' and 'off'—it is in fact much more *restricted*, as discussed under (67). A constraint cannot hold in one language and simply disappear in another; it can only be subordinated to other, conflicting, universal constraints. In OT, given the universal well-formedness principles, there is *no* further freedom in how languages may vary.

(69) **"The lexicon is the best locus for crosslinguistic variation because it has to be learned anyway."**

Clearly, no one would take seriously the proposal that the grasping system is the best locus for crosslinguistic variation because children need to learn to grasp anyway. A learning problem does not get solved, or even get easier, when it is moved under the heading of some other learning problem. In the case of the lexicon, what "has to be learned anyway" is the *arbitrary phonological shape* of morphemes. It hardly follows that learning language-particular grammatical information is suddenly no additional learning burden, or merely more of the same, when put under the heading 'lexicon'.

[45] Grimshaw and Samek-Lodovici (1998, 197) provide the following contrast: *questa mattina,* ***Gianni***$_i$ *ha visitato la mostra; più tardi,* e_i/??***lui***$_i$ *ha visitato l'università* 'this morning, John$_i$ visited the exhibition; later on, he$_i$ visited the university' versus *questa mattina, la mostra è stata visitat da* ***Gianni***$_i$*; più tardi,* *e_i/***lui***$_i$ *ha visitato l'università* 'this morning, the exhibition was visited by John$_i$; later on, he$_i$ visited the university'. In the first case, 'he$_i$' refers to the topic (the subject of the previous sentence: *Gianni*$_i$). Here, the null subject e_i is required; an overt pronoun *lui* is much less acceptable ('??'). DROPTOP renders lower-ranked SUBJ inactive. But in the second case, 'he$_i$' refers not to the topic (the subject *la mostra* 'the exhibition') but to a less salient entity, *Gianni*$_i$, the object of the preposition *da* 'by'. Now that DROPTOP does not apply to 'he$_i$', lower-ranked SUBJ emerges decisively, requiring the overt pronoun *lui*$_i$ and forbidding the null pronoun e_i.

Suppose, for instance, that a child must learn whether *wh*-elements in her language bear a strong or a weak feature.[46] Now, is learning this just like learning that the lexical entry for *DOG* is /dɔg/? As pointed out in Legendre, Smolensky, and Wilson 1998 (see Section 16:5.3 of this book), this learning problem can be formalized within an OT perspective as learning the relative ranking of two constraints: (i) NOTRACE (or STAY (Grimshaw and Samek-Lodovici 1995), analogous to Procrastinate), and (ii) CHECK([*wh*]), which asserts that specifier-head agreement with an overt element is preferred to specifier-head agreement with a silent trace, which in turn is preferred to no agreement at all. To say [*wh*] is a 'strong' feature is literally to say that the constraint CHECK([*wh*]) is stronger (higher ranked) than the economy-of-movement constraint NOTRACE. This problem is utterly unlike learning /dɔg/, but completely parallel to all other grammar-learning problems in OT: learning language-particular constraint ranking.

As discussed in Section 1.6, in OT, the inventories found in the lexicon of a lan-

[46] That is, 'Learn whether *wh*-elements are fronted', in the terminology of Chomsky's theory of the 1990s, the Minimalist Program. As discussed at length in Chapter 16, according to Chomskyan syntax, some languages like English require a *wh*-phrase like *what* to move to the front of a sentence, where it is pronounced (*what$_i$ has John said t$_i$?*); other languages like Chinese also require a *wh*-phrase to move, but this occurs "after" pronunciation is determined: *what* is pronounced in its base position (*has John said what?*) and "then" it moves to the front for semantic interpretation at the level of Logical Form (LF; Huang 1982). On this view, it is universally true that *wh*-elements are fronted at LF: in some languages, like English, this fronting occurs "early" enough to affect pronunciation; in other languages, like Chinese, fronting occurs too "late," affecting LF but not pronunciation.

In the terminology of the Minimalist Program, in English, the feature [*wh*] on *what* entails that *what* must move before pronunciation is determined: [*wh*] is a **strong feature**. The principle called **Procrastinate** requires movement to be "delayed" as long as possible, so that unless [*wh*] is strong—and in Chinese it is *weak*—Procrastinate will postpone movement until after pronunciation. Thus, whether a language pronounces *wh*-phrases at the front of a question or not is determined by the "parameter" declaring whether a language moves [*wh*] early or late, before or after pronunciation is determined—that is, whether [*wh*] is marked *strong* or *weak* in the functional lexicon. (Equivalently, [*wh*] could be marked 'Move me' or 'Don't move me'.)

The minimalist mechanism for movement requires that the [*wh*] of *what* be 'checked' with another [*wh*], the two features being structurally related as specifier and head of the same XP; this is like requiring **specifier-head agreement** in which a feature like [plural] on the subject in SpecVP must agree with a matching feature on the verb in V (see Box 1). The [*wh*] of *what* must be checked by the [*wh*] in C that marks a sentence as an information question; this requires *what* to move to SpecCP—that is, fronting. Now in the OT treatment of *wh*-questions in Legendre, Smolensky, and Wilson 1998, English and Chinese have identical chains linking an overtly pronounced *wh*-phrase and a coindexed silent element. The difference is that in English the pronounced element *what* is at the top of the chain—at the front of the sentence, in SpecCP—while in Chinese it is at the bottom. At the bottom of the English chain is a silent trace; at the top of the Chinese chain is a silent *wh*-operator Q. Thus, in English the [*wh*] in C^0 is checked in SpecCP by an overt *wh*-phrase *what*, while in Chinese it is checked by an empty operator Q. The OT constraint CHECK([*wh*]), as defined below in the text, is best satisfied in the English arrangement (checking with an overt element); it is next-best satisfied in the Chinese configuration, and thoroughly violated if there is no *wh*-chain at all. The work of Procrastinate can be done by NOTRACE, which favors the Chinese configuration in which the overt element *what* (rather than a silent trace) is in its base position at the bottom of the chain. Thus, whether the *wh*-phrase is pronounced at the front of the sentence is determined by the relative ranking of CHECK([*wh*]) and NOTRACE: the 'strong [*wh*]' behavior of English arises when the requirement to CHECK([*wh*]) dominates. (This CHECK([*wh*]) analysis is not the one proposed in Legendre, Smolensky, and Wilson 1998; it is merely an OT formalization of the minimalist conception for comparison. Minimalist-style OT syntax is advocated in Heck and Müller 2000; Müller 2002, 2003.)

guage cannot be stipulated: they must be derived from the same constraint ranking that constitutes the grammar. The grammar and lexicon are not independent—and it is the grammar that is primary. The fundamental principle of OT—Richness of the Base—asserts that there are no systematic language-particular regularities in the base of inputs to the grammar, including the lexicon; this base is universal. So suppose a language's inventory lacks a given element γ—say, an expletive subject like English *it,* or a round front vowel. In OT, this must be because a constraint ℂ violated by γ is relatively highly ranked, filtering it out of all optimal expressions.

Now grammars *must have* constraints like ℂ that govern the distribution of resumptive pronouns, expletives, null elements, the features [front], [round], etc. Given these constraints as ranked in the OT grammar of a particular language, it is *determinate* whether optimal structures in the language will or will not exist with null subjects, resumptive pronouns, [front, round] vowels, etc. If such elements exist in optimal structures, *ipso facto they are part of the language's inventory.* There is simply no *room* for the language's 'lexicon' or whatever to decide whether the language has a resumptive pronoun, expletive subject, etc.[47] The matter has already been decided by the grammar, via machinery that is independently required for the functioning of the grammar. (All that remains for the lexicon to determine is the arbitrary phonological shape of the expletive, etc.) *All* crosslinguistic variation is determined by the one degree of freedom available to grammars: ranking.

(70) **"It cannot be that all constraints are universal, given the many idiosyncratic language-specific phonological alternations, as well as constraints specific to individual morphemes, which are obviously language particular."**

Like any other scientific hypothesis, the OT principle of constraint universality must be understood within the context of the scientific enterprise. In effect, this principle claims that where there *are* universal grammatical patterns to be explained, these are best explained by reranking of universal constraints. Presumably, grammars contain a certain irreducible amount of unprincipled variation; part of this variation is treatable within OT via language-particular constraints. But such constraints count against OT's theory of crossinguistic variation only to the extent that these ad hoc constraints are failing to explain systematic crosslinguistic variation that can be explained by some alternative to OT's theory of variation. Formally describing an individual grammar via a ranking that includes language-particular constraints is not an explanatory failure of OT if the effect of the ad hoc constraints cannot be satisfactorily analyzed, within OT or any other framework, as part of a systematic pattern of crosslinguistic variation. One might say that the OT principle 'Constraints are universal' is a violable metaconstraint on the explanatory value of substantive linguistic

[47] As observed in Chapter 4, under the ranking yielding English-like $\mathcal{L}'_1$ (31), with SUBJ ≫ FULLINT, expletive or dummy *it* is optimal in subject position in *it rains*; with the reverse ranking of Italian-like $\mathcal{L}'_2$ (32), the optimal output is simply *rains*: a null subject, rather than an expletive subject, appears. In OT, the contrast in whether the functional lexicon contains an expletive subject or a null subject *follows from the ranking*; it is not an independent choice of the lexicon. Regarding resumptive pronouns, see Chapter 16.

theories, the most explanatory theory of some domain being the one that best satisfies the universality constraint.[48] OT's theory of crosslinguistic variation is to be judged less explanatory than a competitor only if the competitor better satisfies the metaconstraint demanding that the grammars of the world be all and only those that can be assembled from a given stock of universal elements.

(71) **"Ranked violable constraints can always be replaced by (unranked) inviolable constraints."**

This may be true in principle. A hierarchy such as A $\gg$ B $\gg$ C can be **compiled** into a set of inviolable constraints such as "A must be satisfied, except when no candidate satisfies it," and "B must be satisfied, except when no candidate satisfies it, or except when violating A is necessary to satisfy B," and "C must be satisfied, except when no candidate satisfies it, or except when violating A or B is necessary to satisfy C." (Note that when constraints can be multiply violated—nearly always the case—or when constraint violations fall on a nonbinary scale, such compiled constraints become much more complex.)

Compilation of this sort may in fact be useful for performance theory—say, for efficient computing with a particular grammar, either in man or in machine. However, it has severe drawbacks with respect to competence theory. (i) Compilation does not preserve universality: if the violable constraints are universal, the inviolable ones will not be, since the ranking has been compiled into the inviolable constraints, and the ranking is exactly what varies across languages. (ii) Compilation preserves neither perspicuity nor modularity. If the violable constraints are simple, and each refers to a separate dimension of well-formedness, this will *not* be true of the compiled

[48] In a still more speculative vein: OT more generally may have a contribution to make to the philosophy of science by conceptualizing how to compare competing theories on the basis of 'universal' desiderata—**metaconstraints**. Perhaps some scientific revolutions can be understood as the result of a new theory entering a candidate set of theories, making it possible for the first time to satisfy a metaconstraint that, although always high ranked, had never before been active because no candidate theory satisfied it. And perhaps the cultural differences across scientific communities can be profitably modeled as constraint reranking, since the desiderata clearly conflict and their conflict does not seem to be resolved in the same way across communities. The model-centered versus principle-centered distinction of Chapter 3 might be characterizable in terms of different rankings of metaconstraints such as 'A theory must be specified so as to allow computer implementation', 'A theory must provide an empirically adequate account of data *X*', 'A theory must be a set of simple, general, principled commitments from which empirical predictions follow logically', and so on. It may be that scientists share all these desiderata, but by ranking them differently, distinct scientific cultures may end up selecting different theories as optimal. Of particular note in cognitive science is that there are multiple metaconstraints requiring 'empirical adequacy with respect to data *X*': *X* may be crosslinguistic patterns of linguistic inventories, or reaction times during online language processing, or the computational complexity of aspects of human language. Everyone would prefer a theory that satisfies all these constraints, but in the current candidate set, none does, so these constraints conflict. Differences in ranking among such constraints may play a major role in distinguishing the cultures of theoretical linguistics, psycholinguistics, and computational linguistics. It is perhaps only within each community—where a ranking has been fixed—that competition among theories of the same basic type must be adjudicated by more fine-grained constraints (including more fine-grained values of *X*), constraints evaluating the extent to which a given theory provides an 'empirically adequate account of data *X*'. Reranking of the more fine-grained constraints may be what distinguishes the 'dialects' of a single culture: subcommunities favoring a particular theory.

constraints: the consequences of constraints on dimensions X, Y, and Z have been compiled into constraints on dimension W. (iii) Without ranking, complexity in the resulting inviolable constraints is purely stipulative. Such cross-dimensional interaction is *restricted* and *explained* in OT by ranking; it must be *stipulated* inside the complex compiled constraints. Why the *particular* 'except when ...' types of codicils in the inviolable constraints, rather than any other form of comparable complexity?

5 CONCLUSION

Optimality Theory offers a grammar formalism that enables us to embark on Jakobson's program for a Grand Unified Theory of language based upon the unifying concept of markedness. Several new grammatical principles make this possible: FAITHFULNESS, which combines with MARKEDNESS to yield Harmony; universal violable constraints combining markedness dimensions via language-specific rankings; and explicit competition for optimality.

OT research has, from its earliest days, explicitly pursued answers to all four of Chomsky's million-dollar questions for the cognitive science of language (1). OT research concerning the structure, use, acquisition, and neural realization of knowledge of language has pursued an aggressively grammar-centered agenda, trying, in the spirit of Jakobson, to extract as much insight and explanation as possible from the theory of grammar proper for problems outside the scope of the theory of grammar proper, as this scope has come to be narrowly defined in the last half-century. Four goals for such a grammar-centered research program—each addressing one of Chomsky's questions—were formulated in (2). They are repeated in (72), each with a synoptic reprise of the relevant themes of this chapter.

(72) Goals for a strongly grammar-centered cognitive science of language

a. *Inherent typology.* A grammatical formalism $\mathcal{G}$ in which language-particular grammatical analysis consists in identifying the interaction of universal principles that formally determine a typology of possible human grammars; inherent in any analysis of some phenomenon Φ in some language $\mathcal{L}$ is a theory of Φ in all the world's languages.

✦ A language-particular analysis of Φ in OT must specify a set of structural descriptions, well-formedness constraints over these structures, and a ranking of these constraints. The inescapable claim made by such an analysis is that these structural descriptions and constraints are the same in all other languages, that the typological space of all possible human Φ-grammars is exactly that generated by all rankings of those constraints. (Section 1)

b. *General processing theory.* A general theory $\mathcal{P}$ for computing the generation and interpretation functions determined by any $\mathcal{G}$-grammar; inserting a particular grammar G into $\mathcal{P}$ directly yields algorithms for processing with G.

- ✦ There are a number of explicit processing algorithms for computing optimal forms that are applicable to any OT grammar in a large space of grammars. The limits of this space vary across algorithms, but mostly these limits are inherently computational, not linguistic. The formal structure that all OT grammars share is the essential contribution of linguistic theory; a number of general algorithms can then be applied to this structure, their limits being set not by the generality of the linguistics but by the generality of the computational methods. (Section 2)

c. *General learning theory.* A general theory $\mathcal{L}$ for acquiring an individual grammar within any typology $\mathcal{T}$ of $\mathcal{G}$-grammars; inserting into $\mathcal{L}$ the particular set of universal principles determining $\mathcal{T}$ directly yields learning algorithms for finding any target grammar G in $\mathcal{T}$ on the basis of positive data from the language determined by G.

- ✦ OT learning algorithms, like the processing algorithms of (72b), operate on the basis of the shared structure of all OT grammars, and learn from positive data. Formal analyses of these algorithms yield significant learnability results; the limitations of the algorithms derive from the limitations of overt information explicitly available to the learner. Experimental results are promising in learning settings for which there are not yet formal results. (Section 3)

d. *General theory of neural (genetic) realization.* A general theory $\mathcal{N}$ for realizing the universal principles of a $\mathcal{G}$-typology $\mathcal{T}$ in a neural network; inserting the particular principles of $\mathcal{T}$ into $\mathcal{N}$ directly yields a network $\mathcal{N}$ that can be configured to realize any grammar G in $\mathcal{T}$ (i.e., compute the functions determined by G) and can learn this configuration on the basis of positive data from the language determined by G. Also, a general theory $\mathcal{M}$ for encoding the universal principles of any $\mathcal{G}$-typology $\mathcal{T}$ in a genome $\mathcal{M}$ that governs the growth and operation of the neural networks of $\mathcal{N}$.

- ✦ (Not addressed in this chapter; the relevant discussion is distributed over many other chapters of the book.) The optimization character central to all OT grammars can be formally analyzed as the high-level consequence of low-level representational and dynamic properties of model neural networks; however, the same cannot be said of strict domination at this point. The current limitations are many, including the complexity of the realizable constraints and the avoidance of network states that are not interpretable symbolically. Learning results are limited to networks with local representations, and the first results concerning genomic encoding are limited to a particular substantive theory in the OT framework, CVT. But these methods enable construction of a tiny demonstration model of a neurally realized, genomically encoded

Chomsky-style Language Acquisition Device for a significant typological space of OT grammars (Chapter 21).

Since the early days of generative linguistics (e.g., Chomsky 1965), it has been asserted that linguistic theory can contribute to understanding the human language faculty by characterizing precisely the system of representations and rules/constraints that constitutes a possible human language—not merely by describing individual languages, but by formally characterizing the boundary separating possible from impossible human languages, and by explaining how implicit knowledge of this boundary enables the child to learn a complex language despite the inadequacies of linguistic learning data. Yet despite much progress, this objective has largely remained out of reach. What is relevant here is not the observation that we are uncertain about the exact form of the representations and rules/constraints—it would indeed be unreasonable to expect otherwise at this early stage of linguistic research. What is relevant is that we have lacked a highly general, but richly articulated, typological formalism that strongly characterizes the *kind* of structure that distinguishes the space of possible human languages—a general formalism within which it is possible to formally state particular alternative substantive hypotheses concerning the precise representations and rules/constraints, and to formally deduce their consequences, so these predictions may be put to the empirical test.

But OT offers significant progress toward developing such a typological formalism. OT is not a theory of syntax or phonology: it is not defined by substantive principles (63)–(64). OT is a general theory of crosslinguistic variation, a hypothesis proposing a formal structure pervading all modules of UG. OT does not merely *offer* a fully general formalism for stating precise hypotheses about universal typology: it *imposes* upon its user the *obligation* to formulate such hypotheses—for there is simply no other way to do an OT analysis (65). This is the force of the notion of inherent typology (72a).

OT's formal characterization of the structure of the space of possible human grammars, applying to all linguistic domains, is not merely a hoped-for source of explanation for how grammar learning is possible. There are already formal proofs that provide a strong start to demonstrating the benefit for learning provided by knowledge of this structure (67)—meaningful progress toward a general learning theory (72c).

OT's theory of crosslinguistic variation is not a notational variant of the Principles-and-Parameters framework (68); it is not inherently less perspicuous than theories that locate variation in the lexicon (69); and it is not explanatorily equivalent to inviolable constraints (71).

OT is not trivially inadequate because it predicts only a single grammatical form (59), inherently inadequate because it cannot employ serial derivation (60), or inherently incapable of explaining putatively derivational effects such as phonological opacity (61). It is not trivially psychologically implausible because of optimization over an infinite candidate set (62); indeed, algorithms for computing with OT gram-

Box 2

mars have existed since virtually the inception of the theory, and their formal properties of efficiency and correctness are already well on the way to being rigorously understood — a solid start toward a general processing theory (72b).

Of course, there remain important open questions about the OT framework itself, and enormous challenges for developing formally precise, empirically adequate substantive OT theories of crosslinguistic typology in phonology, syntax, and semantics — and integrating such theories into computationally and empirically adequate formal theories of grammar learning and processing. The claim is certainly not that OT has successfully completed this research program. The claim is that OT has shown considerable initial promise for advancing it.[49]

[49] The material of Section 4 was presented in 1995 by the first author at the Royaumont Conference on Current Trends in Phonology and linguistics colloquia at the University of Maryland at College Park, the University of Southern California, and Stanford University. For helpful discussion, thanks to members of those audiences, and especially to Alan Prince, Bruce Hayes, and Paul Kiparsky. Haruka Fukazawa and Mafuyu Kitahara's thoughtful work on the Japanese translation is deeply appreciated.

References

ROA = Rutgers Optimality Archive, http://roa.rutgers.edu

Aarts, E. H. L., J. H. M. Korst, and P. J. Zwietering. 1996. Deterministic and randomized local search. In *Mathematical perspectives on neural networks*, eds. P. Smolensky, M. C. Mozer, and D. E. Rumelhart. Erlbaum.

Aissen, J. 1999. Markedness and subject choice in Optimality Theory. *Natural Language and Linguistic Theory* 17, 673–711.

Aissen, J. 2003. Differential object marking: Iconicity vs. economy. *Natural Language and Linguistic Theory* 21, 435–83.

Alderete, J., and B. B. Tesar. 2002. Learning covert phonological interaction: An analysis of the problem posed by the interaction of stress and epenthesis. Technical report RuCCS-TR-72, Rutgers Center for Cognitive Science, Rutgers University. ROA 543.

Anderson, J. R., and C. J. Lebiere. 1998. *The atomic components of thought*. Erlbaum.

Anderson, S. R. 1993. Wackernagel's revenge: Clitics, morphology and the syntax of second position. *Language* 69, 68–98.

Anderson, S. R. 1996. How to put your clitics in their place or why the best account of second-position phenomena may be something like the optimal one. *The Linguistic Review* 13, 165–91.

Anderson, S. R. 2000. Towards an optimal account of second position phenomena. In *Optimality Theory: Phonology, syntax, and acquisition*, eds. J. Dekkers, F. van der Leeuw, and J. van de Weijer. Oxford University Press.

Baker, C. L. 1979. Syntactic theory and the projection problem. *Linguistic Inquiry* 10, 533–81.

Barbosa, P., D. Fox, P. Hagstrom, M. McGinnis, and D. Pesetsky, eds. 1998. *Is the best good enough? Optimality and competition in syntax*. MIT Press and MIT Working Papers in Linguistics.

Battistella, E. L. 1990. *Markedness: The evaluative superstructure of language*. State University of New York Press.

Battistella, E. L. 1996. *The logic of markedness*. Oxford University Press.

Beckman, J. 1997. Positional faithfulness, positional neutralization, and Shona vowel harmony. *Phonology* 14, 1–46.

Beckman, J., L. Walsh Dickey, and S. Urbanczyk, eds. 1995. *University of Massachusetts occasional papers in linguistics 18: Papers in Optimality Theory*. Graduate Linguistic Student Association, University of Massachusetts at Amherst.

Belletti, A. 1990. *Generalized verb movement*. Rosenberg & Sellier.

Benua, L. 1995. Output-output faithfulness. In *University of Massachusetts occasional papers in linguistics 18: Papers in Optimality Theory*, eds. J. Beckman, L. Walsh Dickey, and S. Urbanczyk. Graduate Linguistic Student Association, University of Massachusetts at Amherst. ROA 60.

Benua, L. 1997. Phonological relations between words. Ph.D. diss., University of Massachusetts at Amherst. ROA 259. Published by Garland, 2000.

Berwick, R., S. Abney, and C. Tenny, eds. 1991. *Principle-based parsing: Computation and psycholinguistics*. Kluwer.

Black, A. 1993. Constraint-ranked derivation: Truncation and stem binarity in Southeastern Tepehuan. Ms., University of California at Santa Cruz.

Blutner, R. 2001. Some aspects of optimality in natural language interpretation. *Journal of Semantics* 17, 189–216.

Blutner, R., and H. Zeevat, eds. 2003. *Pragmatics in Optimality Theory*. Palgrave Macmillan.

Boersma, P. 1998. *Functional phonology: Formalizing the interactions between articulatory and perceptual drives*. Holland Academic Graphics.

Boersma, P., and B. Hayes. 2001. Empirical tests of the gradual learning algorithm. *Linguistic Inquiry* 32, 45–86. ROA 348.

Bresnan, J., ed. 1982. *The mental representation of grammatical relations.* MIT Press.

Bresnan, J. 1996. LFG in an OT setting: Modelling competition and economy. In *Proceedings of the First LFG Conference.*

Bresnan, J. 2000. Optimal syntax. In *Optimality Theory: Phonology, syntax and acquisition,* eds. J. Dekkers, F. van der Leeuw, and J. van de Weijer. Oxford University Press.

Bresnan, J. 2001. *Lexical-Functional Grammar.* Blackwell.

Buchwald, A., O. Schwartz, A. Seidl, and P. Smolensky. 2002. Recoverability Optimality Theory: Discourse anaphora in a bi-directional framework. In *Proceedings of the 6th Workshop on the Semantics and Pragmatics of Dialogue (EDILOG 2002).*

Burzio, L. 1994. *Principles of English stress.* Cambridge University Press.

Campbell, L. 1980. The psychological and sociological reality of Finnish vowel harmony. In *Issues in vowel harmony,* ed. R. M. Vago. Benjamins.

Chomsky, N. 1965. *Aspects of the theory of syntax.* MIT Press.

Chomsky, N. 1970. Remarks on nominalization. In *Readings in English transformational grammar,* eds. R. Jacobs and P. Rosenbaum. Ginn.

Chomsky, N. 1981. *Lectures on government and binding.* Foris.

Chomsky, N. 1986. *Barriers.* MIT Press.

Chomsky, N. 1988. *Language and problems of knowledge: The Managua lectures.* MIT Press.

Chomsky, N. 1995. *The Minimalist Program.* MIT Press.

Cinque, G. 1999. *Adverbs and functional heads: A cross-linguistic perspective.* Oxford University Press.

Clahsen, H., ed. 1999. *Generative perspectives on language acquisition: Empirical findings, theoretical considerations and crosslinguistic comparisons.* Benjamins.

Clements, G. N. 2000. In defense of serialism. *The Linguistic Review* 17, 181–98.

Clements, G. N., and S. J. Keyser. 1983. *CV phonology: A generative theory of the syllable.* MIT Press.

Coetzee, A., A. Carpenter, and P. de Lacy, eds. 2002. *University of Massachusetts occasional papers in linguistics 26: Papers in Optimality Theory II.* Graduate Linguistic Student Association, University of Massachusetts at Amherst.

Costa, J. 2001. Emergence of the unmarked word order. In *Optimality-theoretic syntax,* eds. G. Legendre, S. Vikner, and J. Grimshaw. MIT Press.

Crain, S., and D. Lillo-Martin. 1999. *An introduction to linguistic theory and language acquisition.* Blackwell.

Davidson, L. 2001. Hidden rankings in the final state of the English grammar. In *RuLing papers II,* eds. G. Horwood and S.-K. Kim. Department of Linguistics, Rutgers University.

Davidson, L., and G. Legendre. 2003. Defaults and competition in the acquisition of functional categories in Catalan and French. In *A Romance perspective on language knowledge and use: Selected papers from the 2001 Linguistic Symposium on Romance Languages (LSRL),* eds. R. Nuñez-Cedeño, L. López, and R. Cameron. Benjamins.

Dekkers, J., F. van der Leeuw, and J. van de Weijer, eds. 2000. *Optimality Theory: Phonology, syntax, and acquisition.* Oxford University Press.

Demuth, K. 1995. Markedness and the development of prosodic structure. In *Proceedings of the North East Linguistic Society* 25. ROA 50.

Dresher, B. E., and J. Kaye. 1990. A computational learning model for metrical phonology. *Cognition* 34, 137–95.

Eisner, J. 1997. Efficient generation in primitive Optimality Theory. In *Proceedings of the Annual Meeting of the Association for Computational Linguistics* 35. ROA 206.

Eisner, J. 2000. Easy and hard constraint ranking in Optimality Theory: Algorithms and complexity. In *Finite-state phonology: Proceedings of the Fifth Workshop of the ACL Special Interest Group in Computational Phonology (SIGPHON)*, eds. J. Eisner, L. Karttunen, and A. Thériault.

Ellison, T. M. 1994. Phonological derivation in Optimality Theory. In *Proceedings of the International Conference on Computational Linguistics 15*. ROA 75.

Féry, C., and R. van de Vijver, eds. 2003. *The syllable in Optimality Theory*. Cambridge University Press.

Flemming, E. 2001. Scalar and categorical phenomena in a unified model of phonetics and phonology. *Phonology* 18, 7–44.

Frank, R., and G. Satta. 1998. Optimality Theory and the generative complexity of constraint violability. *Computational Linguistics* 24, 307–15. ROA 228.

Frazier, L. 1978. On comprehending sentences: Syntactic parsing strategies. Indiana University Linguistics Club.

Garey, M. R., and D. S. Johnson. 1979. *Computers and intractability: A guide to the theory of NP-completeness*. W. H. Freeman.

Gazdar, G., E. Klein, G. Pullum, and I. Sag. 1985. *Generalized Phrase Structure Grammar*. Harvard University Press.

Gerdts, D. 1993. Mapping transitive voice in Halkomelem. In *Proceedings of the Berkeley Linguistics Society 19*.

Gibson, E., and K. Broihier. 1998. Optimality Theory and human sentence processing. In *Is the best good enough? Optimality and competition in syntax*, eds. P. Barbosa, D. Fox, P. Hagstrom, M. McGinnis, and D. Pesetsky. MIT Press and MIT Working Papers in Linguistics.

Gibson, E., and K. Wexler. 1994. Triggers. *Linguistic Inquiry* 25, 407–54.

Gnanadesikan, A. 1995. Markedness and faithfulness constraints in child phonology. Ms., University of Massachusetts at Amherst. ROA 67.

Goldrick, M. 2000. Turbid output representations and the unity of opacity. In *Proceedings of the North East Linguistic Society 30*.

Goldsmith, J. A. 1976. Autosegmental phonology. Ph.D. diss., MIT.

Goldsmith, J. A. 1993. Harmonic Phonology. In *The last phonological rule*, ed. J. A. Goldsmith. University of Chicago Press.

Goldwater, S., and M. Johnson. 2003. Learning OT constraint rankings using a maximum entropy model. In *Proceedings of the Stockholm Workshop on Variation within Optimality Theory*.

Greenberg, J. 1978a. Some generalizations concerning initial and final consonant clusters. In *Universals of human language*. Vol. 2, *Phonology*, ed. J. Greenberg. Stanford University Press.

Greenberg, J. 1978b. *Universals of human language*. Vol. 2, *Phonology*. Stanford University Press.

Grimshaw, J. 1991. Extended projection. Ms., Brandeis University.

Grimshaw, J. 1993. Minimal projection, heads, and optimality. Technical report RuCCS-TR-4, Rutgers Center for Cognitive Science, Rutgers University. ROA 68.

Grimshaw, J. 1997. Projection, heads, and optimality. *Linguistic Inquiry* 28, 373–422.

Grimshaw, J., and V. Samek-Lodovici. 1995. Optimal subjects. In *University of Massachusetts occasional papers in linguistics 18: Papers in Optimality Theory*, eds. J. Beckman, L. Walsh Dickey, and S. Urbanczyk. Graduate Linguistic Student Association, University of Massachusetts at Amherst.

Grimshaw, J., and V. Samek-Lodovici. 1998. Optimal subjects and subject universals. In *Is the best good enough? Optimality and competition in syntax*, eds. P. Barbosa, D. Fox, P. Hagstrom, M. McGinnis, and D. Pesetsky. MIT Press.

Grosz, B., A. Joshi, and S. Weinstein. 1995. Centering: A framework for modelling the local coherence of discourse. *Computational Linguistics* 21, 203–25.

Gussenhoven, C., and R. Kager, guest eds. 2001. Thematic issue on phonetics in phonology. *Phonology* 18, 1–197.

Hale, J., and G. Legendre. 2004. Minimal links, remnant movement, and (non-)derivational grammar. In *Minimality effects in syntax*, eds. A. Stepanov, G. Fanselow, and R. Vogel. Mouton de Gruyter.

Hale, M., and C. Reiss. 1997. Grammar optimization: The simultaneous acquisition of constraint ranking and a lexicon. Ms., Concordia University. ROA 231.

Hammond, M. 1999. *The phonology of English: A prosodic optimality-theoretic approach*. Oxford University Press.

Hayes, B. 1994. *Metrical stress theory: Principles and case studies*. University of Chicago Press.

Hayes, B. 1999. Phonetically driven phonology: The role of Optimality Theory and inductive grounding. In *Functionalism and formalism in linguistics*. Vol. 1, *General papers*, eds. M. Darnell, E. Moravcsik, M. Noonan, F. Newmeyer, and K. Wheatly. Benjamins.

Hayes, B. 2004. Phonological acquisition in Optimality Theory: The early stages. In *Constraints in phonological acquisition*, eds. R. Kager, J. Pater, and W. Zonneveld. Cambridge University Press. ROA 327.

Hayes, B., R. Kirchner, and D. Steriade, eds. 2004. *Phonetically based phonology*. Cambridge University Press.

Heck, F., and G. Müller. 2000. Successive cyclicity, long-distance superiority, and local optimization. In *Proceedings of the West Coast Conference on Formal Linguistics 19*.

Hendriks, P., and H. de Hoop. 2001. Optimality theoretic semantics. *Linguistics and Philosophy* 24, 1–32.

Hermans, B., and M. van Oostendorp, eds. 1999. *The derivational residue in phonological Optimality Theory*. Benjamins.

Hewitt, M., and M. J. Crowhurst. 1996. Conjunctive constraints and templates. In *Proceedings of the North East Linguistic Society 26*.

Holt, D. E., ed. 2003. *Optimality Theory and language change*. Kluwer.

Horwood, G. 2001. Anti-faithfulness and subtractive morphology. Ms., Rutgers University. ROA 466.

Huang, C.-T. J. 1982. Logical relations in Chinese and the theory of grammar. Ph.D. diss., MIT.

Hyams, N. 1986. *Language acquisition and the theory of parameters*. Reidel.

Itô, J., and R. A. Mester. 1995. The core-periphery structure of the lexicon and constraints on reranking. In *University of Massachusetts occasional papers in linguistics 18: Papers in Optimality Theory*, eds. J. Beckman, L. Walsh Dickey, and S. Urbanczyk. Graduate Linguistic Student Association, University of Massachusetts at Amherst.

Itô, J., and R. A. Mester. 1998. Markedness and word structure: OCP effects in Japanese. Ms., University of California at Santa Cruz, ROA 255.

Jackendoff, R. 1977. *X-bar syntax: A theory of phrase structure*. MIT Press.

Jackendoff, R. 2002. *Foundations of language: Brain, meaning, grammar, evolution*. Oxford University Press.

Jakobson, R. 1941/1968. *Child language, aphasia and phonological universals*. Mouton.

Jakobson, R. 1962. *Selected writings I: Phonological studies*. Mouton.

Kager, R., J. Pater, and W. Zonneveld, eds. 2004. *Constraints in phonological acquisition*. Cambridge University Press.

Karttunen, L. 1998. The proper treatment of optimality in computational phonology. In *Proceedings of the International Workshop on Finite-State Methods in Natural Language Processing*. ROA 258.

Kaye, J. 1989. *Phonology: A cognitive view*. Erlbaum.

Kayne, R. S. 1994. *The antisymmetry of syntax*. MIT Press.

Kenstowicz, M. 1993. *Generative phonology*. Blackwell.

Kenstowicz, M., and C. W. Kisseberth. 1977. *Topics in phonological theory*. Academic Press.

Kenstowicz, M., and C. W. Kisseberth. 1979. *Generative phonology*. Academic Press.

Kingston, J., and R. L. Diehl. 1995. Intermediate properties in the perception of distinctive feature values. In *Papers in laboratory phonology IV: Phonology and phonetic evidence*, eds. B. Connell and A. Arvaniti. Cambridge University Press.

Kiparsky, P. To appear. *Paradigms and opacity*. CSLI Publications.

Kisseberth, C. 1970. On the functional unity of phonological rules. *Linguistic Inquiry* 1, 291–306.

Kreps, D. M. 1988. *Notes on the theory of choice*. Westview.

Kurisu, K. 2002. The phonology of morpheme realization. Ph.D. diss., University of California at Santa Cruz. ROA 490.

Leben, W. 1973. Suprasegmental phonology. Ph.D. diss., MIT.

Legendre, G. 1998. Second position clitics in a V2 language: Conflict resolution in Macedonian. In *Proceedings of the 1997 Eastern States Conference on Linguistics*.

Legendre, G. 1999. Morphological and prosodic alignment at work: The case of South-Slavic clitics. In *Proceedings of the West Coast Conference on Formal Linguistics 17*.

Legendre, G. 2000a. For an OT conception of a parallel interface: Evidence from Basque V2. In *Proceedings of the North East Linguistic Society 30*.

Legendre, G. 2000b. Morphological and prosodic alignment of Bulgarian clitics. In *Optimality Theory: Phonology, syntax, and acquisition*, eds. J. Dekkers, F. van der Leeuw, and J. van de Weijer. Oxford University Press.

Legendre, G. 2000c. Optimal Romanian clitics: A cross-linguistic perspective. In *Comparative studies in Romanian syntax*, ed. V. Motapanyane. Elsevier.

Legendre, G. 2000d. Positioning Romanian verbal clitics at PF: An optimality-theoretic analysis. In *Clitics from different perspectives*, eds. B. Gerlach and J. Grijzenhout. Benjamins.

Legendre, G. 2001. Masked V2 effects and the linearization of functional features. In *Optimality-theoretic syntax*, eds. G. Legendre, S. Vikner, and J. Grimshaw. MIT Press.

Legendre, G., P. Hagstrom, J. Chen-Main, L. Tao, and P. Smolensky. 2004. Deriving output probabilities in child Mandarin from a dual-optimization grammar. *Lingua* 114, 1147–85.

Legendre, G., P. Hagstrom, L. Tao, J. Chen-Main, and L. Davidson. 2001. A preliminary look at the acquisition of aspect in Mandarin Chinese in OT. In *Proceedings of the 3rd International Conference on Cognitive Science*.

Legendre, G., P. Hagstrom, A. Vainikka, and M. Todorova. 2000a. Evidence for syntactic competition during acquisition of tense and agreement in child French. In *Proceedings of* the Chicago Linguistic Society 36.

Legendre, G., P. Hagstrom, A. Vainikka, and M. Todorova. 2000b. An optimality-theoretic model of acquisition of tense and agreement in French. In *Proceedings of the Cognitive Science Society 22*.

Legendre, G., W. Raymond, and P. Smolensky. 1993. An optimality-theoretic typology of case and grammatical voice systems. In *Proceedings of the Berkeley Linguistics Society 19*. ROA 3.

Legendre, G., P. Smolensky, and C. Wilson. 1998. When is less more? Faithfulness and minimal links in *wh*-chains. In *Is the best good enough? Optimality and competition in syntax*, eds. P. Barbosa, D. Fox, P. Hagstrom, M. McGinnis, and D. Pesetsky. MIT Press and MIT Working Papers in Linguistics. ROA 117.

Legendre, G., A. Vainikka, P. Hagstrom, and M. Todorova. 2002. Partial constraint ordering in child French syntax. *Language Acquisition* 10, 189–227.

Legendre, G., S. Vikner, and J. Grimshaw, eds. 2001. *Optimality-theoretic syntax*. MIT Press.

Levelt, C. 1995. Unfaithful kids: Place of articulation patterns in early child language. Talk presented at the Department of Cognitive Science, Johns Hopkins University.

Levelt, C., and R. van de Vijver. 1998. Syllable types in cross-linguistic and developmental grammars. ROA 265.

Lisker, L. 1957. Closure duration and the intervocalic voiced-voiceless distinctions in English. *Language* 33, 42–9.

Lombardi, L., ed. 2001. *Segmental phonology in Optimality Theory: Constraints and representations.* Cambridge University Press.

Łubowicz, A. 2002. Derived environment effects in Optimality Theory. *Lingua* 112, 243–80. ROA 239.

Lust, B. C., G. Hermon, and J. Kornfilt, eds. 1994. *Syntactic theory and first language acquisition: Cross-linguistic perspectives.* Vol. 2, *Binding, dependencies, and learnability.* Erlbaum.

Lust, B. C., M. Suñer, and J. Whitman, eds. 1994. *Syntactic theory and first language acquisition: Cross-linguistic perspectives.* Vol. 1, *Heads, projections, and learnability.* Erlbaum.

Marr, D. 1982. *Vision.* W. H. Freeman.

McCarthy, J. J. 1979. Formal problems in Semitic phonology and morphology. Ph.D. diss., MIT.

McCarthy, J. J. 1981. A prosodic theory of nonconcatenative morphology. *Linguistic Inquiry* 12, 373–418.

McCarthy, J. J. 1986. OCP effects: Gemination and antigemination. *Linguistic Inquiry* 17, 207–63.

McCarthy, J. J. 1999a. Harmonic serialism and parallelism. In *Proceedings of the North East Linguistic Society 30.* ROA 357.

McCarthy, J. J. 1999b. Sympathy and phonological opacity. *Phonology* 16, 331–99.

McCarthy, J. J. 2002a. Comparative markedness. Ms., University of Massachusetts at Amherst. ROA 489.

McCarthy, J. J. 2002b. *A thematic guide to Optimality Theory.* Cambridge University Press.

McCarthy, J. J., ed. 2004. *Optimality Theory in phonology: A reader.* Blackwell.

McCarthy, J. J., and A. Prince. 1993a. Generalized alignment. In *Yearbook of morphology,* eds. G. Booij and J. van Marle. Kluwer.

McCarthy, J. J., and A. Prince. 1993b. Prosodic Morphology I: Constraint interaction and satisfaction. Technical report RuCCS-TR-3, Rutgers Center for Cognitive Science, Rutgers University, and University of Massachusetts at Amherst. ROA 482, 2001.

McCarthy, J. J., and A. Prince. 1995. Faithfulness and reduplicative identity. In *University of Massachusetts occasional papers in linguistics 18: Papers in Optimality Theory,* eds. J. Beckman, L. Walsh Dickey, and S. Urbanczyk. Graduate Linguistic Student Association, University of Massachusetts at Amherst. ROA 60.

Misker, J. M. V., and J. R. Anderson. 2003. Combining Optimality Theory and a cognitive architecture. In *Proceedings of the Fifth International Conference on Cognitive Modeling.*

Müller, G. 1997. Partial *wh*-movement and Optimality Theory. *The Linguistic Review* 14, 249–306.

Müller, G. 2002. Harmonic alignment and the hierarchy of pronouns in German. In *Pronouns: Grammar and representation,* eds. H. Wiese and H. Simon. Benjamins.

Müller, G. 2003. Local vs. global optimization in syntax: A case study. In *Proceedings of the Stockholm Workshop on Variation within Optimality Theory.* ROA 598.

Pater, J., and J. Paradis. 1996. Truncation without templates in child phonology. In *Proceedings of the Boston University Conference on Language Development 20.*

Pollard, C., and I. A. Sag. 1987. *Information-based syntax and semantics.* Vol. 1, *Fundamentals.* CSLI Publications and University of Chicago Press.

Pollard, C., and I. A. Sag. 1991. *Information-based syntax and semantics.* Vol. 2, *Agreement, binding, and control.* CSLI Publications and University of Chicago Press.

Pollock, J.-Y. 1989. Verb movement, Universal Grammar, and the structure of IP. *Linguistic Inquiry* 20, 365–424.

Prince, A. 1993. Minimal violation. Talk presented at the Rutgers Optimality Workshop-1.

Prince, A. 1997. Endogenous constraints on OT constraints. Talk presented at the Hopkins Optimality Theory Conference/Maryland Mayfest.

Prince, A. 1999. Pāṇinian relations. Talk presented at the University of Marburg.

Prince, A. 2000. Comparative tableaux. Ms., Rutgers University. ROA 376.

Prince, A. 2002a. Arguing optimality. In *University of Massachusetts occasional papers in linguistics 26: Papers in Optimality Theory II.* Graduate Linguistic Student Association, University of Massachusetts at Amherst.

Prince, A. 2002b. Entailed ranking arguments. Ms., Rutgers University. ROA 500.

Prince, A., and P. Smolensky. 1991a. Notes on connectionism and Harmony Theory in linguistics. Technical report CU-CS-533-91, Computer Science Department, University of Colorado at Boulder.

Prince, A., and P. Smolensky. 1991b. Optimality. Talk presented at the Arizona Phonology Conference.

Prince, A., and P. Smolensky. 1993/2004. *Optimality Theory: Constraint interaction in generative grammar.* Technical report, Rutgers University and University of Colorado at Boulder, 1993. ROA 537, 2002. Revised version published by Blackwell, 2004.

Prince, A., and P. Smolensky. 2003. Optimality Theory in phonology. In *International encyclopedia of linguistics*, ed. W. J. Frawley. Oxford University Press.

Prince, A., and B. B. Tesar. 1999. Learning phonotactic distributions. Ms., Rutgers University. ROA 353.

Prince, A., and B. B. Tesar. 2004. Learning phonotactic distributions. In *Constraints in phonological acquisition*, eds. R. Kager, J. Pater, and W. Zonneveld. Cambridge University Press. ROA 353.

Pulleyblank, D., and W. J. Turkel. 1998. The logical problem of language acquisition in Optimality Theory. In *Is the best good enough? Optimality and competition in syntax*, eds. P. Barbosa, D. Fox, P. Hagstrom, M. McGinnis, and D. Pesetsky. MIT Press and MIT Working Papers in Linguistics.

Ritter, N. A., ed. 2000. Special issue: A review of Optimality Theory. *The Linguistic Review* 17, numbers 2-4.

Samek-Lodovici, V. 1992. Universal constraints and morphological gemination: A cross-linguistic study. Ms., Brandeis University.

Samek-Lodovici, V. 1996. Constraints on subjects: An optimality theoretic analysis. Ph.D. diss., Rutgers University. ROA 148.

Samek-Lodovici, V., and A. Prince. 1999. Optima. ROA 363.

Samek-Lodovici, V., and A. Prince. 2002. Fundamental properties of harmonic bounding. Technical report RuCCS-TR-71, Rutgers Center for Cognitive Science, Rutgers University.

Sells, P., ed. 2001. *Formal and empirical issues in optimality-theoretic syntax*. CSLI Publications.

Smolensky, P. 1993. Harmony, markedness, and phonological activity. Handout of talk presented at the Rutgers Optimality Workshop–1. ROA 87.

Smolensky, P. 1995. On the internal structure of the constraint component *Con* of UG. Talk presented at the UCLA Linguistics Department. ROA 86.

Smolensky, P. 1996a. Generalizing optimization in OT: A competence theory of grammar "use." Talk presented at the Stanford Workshop on Optimality Theory.

Smolensky, P. 1996b. The initial state and 'Richness of the Base' in Optimality Theory. Technical report JHU-CogSci-96-4, Cognitive Science Department, Johns Hopkins University. ROA 154.

Smolensky, P. 1996c. On the comprehension/production dilemma in child language. *Linguistic Inquiry* 27, 720–31. ROA 118.

Smolensky, P. 1997. Constraint interaction in generative grammar II: Local conjunction (or, Random rules in Universal Grammar). Talk presented at the Hopkins Optimality Theory Conference.

Smolensky, P. 1998. Why syntax is different (but not really): Ineffability, violability and recoverability in syntax and phonology. Talk presented at the Stanford University Workshop: Is syntax different?

Smolensky, P. 1999. Optimality Theory. In *MIT encyclopedia of the cognitive sciences*, eds. R. A. Wilson and F. C. Keil. MIT Press.

Smolensky, P. 2001. Optimality Theory: Frequently asked 'questions'. *Gengo*. [In Japanese.]

Smolensky, P. 2002. Optimality Theory: Frequently asked 'questions'. *Phonological Studies* 5, 91–8.

Smolensky, P., and C. Wilson. 2000. The architecture of the grammar: Optimization in phonology, syntax, and interpretation. Talk presented at the Utrecht Optimization of Interpretation Conference.

Spaelti, P. 1997. Dimensions of variation in multi-pattern reduplication. Ph.D. diss, University of California at Santa Cruz. ROA 311, 1999.

Speas, M. 1997. Optimality Theory and syntax: Null pronouns and control. In *Optimality Theory: An overview*, eds. D. Archangeli and D. T. Langendoen. Blackwell.

Steedman, M. 2000. *The syntactic process*. MIT Press.

Stemberger, J. P., and B. H. Bernhardt. 1998. *Handbook of phonological development from the perspective of constraint-based nonlinear phonology*. Academic Press.

Tesar, B. B. 1994. Parsing in Optimality Theory: A dynamic programming approach. Technical report CU-CS-714-94, Computer Science Department, University of Colorado at Boulder.

Tesar, B. B. 1995a. Computational Optimality Theory. Ph.D. diss., University of Colorado at Boulder. ROA 90.

Tesar, B. B. 1995b. Computing optimal forms in Optimality Theory: A basic syllabification. Technical report CU-CS-763-95, Computer Science Department, University of Colorado at Boulder. ROA 52.

Tesar, B. B. 1996. Computing optimal descriptions for Optimality Theory grammars with context-free position structures. In *Proceedings of the Annual Meeting of the Association for Computational Linguistics 34*.

Tesar, B. B. 1997. An iterative strategy for learning metrical stress in Optimality Theory. In *Proceedings of the Boston University Conference on Language Development 21*. ROA 177.

Tesar, B. B. 1998a. Error-driven learning in Optimality Theory via the efficient computation of optimal forms. In *Is the best good enough? Optimality and competition in syntax*, eds. P. Barbosa, D. Fox, P. Hagstrom, M. McGinnis, and D. Pesetsky. MIT Press and MIT Working Papers in Linguistics.

Tesar, B. B. 1998b. An iterative strategy for language learning. *Lingua* 104, 131–45. ROA 177.

Tesar, B. B. 1999. Robust interpretive parsing in metrical stress theory. In *Proceedings of the West Coast Conference on Formal Linguistics 17*. ROA 262.

Tesar, B. B. 2000a. On the roles of optimality and strict domination in language learning. In *Optimality Theory: Phonology, syntax, and acquisition*, eds. J. Dekkers, F. van der Leeuw, and J. van de Weijer. Oxford University Press.

Tesar, B. B. 2000b. Using inconsistency detection to overcome structural ambiguity in language learning. Technical report RuCCS-TR-58, Rutgers Center for Cognitive Science, Rutgers University. ROA 426.

Tesar, B. B. 2002. Enforcing grammatical restrictiveness can help resolve structural ambiguity. In *Proceedings of the West Coast Conference on Formal Linguistics 21*. ROA 262.

Tesar, B. B. 2004. Using inconsistency detection to overcome structural ambiguity. *Linguistic Inquiry* 35, 219–253.

Tesar, B. B., J. Alderete, G. Horwood, N. Merchant, K. Nishitani, and A. Prince. 2003. Surgery in language learning. In *Proceedings of the West Coast Conference on Formal Linguistics 22*.

Tesar, B. B., and A. Prince. To appear. Using phonotactics to learn phonological alternations. In *Proceedings of the Chicago Linguistic Society 39*. Vol. 2, *The panels*.

Tesar, B. B., and P. Smolensky. 1993. The learnability of Optimality Theory: An algorithm and some basic complexity results. Technical report CU-CS-678-93, Computer Science Department, University of Colorado at Boulder. ROA 2.

Tesar, B. B., and P. Smolensky. 1996. Learnability in Optimality Theory (long version). Technical report JHU-CogSci-96-3, Cognitive Science Department, Johns Hopkins University. ROA 156.

Tesar, B. B., and P. Smolensky. 1998. Learnability in Optimality Theory. *Linguistic Inquiry* 29, 229–68.

Tesar, B. B., and P. Smolensky. 2000. *Learnability in Optimality Theory*. MIT Press.

Trubetzkoy, N. 1939/1969. *Principles of phonology* (translation of *Grundzüge der Phonologie*). University of California Press.

Turk, A. E. 1994. Articulatory phonetic clues to syllable affiliation: Gestural characteristics of bilabial stops. In *Papers in laboratory phonology III: Phonological structure and phonetic form*, ed. P. Keating. Cambridge University Press.

Vennemann, T. 1988. *Preference laws for syllable structure and the explanation of sound change*. Mouton de Gruyter.

Walker, M. A., A. Joshi, and E. Prince. 1998. Centering in naturally occurring discourse: An overview. In *Centering theory in discourse*, eds. M. A. Walker, A. Joshi, and E. Prince. Clarendon Press.

Wareham, H. T. 1998. Systematic parameterized complexity analysis in computational phonology. Ph.D. diss., University of Victoria. ROA 318.

Wexler, K., and R. Manzini. 1987. Parameters and learnability in binding theory. In *Parameter setting*, eds. T. Roeper and E. Williams. Reidel.

Wilson, C. 1995. Optimality-theoretic constraints on pronouns and reflexive predicates. Ms., Johns Hopkins University.

Wilson, C. 2000. Targeted constraints: An approach to contextual neutralization in Optimality Theory. Ph.D. diss., Johns Hopkins University.

Wilson, C. 2001a. Bidirectional optimization and the theory of anaphora. In *Optimality-theoretic syntax*, eds. G. Legendre, S. Vikner, and J. Grimshaw. MIT Press.

Wilson, C. 2001b. Consonant cluster neutralisation and targeted constraints. *Phonology* 18, 147–97.

Yip, M. 1993. Cantonese loan word phonology and Optimality Theory. *Journal of East Asian Linguistics* 2, 261–91.

Zeevat, H. 2000. The asymmetry of OT syntax and semantics. *Journal of Semantics* 17, 243–62.

Index

Italic numbers refer to Volume 2. **Boldface** locates principal introductions of key terms.

D

H

I

N

S